THE Texture OF Life

Occupations and Related Activities

5TH EDITION

Edited by

Marie-Louise Blount, AM, OT, FAOTA

Paula Kramer, PhD, OTR, FAOTA

With Wesley Blount, SHRM–CP

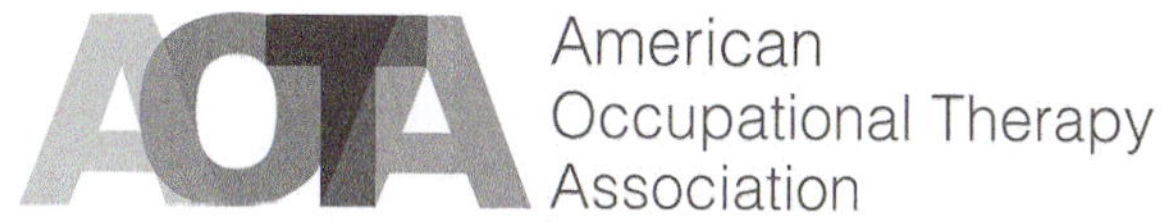

American Occupational Therapy Association

AOTA Vision 2025
As an inclusive profession, occupational therapy maximizes health, well-being, and quality of life for all people, populations, and communities through effective solutions that facilitate participation in everyday living.

Mission Statement
The American Occupational Therapy Association advances occupational therapy practice, education, and research through standard-setting and advocacy on behalf of its members, the profession, and the public.

AOTA Staff
Sherry Keramidas, *Executive Director*
Matthew Clark, *Chief Officer, Innovation & Engagement*

Elizabeth Dooley, *Vice President, Strategic Marketing & Communications*
Laura Collins, *Director of Communications and Publications*
Ashley Hofmann, *Acquisitions & Development Manager, AOTA Press*
Amy Ricci, *Product Manager & Business Analyst, AOTA Press*

Rebecca Rutberg, *Director, Marketing*
Amanda Goldman, *Marketing Manager*
Jennifer Folden, *Brand Designer*

American Occupational Therapy Association, Inc.
6116 Executive Boulevard, Suite 200
North Bethesda, MD 20852-4929
Phone: 301-729-AOTA (2682)
Fax: 301-652-7711
www.aota.org
To order: 1-877-404-AOTA or store.aota.org

Printed in the United States of America.

Disclaimers
This publication is designed to provide accurate and authoritative information in regard to the subject matter covered. It is sold or distributed with the understanding that the publisher is not engaged in rendering legal, accounting, or other professional service. If legal advice or other expert assistance is required, the services of a competent professional person should be sought.
—From the Declaration of Principles jointly adopted by the American Bar Association and a Committee of Publishers and Associations

It is the objective of the American Occupational Therapy Association to be a forum for free expression and interchange of ideas. The opinions expressed by the contributors to this work are their own and not necessarily those of the American Occupational Therapy Association.

ISBN: 978-1-56900-615-3
eBOOK ISBN: 978-1-56900-616-0
Library of Congress Control Number: 2022949967

Cover design by Steve Parrish, AOTA, North Bethesda, MD
Composition by Manila Typesetting Company, Manila, Philippines
Printed by Automated Graphic Services, Inc., White Plains, MD

Contents

Acknowledgements

First and foremost, we wish to thank Jim Hinojosa for his vision in developing the first four editions of *The Texture of Life*. We would not be writing a fifth edition without his original ideas and plan. We are very grateful to all the authors who contributed to this book. We know that they put much time and effort into their work and that is what makes this book so rich. Ashley Hofmann, Acquisitions & Development Manager for AOTA Press, has been with us every step of the way and has been an amazing support throughout this process. We are very grateful for her involvement and assistance throughout this project. We are very appreciative to all the wonderful people who allowed us to use their pictures and pictures of their children. They make this book more fun to read.

Marie-Louise Blount is celebrating her 65th year of a wonderful career as an occupational therapist. Her son, Wesley; her daughter, Elena, as well as her son-in-law, Barry; and her three grandsons Meyer, Ari, and Guy, give her joy, love, and support every day.

Paula Kramer is grateful that Marie-Louise Blount asked her to be part of this edition. Paula is very thankful for her husband, David L. Hunt, who supports her in everything she does, including all her professional efforts and the time they take away from other activities; Andrew L. K. Hunt, who is a kind and wonderful son; and Phaeton Hunt, who sat at feet throughout the writing and editing of this book.

Wesley Blount is extremely appreciative of the opportunity to work with such thoughtful, intelligent, and caring occupational therapy practitioners, educators, writers, and thinkers, especially the co-editors of this edition and the staff of AOTA Press. He is also grateful for the support and encouragement of numerous friends, family, and coworkers at a transformational personal moment.

Finally, we are grateful for all of our clients who help us learn more about the value of occupation every day.

About the Editors

Marie-Louise Blount, AM, OT, FAOTA, is an occupational therapist with clinical experience and a long career as an educator. She has been an occupational therapist for over 65 years. Retired from the position of professional program director at the Department of Occupational Therapy at the Steinhardt School of Culture, Education, and Human Development at New York University, she held the rank of clinical professor. She has been a co-editor of all five editions of this text.

Previously, Ms. Blount held faculty positions at three other universities. In the past, she served on the American Occupational Therapy Association's (AOTA's) Representative Assembly as the representative from Maryland. She served for 22 years as co-editor of the journal *Occupational Therapy in Mental Health.*

Paula Kramer, PhD, OTR, FAOTA, is Professor Emerita of St. Joseph's University (formerly University of the Sciences). She has been an occupational therapist for almost 50 years, practicing primarily in pediatrics, and an educator for almost 40 years. Dr. Kramer is a Fellow of AOTA; a recipient of the A. Jean Ayres Award from the American Occupational Therapy Foundation; and a recipient of the AOTA Award of Merit, the highest award of the Association. She has co-authored and co-edited 11 books and over 90 chapters.

Wesley Blount, SHRM–CP, is a graduate of Hamilton College, with a degree in writing. His interest in criticism and politics led him to blogging, where he has written extensively on health care policy among a wide swath of topics. This, in addition to growing up around occupational therapy and academia, made the chance to participate in the original edition of *Texture of Life* a natural fit. He has since contributed to, revised, and copyedited parts of each subsequent edition, leading to the junior editor role in this edition. Professionally, Mr. Blount is a certified human resources professional, advising small businesses on matters of policy and practice from his home in New York.

Contributors

Marie-Louise Blount, AM, OT, FAOTA
Retired Clinical Professor
Department of Occupational Therapy
Steinhardt School of Culture, Education, and Human Development
New York University
Formerly Co-Editor, *Occupational Therapy in Mental Health*
Croton-on-Hudson, NY

Wesley Blount, SHRM–CP
Writer and Assistant Editor
Human Resource Business Partner
Paychex, Inc.
Rochester, NY

Karen A. Buckley, MA, OT/L
Retired Clinical Assistant Professor
Department of Occupational Therapy
Steinhardt School of Culture, Education, and Human Development
New York University
New York, NY

Jyothi Gupta, PhD, OTR/L, FAOTA
Academic Consultant
Austin, TX

Kristine Haertl, PhD, OTR/L, FAOTA, ACE
Professor
Department of Occupational Therapy
St. Catherine University
St. Paul, MN

Tsu-Hsin Howe, PhD, OTR, FAOTA
Associate Professor and Department Chair
Department of Occupational Therapy
Steinhardt School of Culture, Education, and Human Development
New York University
New York, NY

Paula Kramer, PhD, OTR, FAOTA
Professor Emerita
Department of Occupational Therapy
St. Joseph's University, University City Campus
Philadelphia, PA

Susan Lin, ScD, OTR/L, FAOTA, FACRM
Affiliate Faculty
Marymount University Center for Optimal Aging
Arlington, VA

Heidi MacAlpine, OTD, MEd, OTR/L
Adjunct Instructor and Clinical Educator
Occupational Therapy Program
Touro University
Central Islip, NY
Owner
W.E.L.L. Alignment
East Moriches, NY

Wanda Mahoney, PhD, OTR/L
Associate Professor
Program in Occupational Therapy
Washington University School of Medicine
St. Louis, MO

Peggy Martin, PhD, OTR/L
Director, Occupational Therapy
University of Minnesota
Minneapolis, MN

Julie Ann Nastasi, ScD, OTD, OTR/L, SCLV, CLA, FAOTA
Associate Professor,
Department of Occupational Therapy
University of Scranton
Scranton, PA

Vikram Pagpatan, OTR/L, ATP, BCP, CLA
Assistant Professor and Admissions Coordinator
Occupational Therapy Program
State University of New York at Downstate
Brooklyn, NY

Anita Perr, PhD, OT/L, FAOTA
Clinical Professor
Department of Occupational Therapy
Steinhardt School of Culture, Education, and Human Development
New York University
New York, NY

Christine O. Peters, PhD, OTR/L, FAOTA
Independent Occupational Therapy Historian
Indio, CA

Sally E. Poole, OTD, OT/L, CHT
Clinical Assistant Professor
Department of Occupational Therapy
Steinhardt School of Culture, Education, and Human Development
New York University
New York, NY

Krystal Robinson-Bert, OTD, OTR/L, CSRS, C/NDT, CBIS, CKTP, CAPS
Assistant Professor
Department of Occupational Therapy
Messiah University
Mechanicsburg, PA
Staff Occupational Therapist
Helen M. Simpson Rehabilitation Hospital
Harrisburg, PA

Jeff Snodgrass, PhD, MPH, OTR, FAOTA
Associate Dean of Academic Affairs (Interim)
College of Clinical and Rehabilitative Health Sciences
Professor of Rehabilitative Sciences
East Tennessee State University
Johnson City, TN

Carolyn Unsworth, PhD, BAppSci(OccTher), GCTE, OTR, MRCOT, FOTARA
Professor and Discipline Lead, Occupational Therapy
Institute of Health and Wellbeing
Federation University
Churchill, Australia

Sheri Wadler, MS, OTR/L
Adjunct Instructor
Department of Occupational Therapy
Steinhardt School of Culture, Education, and Human Development
New York University
New York, NY

Wendy E. Walsh, PhD, OTR/L, FAOTA
Associate Professor and Chair
Department of Occupational Therapy
Saint Joseph's University, University City Campus
Philadelphia, PA

Judith Wilson, MA, OTR
Assistant Director of Occupational Therapy
Bellevue Hospital of New York University
New York, NY

Diana Chen Wong, OTD, OTR/L, CAPS
Clinical Adjunct Instructor
Department of Occupational Therapy
Steinhardt School of Culture, Education, and Human Development
New York University
New York, NY

Figures, Tables, Exhibits, Case Examples, and Appendixes

FIGURES

TABLES

EXHIBITS

CASE EXAMPLES

APPENDIXES

1

Occupation and Occupational Therapy

PAULA KRAMER, PhD, OTR, FAOTA;
MARIE-LOUISE BLOUNT, AM, OT, FAOTA;
AND WESLEY BLOUNT, SHRM-CP

CHAPTER HIGHLIGHTS

- Importance of occupation in practice
- Evolving, inclusive terms
- Terms developed over time
- Reviewing theoretical concepts: Activity analysis
- Frames of reference and legitimate tools
- Holistic approaches: Ecology of Human Performance and client-centered care
- Learning and adaptive models
- *Occupational Therapy Practice Framework, 4th Edition*
- Interventions in practice
- Further goals of this edition of *Texture of Life*

KEY TERMS AND CONCEPTS

• activity • activity analysis • *AOTA 2020 Occupational Therapy Code of Ethics* • client • client factors • context • co-occupations • Ecology of Human Performance • environmental factors • frames of reference • legitimate tools • occupation • occupational behavior • occupational justice • occupational science • occupational therapy • *Occupational Therapy Practice Framework* • outcome measures • Person–Environment–Occupation model • personal factors

Introduction

Occupation—what a complex concept! To most people, it means their job, their work. To occupational therapy practitioners, however, it means something entirely different. The definition of *occupation* has changed and evolved over the years, and various theorists have defined it slightly differently. Overall, the definition we use in this book is taken from the *Occupational Therapy Practice Framework: Domain and Process* (4th ed.; *OTPF–4;* American Occupational Therapy Association [AOTA], 2020b). We believe that ***occupation*** refers to "the everyday activities that people do as individuals, in families and with communities to occupy time and bring meaning and purpose to life. Occupations include things people need to, want to and are expected to do" (World Federation of Occupational Therapists, as cited in AOTA, 2020b, p. 7). AOTA (2020b) currently lists the various categories of occupation as

- activities of daily living (ADLs),
- instrumental activities of daily living (IADLs),
- health management,
- rest and sleep,
- education,
- work,

- play,
- leisure, and
- social participation (p. 30).

From our perspective, the key factor to keep in mind is that occupations and activities are personalized; what is important to one person, family, or community may not be what is important to another. For example, getting together for a weekly family dinner may be very important to some people, but a weekly phone call, video call, or text might be more important to others.

However, activities make up occupations, which raises the question of what constitutes an activity. ***Activity*** is defined as "actions designed and selected to support the development of performance skills and performance patterns to enhance occupational engagement" (AOTA, 2020b, p. 74). This definition may seem more abstract, but to simplify, activities are the things people do regularly that are important to them and that enable them to develop the skills and abilities to engage in occupations. Activities are also personalized; what some people do will be different from what other people do. Many activities make up an occupation. Another term that is frequently seen in the literature is *purposeful activities*. The *OTPF–4* no longer uses this term. The perspective is that all activities should be meaningful to the client; therefore, the phrase *purposeful activities* is redundant. However, it is commonly used in much of the recent literature.

Several examples may make it easier to understand the significant differences between these two concepts. Dressing is an occupation that is an ADL, whereas putting one's arm through a shirtsleeve is an activity. Grocery shopping is viewed as an IADL, but choosing the foods to buy to make dinner is an activity. Shopping may be a leisure occupation for some people, whereas picking out specific clothes for a special occasion is an activity. On a more abstract level, concentrating on a specific academic task may be viewed as an activity, whereas completing a course or program might be viewed as an occupation. The very specific components of an occupation are generally activities.

Occupations and the activities that are part of them define the person. Whereas occupations may be general categories, activities are often very person specific. Occupational therapy practitioners treat both individuals and groups, and it is imperative that practitioners consider their clients' and the particular groups' needs and desires when choosing goals and intervention strategies. Therefore, the activities must be specific to those being served.

In reviewing the professional literature, one can see that these definitions have evolved and changed over the course of the profession, aspects of which we address in this chapter. For the purposes of our overall approach in this book, we use the definitions from the *OTPF–4*.

Importance of Occupation in Practice

In 2015, the profession adopted the following statement: "Occupational therapy's distinct value is to improve health and quality of life through facilitating participation and engagement in occupation, the meaningful, necessary, and familiar activities of everyday life. Occupational therapy is client centered, achieves positive outcomes, and is cost-effective" (AOTA, 2015). It is critical to explore how this focus on occupation is implemented in practice. The *2018 Accreditation Council for Occupational Therapy Education (ACOTE®) Standards and Interpretive Guide* frequently mentions *occupation-based interventions,* which are defined as "client-centered intervention[s] in which the occupational therapy practitioner and client collaboratively select and design activities that have specific relevance or meaning to the client and support the client's interests, needs, health, and participation in daily life" (p. 77). Trombly (1995) identified both occupation as means and occupation as ends. *Occupations as means* refers to the process of the intervention, and *occupation as ends* refers to the goals or the outcomes of the intervention. Although this distinction was made some time ago, the idea still holds true today.

Theoretical and Historical Issues Related to Occupation-Based Intervention

Occupational therapy practitioners strive to use occupation-based interventions, but for many reasons it is not always possible. Quite a few theoretical approaches, models, and frames of reference use interventions that are not necessarily occupation based, and there are several areas of practice in which the client cannot engage collaboratively with the occupational therapy practitioner. Throughout the history of the profession, occupational therapy has shifted between a biomedical model approach and an occupation-based approach (Gillen, 2013). At the profession's inception, occupation was clearly the focus, and then from the 1940s to the 1970s, with the exception of a few theorists, the profession moved closer to a biomedical model, using many assessments and techniques from other professions (Gillen, 2013). A few prominent voices, such as Reilly (1962) and Kielhofner and Burke (1980), reminded occupational therapy practitioners of the importance of occupation. Their contributions were followed by many other important ones, including but not limited to, those of Christiansen and Baum (1991), Dunn et al. (1994), and Law (1998).

However, occupational therapy still includes many approaches—such as the biomechanical and neurodevelopmental approaches, for example—that are not necessarily occupation based, nor do they necessarily involve collaboration with the client. Making a splint can certainly be part of occupation as ends, but it is not an occupation-based activity. The domain of the profession is large and varied, and even with the breadth of its models and frames of reference, it behooves practitioners to strive to be occupation based and make the connection between interventions and real occupations. It is incumbent on practitioners to make the connection for themselves and for their clients and to explain how any intervention relates to an occupation.

Moreover, although it is best to collaborate with clients, this is not always possible. Some examples of clients who are not capable of collaborative discussions about intervention are infants in neonatal intensive care, younger children, people with cognitive impairment, and people experiencing dementia. In these cases, the practitioner can collaborate with parents, caregivers, or significant others. Diamantis (2010) proposed that although many pediatric approaches follow a biomedical model that is not necessarily occupation based, it is incumbent on practitioners to focus on the occupational nature of the goals and intended outcomes of the intervention rather than on whether the specific interventions are occupation based. He also proposed that focusing on occupational outcomes supports the uniqueness and importance of occupational therapy.

Studies Related to Occupation-Based Intervention in Clinical Settings

There have been quite a few studies on the use of occupation-based interventions in various clinical settings. Here we discuss just a few to give readers an idea of the breadth of settings and findings. A study of the use of occupation with clients receiving occupational therapy after a hip fracture (Wong et al., 2018) identified that the use of an occupation-based approach did not always fit well with the biomedical model used in hospital or rehabilitation settings—the typical settings in which interventions with these clients occur. The appropriate facilities for an occupation-based approach were often not available. This approach is also difficult to use with an electronic medical record. However, the study found that it was quite effective, especially in preparing clients for discharge and engagement in their lives after discharge (Wong et al., 2018).

A systematic review of occupation-based interventions with people with addictive disorders was conducted; it found that such interventions were often used in the areas of work, leisure, and social participation. Although a limited number of publications fit both the diagnostic criteria and the specified type of intervention, the systematic review found that occupation-based interventions in the area of social participation had better outcomes than control or comparison interventions (Wasmuth et al., 2016).

Another systematic review was conducted to determine the effectiveness of occupation- and activity-based interventions for children ages 5 to 21 years (Laverdure & Beisbier, 2020). The results showed that both can effectively improve outcomes related to ADLs, play, and leisure; however, the authors identified quite a few areas for practitioners to consider with such interventions. These areas included the importance of collaborating with clients and caregivers; the need to provide caregivers with training and feedback for support; the importance of embedding occupations in natural routines and environments; the need to structure the intervention; the use of video modeling and gaming activities to support participation and performance; and instruction for parents and caregivers in practice, coaching, and feedback skills for ADL activities (Laverdure & Beisbier, 2020).

Jack and Estes (2010) found that occupation-based interventions led to enhanced outcomes in hand therapy. However, a survey of hand therapists on the use of occupation-based interventions found that although more than 50% of those surveyed used occupation-focused assessments, their interventions were frequently not occupation based, and the primary reason cited for this was time constraints (Grice, 2015).

Gartz et al. (2021) used an exploratory case-study method to compare component-based interventions with occupation-based interventions for a person with visual deficits. They used a component-based approach, an occupation-based approach, and a combination of both approaches. Each intervention was measured by means of pre- and posttest administration of the Assessment of Motor and Process Skills (Fisher & Jones, 2012). Although there are limitations to the conclusions that can be drawn from a case study, the authors determined that use of both a component-based and an occupation-based approach resulted in the most improvement.

Although the use of occupation-based interventions is becoming more popular, and educational programs are focusing more on the importance of occupation-based interventions, it is important to recognize that many occupational therapy models and frames of reference, as well as intervention settings, are still component driven. As Diamantis (2010) suggested, it is important for practitioners to focus on the occupational nature of goals and to strive to have occupational outcomes for clients, regardless of the nature of the setting.

Evolving, Inclusive Terms

Over four editions and 20 years, *The Texture of Life* has laid a framework for translating ideas and theoretical concepts into practice. Drawing from the work of prominent theorists and the professional guidance provided by AOTA, we have worked to develop a common set of terms to serve as the basis for an in-depth examination of approaches to practice. From the beginning, we have acknowledged the challenges in an evolving landscape of new ideas and a wide array of methodologies. "No one universally accepted way exists in which occupational therapy practitioners conceptualize practice. . . . We accept that many scholars use different organizational structures and view practice differently" (Hinojosa & Blount, 2000, p. 5). Even as we centered our focus on purposeful activities, we were mindful that both words—the sense of purpose or meaning, coupled with the use of specific activities in a treatment setting—were topics of thoughtful exploration and debate (Hinojosa & Blount, 2004).

In this book, our approach has been to use broad, inclusive terms, encompassing many of the theoretical ideas and structures put forward since occupational therapy began. This is not meant to suggest a sense that anything fits; instead, we believe that although some word choices may differ, the principles and concepts underlying each term we use are drawn from, and refer back to, much of the work done by thinkers and scholars across the profession and across time. By focusing on terms that suggest a broadly inclusive approach, and using that inclusive mindset, students can see the application of a wide spectrum of theoretical approaches and ways to apply theoretical concepts in similarly inclusive ways to provide a comprehensive approach to practice.

Hinojosa and Blount (2009) said, "We believe that activities represent the core and the texture of people's daily lives" (p. 4). And, although ideas within the profession continue to evolve and change, its underlying foundation is based on consistent concepts. Conceptions of what define *activity* and *occupation* may continuously evolve, but understanding that human occupation plays an important role in overall well-being remains a foundational principle. The choice of what activities and interventions to use to aid others in a health care setting continues to develop, but the potential impact of the right intervention to improve overall occupational performance remains a core value of occupational therapy.

Terms Developed Over Time

The development of concepts and theories around activity, occupation, and the use of activities in therapeutic intervention are still evolving, as demonstrated over four previous editions of this text. Occupational therapy practitioners continually adapt and respond to client needs with new ideas in practice, and these new practices can and will lead to redefining what constitutes activity, occupation, and so on. Similarly, changes in society as a whole, and in the specific arena of health care, also serve to change the environment and the ways in which occupational therapy is practiced, and occupational therapy will respond and adapt to continue to be viable.

As we worked on this edition, the world was adjusting to many remarkable shifts: some resulting from the worldwide coronavirus pandemic, some resulting from cultural shifts in communities in the United States and around the world. We continue to see changes to the kinds of activities people do and the ways in which they do them as a result of the ever-shifting world of the Internet and online technologies. Throughout the quarantine and home confinement period, we have seen changes in how people work, how they communicate, and how they support one another. These shifts will help shape and reshape a continuing discussion of the terms we discuss here. Many of these shifts will remain permanent and others will not, but as we adapt and evolve, we need to approach new ideas with an open mind and a goal of inclusivity. By being open to new and changing ideas, we will be able to put them into occupational therapy practice successfully.

Chapter 2 of this edition updates the historical perspective to describe different theories and approaches, and it reexamines how those ideas developed over time. Just as the profession has grown and evolved, the theories and concepts used to define occupational therapy have grown and evolved and deepened our understanding of not just how occupational therapy works, but why.

The work of many important theorists also helped to shape the work of the current ***Occupational Therapy Practice Framework,*** the *OTPF–4,* which is meant to serve as the most comprehensive and inclusive definition of occupational therapy for practitioners. Here, we briefly summarize some of the important theoretical concepts, although "nothing can substitute for reading the works of these distinguished contributors in their original form" (Hinojosa & Blount, 2009, p. 22). We then conclude with a review of important aspects of the *OTPF–4.*

Reviewing Theoretical Concepts: Activity Analysis

For our definitional purposes, we think it is important to start with some of the earliest occupational therapy theoretical concepts. Gail Fidler's early work, grounding the still-nascent profession after World War II, advanced the idea of ***activity analysis,*** that is, looking at and breaking down activities so that their application and usefulness to the client's objectives could be best understood and applied in the context of therapeutic intervention (Fidler, 1948). Over time, Fidler, in partnership with her husband, showed the application of occupational therapy activities in the mental health setting, establishing how therapeutic intervention "impels the person to develop skills through an action-oriented learning experience (Fidler & Fidler, as cited in Hinojosa & Blount, 2009, p. 23). As with the work of many theorists, Fidler's work evolved into more comprehensive and holistic views of how occupational therapy affected individuals in treatment, models that have informed the *OTPF–4*'s approach as well.

Occupational Behavior and a Model of Human Occupation

Establishing the value of activity in the therapeutic setting was important; the challenge for occupational therapy is tying the use of activity to larger notions of the role of occupation in the overall human experience. Mary Reilly, a seminal thinker in the profession, provided that grounding by advancing the idea of ***occupational behavior*** (Reilly, 1962), suggesting that using activity in a therapeutic setting was not enough; the activity also needed to enhance individual human productivity. Reilly (1962) pointed out that productivity provides the most life satisfaction. This widely encompassing approach is also important because it incorporates notions of not just work as occupation but also play and school, which supported the theories underlying pediatric occupational therapy.

Using Reilly's (1962) concepts of occupational behavior, her occupational therapy students Gary Kielhofner and Janice Burke (1980) developed the Model of Human Occupation, which sought to provide a comprehensive framework for observing, analyzing, and classifying human behavior in a holistic context. Using this model, Kielhofner broadened the notion of how to look at human activity in the most encompassing and inclusive way, covering aspects of work and leisure, the mental and the physical, and the therapeutic value of learning and feedback. Defining human beings as an open system, he showed that the value of therapeutic interventions was in the individual's capacity to learn and adapt. In developing, refining, and evolving the model, Kielhofner and his collaborators (1980, 1985, 1992, 1995, 2007, 2009) provided an open framework for thinking about human activity on multiple levels and in many aspects and different settings that serves as a conceptual basis for many of the widely inclusive notions seen in the *OTPF–4*.

Frames of Reference and Legitimate Tools

Anne Mosey (1971) provided important concepts for looking at the ***frames of reference*** a practitioner uses to evaluate the use of appropriate therapeutic interventions. In part, developing frames of reference expands on Fidler's (1948) notions of activity analysis—that is, once an activity's therapeutic benefits are understood, the practitioner can then determine which activity will provide the greatest therapeutic benefit. Mosey posited that these therapeutic interventions serve as ***legitimate tools***—the tools of a professional, which may be similar, even shared, with others—that are used specifically by the occupational therapy practitioner to achieve defined goals. The key to Mosey's approach was her insistence on a shared nomenclature—that is, a shared set of concepts and terms that allowed the profession to develop a common language around practice and treatment.

In 1981, Mosey defined six legitimate tools of the profession. However, in 2001 in personal communication with Jim Hinojosa, she expanded that list to include the following legitimate tools:

- *conscious use of self*—preplanned verbal and nonverbal responses to a person
- *activities*—tasks or interactions in which people typically engage
- *activity groups*—types of primary groups that involve participation in activities or discussion of anticipated or current involvement in activities
- *stimulus-response interactions*—specific sensory input with a predictable motor response
- *atmospheric elements*—aspects of the physical environment that can be modified
- *assistive technologies*—devices, equipment, or systems specifically designed or adapted to prevent or remediate dysfunction to maintain or improve function
- *physical agent modalities*—properties of temperature, light, sound, water, and electricity that produce selected effects on soft tissue.

Although Mosey's list of tools is meant to be comprehensive, it cannot be seen as the last word; the framework she provided is meant to evolve and adapt as new legitimate tools are identified. For instance, if one looks at the ongoing development of tools and technologies in virtual space, it is clear that virtual reality is developing into a new legitimate tool. It is just this kind of dynamism around new technologies that makes Mosey's approach broadly applicable across the wide range of practice, underpinned by the notion that it is this shared nomenclature that serves to provide the profession's frames of reference.

Holistic Approaches: Ecology of Human Performance and Client-Centered Care

Theories, models, and frames of reference exist in terms of viewing both the individual's use of activity and occupation and the profession's use of activities and other tools in therapeutic intervention. The remaining theoretical piece is the relationship between practitioner and client—in other words, once an activity has been analyzed and its use as a legitimate tool is established, how does the practitioner choose the right intervention for the client? Or, for the client, how is a need for therapeutic intervention communicated and understood, and what constitutes a successful intervention? In part, the focus on communication with the client reflects a growing understanding of the collaborative, interpersonal nature of the therapeutic interaction as well as the implications raised by many theorists about seeing the ***client*** as a whole person and, thus, able to participate, constructively, in treatment, rather than the biomedical model of a patient as a passive agent being acted upon.

Winnie Dunn and colleagues developed the ***Ecology of Human Performance*** (EHP), "a framework of context to explain the way in which a person and the tasks the person does fit into the environment" (Dunn et al., 1994, 2003). The role of activity and occupation in an intervention, although important, becomes part of a larger context, taking in the environment around the person receiving treatment, so that treatment is beneficial, not just to the individual, but also to how the individual interacts and performs within a larger context or environment (e.g., in the home or the workplace). Thinking holistically, the EHP moves the profession into thinking more broadly about the benefits of therapeutic intervention and the role it can play once the individual leaves a rehabilitation setting.

Another holistic element of practice is thinking more broadly about the person receiving treatment. The ***Person–Environment–Occupation model*** put forth by Mary Law et al. (1994, 1998) and a team of Canadian occupational therapists attempts to define the variety of factors a practitioner needs to consider for a successful intervention meant to improve the client's occupational performance. Often referred to as the *Canadian model,* it considers the needs of not just the client, but the environment around the client—factors such as living situation, availability of support, and other extrinsic factors that may play a role in selecting an appropriate intervention. The model also asks the provider to consider the role the particular occupation plays in the client's overall life: Is the occupation intrinsic to the client's quality of life? Is the client able to adapt to a new working role and thus attempt a different occupation than before?

The client-centered approach also brings in a more complex understanding of *client* as a term itself—acknowledging the role of the caregiver or other family members as also being a part of the therapeutic relationship and being a part of the overall outcome of a successful intervention. Law's (1998) work to define a context for the therapeutic intervention—beyond the basics of using an activity to achieve a goal related to occupation—serves an important role in the development of a framework such as the *OTPF–4*. By introducing the complexities that most people face—the need for treatment that involves where and how they live, work, and participate in leisure activities—the therapeutic intervention becomes personal, targeted, and individualized. No therapeutic intervention should be seen as a one-size-fits-all approach to care. The most effective therapy is tailored to the client, addresses a specific need, and provides an outcome that benefits not just the individual, but also the others involved—often very involved—in a friend or family member's care.

Learning and Adaptive Models

Other recent developments in theoretical models may involve more targeted aspects of the occupational therapy practitioner's role. Learning theories have become more prominent as researchers explore how people learn and how best to develop approaches that aid in development and adaptation. The more we can understand how people learn—as children (Rodger & Ziviani, 2006) and as adults—the more we can grasp how therapeutic intervention can be used to provide growth and ease common human fears of change.

Moreover, if researchers want to fully understand the role of occupation for people, not just in the therapeutic context but more broadly in society, it may be necessary to separate that study from occupational therapy as we have come to understand it. ***Occupational science*** focuses on taking theories of occupation and looking at them broadly, often beyond the therapeutic context, to better understand the overall role of occupation in the wide scope of human activity. Originally developed at the University of Southern California, led by Florence Clark, occupational science sees the therapeutic use of occupation as just part of a larger investigation into understanding occupation. Clark et al. (1991) defined *occupation* as "chunks of culturally and personally meaningful activity in which humans engage that can be named in the lexicon of culture" (p. 301). Encompassing anthropological as well as sociological aspects, occupational science can provide wider academic and societal understanding of occupation and better inform the understanding of how to apply occupation in therapeutic settings.

However, for our purposes, as the ideas and theories of occupational therapy have developed, we see increasing complexity, layers of understanding, and the development of terminology that speaks to a broad scope of possibilities for using activity as an intervention that improves function and performance related to an individual's occupation. As we see how these ideas developed over time, we can examine how they come together in a framework that seeks to describe, in broadly inclusive terms, how these ideas are integrated into practice.

OTPF–4

This edition of *The Texture of Life* discusses various aspects of occupational therapy practice in depth. As part of this, we provide an overview of the latest *OTPF* (AOTA, 2020b). Here, we provide a discussion of the *Framework*'s domain and process. *The Texture of Life* applies the *OTPF–4* and provides examples that show its application in many situations.

The *OTPF–4* takes a broad, inclusive approach to the role of occupational therapy and the role of the practitioner in practice. For many practitioners, this approach may seem overly broad and to lack specificity. Over time, practitioners tend to specialize and do not necessarily have in-depth knowledge in other areas of practice. Not every practitioner with a pediatric practice will be fully versed in the day-to-day needs of elderly nursing home patients. Students and beginning practitioners start out applying the broad, general knowledge in the *OTPF–4* holistically but need to consider the specific requirements of treating each individual client in their particular context and environment.

The *OTPF–4* is the fourth in a line of documents from AOTA that describe the sphere of occupational therapy and how the occupational therapy practitioner applies it. The third version of the *Framework* (the *OTPF–3;* AOTA, 2014) has a similar structure, but the current edition has notable changes. The definition of ***occupational therapy,*** right at the outset, is briefer and somewhat altered:

> *Occupational therapy* is defined as the therapeutic use of everyday life occupations with persons, groups, or populations for the purpose of enhancing or enabling participation. (AOTA, 2020b, p. 1)

This definition is more succinct than the *OTPF–3* definition. It emphasizes prevention of illness and disability as well as intervention when such conditions have already occurred. Those who are qualified to offer these services are still designated as *occupational therapy practitioners,* which encompasses occupational therapists and occupational therapy assistants. *Clients* broadly includes individuals, groups, and populations. Both the *OTPF–3* (AOTA, 2014) and the *OTPF–4* (AOTA, 2020b) discuss how these documents developed over time.

The *OTPF* is an official AOTA document and is considered to be one that continually changes or evolves over time. It is important to note that students and practitioners should be prepared for new versions of the document in the future; AOTA requires that all Association documents undergo review every 5 years. The intent is to view changes in society and culture and how they affect service delivery and health care in general. These changes could include institutional as well as governmental developments and technology as well as trends in daily living and environment. These areas are not exhaustive but may serve as indicators of the breadth of circumstances that could affect occupational therapy practice in the future. To remain relevant, professions must evolve and be responsive to changes in society.

Occupational Therapy's Domain

The *OTPF–4,* like previous *Framework* documents, concentrates on the domain of occupational therapy (the profession's purview and the areas in which practitioners have knowledge and expertise). The domain, as indicated earlier, changes over time. In addition, the document addresses the occupational therapy process, which is the series of steps taken by practitioners to apply their expertise in the domain. These steps include evaluation, intervention, and measurement of outcomes (AOTA, 2020b), and they require collaboration among the occupational therapist, occupational therapy assistant, and client.

Definitions of terms used by practitioners are a major concern of *Framework* documents, to provide a shared nomenclature for the profession. Thus, the *OTPF–4* presents a list of terms and domain specifications that are new to this edition or are altered within it. Also, the *OTPF–4* includes new illustrations and tables to depict and clarify the precepts it is addressing. It may seem confusing, but *OTPF–4* firmly states that the document is not a taxonomy, a theory, or a model for occupational therapy. This, too, reflects the determination to make the framework broadly inclusive—setting up a structure that draws on the potential for a variety of models, theories, and approaches. The overall intent of the document is to provide a structure for practice.

A complete discussion of occupations always includes the term *activities.* As noted earlier in the chapter, activities are parts of occupations, and occupations often include many activities. For the practitioner, the key here is that in the *OTPF–4* both occupations and activities can be used as interventions. The *Framework* stresses the value of occupation (what people do every day) to human life and the centrality of the therapeutic relationship between practitioner and client in addressing needs and methods of intervention. The structure of the profession is compared with the structure of a building. So, for example, the profession is based on "cornerstones" (AOTA, 2020b): (1) core values and beliefs, (2) expertise in the therapeutic use of occupations, (3) professional (ethical) behavior, and (4) therapeutic use of self.

The cornerstones are influenced by what the *OTPF–4* calls "contributors" (AOTA, 2020b, p. 6). The list of contributors includes 16 items, which are also noted as not exhaustive. Many of these contributors are discussed in this edition of *Texture of Life;* for example, client-centered practice, clinical and professional reasoning, ethics, evidence-informed practice, professionalism, professional advocacy, and theory-based practice.

The domain of occupational therapy did not change much in the *OTPF–4*. In the *OTPF–4*'s Exhibit 1 (AOTA, 2020b, p. 7), the order of the domains differs from that depicted in the *OTPF–3,* but the most notable wording change is that the contexts are now divided into environmental factors and personal factors. Otherwise, it is unchanged. Relevant occupations are still ADLs, IADLs, rest and sleep, education, work, play, leisure, and social participation, with, as Amini (2021) noted, the addition of health management. Performance patterns are still listed as habits, routines, roles, and rituals. Performance skills are motor skills, process skills, and social interaction skills. ***Client factors*** are values, beliefs, and spirituality; body functions; and body structures.

Client factors, as well as the interests and valued occupations of an individual client, interact with occupations themselves. So, for one client, playing golf may be a preferred leisure occupation, but a professional golfer probably sees it as work. The *OTPF–4* presents many aspects of occupations and how they interact with time allocation and constraints, life and societal contexts, and healthy choices and traumatic influences. There is considerable literature on so-called unhealthy occupations and also unhealthy engagement in otherwise healthy occupations (Robinson Johnson & Dickie, 2019; Twinley, 2021). A ballet dancer whose body image issues contribute to an eating disorder is an example of how a healthy occupation can affect an unhealthy behavior.

Occupations are also frequently shared or performed with or for others. Such occupations are designated as ***co-occupations*** (Pierce, 2009). There are many examples of such co-occupations, and they represent the most interactive of daily or periodical occupations. In this edition of *The Texture of Life,* when chapters deal with caring for others, they are not addressing independence as a goal so much as interdependence.

As noted, the order in which the *OTPF–4* discusses aspects of the profession's domain has changed, which changes the emphasis placed on the topics included. After occupations, it discusses context. ***Context*** includes both environmental and personal factors that "influence engagement and participation in occupations" (AOTA, 2020b, p. 9). ***Environmental factors*** are also further delineated in *OTPF–4*. They include natural and human changes to the environment, human products and technology, relationships with people and other animals, a wide range of human beliefs and practices, and related structures and limitations.

Personal factors are, in part, unique to the clients themselves. They include things that are usually readily identifiable as part of each person's presentation of themself to the world, such as age, gender, and race. It is also obvious, however, that any of these characteristics might be intentionally or unknowingly obscured. For example, a woman with a deep voice might be mistaken for a man when answering the telephone. Other personal factors, such as amount of education or professional identity, might not be immediately evident on first contact. Personal factors might also be those that are shared with others in a group (e.g., a sports team) or population (e.g., nationality). Group members may have some similar characteristics but not others, and even more similarities and differences will occur in populations.

In the process of occupational therapy, caring for others raises ethical issues, such as equity and fairness. As such, the *OTPF–4* closely relates the concept of ***occupational justice*** to personal factors. Occupational justice is "a justice that recognizes occupational right to inclusive participation in everyday occupations for all persons in society regardless of age, ability, gender, social class, or other differences" (Nilsson & Townsend, 2010, p. 58).

The next domain category, according to the *OTPF–4*, is performance patterns—habits, routines, roles, and rituals. *Habits* are regular behaviors, and they may be healthy or unhealthy. *Routines* are regular sequences of occupations. *Roles* are "pattern(s) of behavior . . . structured around . . . particular statuses" (Theodorson & Theodorson, 1969, p. 352). *Rituals* are repeated sets of behaviors that fit into many different aspects of life. They may be expressed during holiday seasons or spiritual practices and reflect beliefs and values. They can also be seen in daily life activities; for example, the sequence of activities that people do when they wake up in the morning. They may also, however, be expressions of pathology and can be found in many areas of daily living. For example, people with obsessive–compulsive disorder may repeatedly check to see that a door is locked even after they have just locked it.

Performance skills may be motor, process, or social interaction. They can be considered a part of a client's initial and continuing occupational therapy evaluation. They are evaluated both for individuals and for groups, and when problem areas are assessed, occupational therapy practitioners consider why the problems are occurring and what interventions might be required.

According to the *OTPF–4*, the last part of occupation is client factors, which include both body structures and body functions; however, they are also, for the individual client, related directly to the individual's values and beliefs and encompass spirituality.

Occupational Therapy Process

The occupational therapy process itself involves all the factors previously discussed. The *OTPF–4* presents an extensive list (see Exhibit 2 of the *OTPF–4*) of how this process plays out. The first part of the process (evaluation), the occupational profile, epitomizes collaboration with clients to determine their own assessment of the need for services. The occupational profile is frequently used as a starting point in the evaluation of clients, and AOTA (2020a) has produced the Occupational Profile Template to assist practitioners in summarizing the findings of the occupational profile. Standardized and other evaluations are also used during the process (see Chapter 4, "The Occupational Profile," for further information).

The occupational therapist then moves on to the analysis of the client's occupational performance and finally synthesizes the entire evaluation process. Occupational or activity analysis becomes a part of this process (see Chapter 3, "Occupational and Activity Analysis"). It is preceded by an identification of the occupations that are important or crucial to the client. Information from various assessments that have been administered will include client factors, performance skills, patterns, and deficits. The contexts within which the client usually functions must be considered, as well as the impacts of each of these factors.

For the occupational therapy practitioner, the development of clinical or professional reasoning (see Chapter 6, "Professional Reasoning and Reflective Practice," and Unsworth & Baker, 2016) is crucial to understanding and mastering effective intervention. The practitioner's abilities develop over time and are nurtured through clinical internship, mentoring, and clinical experience. This is critical to effective use of the *OTPF–4*.

Interventions in Practice

The initial evaluation itself may take greatly varying amounts of time, which is partly dependent on the setting or settings where it takes place. Once these initial steps are completed and goals have been developed, the practitioner, if appropriate, is prepared to enter the ***intervention*** stage of the process, in collaboration with others, including the client. The intervention requires collaborative planning; estimates of the time required for the intervention, including probable discharge; and recommendations or referrals to other professionals. Interventions are selected on the basis of the analysis and may include

- therapeutic application of occupations and activities;
- interventions supporting occupations (including assistive devices);
- education;
- establishment of new routines;
- advocacy recommendations, including those that strengthen advocacy for oneself;
- group activities; and
- virtual approaches.

As the intervention proceeds, continuous reevaluation occurs, and changes are made as needed. When the entire process has been completed, ***outcome measures*** can be reviewed and evaluated. They should include an assessment of how effectively the client's goals have been met. Outcome measures should be carefully selected to meet standards that provide adequate evidence and should be appropriately sensitive to changes. Results should help clients and other health care providers to plan realistically for the future.

Considering the occupational therapy process carefully, it may also be necessary to look at or include others in the client's environment and issues that may be beyond the interaction of the individual practitioner and the individual client. For example, sometimes families are involved in planning and intervention, and sometimes larger entities such as housing facilities or school systems may be involved. This is particularly true when the client is a child or someone who requires individual or institutional guardians because of problems with judgment, infirmity, or other limitations.

As the client moves on from intervention, the occupational therapy practitioner has a role in making the transition to previous daily living or to new environments (e.g., other living facilities, school, new interventions, new relationships) smooth and less stressful. Establishing clear goals from the start allows the goals themselves to help set the tone and the progress of intervention, however long, and lead smoothly to the end or discontinuation of this phase of the intervention process and the successful completion of the initial plan.

The *OTPF–4* seeks to widen the scope of practice, enabling practitioners to apply their knowledge and skills to a broader range of individual problems and to problems beyond the scope of the immediate therapeutic relationship. Aspects of life beyond the immediate need, aspects that may involve the client's circle of associations and relationships and the environment in which the client functions, should be considered. For the practitioner, however, the salient issues are those raised by the client and will, for most part, provide the guidelines and intensity of the individual therapeutic relationship. The *OTPF–4* is replete with examples of how all of the concepts discussed apply to cases that are often seen in practice.

The ***AOTA 2020 Occupational Therapy Code of Ethics*** (AOTA, 2020a) is integral to all parts of the process. It is applicable from initial selection of students through the learning process to the behavior of seasoned practitioners, and it stresses the caring, scientific rigor, fairness, and knowledge undergirding all professional activities. Collaboration is an essential part of the practitioner's role, and the skills required of an effective collaborator apply to all parts of the process. Knowing oneself and one's limitations helps one to develop new and better approaches to others and the therapeutic process, and ethics are no different. Practitioners sharing ethical approaches, and holding one another accountable, are key to this process as well.

Further Goals of This Edition

We are acutely aware of how society and social life change as outside or unexpected forces arise to disrupt and change one's way of life. Pandemics, climate change, political realities, and loss of employment opportunities deeply affect not only how people see the world but also how they act within it. Health care has clearly been affected by some of these large-scale developments, and the role of the occupational therapy practitioner has changed as well. This edition of *The Texture of Life* takes these changes into consideration and suggests not only how such changes affect practice but also stimulates further thinking about planning for the future when change provides disruption but also room for growth and development.

As occupational therapy practitioners' roles change in tandem with societal changes, we need to continually reassess those roles and how we respond. The *OTPF–4* aims to do this in a way that incorporates broader and more comprehensive roles, and, considering the breadth of practice, leads practitioners to expand their view of possible clients, the contexts in which they operate, and the changing environment—all of which require frequent readjustment. We can begin to see how uneven responses to societal challenges affect our daily lives, and perhaps our realization of how the connections between all human life, and the planet we share, affect our choices and those of the people we work with.

As *The Texture of Life* moves from ideas into practice in subsequent chapters, we encourage you to think broadly and inclusively about the possibilities of occupational therapy for you as a practitioner and, ultimately, the benefit provided to those who receive care. At a moment of enormous change, we see the value of both respecting and drawing from the long line of theory and ideas developed over time within occupational therapy practice, while broadening the sense of how these ideas, applied in practice, can provide benefits we may not fully see at this moment.

References

Accreditation Council for Occupational Therapy Education. (2018). 2018 Accreditation Council for Occupational Therapy Educational (ACOTE®) Standards and interpretative guide (effective July 31, 2020). *American Journal of Occupational Therapy, 72*(Suppl. 2), 7212410005. https://doi.org/10.5014/ajot.2018.72S217

American Occupational Therapy Association. (2014). Occupational therapy practice framework: Domain and process (3rd ed.). *American Journal of Occupational Therapy, 68*(Suppl. 1), S1–S48. https://doi.org/10.5014/ajot.2014.682006

American Occupational Therapy Association. (2015). *Articulating the distinct value of occupational therapy.* https://aota.org/publications-news/aotanews/2015/distinct-value-of-occupational-therapy.aspx

American Occupational Therapy Association. (2020a). AOTA 2020 Occupational Therapy Code of Ethics. *American Journal of Occupational Therapy, 74*(Suppl. 3), 7413410005. https://doi.org/10.5014/ajot.2020.74s3006

American Occupational Therapy Association. (2020b). Occupational therapy practice framework: Domain and process (4th ed.). *American Journal of Occupational Therapy, 74*(Suppl. 2), 7412410010. https://doi.org/10.5014/ajot.2020.74s2001

Amini, D. (2021). The *OTPF–4:* Continuing our professional journey through change. *OT Practice, 26*(2), 34–42.

Christiansen, C., & Baum, C. (1991). Occupational therapy interventions for life performance. In C. Christiansen & C. Baum (Eds.)

Occupational therapy: Overcoming human performance deficits (pp. 3–43). Slack.

Clark, F., Parham, A., Carlson, M., Frank, G., Jackson, J., Pierce, D., . . . Nemke, R. (1991). Occupational science: Academic innovation in the service of occupational therapy's future. *American Journal of Occupational Therapy, 45,* 300–310. https://doi.org/10.5014/ajot.45.4.300

Diamantis, A. (2010). Defending occupation in pediatric practice. *British Journal of Occupational Therapy, 73,* 343. https://doi.org/10.4276/030802210x12813483277026

Dunn, W., Brown, C., & McGuigan, A. (1994). The Ecology of Human Performance: A framework for considering the effect of context. *American Journal of Occupational Therapy, 48,* 595–607. https://doi.org/10.5014/ajot.48.7.595

Dunn, W., Brown, C., & Youngstrom, M. J. (2003). Ecological model of occupation. In P. Kramer, J. Hinojosa, & C. B. Royeen (Eds.), *Perspectives in human occupation: Participation in life* (pp. 223–263). Lippincott Williams & Wilkins.

Fidler, G. S. (1948). Psychological evaluation of occupational therapy activities. *American Journal of Occupational Therapy, 2,* 284–287.

Fisher, A. G., & Jones, K. B. (2012). *Assessment of Motor and Process Skills: Development, standardization and administration manual* (7th ed.). Three Star Press.

Gartz, R., Dickerson, A., & Radloff, J. C. (2021). Comparing component-based and occupation-based interventions of a person with visual deficits' performance. *Occupational Therapy in Health Care, 35*(1), 40–56. https://doi.org/10.1080/07380577.2020.1862443

Gillen, G. (2013). Eleanor Clarke Slagle Lecture—A fork in the road: An occupational hazard? *American Journal of Occupational Therapy, 67,* 641–652. https://doi.org/10.5014/ajot.2013.676002

Grice, K. O. (2015). The use of occupation-based assessments and intervention in the hand therapy setting: A survey. *Journal of Hand Therapy, 28,* 300–306. https://doi.org/10.1016/j.jht.2015.01.005

Hinojosa, J., & Blount, M.-L. (2000). Purposeful activities within the context of occupational therapy. In J. Hinojosa & M.-L. Blount (Eds.), *The texture of life: Purposeful activities in occupational therapy* (pp. 1–15). American Occupational Therapy Association.

Hinojosa, J., & Blount, M.-L. (2004). Purposeful activities within the context of occupational therapy. In M.-L. Blount & J. Hinojosa (Eds.), *The texture of life: Purposeful activities in occupational therapy* (2nd ed., pp. 1–16). AOTA Press.

Hinojosa, J., & Blount, M.-L. (2009). Occupation, purposeful activities, and occupational therapy. In J. Hinojosa & M.-L. Blount (Eds.), *The texture of life: Purposeful activities in occupational therapy* (3rd ed., pp. 1–19). AOTA Press.

Jack, J., & Estes, R. D. (2010). Documenting progress: Hand therapy treatment shift from biomedical to occupational adaptation. *American Journal of Occupational Therapy, 64,* 82–87. https://doi.org/10.5014/ajot.64.1.82

Kielhofner, G. (Ed.). (1985). *A Model of Human Occupation: Theory and application.* Lippincott Williams & Wilkins.

Kielhofner, G. (1992). *Conceptual foundations of occupational therapy.* F. A. Davis.

Kielhofner, G. (Ed.). (1995). *A Model of Human Occupation: Theory and application* (2nd ed.). Lippincott Williams & Wilkins.

Kielhofner, G. (Ed.). (2007). *A Model of Human Occupation: Theory and application* (4th ed.). Lippincott Williams & Wilkins.

Kielhofner, G. (2009). *Conceptual foundations of occupational therapy practice* (4th ed.). F. A. Davis.

Kielhofner, G., & Burke, J. (1980). A Model of Human Occupation, Part 1: Conceptual framework and content. *American Journal of Occupational Therapy, 34,* 572–581. https://doi.org/10.5014/ajot.34.9.572

Laverdure, P., & Beisbier, S. (2020). Occupation- and activity-based interventions to improve performance of activities of daily living, play, and leisure for children and youth ages 5 to 21: A systematic review. *American Journal of Occupational Therapy, 75,* 7501205050. https://doi.org/10.5014/ajot.2021.039560

Law, M. (Ed). (1998). *Client-centered occupational therapy.* Slack

Law, M., Baptiste, S., Carswell, A., McColl, M. A., Polatajko, H., & Pollock, M. (1994). *Canadian Occupational Performance Measure* (2nd ed.). CAOT Publications.

Mosey, A. C. (1971). *Three frames of reference for mental health.* Slack.

Mosey, A. C. (1981). *Occupational therapy: Configuration of a profession.* Raven Press.

Nilsson, I., & Townsend, E. (2010). Occupational justice—Bridging theory and practice. *Scandinavian Journal of Occupational Therapy, 17,* 57–63. https://doi.org/10.3109/11038120903287182

Pierce, A. (2009). Co-occupations: The challenges of defining concepts original to occupational science. *Journal of Occupational Science, 16,* 203–207. https://doi.org/10.1080/14427591.2009.9686663

Reilly, M. (1962). A psychiatric occupational therapy program as a teaching model. *American Journal of Occupational Therapy, 22,* 221–225.

Robinson Johnson, K., & Dickie, V. (2019). What is occupation? In B. A. B. Schell & G. Gillen (Eds.), *Willard & Spackman's occupational therapy* (13th ed., pp. 320–333). Wolters Kluwer.

Rodger, S., & Ziviani, J. (Eds). (2006). *Occupational therapy with children: Understanding children's occupations and enabling participation.* Blackwell.

Theodorson, G. A., & Theodorson, A. G. (1969). *Modern dictionary of sociology.* Thomas Y. Cromwell.

Trombly, C. A. (1995). Occupation: Purposefulness and meaningfulness as therapeutic mechanisms. *American Journal of Occupational Therapy, 49,* 960–972. https://doi.org/10.5014/ajot.49.10.960

Twinley, R. (2021). *Illuminating the dark side of occupation: International perspectives from occupational therapy and occupational science.* Routledge.

Unsworth, C. A., & Baker A. (2016). A systematic review of professional reasoning literature in occupational therapy. *British Journal of Occupational Therapy, 79*(1), 5–16. https://doi.org/10.1177/0308022615599994

Wasmuth, S., Pritchard, K., & Kaneshiro, K. (2016). Occupation-based intervention for addictive disorders: A systematic review. *Journal of Substance Abuse Treatment, 62,* 1–9. https://doi.org/10.1016/j.jsat.2015.11.011

Wong, C., Fagan, B., & Leland, N. E. (2018). Occupational therapy practitioners' perspectives on occupation-based interventions for clients with hip fracture. *American Journal of Occupational Therapy, 72,* 7204205050. https://doi.org/10.5014/ajot.2018.026492

2

Developing Occupational Therapy Over Time: A Historical Perspective

CHRISTINE O. PETERS, PhD, OTR/L, FAOTA;
WANDA MAHONEY, PhD, OTR/L;
AND PEGGY MARTIN, PhD, OTR/L

CHAPTER HIGHLIGHTS

- Historical overview
- Pre–World War I (1756–1917)
- World War I
- Reprieve between wars
- World War II
- Postwar-era medicalization of occupational therapy
- Expanding practice
- Becoming authentic

KEY TERMS

• clinical reasoning • Community Mental Health Centers Act • Consolation House • cultural aspects • Education for All Handicapped Children Act of 1975 • National Society of the Promotion of Occupational Therapy • occupational justice • occupational movement • occupational science • occupational therapy • occupational therapy models • *Occupational Therapy Practice Framework: Domain and Process* • Pennsylvania Hospital • physical medicine and rehabilitation • reconstruction aides • reconstruction hospitals • rehabilitation • Social Security Amendments of 1965 • Uniform Terminology for Reporting Occupational Therapy Services

Introduction

Understanding the past gives us great insight into the present. Occupation was a primary focus of the founders of the profession. Early occupational therapists were White, middle- and upper middle-class, educated women, and some men, with privilege or status who recognized the value of occupation in treating long-term illness, and many knew from personal experience the meaning of occupation or engagement. Occupational therapy was founded on the principle that occupation is essential to health. ***Occupational therapy*** was defined in 1923 as "any activity, mental or physical, definitely prescribed and guided for the distinct purpose of contributing to or hastening recovery from disease or injury" (Jenkins, 1923, p. 1).

Focused primarily on the doing—putting the "active" in *activity* rather than defining the exact nature of therapeutic benefit or creating a nomenclature of occupation versus activity—occupational therapy's paradoxes start from its beginnings, where a new kind of patient—one who had survived an illness or injury previously considered fatal or permanently disabling—met a group of individuals determined to provide practical solutions to everyday problems. What was immediately clear to patient and practitioner—that resuming everyday activities and usefulness provides a therapeutic benefit—was unfamiliar to the world of medicine and the culture of the day, and helped to create a new notion of health. It is perhaps no wonder that it took a while for the words to catch up to the reality. "Occupational therapy can be one of the great ideas of 20th century medicine," Mary Reilly (1962, p. 1) proclaimed in her 1961 Eleanor Clarke Slagle Lecture to the American Occupational Therapy Association (AOTA). Indeed, in the literal doing, it was. In theory, occupation as therapy is still an idea in progress.

Historical Overview

Occupational therapy as a form of treatment began in houses, some modest structures, others grand private estates; large institutions; and new places in the community. Immigrants, many living and working in overcrowded conditions, changed the nature of urban life; these changes led to needed social and legal reform as part of the settlement house movement. Early occupation workers employed or volunteered at settlement houses teaching new skills. Occupational therapy responded as engineers conceptualized "scientific efficacy," methodically studying how to streamline mechanical production costs and time. Scientific efficiency became central to the efforts of the ***National Society of the Promotion of Occupational Therapy*** (NSPOT), the first professional organization of occupational therapists, as Lillian Gilbert—an efficiency expert and engineer widowed from her partner and husband Frank—sought to apply their efficiency studies to everyday tasks. Consequently, occupational therapy founders and practitioners adopted a scientific mentality, prescribing simple to more complex work or task projects. Early occupational therapy influencer Adolf Meyer (1922) viewed work philosophically, proposing a balance among work, play, and rest. Occupation as therapy, elementally rooted in the American arts and crafts movement and steeped in upper-class culture, influenced knowledge and delivery of the developing practice.

Advances in medical care during the Industrial Revolution meant that by World War I, many who would previously have died from illness and injury survived with disability. These survivors now came seeking specialized treatment after war, industrial factory injuries, and disease pandemics such as polio and tuberculosis. Before the 1950s, patients spent months or years in tuberculosis hospitals or sanatoriums because of the infectious nature of the disease and the lack of effective treatments beyond bed rest (Hudson & Fish, 1944; Mellinger, 1963). Occupational therapists provided graded activities in sanatoriums, which provided much-needed opportunities for purpose and usefulness, eventually allowing many recovered patients to return to the community. Occupational therapy in early hospitals practiced "the science of organized work for invalids . . . [effectively hastening] recovery from diseases or injury under medical supervision" (Slagle, 1930, p. 299).

Medicalization meant science, prescriptive care, and occupational therapy's pushback against unsuccessful takeover attempts by physiatrists practicing physical medicine. Occupational therapy experienced other changes in these years, including an increase in the qualified workforce and a response to multiple war demands. Hospitals influenced occupational therapy practice, not all for the good. What could be measured—physical change and improved function—overtook the obvious benefits of a less quantifiable increased sense of purpose and usefulness that had driven so many to use occupation as therapy from the start. What the focus on physical wellness neglected was mental health.

Institutionalization of people with mental illness hid mental illness from the masses and increased the need for professionals who could care for those inside. As part of this, occupational therapy (now part of the health professions) added the occupational therapy assistant as a simpler role that required less training. Occupational therapists seeking new ways of practice worked in community mental health centers called *clubhouses* in the 1960s and in public schools in the 1970s, successfully negotiating disability rights and legislative change. With a new lens on disability equity in the 1990s, occupational therapists joined city planners and architects in making neighborhoods and homes accessible to people with physical and mental illness. Occupational therapy knowledge grew, linking theory to practice and research to reflect societal needs. A uniform language or terminology was created, and practitioners discussed varied practice specialties, including preventive health care. Some traditional healing centers in hospitals and nursing homes remained in place, but new reimbursement structures led to shorter lengths of stay. Occupational science, a discipline that studies occupation, emerged in the late 1980s, and occupational scientists, concerned with social disparities and injustices, examined in new ways inequities similar to those that reformers had addressed in the U.S. settlement movement in the early 1900s, including poverty, insufficient health care, and feeding homeless people in soup kitchens.

The changing nature of practice, the democratization of postwar society, and the development of an ever-expanding body of knowledge have helped guide the transformations of occupational therapy: never completely losing sight of the forces that willed the profession into being, but continually transforming and evolving as notions of occupation, activity, therapy, and purpose have changed over time. "In every phase of life, the will to do brings about accomplishment of anything. The selection of an occupation should be one's own initiative" (Dunton, 1919, p. 194; see Figure 2.1).

The ***occupational movement,*** termed *work-cure, diversional occupation,* or *occupational therapy,* was an effort to create balance and normalize daily lives (Hall, 1910; Slagle, 1914). Specifically designed occupational therapy treatment began in healing houses, directed by leaders of the occupational movement and future founders of the occupational therapy profession: for example, Marblehead or the Devereux Mansion (Herbert James Hall), Hull House (Eleanor Clarke Slagle), and Consolation House (George Edward Barton). Locations varied, ranging from overpopulated cities such as New York,

FIGURE 2.1. Healing in a house: Stitch by stitch.

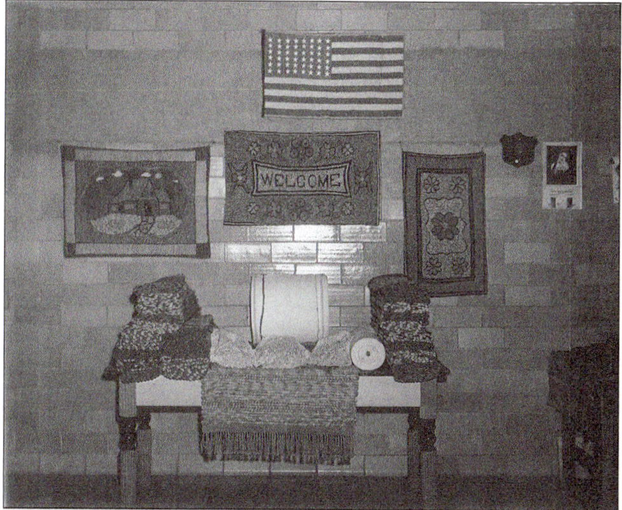

Note. Examples of occupational therapy craft samplers (no date).
Source. Courtesy of the Archives of the American Occupational Therapy Association, Inc., North Bethesda, MD.

Chicago, and Philadelphia to the rural, isolated country homes of wealthy patrons and benefactors.

Healing houses where occupation occurred "diverted attention from problems" (Slagle, 1930) and "recreated the play spirit" that Jane Addams, the founder of Hull House, described as "tarnished in the urban environment that leads to fatal passivity and social deviations" (Slagle, 1922, p. 16). Slagle (1922), an occupational therapy founder and social worker, characterized the "seeds of occupational therapy being sown for humanitarian, social, charitable, custodial, correctional and dependent problems of the time" (p. 11). These seeds aligned occupational therapy with the settlement movement in common leadership, training models, and a shared purpose to serve those who were poor, disenfranchised, sick, or marginalized.

Samuel A. Barnett, the vicar of Whitechapel Parish in London's East End, opened Toynbee Hall in 1884. Toynbee Hall, credited as the first settlement house, was modeled after the university or college settlements used for social and educational enrichment. Hull House opened a few years later in Chicago in 1889, after Jane Addams traveled to Toynbee Hall with Ellen Gates Starr. Hull House assisted immigrants and people with mental illness, addressed child labor laws, and provided "a safer place for gatherings" (Loomis, 1992, p. 34). To expand her studies in social work, Eleanor Clarke Slagle attended a training class in 1911 covering occupations and amusements for attendants at Hull House, which operated the Chicago School of Civics and Philanthropy as a way to develop professionals. Physician Adolf Meyer, then at Kankakee State Hospital in Illinois, who consulted and supported the Hull House occupations course, knew of Slagle's involvement, later recruiting Slagle to direct a new occupational therapy program for psychiatric patients when he relocated to the Phipps Clinic in Baltimore in 1913.

There, Slagle perfected the new "habits training" treatment approach for adults, using handwork, games, and organized play as part of a 24-hour schedule of regulated activities. Slagle then returned to Chicago to start the Favill School of Occupations at Hull House in 1915, a 5-month occupational therapy training program to "prepare students to treat persons with physical or mental illness, soldiers with disabilities and school-age children with learning disabilities" (Loomis, 1992, p. 36). The curriculum was divided into two parts. The first part consisted of theoretical lecture courses, including "Administration of Charitable Institutions, Industrial and Public Hygiene and Case Work." The second part, technical courses, required 8 to 10 hours per week of practical training in which kinesiology was juxtaposed with folk dancing (Loomis, 1992). With no program supervisor or applicant replacement, the Favill School of Occupations closed in 1920 when Slagle resigned to take a new position in New York. Complicating the situation, other academic occupational therapy educational programs with more rigorous requirements were opening by 1918, and the settlement house movement became a less viable location for a training program.

By 1930, the National Federation of Settlements in the United States represented 160 settlements, with 1,500 staff and 7,500 volunteers and assistants. Settlement houses, run by "well to do young men and women" (Loomis, 1992, p. 34), took on the cause in their area and developed them in stages. First, they selected neighborhoods and social and educational programs. Then they added institutional rooms, an assembly hall, gymnasium, social–recreational activities, and a more extensive physical plant that housed handwork, education, social activities, drama, swimming, and homemaking. Health work included health education, personal hygiene training, and training in good mental habits (Loomis, 1992). Reformers in the New York settlement house movement initiated a tenements rights protest against immigrant overcrowding and poor health conditions.

Herbert James Hall (1870–1923), a physician and an AOTA president (1920–1923), believed finely crafted arts both educated and were therapeutic. Starting in 1905, Hall, a Harvard Medical School graduate, designed a small industrial workshop in a home in Marblehead, Massachusetts, for patients with neurasthenia (characterized as a nonspecific emotional disorder that included insomnia, headache, fatigue, and depression) or nervous exhaustion (Gosling, 1987). He secured $1,000 from the Proctor Fund at Harvard University "to assist in the study of the treatment of neurasthenia by progressive and graded manual occupation" (Hall, 1910, p. 13). "Artistic crafts" were selected because their "essential dignity and proficiency is well valued by anyone, whatever the education or position in life may be" (Hall, 1910, p. 12). Hall employed educated artists to work with patients at Marblehead. In July 1905, Hall conceptualized Marblehead as "set apart from the sanatorium" and as a practical industrial workshop for patients to apprentice and train, with future opportunities.

Hall's workshop moved to Devereux Mansion in 1912, a former country club estate. Patients lived in the mansion house at the Devereux Mansion (Devereux Sanitarium) and did their craft work in adjacent buildings. Hall justified this treatment by saying, "If a young woman comes complaining of sleeplessness, fear, nervous weakness the patient should be sent to some medical workshop. She will forget and leave behind such symptoms" (Hall & Buck, 1915, p. xxiii). Marblehead and Devereux Mansion, situated in beautiful locations and primarily intended for women of means with nervous exhaustion, represented an occupation treatment model that informed other healing houses at the time (see Figure 2.2).

Consolation House, opened by George Edward Barton in Clifton Springs, New York, in March 1914, was an important occupational therapy healing house because it was here, from March 15 to 17, 1917, that the founders formally conceptualized and defined *occupation* and founded the NSPOT (Barton, 1917).

FIGURE 2.2. Healing in a house: Restorative childhood occupation.

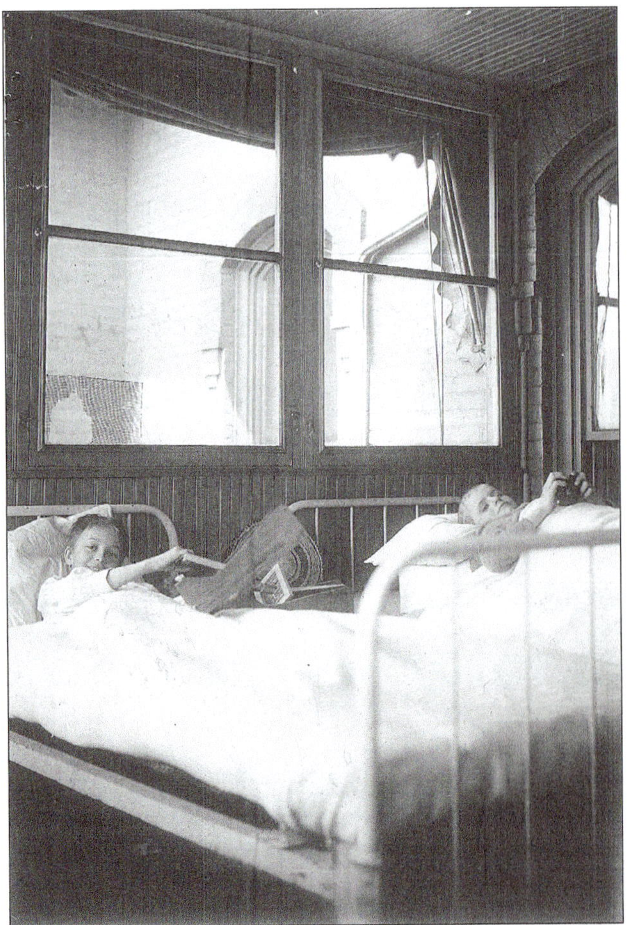

Note. Children with active tuberculosis rest on the porch and get some fresh air and nutrition before the advent of surgery or medication (ca. 1920). *Source.* Courtesy of the Archives of the American Occupational Therapy Association, North Bethesda, MD.

Letters exchanged among Barton, Dunton, and Slagle from 1914–1917 discuss quandaries about naming the organization and profession and determining the first meeting location and founding officers, grounding initial discussions in professional identity that would remain an ongoing occupational therapy interest (Bing, 1992; Nelson, 1997). In a historical analysis, Breines (1995) argued that in deliberating a mediating professional name, the ambiguity and comprehensiveness of the term *occupation* served the profession's mental and physical treatment focus. Barton, the first president of NSPOT, is particularly interesting, not only for his conceptualization of Consolation House, teaching about occupations, and his marriage to Isabel Barton (also a founder of NSPOT), but for his influence as an occupational therapy patient. Because of this, it is important to understand both the healing house and the man.

Barton's patient history is unclear, but in 1913, he responded to an advertisement for convalescence at the progressive Clifton Springs Sanitarium, or "Old San," to recover from tuberculosis, paralysis, and two amputated toes (Wemett, 2017). "No one can doubt that Mr. Barton is the most convincing example of all that re-education can do for a sick man" (Newton, 1917, p. 326). Isabel Barton described her future husband's struggles:

> He spent twenty-seven percent of his life in hospitals. His last collapse had apparently robbed him of everything which made life worth living: he seemed hopelessly down and out. The Rev. Elwood Worcester convinced him . . . [to] get well for the sake of the other fellow. (Newton, 1917, p. 321)

Barton, working with others, lived his beliefs about healing occupations.

Consolation House "was not an institution, but a movement to get away from institutional life towards [being] self-supporting" (Newton, 1917, p. 321; see Figure 2.3). The house was conceptualized as a "school-workshop and vocational bureau for convalescents" in "raising hospital occupations out of the place of amusement" (Bing, 1992, p. 30). Barton, a proponent of re-education, physical restoration, and craftwork for employment, did not support the arts and crafts movement for aesthetics and criticized Hall for using crafts for the wealthy, although Barton himself was raised in comfort (Bing, 1992). Barton opened Consolation House to carry out his "new purpose in life" (Barton, 1968, p. 340). Converting an old red barn, Barton created an industrial workshop. Barton, advocating occupation, labored in the workshop and garden regularly and even regained more motion in his left hand and arm over time (Barton, 1968). A retired architect, Barton designed wheelchair accommodations using the downstairs dining room as his bedroom with an additional full bath. His occupational therapy office was the former first floor front parlor, which held NSPOT's first occupational therapy library, including a glass case exhibiting items made at the workshop (see Figure 2.4).

Like glazed pottery made at Marblehead, fabric woven and displayed at the Labor Museum in Hull House, or a solid chair made at Consolation House and placed in the society's

FIGURE 2.3. Healing in a house—an occupations movement: Consolation House (a) and shop and studio (b).

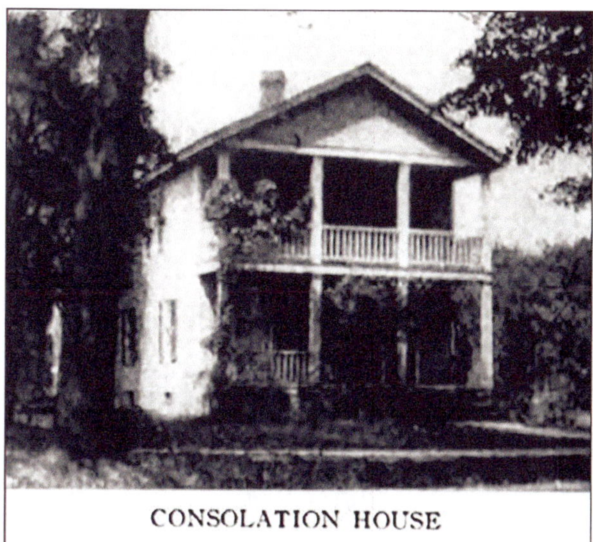

CONSOLATION HOUSE

(a)

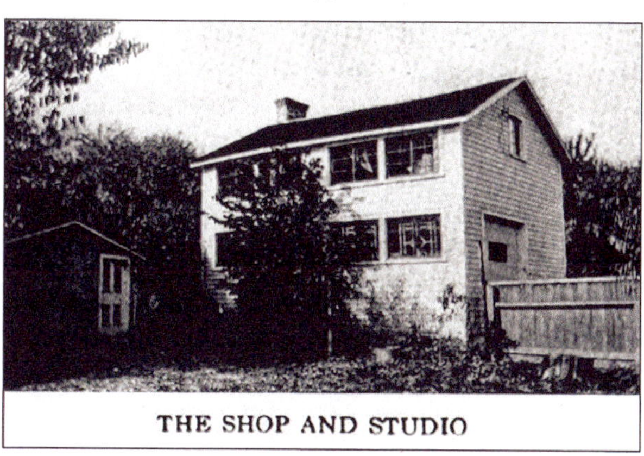

THE SHOP AND STUDIO

(b)

Source. From "Consolation House," by I. G. Newton, 1917, *Trained Nurse and Hospital Review, 59,* 321–326. In the public domain.

library, these crafts are tangible reminders that those who are ill, young or old, needy or privileged, become healthier when occupied.

As hospitals grew in size, scope, and number across the United States, so did occupational therapy. Hospitals—military and civilian—increasingly became the main source of health care for millions as the United States invested in returning people with injuries, disease, and disability to productive roles in society; they became places where physicians practiced with science and people healed. Wars spurred new technologies, and rehabilitation practices strengthened the role of occupational therapy in medicine. Medicine became synonymous with health care. Patients' move toward independent and self-reliant living and occupational therapy's independence from physical medicine helped transform both the profession and the nature of rehabilitative care.

FIGURE 2.4. George Barton taking a dose of his own occupational medicine.

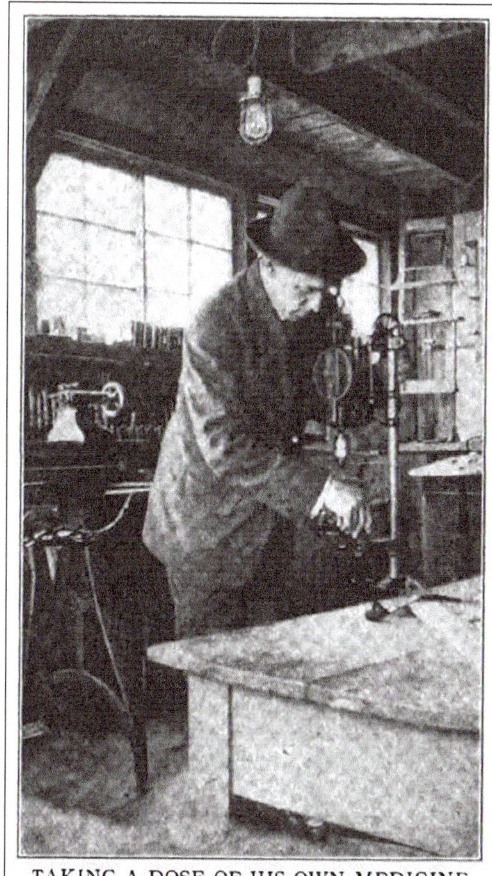

TAKING A DOSE OF HIS OWN MEDICINE
THE DIRECTOR TRAINING HIMSELF IN CO-ORDINATION WITH THE BENCH DRILL-PRESS

Note. From "Consolation House," by I. G. Newton, 1917, *Trained Nurse and Hospital Review, 59,* 321–326. In the public domain.

Pre–World War I (1756–1917)

The Philadelphia-located ***Pennsylvania Hospital*** claims to be the first hospital with the sole intent of curing the "sick poor" (Penn Medicine, n.d.-b; Ransom, 1943). The Pennsylvania Hospital first admitted patients in 1756 with a basement reserved for "persons 'distempered' in mind and deprived of their rational faculties" (Slagle, 1914, p. 14). The hospital cared for soldiers from the Revolutionary War, the Spanish–American War, the War of 1812, and the Civil War (Ransom, 1943). Dr. Benjamin Rush, later known as the father of psychiatry, served on staff (1783–1813) and was a known early advocate of occupations and the work cure ("Benjamin Rush [1745–1813]," 1945), and he regularly encouraged "patients to sew, garden, listen to music, or exercise during the day" (Penn Medicine, n.d.-a). By 1832, a separate asylum was created "for our insane patients with ample space for their proper seclusion, classification and employment" (Penn Medicine, n.d.-b), and by 1841 the number of insane patients at the Pennsylvania Hospital was double the number of those with physical diagnoses (Penn Medicine, n.d.-b). This proportion would change by the mid-1900s.

In the 1800s, most Americans seldom saw a doctor. Rather, their medical care was primarily performed by family members at home or in private rest homes. Hospitals were regarded as places of last resort, with public hospitals most aligned with poverty and plagues (Hirsh, 1954). Wealthy Americans received private care at home and paid for this service in cash. In 1850, only three major hospitals served New York City, one voluntary (St. Luke's Hospital, privately endowed), one public (Bellevue), and one a Catholic hospital (St. Vincent's Hospital of the City of New York) that was newly opened in this rapidly growing city with a large immigrant population and was funded by modest payments and church fundraisers (Hirsh, 1954).

A surge of private or donor-supported hospitals emerged in response to a growing immigrant population, and ward (inpatient) care was free of charge to the patient (Hirsh, 1954). This meant that hospitals were in a perpetual deficit that only increased as the population rapidly expanded as a result of waves of immigrants in the late 1800s. The number of hospitals grew rapidly from 149 in 1873 to 7,269 in 1929, including general hospitals (public and voluntary or private), sanatoriums, surgical hospitals, industrial hospitals, and hospitals in which special populations could convalesce, such as those for infectious disease, cancer, and mental or nervous disorders. Hospital stays decreased from an average of 20 days to 11 to 12 days (Hall & Ellis, 1930). Health care became increasingly hospital based, with quality hospitals associated with the use of laboratories and specialized equipment.

World War I (1917–1918)

Technological advances revolutionized American hospitals, now synonymous with health care, when the United States entered World War I in April 1917. Hospital cost deficits were extreme, with public institutions predominantly serving the poor, and privately funded voluntary institutions serving the wealthy. New health profession societies emerged, including NSPOT (March 15, 1917), the American Association of Hospital Social Workers (1918; Cowles & Fort, 2003), and the American Physical Therapy Association (1921). A year later, hospital deficits jumped another 25% (Hirsh, 1954).

Reconstruction Hospitals

Hospitals organized overseas units, provided medical and surgical services to enable servicemen to be fit for duty, cared for military families, and set up rehabilitation units for returning injured servicemen. ***Reconstruction hospitals*** were located within the United States and were administered by medical officers who prescribed occupational therapy for patients (McDaniel, 1968; see Figure 2.5). Two types of ***reconstruction aides*** served in World War I: (1) physiotherapy aides and (2) occupational therapy aides (Linker, 2011). Physiotherapy aides used techniques such as massage, exercise, electrotherapy, hydrotherapy, and mechanotherapy to enhance physical health, whereas occupational therapy aides used crafts, industrial activities, and prevocational activities to enhance overall convalescence, improve self-confidence, and reduce the effects of a new condition, shell shock (Dunton, 1919; Linker, 2011). The first supervisor of reconstruction aides in occupational therapy and physical therapy, Marguerite Sanderson, was appointed in January 1918 to recruit and train persons into four classifications of personnel: craft teachers, academic teachers, medical social workers, and office workers (McDaniel, 1968).

FIGURE 2.5. Healing in hospitals: Basic skills.

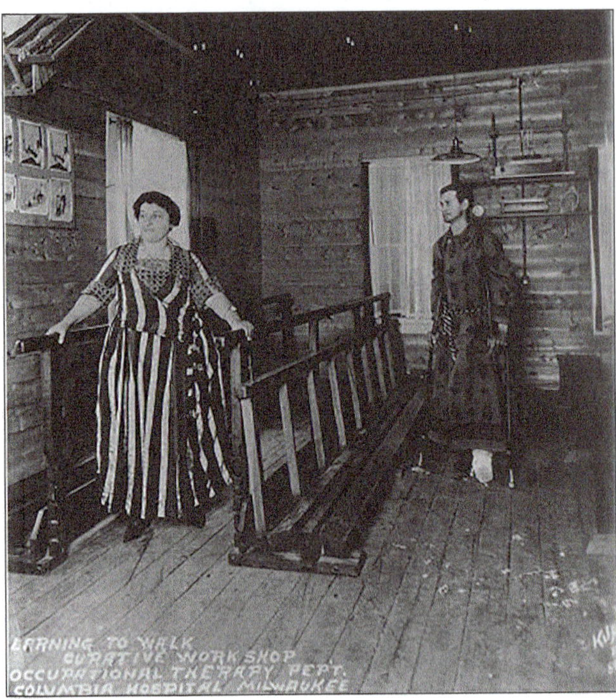
LEARNING TO WALK
CURATIVE WORKSHOP
OCCUPATIONAL THERAPY DEPT.
COLUMBIA HOSPITAL MILWAUKEE

Note. This was occupational therapy as carried out in 1919 in a small cottage on the grounds of the Columbia Hospital in Milwaukee, Wisconsin, in a program that eventually became the well-known Workshop of Milwaukee. *Source.* Courtesy of the Archive of the American Occupational Therapy Association, North Bethesda, MD.

Occupational therapy aides' function was associated with that of a craft teacher. At this time, occupational therapy was classified differently from physical therapy and separated into ward occupations, workshop, and farm work (McDaniel, 1968). Occupational therapy aides generally administered ward occupations and trade and farm occupations, originally taught by male instructors who also supervised curative workshops, which were gradually managed by occupational therapists (McDaniel, 1968, p. 71; see Figure 2.6).

Postwar Occupational Therapy

The goal of postwar occupational therapy was to return recovered civilian soldiers to productive work, thereby minimizing the economic burden of nonworking people on society, which,

FIGURE 2.6. Healing in hospitals: The World War I weavers.

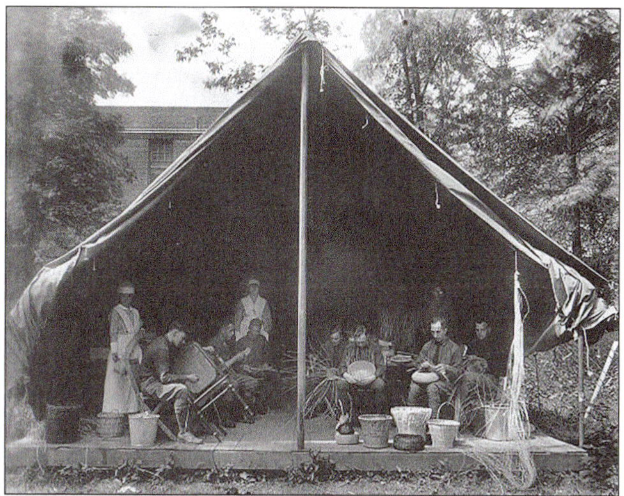

Note. Occupational therapy basketry and chair caning workshop. U.S. General Hospital No. 38, Eastview, NY (ca. 1919).
Source. Courtesy of the Archives of the American Occupational Therapy Association, North Bethesda, MD.

although theoretically in line with the client's desired outcome, had no real connection to determining patients' needs or desires after therapy. The U.S. Senate, in response to a 1918 study conducted by the Federal Board for Vocational Education, directed that ***rehabilitation*** programs be established for the "rehabilitation and vocational reeducation of crippled soldiers and sailors" (U.S. Federal Board for Vocational Education, 1918, p. 3). This document defined *rehabilitation* using the words *invalid or bedside occupations, occupational therapy, curative workshop,* and *vocational education* (p. 11) and, more important, described the process of rehabilitation (Table 2.1). Treatment by occupation was diversional, which was found to influence the mind and spirit, resulting in favorable physical changes. "It was frequently observed that, while the patient's mind was absorbed in mastering an occupation in the hospital workshop, his interest was awakened, his ambition stimulated, his morbid and brooding thoughts eliminated, and his hope and self-confidence were restored" (U.S. Federal Board for Vocational Education, 1918, p. 35). The U.S. Federal Board for Vocational Education (1918) described the aims of occupational therapy as

> first to create a wholesome interest in something outside the patient's morbid interest in himself and his symptoms; second, to fill the unoccupied portions of the patient's day; third, to prepare his mental attitude so that he may adjust himself to normal demands and environment after hospital discharge; and fourth, to facilitate medical treatment by regulated exercise. (p. 50)

Few hospitals outside of the military had the equipment to provide curative intervention in hospitals; more supported teaching invalid occupations (U.S. Federal Board for Vocational Education, 1918). The newly formed NSPOT readily reacted to the news of the rehabilitation plan; then-President W. R. Dunton (1918) wrote, "We have been informed by one person that the Surgeon-General's office has perfected very elaborate plans for the care of the war cripple" (p. 55). He went on to report that Eleanor Clarke Slagle would remain in Chicago, "which she considers the normal center of America and the natural receiving station for the armies of wounded soldiers which will soon begin arriving from the front" (U.S. Federal Board for Vocational Education, 1918, p. 56). When asked by the Surgeon General's office to direct a national effort in occupational therapy, Slagle stipulated that the headquarters of the movement be in Chicago (Dunton, 1918). Occupational therapy, as a medical veteran's service, began in February 1918 on the orthopedic wards at Walter Reed General Hospital in Washington, DC, with three unpaid occupational therapy aides, followed soon thereafter by reconstruction programs at several other Army hospitals (McDaniel, 1968). At first originally organized under education, occupational therapy soon joined physical therapy as being located within reconstruction programs (McDaniel, 1968).

War training courses for reconstruction aides emerged, with philanthropic organizations funding many such courses

TABLE 2.1. STAGES OF REHABILITATION IN WORLD WAR I

STAGE	PATIENT	OCCUPATIONAL THERAPY INTERVENTION
Acute convalescing	Injured or ill men unable to go to curative workshop and in bed	Invalid bedside occupations to help wounded men feel productive and prevent self-pity and brooding
General convalescing	Men unable to return to the field, but able to work	Curative workshop: "the science of healing by occupation" (U.S. Federal Board for Vocational Education, 1918, p. 12) Prevocational preparation Common conditions: general debility, heart trouble, nerve disorders, tuberculosis, rheumatism, injuries with orthopedic care
Vocational reeducation	Men returning to same vocation or who must learn a new vocation	Supported work in natural setting

Source. Adapted from U.S. Federal Board for Vocational Education (1918).

(Hirsh, 1954). The U.S. government's reconstruction hospitals for disabled persons required all occupational therapy practitioners to first qualify by completing a short intensive training course no more than 4 weeks long to learn about the medical and social problems of the disabled soldiers and to receive necessary practical experience. These early occupational therapy practitioners were recruited from manual training teachers, men who had technical knowledge in the teaching profession, and from skilled workmen (U.S. Federal Board for Vocational Education, 1918). Through readings, lectures, and exams, students were expected to learn about the psychology of the disabled soldier, occupational therapy in relation to orthopedic treatment, occupational therapy for mental and nervous disorders, general techniques of occupational therapy, therapeutic value of occupations, methods of teaching, and the workings of a curative workshop. Work, or being productive, was highly valued, and work was evaluated and reinforced in hospital-based workshops. The presence of productive and meaningful work was highly valued as a therapeutic agent.

The adoption of occupational therapy's core ideas about occupation, use of activity, and expectation of beneficial results by government and society as a whole, and as a necessary component of postwar care, was a key step for the profession; at the same time, the binary notion of disability (in terms of usefulness to society) and lack of a nuanced—never mind individualized—approach to care pointed to the growing pains of achieving mass acceptance. Leaving behind the smaller scale, if more bourgeois, notions of settlement house care resulted in trade-offs that continue to animate debates central to the profession and the approaches to care.

Reprieve Between World Wars

After World War I, health care shifted from a focus on hospitals to a focus on alternative forms of delivery, in part because hospitals were "overage, outmoded, overcrowded and understaffed" (Hirsh, 1954, p. 41). In 1921, the Veterans Bureau was formed, and veterans homes and programs transitioned into Veterans Bureau hospitals designed to treat the new types of injuries resulting from the new forms of mechanized warfare seen in World War I (VA History Office, n.d.). Fees were introduced to help cover costs, and by 1924 the Cornell University Medical College reported that within the first 6 months of the introduction of fees, 13,072 people visited the clinic for a total of 53,387 visits at $1.00 per visit. New services were introduced, including well-baby care, maternity care, regular physical exams, and services for people who were emotionally disturbed or ill (Hirsh, 1954), and patients started to pay for their services.

After World War I, demand for ward and outpatient services sharply increased, with an equally large decrease in paying patients (Hirsh, 1954). A 1934 survey of all 329 New York City hospitals found that they were poorly equipped or funded to meet growing health care needs, particularly to care for persons affected by "tuberculosis, the mentally ill, and patients with acute communicable diseases" (Hirsh, 1954, p. 58). A key recommendation from the survey was to expand social services and to use a form of insurance to fund these expanded services by allowing wage earners to spread the risk of hospital expenses by prepaying hospital costs (Hirsh, 1954, p. 61).

Occupational therapists focused on grading activities as interventions for convalescing tuberculosis patients and applying scientific principles to the large influx of rehabilitation needs resulting from war injuries and conditions. Occupational therapists based physical intervention on biomechanical principles of muscle strength and joint range. Medicalization of occupational therapy stemmed from the belief that removing impairments would sufficiently rehabilitate people to return to daily life.

World War II

World War II resulted in another surge of demand for occupational therapists (Dunton, 1947; U.S. War Department, 1944). Dunton, in his history of occupational therapy in the first Willard and Spackman occupational therapy textbook, reported, "With the opening of World War II . . . the total number of practicing therapists was less than that required by the military hospitals alone" (Dunton, 1947, p. 8). Major Wilma West (1966) reported that in 1943, the U.S. Surgeon General established occupational therapy departments in U.S. Army general hospitals while describing occupational therapy as "a valuable adjunct to medical treatment" (p. 651). New York voluntary hospitals released more than 10,000 doctors, nurses, and others to the armed forces. At the same time, they struggled to retain a health care workforce to care for civilians at home. Occupational therapists were in demand. The five original occupational therapist training programs at the end of World War I continued to be the only available training programs in 1944 and graduated fewer than 100 graduates per year (West, 1966). Of these, the majority of occupational therapists (99% female civilians) were employed by large state psychiatric hospitals, limiting the number of occupational therapists available to serve war needs, and on December 7, 1941, when Pearl Harbor was attacked, only 12 occupational therapists were on duty in 13 Army hospitals across the United States (West, 1966; see Figure 2.7).

Army psychiatrists particularly supported the need for qualified occupational therapy personnel because "occupational therapy had its beginnings, earliest recognition, and most extensive use in treatment programs for the mentally ill" (West, 1966, p. 651), and many psychiatrists, commissioned in the Medical Corps from civilian hospitals, were familiar with occupational therapy's contributions to psychiatric treatment. To help meet the demand, the Red Cross hired "recreation workers, volunteer Gray Ladies with some craft training, and volunteer members of the Arts and Skills Corps" (West, 1966, p. 652) who were outstanding artists and craftsmen to contribute their time to offer diversional crafts to hospital

FIGURE 2.7. Healing in hospitals: Hands-on victory after World War II.

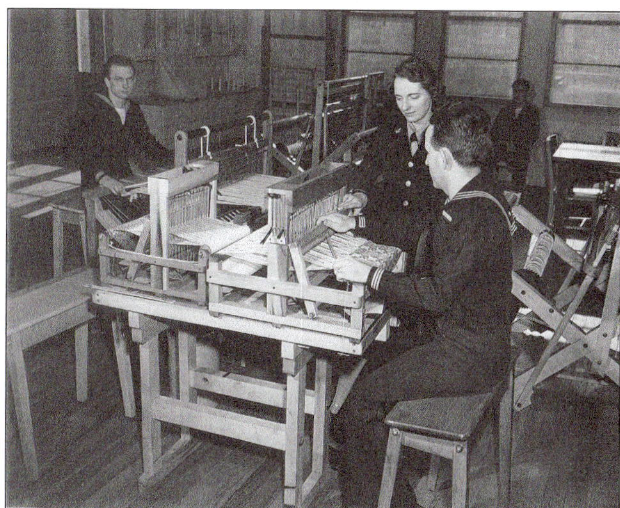

Note. Occupational therapy building at U.S. Naval Hospital at St. Albans, Long Island, NY. Here, wounded men of the Navy exercise injured muscles and find mental relaxation at looms and printing presses and in pottery making and other useful occupations (ca. 1940s).
Source. Courtesy of the Archive of the American Occupational Therapy Association, North Bethesda, MD.

patients and who were under the supervision of occupational therapists (U.S. War Department, 1944). Irene Hollis, occupational therapist, recounted a personal experience in her 1979 Eleanor Clarke Slagle lecture titled "Remember":

> In 1944 I was happily teaching high school home economics only 30 miles from a large Army Hospital in central Texas. World War II was raging. There was an announcement in the local paper asking for volunteers to help thread looms in the Occupational Therapy Department of this Army hospital. . . . While threading looms, I observed other activities and was intrigued . . . the Army was setting up war emergency courses to help relieve the shortage of occupational therapists, I applied and was accepted. (p. 494)

Military-serving occupational therapists also struggled with adapting traditionally feminine occupations to those with a more masculine appeal. Occupational therapy modalities expanded to include plastics, electricity, and radio repair (West, 1966). Existing hospitals were remodeled, and new hospitals were built to include workshop space for occupational therapy. By 1945, 18 of 21 war training courses were accredited to help meet the demand (Dunton, 1947). West (1968, p. 684) stated,

> [Pre–World War II] occupational therapy consisted largely of understaffed, overcrowded, activity-centered programs for female patients or for deteriorated, chronic male "psychotics." Weaving and basketry were the symbols of practice. Increasingly, today, occupational therapy is an integral part of admission and acute treatment services, of day and night hospitals, of halfway homes, and of mental hygiene clinics and other outpatient facilities. More specific individual and group techniques are demanded by the psychiatrist, and a more realistic scope of vocationally related activities characterizes the modern treatment program. (p. 684)

Occupational therapy programs differed on the basis of the type of World War II hospital: general, convalescent, regional, station, and specialty (West, 1966). General hospitals were designated to serve psychiatric patients, who typically received occupational therapy daily, both individually and in groups (West, 1966, p. 663). Occupational therapy restored physical function to muscles and joints, provided controlled activity for those with nervous and mental disorders, helped soldiers readjust to chronic conditions, reeducated soldiers with permanent disabilities, and ensured that patients used their time in the hospital purposefully (U.S. War Department, 1944). Goals of occupational therapy were to prevent mental and physical deterioration, encourage socialization and feelings of group identification, simulate creative imagination and expression, reduce poverty of ideation, and provide self-confidence and a sense of security (West, 1966, p. 663). Interventions were delivered to individuals, groups, and populations of soldiers.

One overarching goal of rehabilitation during World War II was to facilitate the employment of disabled soldiers (U.S. War Department, 1944). Industrial therapy, the final phase of occupational therapy, was prescribed to reduce psychosomatic symptoms, grade work situations, provide vocational exploration, or practice work habits. Jobs were first analyzed on the basis of personal requirements, physical and environmental demands, and their hazards or risks (West, 1966, p. 668). Specific military convalescent hospitals mimicked Army field units with patients who were dressed in duty uniforms and largely independent in their care. These soldiers participated in reconditioning programs, educational classes, medical counseling, social work, and occupational therapy as needed to develop ego strength and group social skills (West, 1966). Patients worked independently in specific settings such as machine shops, quiet shops, and art studios to develop a variety of occupations (West, 1966). Referrals to vocational reeducation were partially based on screening by the occupational therapists who managed these prevocational industrial experiences. As with World War I, expected outcomes were simplistic and generalized; however, far more Americans had been wounded or traumatized, and the dominance of medical doctors over health care was firmly in place. This environment, combined with the successes of rehabilitation for veterans, was the force that shaped the modern, postwar occupational therapy profession, in which experienced military therapists, such as West, assumed a major role in guiding the profession forward.

Postwar Era Medicalization of Occupational Therapy

> Our responsibility is to read widely and observe, to think and bring to the doctor's attention those things which might affect the patient. (Rood, 1958, p. 328)

By the end of World War II, rehabilitation was a respected area of medical intervention for both returning veterans and those with industrial disabilities. Occupational therapy required a physician's prescription, as did other medical interventions, but questions arose about where occupational therapy best fit within the growing number of medical specializations. A committee of physicians recommended that ***physical medicine and rehabilitation*** (PM&R) teaching and research centers be located in medical schools and hospitals across the United States and that occupational therapy and physical therapy be located under PM&R (Colman, 1992; Krusen, 1944). By 1945, the year World War II ended, the American Medical Association had established a section for PM&R, and by 1946, 25 hospitals had PM&R residencies and 12 universities had training and research funding for PM&R (American Academy of Physical Medicine and Rehabilitation, n.d.). One of the subcommittees specifically focused on occupational therapy recommended that occupational therapy be part of the course of study in medical schools and that "all of the centers for physical medicine promote a program for better coordination of physical therapy, occupational therapy, physical rehabilitation and spa therapy" (Krusen, 1944, p. 1095). Occupational therapy was described as providing "a graded program of activity to restore maximal physical and mental function or [seeking] to divert a person and improve morale by arousing his interest, courage and confidence" (Krusen, 1944, p. 1094). In this context, occupational therapy focused primarily on restoring function.

In response to the recommendation that occupational therapy be located under PM&R, AOTA (1948) stated, "The American Occupational Therapy Association believes that the scope of occupational therapy, its interest and efforts are considerably broader than at present indicated by physical medicine." AOTA set the stage so that occupational therapy could retain its mental health roots in psychiatry rather than be focused predominantly on rehabilitation of physical dysfunction, which would likely have occurred if organizationally located under PM&R. This decision by AOTA in part enabled the occupational therapy profession's current movement into primary care and the ability to practice without a medical prescription (Figure 2.8).

FIGURE 2.8. Healing in hospitals: Building strength.

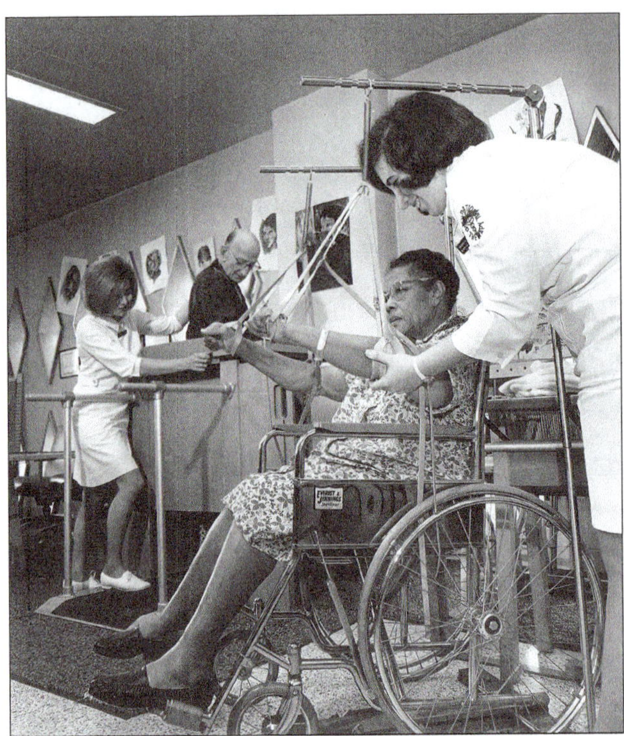

Note. Occupational therapists working in hospitals in the 1960s adhered to a prescribed physician-driven model. This figure exemplifies a treatment session in a physical rehabilitation setting, in which goals included strengthening and mobility.
Source. Courtesy of the Archives of the American Occupational Therapy Association, North Bethesda, MD.

At this same time, medicine was focusing on using consistent interventions and outcome measures to increase its use of science in practice. When Sidney Licht delivered his speech "The Objectives of Occupational Therapy" to the New York Society of Physical Medicine on November 6, 1946, occupational therapy was described as a "medically prescribed activity for therapeutic objectives" (Licht, 1947, p. 17). In an effort to apply the scientific method to occupational therapy, Licht (1947) identified four measurable outcomes of occupational therapy, each with subobjectives, as described in Exhibit 2.1. By purposefully selecting the word *kinetic* to replace *functional,* Licht made sure that physicians would not misinterpret its meaning; in medical culture, the word *functional* meant "unable to find the impairment." Licht felt that this was important because

> the recent publicity given this type of treatment [occupational therapy] has stressed the by-products rather than the objective. Displays of patients' craftwork have led the public and many physicians to think in terms of design and merchandise rather than the basic philosophy of this form of treatment. (Licht, 1947, p. 18)

The replacement of *graded* with *metric* emphasized the importance of measuring the increase or decrease in resistance or another physical property to grade the activity. Licht translated the word *activities* to *modalities* and identified six main modalities of occupational therapy: agriculture, arts, crafts, education, industry and maintenance, and recreational therapy. *Industrial therapy* referred to hospital maintenance work (e.g., mechanical, administrative, and custodial; Licht, 1947).

The belief that occupation was central to maintaining health and well-being eroded with the increased pressure to apply interventions to reduce impairments (Friedland, 1998). Physical intervention applied anatomy and kinesiology to understand and improve movement. For example, Berta Bobath (1948) altered the course of therapy for children diagnosed with cerebral palsy and adults with hemiplegia when she and her husband proposed a method of intervention that, through handling, replaced impaired movement patterns with

EXHIBIT 2.1. Proposed Taxonomy and Objectives for Occupational Therapy, 1946

1. Kinetic (old word: *functional*) used to restore or improve
    a. muscle strength
    b. joint mobilization
    c. coordination.
2. Metric (old word: *graded*) used to
    a. improve work tolerance and
    b. measure progress of tolerance.
3. Tonic (old word: *diversional*) used to improve and maintain
    a. muscle tone
    b. mental tone.
4. Psychiatric: used to favorably influence
    a. psychomotor activity
        i. stimulation
        ii. sedation
    b. emotional disturbance
        i. emotional stability (contentment)
        ii. mood
    c. behavior
        i. behavior (habit) training
    d. abnormal mental content
        i. guilt complex
        ii paranoid trends
    e. psychosocial activity
        i. socialization
        ii. obtainable objectives
    f. diagnosis
        i. reaction to situation in clinic
        ii. identification of problem (in psychodrama)
        iii. determination of limit of intellectual work capacity
        iv. prevocational exploration
    g. mental hygiene
        i. overcome restlessness
        ii. promote good work and play habits.

Source. Licht (1947).

those considered more "normal." Proprioceptive neuromuscular facilitation, introduced by Margaret Knott and Dorothy Voss in 1965, combined movement patterns that were both spiral and diagonal and facilitated by stretch. The second edition of Willard and Spackman's (1954) *Principles of Occupational Therapy* expanded to include more content about the basic principles of treatment for physical disabilities.

Hospitals—public and private, military and veteran—directly contributed to the development of occupational therapy as a profession. Occupational therapy, which had been used as a medical service intrinsic to the health and well-being of injured, impaired, and convalescing individuals with the goal to return people to useful, functional living (see Figure 2.5), returned to its civilian context. The expansion of occupational therapy was supported in wartime, with consistent military commitment and funding to support its role in the rehabilitation of those with physical, mental, or emotional injuries, and this commitment ensured that, after the war, occupational therapy treatment moved into the mainstream of rehabilitative care. By the 1940s, the definition of *rehabilitation* had expanded beyond the vocational training and placement that was a focus in the early years of occupational therapy. The National Council on Rehabilitation adopted a definition of *rehabilitation* as "restoration of the handicapped to the fullest physical, mental, social, vocational and economic usefulness of which they are capable" (as cited in Hudson, 1947, p. 313).

Although hospital-based services helped to substantiate occupational therapy in the 1920s through the 1950s, discussions continued about ensuring occupational therapy's status as a true profession (Yerxa, 1967, p. 1). From the 1960s through the early 2000s, occupational therapy leaders looked beyond the medical model of hospital-based services to build an occupational therapy profession aimed more directly at community needs. Occupational therapy redefined itself as an act of professional autonomy, moving past relying on physicians or other external stakeholders for definition (Gillette & Kielhofner, 1979; Yerxa, 1967). This self-definition involved expanding areas of practice beyond the medical model, such as developing a common language, theoretical explanations, and research to encompass all areas of occupational therapy practice. Adapting notions of occupation, activity, and the role of therapeutic intervention was key to addressing these more contemporary issues.

Expanding Practice

> Our responsibility as a profession is to implement a broader perspective of healthcare delivery—one that places its value on individuals as they accept the responsibility for their own health status. (Baum, 1980, p. 505)

By the late 20th century, occupational therapy practice in the United States focused on mental health, physical disabilities, and pediatrics. In the late 1970s, AOTA created the first Special Interest Groups in recognition of the increasing specialization among occupational therapy practitioners. The five groups were Mental Health, Physical Disabilities, Gerontology, Developmental Disabilities, and Sensory Integration. However, the debate about the pros and cons of specialization continued (Gillette & Kielhofner, 1979). Changing federal legislation and consumer movements helped occupational therapy practitioners consider how to develop emerging areas of practice and expand traditional areas of practice beyond hospitals and other institutional care settings. Opportunities and discussions about further specialization, especially in the 1970s, also affected occupational therapy's expansion into emerging areas of practice.

Mental Health

The passage of the ***Community Mental Health Centers Act*** (P. L. 88-164) in 1963 led to mental health services shifting from hospitals to halfway houses and community mental health centers (Ethridge, 1976; Finn, 1972). Occupational

FIGURE 2.9. Building occupational houses: Practical steps.

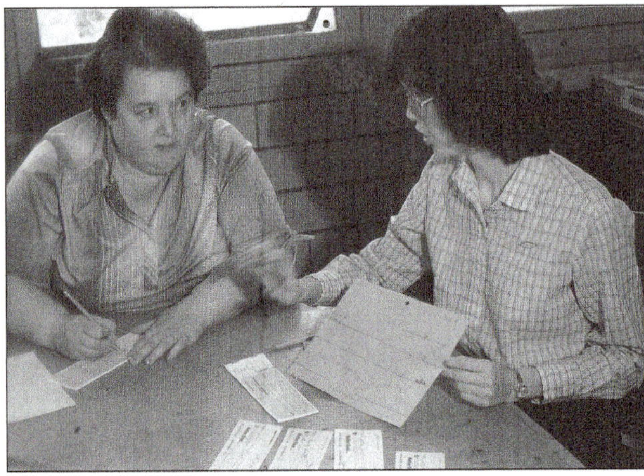

Note. Mental health clients practice the mechanics of managing a checking account as part of a community readiness program. Real-life situations are simulated to allow clients to prepare for independent living (ca. 1981). Mayview State Hospital, Bridgeville, PA. Photo by Samuel A. Taylor.
Source. Courtesy of the Archives of the American Occupational Therapy Association, North Bethesda, MD.

FIGURE 2.10. Building occupational houses: Accessing the neighborhood.

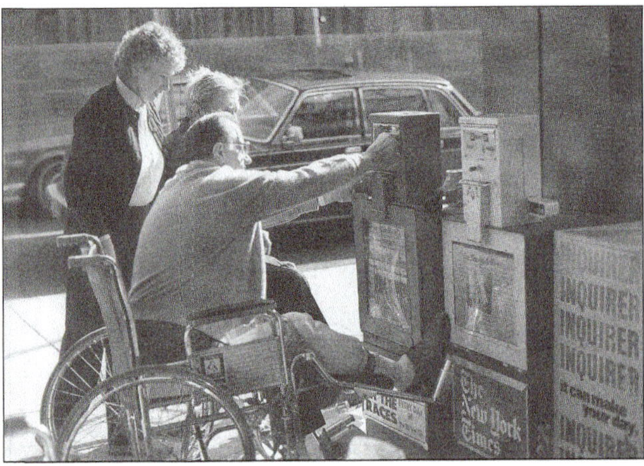

Note. The challenge of carrying out daily activities can be complicated by a physical disability. The occupational therapist accompanies a client as he learns to operate independently in the community (ca. 1984). Magee Rehabilitation Hospital, Philadelphia, PA. Photo by Suzanne Green. Courtesy of the Archive of the American Occupational Therapy Association, Inc.

therapists created centers to assist long-term patients transitioning from acute hospitals to community settings through halfway or even quarter-way houses (Mann, 1976). They also created additional community mental health practice opportunities in the 1960s through 1980s in settings such as jails, homeless shelters, and community mental health clubhouses (Peters, 2011; see Figure 2.9).

Physical Disabilities

The passage of the ***Social Security Amendments of 1965*** (P. L. 89-97) established Medicare and Medicaid, which provided a funding mechanism for occupational therapy to expand traditional physical disability services for a growing geriatric population. Increased focus on prevention in health care prompted calls for occupational therapy to move beyond hospitals into more community settings (Diamond & Laurencelle, 1961; Johnson & Smith, 1966; Wiemer & West, 1970; see Figure 2.10). Occupational therapists could access Medicare funding for home-based care and short-term therapy in skilled nursing facilities, and occupational therapists in rehabilitation centers increased the frequency with which they provided home services (Jackson, 1970; Johnson & Smith, 1966). Rehabilitation in nursing homes with geriatric populations allowed occupational therapy practitioners to integrate their skills working with those with psychosocial and physical disability (Jackson, 1970; Maloney, 1976). Occupational therapy in nursing homes and outpatient clinics had limited federal funding until it became a covered service under Medicare (Fisher, 2017).

The early 1980s brought managed health care and prospective payment systems to hospitals in an attempt to control increasing costs. This led to shorter hospital stays and concerns about decreased job opportunities in occupational therapy (Brachtesende, 2005). In actuality, because occupational therapy practitioners worked in the settings to which patients were discharged, including rehabilitation centers, skilled nursing facilities, and home care, they were already key to the cost efficiencies envisioned in managed care. This was not the case 10 years later when facilities adjusted to new payment restrictions associated with the Budget Enforcement Act of 1990 (P. L. 101-508), designed to counter the growth of Medicare spending in skilled nursing facilities (Brachtesende, 2005; Fisher, 2017). The occupational therapy job market did not recover until 2005, 15 years later (Brachtesende, 2005).

Pediatrics

Occupational therapy's work with children, first in home, medical, and institutional settings and later in community schools (Paisley, 1929), was a key part of the profession and its development over time. The relationship between the federal Maternal and Child Health Bureau and occupational therapy fueled the expansion of pediatric occupational therapy through the 1950s (Colman, 1988). The Maternal and Child Health Bureau supported Title V of the 1935 Social Security Act that created Crippled Children's Services, a state grant program under which occupational therapists provided services to children with orthopedic and other physical disabilities (Colman, 1988; Hanft, 1988).

Occupational therapy's role in public schools was enabled by the ***Education for All Handicapped Children Act of 1975*** (P. L. 94-142), federal legislation that required schools to provide free, appropriate educational services to all children with disabilities. The law required that related services, including occupational therapy, be provided as needed for children to access their education. Schools ensured children's readiness for learning in addition to providing traditional educational content, and occupational therapy contributed meaningful intervention to learning readiness (Colman, 1988; Gilfoyle & Hays, 1979).

Occupational therapists advocated for amendments to the Education for All Handicapped Children Act in the 1980s to further expand occupational therapy's role with young children ages birth to 5 years (Hanft, 1988). In spite of federal cost-cutting measures in the 1980s, the Education for All Handicapped Children Amendments of 1986 (P. L. 99-457) became law by arguing that money spent on services for young children would save money on long-term education and prevent future costs associated with institutionalization (Hanft, 1988). Under the new law, occupational therapy continued as a related service for early childhood, primary, and secondary education for children ages 3 to 21 years and as a primary service for early intervention services for children from birth to age 2 years (Hanft, 1988). Later amendments to the act (i.e., Individuals With Disabilities Education Act of 1990 [P. L. 101-476], Individuals With Disabilities Education Improvement Act of 2004 [P. L. 108-446]) ensured occupational therapy's continued role in public schools (see Figure 2.11).

FIGURE 2.11. Building occupational houses: Finding new ways.

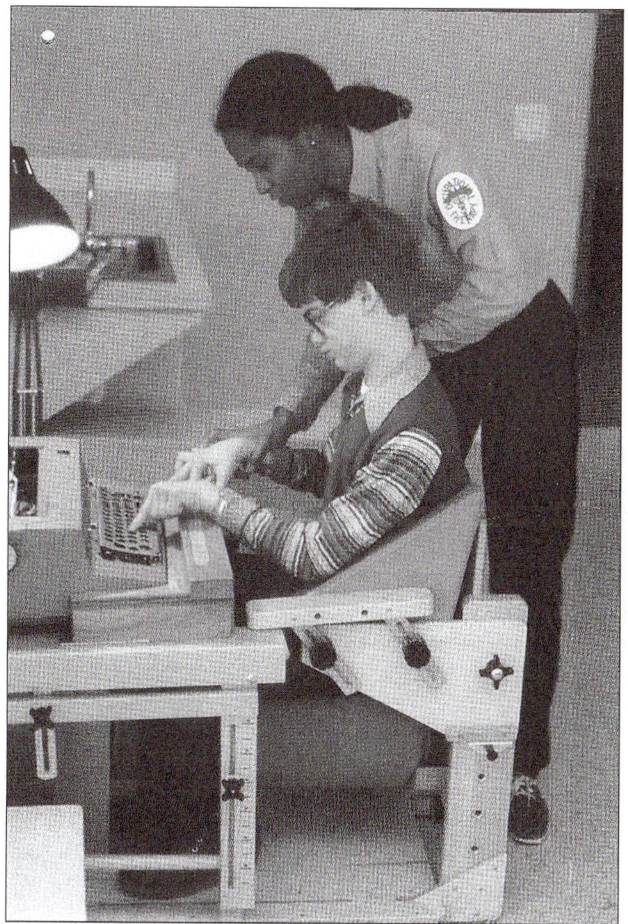

Note. This teenager's disability requires that they develop an alternative means of communication. The occupational therapist has provided an adapted typewriter and chair and training so they may function independently in school (ca. 1981). Norman A. Bleshman School, Paramus, NJ. Photo by Leon A. Butchko. Courtesy of the Archive of the American Occupational Therapy Association, Inc.

Consumer Advocacy

People with disabilities sought to define their own lives and rebelled against a medical system that did not address their needs and often did not see them as capable of independent, productive lives. The independent living movement began in the late 1960s, and advocacy around these issues is ongoing. The independent living movement called for the eradication of institutions, particularly those housing persons with mental impairments. In his landmark book *The Origin and Nature of Our Institutional Models,* Wolfensberger (1975) challenged the claim that institutions separated the deviant from the nondeviant, stating,

> the institution became not a paradise but a purgatory, not a Garden of Eden but an agency of dehumanization; to this day, residents are subjected to physical and mental abuse, to neglect and inadequate care and services, to environmental deprivation, and to restriction of the most basic rights and dignities of a citizen. (p. 60)

In addition to asserting their right to live in community settings, people with disabilities also advocated for reasonable accommodations for work and community access (Peters, 2011; Veltri, 1997; Wolfensberger, 1975). This advocacy led to the Rehabilitation Act of 1973 (P. L. 93-112) and the Americans With Disabilities Act of 1990 (P. L. 101-336; see Figure 2.12). Occupational therapy practitioners expressed support for the independent living movement, especially because it had the potential to further expand the role of occupational therapy in community settings and in emerging areas of practice, such as environmental accessibility (AOTA, 1981, 1993). Given the profession's founding goals of returning individuals to productive, healthy, and fulfilling lives, advocacy for people with disabilities is often intrinsic; however, decades of institutional care also meant broadly rethinking and reshaping the roles of therapeutic intervention for a population no longer isolated from the larger community.

Becoming Authentic

> Professionalism . . . means being able to meet real needs. It means being unique. . . . It also means being "authentic." (Yerxa, 1967, p. 1)

To claim its status as a true profession, occupational therapy needed a unique body of knowledge grounded in research and theory (Mosey, 1968; Yerxa, 1967). Professions, as opposed to trades or semiprofessions, require a unique knowledge base, extensive education, explicit processes of professional

FIGURE 2.12. The Americans With Disabilities Act of 1990: Building community pathways.

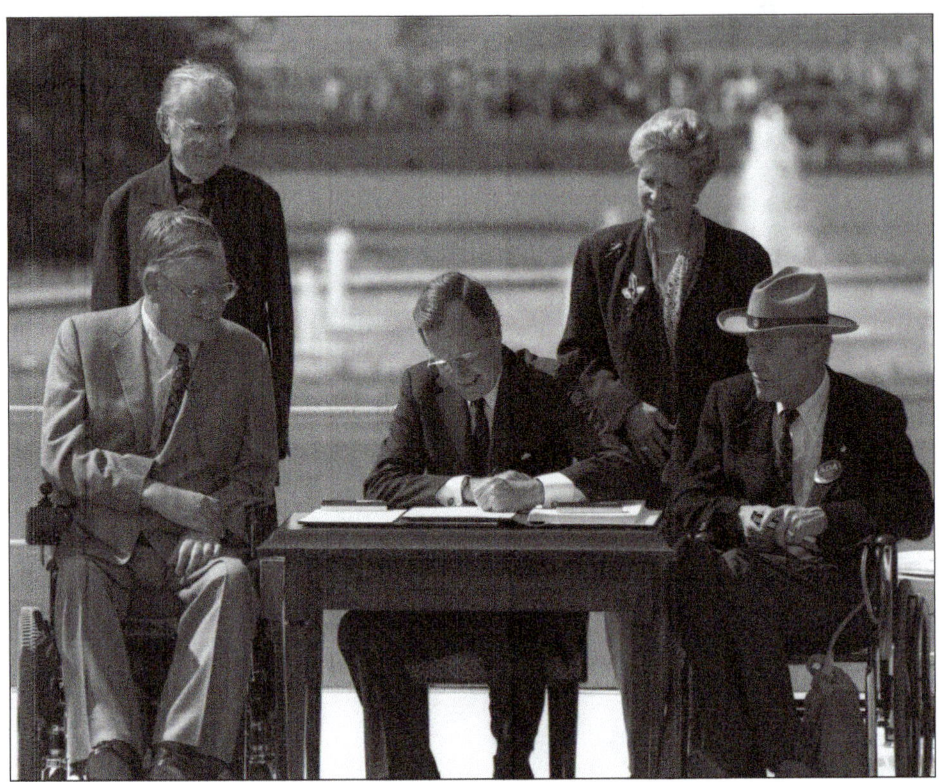

SIGNING OF THE ADA BILL / SOUTH LAWN
JULY 26, 1990 / 10:00 A.M.

THANK YOU. AND WELCOME TO EVERY ONE OF YOU OUT THERE IN THIS SPLENDID SCENE OF HOPE SPREAD ACROSS THE SOUTH LAWN. \\\

THIS IS AN INCREDIBLE DAY -- ESPECIALLY FOR THE THOUSANDS OF PEOPLE ACROSS THE NATION WHO HAVE GIVEN SO MUCH OF THEIR TIME, THEIR VISION AND THEIR COURAGE TO SEE THIS ACT BECOME A REALITY. \\

- 2 -

YOU KNOW, I STARTED PUTTING TOGETHER A LIST OF ALL THE PEOPLE WHO SHOULD BE MENTIONED TODAY -- BUT WHEN THAT LIST STARTED LOOKING LONGER THAN THE SENATE TESTIMONY FOR THE BILL, I DECIDED I'D BETTER GIVE UP OR WE'D NEVER GET OUT OF HERE BEFORE SUNSET.\\ SO I WILL SINGLE OUT ONLY TWO FRIENDS WHO HAVE GUIDED ME TO THIS DAY: EVAN KEMP AND JUSTIN DART. \\

Note. Occupational therapists were among those people present for the signing of the ADA. President George H. W. Bush signs into law the Americans With Disabilities Act of 1990 on the South Lawn of the White House (July 26, 1990). L to R, sitting: Evan Kemp, Chairman, Equal Employment Opportunity Commission; Justin Dart, Chairman, President's Committee on Employment of People With Disabilities. L to R, standing: Rev. Harold Wilke and Swift Parrino, Chairperson, National Council on Disability. Document: Photocopy of speech cards used by President George H. W. Bush at the signing ceremony. Courtesy of the National Archives. In the public domain.

decision making, and recognition of their contribution to society (*Proceedings of Workshop on Graduate Education in Occupational Therapy,* 1963; Yerxa, 1967). Moreover, for occupational therapy, it was necessary for its knowledge and processes to encompass practice across all client populations, settings, and other specializations.

Developing a Common Language

As an initial step toward authentic, professional identity, AOTA (1972) issued an official definition of *occupational therapy* that deliberately broadened the scope of practice to include health promotion. AOTA (1972) described occupational therapy practice as three key programs: "prevention and health maintenance," "remedial programs," and "daily life tasks and vocational adjustment" (p. 204). This shift from medical treatment to comprehensive health care required occupational therapy practitioners to take on new roles in prevention and community health (Llorens, 1973; Wiemer & West, 1970). To prepare students, the 1976 Essentials for Educational Programs specifically required that "experiences must be provided *outside* as well as within the medical model" (AOTA, 1976, p. 474, emphasis added). Although this requirement was not maintained with subsequent standards, occupational therapy educational programs developed partnerships to prepare students for work in community settings, such as daycare centers and community health organizations (Cermak, 1976; Cromwell & Kielhofner, 1976).

AOTA (1989) developed the first ***Uniform Terminology for Reporting Occupational Therapy Services*** in response to amendments to Medicare and Medicaid laws that required uniform reporting systems. Although a key purpose was to provide a common language for occupational therapy in the United States, AOTA selected terms and definitions primarily from a medical perspective (AOTA, 1979/1983, p. 899). The document described major areas of concern, including daily living skills, sensorimotor components, cognitive components, and psychosocial components, and the process of assessment, treatment, and other professional duties (AOTA, 1979/1983). Interestingly, although the document referred to "therapeutic use of activities and the activity process" (AOTA, 1979/1983, p. 899), the term *occupation* does not appear in the document.

Subsequent updates to the uniform terminology document sought "to facilitate the uniform use of terminology and definitions throughout the profession" (AOTA, 1989, p. 808). The second edition of the *Uniform Terminology for Occupational Therapy* more clearly distinguished occupational performance areas from performance components, which were "the functional abilities required for occupational performance" (AOTA, 1989, p. 812), defining *occupational therapy practice* as including "occupational performance areas and occupational performance components" (p. 808). In the third edition, these terms were shortened to *performance areas* and *performance components,* removing the *occupational* label (AOTA, 1994, p. 1047). The first and second editions of the *Uniform Terminology* provided examples of occupational performance areas, but it was not until the third edition that an actual definition of *performance areas* was included: "broad categories of human activity that are typically part of daily life" (AOTA, 1994, p. 1047). The document went on to state that "function in performance areas is the ultimate concern of occupational therapy" (AOTA, 1994, p. 1047). The term *occupation,* as distinct from *occupational performance,* was not specifically included in any of the *Uniform Terminology* versions, even when discussing the person–activity–environment fit that influences the quality of performance (AOTA, 1994, p. 1049). Explicit inclusion of occupation language beyond medical settings was included when the ***Occupational Therapy Practice Framework: Domain and Process*** (*OTPF;* AOTA, 2002) replaced the *Uniform Terminology.*

Although some of this word usage may seem esoteric, the examples discussed in the preceding paragraph illustrate the challenges of settling on common terms around *activity* and *occupation,* providing a sense that terms are interchangeable or that their meanings are vague and overgeneralized. In reality, developing terminology and definitions was complicated, was subject to frequent debate, and is continually evolving—a pattern that goes back to the early days of a profession developed from the therapeutic benefit of activities. Indeed *activity therapy* itself seems more limited and limiting than *occupational therapy,* which takes the use of specific activities to address a more holistic notion of occupation as defining personhood: living, working, and participating fully in society. Most important, to continue to evolve and offer the greatest benefit, occupational therapy needs terms that are broadly inclusive. The conversation continues.

Creating Theoretical Knowledge

Creation and application of theoretical knowledge is one of the hallmarks of a profession (Mosey, 1968; Yerxa, 1967), and occupational therapists have used theories from other professions in addition to creating their own. For example, occupational therapists incorporated developmental theories, including those from psychologists Jean Piaget and Erik Erikson to inform their work with children and from Havighurst to apply with older adults (Cermak, 1976; Llorens, 1970). A. Jean Ayres's development of sensory integration theory increased occupational therapy's work with children with learning disabilities (Ayres, 1963; Kauffman, 1978). Although occupational therapy had developed or applied theoretical knowledge for specific areas of concern, including developmental, sensory, motor control, and psychodynamic issues, there was debate about the benefits of multiple population-specific or issue-specific theories versus grand theoretical explanations that encompassed the entire profession (Mosey, 1986).

Occupation-centered models

Occupational therapy leaders discussed the potential need for new theoretical models to provide an overarching explanation for occupational therapy that bridged specialization areas. In her 1978 Slagle lecture, Lorna Jean King warned,

"Without a unifying theory to ensure cohesiveness, specialization could easily become fragmentation . . . [and] further fragmentation might well be suicidal" (p. 429). Occupational therapy leaders debated the benefits and drawbacks of embracing a comprehensive theory or construct that defined the profession (Mosey, 1985). Proponents of a core or grand theory of occupational therapy suggested adaptation, function, or occupation as an organizing construct (AOTA, 1979; King, 1978; Yerxa, 1967).

Amid this discussion in the 1980s and 1990s, six ***occupational therapy models*** emerged that continue to be cited in the current *OTPF-4* (AOTA, 2020; Table 2.2). Each new model provides an overarching explanation of occupational therapy practice that explains how people engage in occupations, how occupations relate to environments, factors that affect their doing, and ways for occupational therapy to assess and therapeutically incorporate occupations as interventions (see Table 2.2). For example, the Model of Human Occupation, one of the earliest occupation-centered models, focuses on describing the subsystems within the person that affect performance (i.e., volition, habituation, and performance [capacity]) while applying systems theory to occupational therapy (Kielhofner & Burke, 1980). A series of articles introduced the model by describing its parts and how they are connected (Kielhofner, 1980; Kielhofner & Burke, 1980). In contrast, the Occupational Therapy Intervention Process Model, associated with the Assessment of Motor and Process Skills, focuses on explaining the evaluation and intervention process in occupational therapy (Fisher, 1998). Only in the description of the first step of the evaluation process, establishing the "client-centered performance context," were different concepts defined (Fisher, 1998, p. 514). Although each provides a theoretical explanation that covers many aspects of occupational therapy practice, the existence of six (at least—others exist that are not included in the *OTPF*) suggests a plurality of views on how best to structure a comprehensive, all-encompassing view of the profession.

Cultural context

The profession's focus on occupation and occupational performance as a central tenet led to explicit attention to the environment or context. Each of the occupation-centered models listed in Table 2.2 includes social, physical, and ***cultural aspects*** as key considerations for occupational therapy. This consideration of a cultural environment was relatively new to occupational therapy at the time. It was not until its third edition that the *Uniform Terminology* included performance contexts (physical, social, and cultural environments) as part of occupational therapy's domain (AOTA, 1994). Although not a fully comprehensive indicator, the indexes for the *American Journal of Occupational Therapy* from 1947 to 1971 list only three articles under the topic of cultural considerations (Myers, 1973). As well, strong biases remained in these models; although Schultz and Schkade (1992), who developed the Occupational Adaptation Model, explicitly stated that they believed their model's assumptions "to be universal regardless of age, race, culture, gender, condition, or other classifications" (p. 919), there was little effort to check or confirm such assumptions.

As an organization, AOTA recognized the importance of addressing culture with its Multicultural Affairs Program in the 1990s (Black, 2002). Not until the early 2000s did occupational therapy in the United States acknowledge the need to consider other ways to understand the experiences of non-Western clients, such as through the Kawa model (Iwama, 2005) or the participatory occupational justice framework (Townsend & Whiteford, 2005).

Importance of Research

Historically, research focusing on outcomes in occupational therapy has been challenging. Although AOTA encouraged occupational therapy research, there was a significant gap between the need for and the production of research. In 1953, AOTA hosted a Research in Occupational Therapy Institute based on member topic requests because "we, as a whole, have not been trained in science, but rather in the art of healing" (Welch et al., 1954, p. 139). Symbolically, one of the first topics of articles from this institute printed in the *American Journal of Occupational Therapy* was research (Hudson, 1954; Welch et al., 1954). Diamond and Laurencelle (1961) stated, "It is no longer enough that a particular theory in application appears to effect change or movement; now we hope to learn why" (p. 140). The need to train occupational therapists to be consumers and producers of research was a key argument for graduate education, both postprofessional and entry level (*Proceedings of Workshop on Graduate Education in Occupational Therapy,* 1963). This ongoing concern for the need for research to both inform and support occupational therapy practice continued throughout the 20th century (Holm, 2000).

Another question was whether studying occupation was, in fact, a science unto itself. The University of Southern California founded the first occupational science program in 1989 (Yerxa et al., 1990). ***Occupational science*** was defined as "a new scientific discipline . . . [for the] study of the human as an occupational being" (Clark et al., 1991, p. 300). In addition to providing basic science research, Clark et al. (1991) stated that the new discipline could enhance occupational therapy practice and address the need for doctoral-prepared faculty. There was debate and discussion about the value of a separate discipline and the relationship between occupational therapy and occupational science (Clark et al., 1991, 1993; Henderson et al., 1991; Mosey, 1992, 1993; Yerxa et al., 1990). Although discussions continue, scholars of occupational science have generated research about occupation that informs occupational therapy practice (Molke et al., 2004; Zemke & Clark, 1996) and offered an approach for studying occupations outside of the therapeutic context.

Occupational justice is a key concept that emerged from international colleagues in occupational science (Townsend & Wilcock, 2004). ***Occupational justice*** involves recognizing

TABLE 2.2. **OCCUPATION AND CULTURE IN OCCUPATIONAL THERAPY MODELS**

MODEL	INITIAL CITATION YEAR	OCCUPATION AND OCCUPATIONAL PERFORMANCE DEFINITIONS	CULTURE
Model of Human Occupation (MOHO)	1980	"Occupation is the purposeful use of time by humans to fulfill their own internal urges toward exploring and mastering their environment that at the same time fulfills the requirements of the social group to which they belong and personal needs for self-maintenance" (Kielhofner, 1980, p. 659). Occupational behavior or performance is "the output [of the open system] . . . comprised of both information and action" (Kielhofner & Burke, 1980, p. 581).	Cultural setting is one of three aspects of environment. Patterns of developmental change in a person are recognized as culturally determined. Valued goals aspect of volition reflects culture. MOHO "focuses on the psychosocial and cultural aspects of occupation" (Kielhofner & Burke, 1980, p. 573).
Person–Environment–Occupation–Performance (PEOP)	1991	"Occupation is the general term that refers to engagement in activities, tasks, and roles for the purpose of productive pursuits (such as work and education), maintaining oneself in the environment, and for purposes of relaxation, entertainment, creativity, and celebration . . . all goal-oriented behavior related to daily living is occupational in nature" (Christiansen, 1991, p. 26). Occupational performance is "the day-to-day engagement in occupations that organize our lives and meet our needs to maintain ourselves, to be productive, and to derive enjoyment and satisfaction within our environments" (Christiansen, 1991, p. 27).	Cultural influences are one of three aspects of the environment or context of performance.
Occupational Adaptation (OA)	1992	"Occupations are activities characterized by three properties—active participation, meaning to the person, and a product that is the output of a process. The product may be tangible or intangible" (Schkade & Schultz, 1992, p. 831). Level of occupational performance is how relative mastery is assessed on the basis of efficiency, effectiveness, and satisfaction with performance (Schultz & Schkade, 1992).	Cultural subsystem is one of three aspects of the occupational environment. Assumptions of the OA model "are considered to be universal regardless of age, race, culture, gender, condition, or other classifications" (Schultz & Schkade, 1992, p. 919).
Ecology of Human Performance (EHP)	1994	Uses "task" language instead of "occupation." "Task: An objective set of behaviors necessary to accomplish a goal . . . Performance: Both the process and result of the person interacting with context to engage in tasks" (Dunn et al., 1994, p. 606).	Cultural environment is one of three types of environment. Cultural meaning of temporal aspects of context are acknowledged.
Person–Environment–Occupation (PEO) model	1996	Occupation is "groups of self directed, functional tasks and activities in which a person engages over the lifespan . . . those clusters of activities and tasks in which the person engages in order to meet his/her intrinsic needs for self-maintenance, expression and fulfillment" (Law et al., 1996, p. 16). "Occupational performance is the outcome of the transaction of the person, environment and occupation . . . the dynamic experience of a person engaged in purposeful activities and tasks within an environment" (Law et al., 1996, p. 16).	Cultural environment is one of five environmental factors affecting occupational performance. Cultural background is personal attribute that affects occupational performance.

(Continued)

TABLE 2.2. **OCCUPATION AND CULTURE IN OCCUPATIONAL THERAPY MODELS *(Cont.)***

MODEL	INITIAL CITATION YEAR	OCCUPATION AND OCCUPATIONAL PERFORMANCE DEFINITIONS	CULTURE
Occupational Therapy Intervention Process Model (OTIPM)	1998	Occupation is "a noun of action—it is about 'doing!' . . . We must view occupation as . . . activity that is both meaningful and purposeful to the person who engages in it" (Fisher, 1998, p. 511). "Occupational performance unfolds as a transaction between the person and the environment as he or she enacts a task" (Fisher, 1998, p. 514).	Cultural dimension is one of nine aspects of client-centered performance context.

Note. These models were selected because they are the only comprehensive occupational therapy models cited in the *Occupational Therapy Practice Framework: Domain and Process* (4th ed.; American Occupational Therapy Association, 2020).

and supporting occupational rights, such as the "right to experience occupation as meaningful and enriching" and the "right to develop through participation in occupations for health and social inclusion" (Townsend & Wilcock, 2004, p. 80). Social justice concerns around occupation may be tangential to therapeutic approaches, but considering occupation as a justice-based issue does serve to broaden the potential client base for occupational therapy and address population-level issues such as poverty, homelessness, and international displacement (Kronenberg et al., 2005). At a moment at which occupational therapy seeks more than ever to provide the most individualized approach to each client, the opening to also think of occupational therapy on a global scale may seem daunting but does also take note of the connection of the person to the wider world.

Clinical Reasoning

As the profession matured, language integrating research and theory into practice made clear the connections between high-level thinking and new ideas about how to think about the beneficial outcome of therapeutic intervention. Examining ***clinical reasoning*** offered a more nuanced definition of how occupational therapists made decisions when evaluating and intervening with clients. Difficulty articulating one's reasoning was "a particular problem for occupational therapists because, although what they *do* looks simple, what they *know* is quite complex" (Mattingly, 1994, p. 24, emphasis added). In 1986, the American Occupational Therapy Foundation and AOTA funded a clinical reasoning study to "examine the clinical reasoning processes that reflect the occupational therapist's knowledge and use of theory in practice" (Gillette & Mattingly, 1987, p. 399) to inform occupational therapy research and education. Clinical reasoning research "developed a language for understanding and describing practice" (Mattingly & Fleming, 1994, p. 4).

By the early 2000s, occupational therapy had developed a professional identity grounded in the central constructs of occupation, occupational performance, and participation with supporting theoretical and research knowledge. In 2002, AOTA significantly revised the *Uniform Terminology* to create the *OTPF*

> in response to current practice needs . . . to more clearly affirm and articulate occupational therapy's unique focus on occupation and daily life activities and the application of an intervention process that facilitates engagement in occupation to support participation in life. (AOTA, 2002, p. 609)

In the accompanying editorial, Youngstrom (2002) emphasized the need for the new *OTPF* to explicitly connect to both the domain of what occupational therapy addresses and the process of creating change. This is reflected in the overarching focus and outcome of occupational therapy as "engagement in occupation to support participation in context" (AOTA, 2002, p. 611). The document integrates theory, (research) evidence, collaboration with the client, and other specific forms of clinical reasoning into the description of the occupational therapy process (AOTA, 2002).

Moving Forward

> We are living in a time of rapid and unpredictable change. . . . If we do not participate timely and effectively in the decision-making process, we risk being swept aside. (Hinojosa, 2007, pp. 629–630)

The philosophical belief that meaningful engagement in occupations cured or remediated the mind, body, and spirit (Bing, 1981; Nelson et al., 1996; Reed, 1986; Royeen, 2003; Schwartz, 2009) continues to animate the profession as it moves forward. Founding values of empathy or the caring heart applied to interpersonal interactions, complexity, resiliency, and understanding the inner lives of others (Abreu, 2011; Fine, 1991; Peloquin, 2005). The concept of adaptation became a unifying or core framework across select lectures involving caring touch (Huss, 1977), adaptive response to real-life environments (King, 1978), and diverse populations (Grady, 1995). The belief that healing occurred in naturalistic settings such as the neighborhood settlement houses and homelike Marblehead or Consolation House was crucial to adaptation.

Occupational therapy leaders and those working in medically based healing in hospitals directed their attention to function and treatment outcomes for reimbursement and service justification. As Holm (2000) stated, "We are now being judged by the functional outcomes our patients achieve" (p. 576), and practitioners must use evidence-based practice integrating clinical expertise with current evidence to make decisions about care. This focus on function shifted the emphasis from a philosophically based practice to medical models of disease intervention that led to more dialogue about occupational therapy's uniqueness, identity, or legitimacy (Holm, 2000; Reilly, 1962; Yerxa, 1967). Reilly (1962) warned that occupational therapy was "preoccupied with the medical science which supports the application of our craft knowledge to medical conditions . . . and medical science knowledge is . . . not an end in itself" (p. 7). Conforming to a medical model ultimately pushed occupational therapy leaders to argue for autonomy and an "identifiable" or "authentic" profession (Gillen, 2013; Yerxa, 1967). Others debated specialization or generalization, as well as a reductionism that "plagued the profession" (Johnson, 1973) or created "forks in the road" (Gillen, 2013, p. 641)—detours to core occupational therapy values. While some of these debates still continue, Sokolov (1957) reminded us that, "Regardless of our tools . . . we shall bridge the chasm of illness to draw the patient back into the mainstream of active participation which signifies the return to life and hope" (p. 16).

Scholars conceptualized *occupations* as reality-orienting, meaningful, self-initiated, purposeful, and theoretically based (Llorens, 1970; Reilly, 1962; Yerxa, 1967). As Grady (1995) put it, "Occupation provides a context for organizing one's self and one's environment" (p. 307). Occupational performance uncovers a transaction between the person and the environment in which the client takes possession of an aim or reason (Fisher, 1998) or a means to construct meaning in the context of culture, life experience, and disability (Trombly, 1995). Occupation defined not only a purpose but the essence of being: "the mind and will of man are occupied" (Reilly, 1962, p. 2); "the simple things—the commonplace activities that have meaning for the individual that really matter" (Giles, 2018, p. 13). Occupations are key not just to being a person but to being a particular person (Christiansen, 1999). Conclusively, Llorens (1970) offered a compelling pledge about occupation, that "skilled application of activities and relationships . . . assist in closing the gap between expectation and ability. . . . This in my opinion is the promise of occupational therapy" (p. 94).

Summary

It is misleading to conceptualize *occupation* as occupational therapy's exclusive unifying belief, identity, model, or frame of reference because a profession stands on more than one overarching concept. History shows us that sometimes the need to rebuild a profession shores up its foundation. Responding to change is a dynamic rather than static process, and studying those shifts over 100 years of history shows us a profession that is ever evolving, absorbing new ideas and concepts, adapting and learning, and often helping to reshape the culture along the way. Yet it may be necessary to avoid using history to substantiate ideas for current practice because issues change (Mosey, 1985). Those who support using history suggest that it provides an appreciation of context, relationships, and understanding of those leaders who created change (Bing, 1983; Schwartz, 2009). The records and artifacts of this historical writing belong mostly to White women, many of a privileged class, and that story does not reflect occupational therapy's unfolding story of diversity.

Occupational therapists were powerful shapers using daily occupations and promising health and restoration. Occupational therapy developed because of strong and unyielding beliefs (Schwartz, 2009; Stattel, 1956). The statement "Most ideas are really very old. . . . New ideas are rare" (Stattel, 1956, p. 194) also applies to how we think about occupation. The notions of activity and occupation, and of the therapeutic benefit that lies in using them, are in many ways not new. However, the more we broaden the notions of what activity and occupation are, of what they can do, for whom they can do it, the more occupational therapy comes closer, however imperfectly, to fulfilling those early notions that all of us, when occupied, become healthier.

References

Abreu, B. C. (2011). Accentuate the positive: Reflection on empathetic interpersonal interactions. *American Journal of Occupational Therapy, 65,* 623–634. https://doi.org/10.5014/ajot.2011.656002

American Academy of Physical Medicine and Rehabilitation. (n.d.). *A brief history of the establishment of the specialty of PM&R.* https://www.aapmr.org/about-physiatry/history-of-the-specialty

American Occupational Therapy Association. (1948). *Statement of the American Occupational Therapy Association regarding relationship with physical medicine.* Box 23, Folder 156, Archives of the American Occupational Therapy Association, North Bethesda, MD.

American Occupational Therapy Association. (1972). Occupational therapy: Its definition and functions. *American Journal of Occupational Therapy, 30,* 245–263.

American Occupational Therapy Association. (1976). Essentials of an accredited educational program for occupational therapists. *American Journal of Occupational Therapy, 24,* 485–496.

American Occupational Therapy Association. (1979). The philosophical base of occupational therapy (Resolution 531-79). *American Journal of Occupational Therapy, 33,* 785.

American Occupational Therapy Association. (1981). Occupational therapy's role in independent or alternative living situations. *American Journal of Occupational Therapy, 35,* 812–814. https://doi.org/10.5014/ajot.35.12.812

American Occupational Therapy Association. (1983). Uniform terminology for reporting occupational therapy services. In H. L. Hopkins & H. D. Smith (Eds.), *Willard & Spackman's occupational therapy* (6th ed., pp. 899–907). Lippincott. (Original work published 1979)

American Occupational Therapy Association. (1989). Uniform terminology for occupational therapy—Second edition. *American Journal of Occupational Therapy, 43,* 808–815. https://doi.org/10.5014/ajot.43.12.808

American Occupational Therapy Association. (1993). The role of occupational therapy in the independent living movement. *American Journal of Occupational Therapy, 47,* 1079–1080. https://doi.org/10.5014/ajot.47.12.1079

American Occupational Therapy Association. (1994). Uniform terminology for occupational therapy—Third edition. *American Journal of Occupational Therapy, 48,* 1047–1054. https://doi.org/10.5014/ajot.48.11.1047

American Occupational Therapy Association. (2002). Occupational therapy practice framework: Domain and process. *American Journal of Occupational Therapy, 56,* 609–637. https://doi.org/10.5014/ajot.56.6.609

American Occupational Therapy Association. (2020). Occupational therapy practice framework: Domain and process (4th ed.). *American Journal of Occupational Therapy, 74*(Suppl. 2), 7412410010. https://doi.org/10.5014/ajot.2020.74S2001

Americans With Disabilities Act of 1990, Pub. L. 101-336, 42 U.S.C. §§ 12101–12213 (2000).

Ayres, A. J. (1963). Occupational therapy directed toward neuromuscular integration. In H. S. Willard & C. S. Spackman (Eds.), *Occupational therapy* (3rd ed., pp. 358–466). Lippincott.

Barton, G. E. (1917). Leaders in work therapy form society: Conference at Clifton Springs leads to organization of a National Society for the Promotion of Occupational Therapy. *Modern Hospital, 8,* 356–357.

Barton, I. G. (1968). Consolation House, fifty years ago. *American Journal of Occupational Therapy, 22,* 340–345.

Baum, C. (1980). Occupational therapists put care in the health system. *American Journal of Occupational Therapy, 34,* 505–516. https://doi.org/10.5014/ajot.34.8.505

Benjamin Rush (1745–1813). (1945). *Nature, 156,* 743–744. https://doi.org/10.1038/156743d0

Bing, R. K. (1981). Occupational therapy revisited: A paraphrastic journey. *American Journal of Occupational Therapy, 35,* 499–518. https://doi.org/10.5014/ajot.35.8.499

Bing, R. K. (1983). The industry, the art, and the philosophy of history. *American Journal of Occupational Therapy, 37,* 800–801. https://doi.org/10.5014/ajot.37.12.800

Bing, R. K. (1992). Point of departure (a play about founding the profession). *American Journal of Occupational Therapy, 46,* 27–32. https://doi.org/10.5014/ajot.46.1.27

Black, R. M. (2002). Occupational therapy's dance with diversity. *American Journal of Occupational Therapy, 56,* 140–148. https://doi.org/10.5014/ajot.56.2.140

Bobath, B. (1948). The importance of the reduction of muscle tone and the control of mass reflex action in the treatment of spasticity. *Occupational Therapy and Rehabilitation, 27,* 371–383.

Brachtesende, A. (2005, January 24). The turnaround is here. *OT Practice, 23,* 13–29.

Breines, E. B. (1995). Understanding "occupation" as the founders did. *British Journal of Occupational Therapy, 58,* 458–460. https://doi.org/10.1177/030802269505801102

Budget Enforcement Act of 1990, Pub. L. 101-508, 111 Stat. 677.

Cermak, S. A. (1976). Community-based learning in occupational therapy. *American Journal of Occupational Therapy, 30,* 157–161.

Christiansen, C. (1991). Occupational therapy: Intervention for life performance. In C. Christiansen & C. Baum (Eds.), *Occupational therapy: Overcoming human performance deficits* (pp. 26–35). Slack.

Christiansen, C. H. (1999). Defining lives: Occupation as identity: An essay on competence, coherence, and the creation of meaning. *American Journal of Occupational Therapy, 53,* 547–558. https://doi.org/10.5014/ajot.53.6.547

Clark, F. A., Parham, D., Carlson, M. E., Frank, G., Jackson, J., Pierce, D., . . . Zemke, R. (1991). Occupational science: Academic innovation in the service of occupational therapy's future. *American Journal of Occupational Therapy, 45,* 300–310. https://doi.org/10.5014/ajot.45.4.300

Clark, F., Zemke, R., Frank, G., Parham, D., Neville-Jan, A., Hedricks, C., . . . Abreu, B. (1993). Dangers inherent in the partition of occupational therapy and occupational science. *American Journal of Occupational Therapy, 47,* 184–186. https://doi.org/10.5014/ajot.47.2.184

Colman, W. (1988). The evolution of occupational therapy in the public schools: The laws mandating practice. *American Journal of Occupational Therapy, 42,* 701–705. https://doi.org/10.5014/ajot.42.11.701

Colman, W. (1992). Maintaining autonomy: The struggle between occupational therapy and physical medicine. *American Journal of Occupational Therapy, 46,* 63–70. https://doi.org/10.5014/ajot.46.1.63

Community Mental Health Centers Act, Pub. L. 88-164, 42 U.S.C. 2689 *et seq.*

Cowles, L., & Fort, A. (2003). *Social work in the health field: A care perspective.* Haworth Social Work Practice Press.

Cromwell, F. S., & Kielhofner, G. W. (1976). Educational strategy for occupational therapy community service. *American Journal of Occupational Therapy, 30,* 629–633.

Diamond, M. V., & Laurencelle, P. (1961). The role of the occupational therapist in the care of the geriatric patient. *American Journal of Occupational Therapy, 15,* 139–141.

Dunn, W., Brown, C., & McGuigan, A. (1994). The ecology of human performance: A framework for considering the effect of context. *American Journal of Occupational Therapy, 48,* 595–607. https://doi.org/10.5014/ajot.48.7.595

Dunton, W. R. (1918). National Society for the Promotion of Occupational Therapy. *Maryland Psychiatric Quarterly, 7*(3), 55–56.

Dunton, W. R. (1919). *Reconstruction therapy.* W. B. Saunders.

Dunton, W. R. (1947). History and development of occupational therapy. In H. S. Willard & C. S. Spackman (Eds.), *Principles of occupational therapy* (pp. 1–9). Lippincott.

Education for All Handicapped Children Act of 1975, Pub. L. 94-142, renamed the Individuals With Disabilities Education Improvement Act, codified at 20 U.S.C. §§ 1400–1482.

Education for All Handicapped Children Amendments of 1986, Pub. L. 99-457, 100 Stat. 1145.

Ethridge, D. A. (1976). The management view of the future of occupational therapy in mental health. *American Journal of Occupational Therapy, 30,* 623–628.

Fine, S. B. (1991). Resilience and human adaptability: Who rises above adversity? *American Journal of Occupational Therapy, 45,* 493–503. https://doi.org/10.5014/ajot.45.6.493

Finn, G. L. (1972). The occupational therapist in prevention programs. *American Journal of Occupational Therapy, 26,* 59–66.

Fisher, A. G. (1998). Uniting practice and theory in an occupational framework. *American Journal of Occupational Therapy, 52,* 509–521. https://doi.org/10.5014/ajot.52.7.509

Fisher, G. S. (2017). *The effect of Medicare Part B therapy on skilled nursing facility residents* [Doctoral dissertation, University of Illinois Chicago]. ProQuest Dissertation and Theses.

Friedland, J. (1998). Occupational therapy and rehabilitation: An awkward alliance. *American Journal of Occupational Therapy, 52,* 373–380. https://doi.org/10.5014/ajot.52.5.373

Giles, G. M. (2018). Neurocognitive rehabilitation: Skills or strategies? *American Journal of Occupational Therapy, 72,* 7206150010. https://doi.org/10.5014/ajot.2018.726001

Gilfoyle, E. M., & Hayes, C. (1979). Occupational therapy roles and functions in the education of the school-based handicapped student. *American Journal of Occupational Therapy, 33,* 565–576.

Gillen, G. (2013). A fork in the road: An occupational hazard? *American Journal of Occupational Therapy, 67,* 641–652. https://doi.org/10.5014/ajot.2013.676002

Gillette, N., & Kielhofner, G. (1979). The impact of specialization on the professionalization and survival of occupational therapy. *American Journal of Occupational Therapy, 33,* 20–28.

Gillette, N., & Mattingly, C. (1987). Clinical reasoning in occupational therapy. *American Journal of Occupational Therapy, 41,* 399–400. https://doi.org/10.5014/ajot.41.6.399

Gosling, F. G. (1987). *Before Freud: Neurasthenia and the American medical community, 1870–1910.* University of Illinois Press.

Grady, A. P. (1995). Building inclusive community: A challenge for occupational therapy. *American Journal of Occupational Therapy, 49,* 300–310. https://doi.org/10.5014/ajot.49.4.300

Hall, F. S., & Ellis, M. B. (1930). *Social work yearbook.* Russell Sage Foundation.

Hall, H. J. (1905). The systematic use of work as a remedy in neurasthenia and allied conditions. *Boston Medical and Surgical Journal, 112,* 29–32. https://doi.org/10.1056/NEJM190501121520201

Hall, H. J. (1910). Work cure: A report of five years' experience at an institution devoted to the therapeutic application of manual work. *Journal of the American Medical Association, 54,* 12–14. https://doi.org/10.1001/jama.1910.92550270001001d

Hall, H. J., & Buck, M. M. C. (1915). *The work of our hands: A study of occupations for invalids.* Moffat, Yard & Co.

Hanft, B. (1988). The changing environment of early intervention services: Implications for practice. *American Journal of Occupational Therapy, 42,* 724–731. https://doi.org/10.5014/ajot.42.11.724

Henderson, A., Cermak, S., Coster, W., Murray, E., Trombly, C., & Tickle-Degnen, L. (1991). Occupational science is multidimensional. *American Journal of Occupational Therapy, 45,* 370–372. https://doi.org/10.5014/ajot.45.4.370

Hinojosa, J. (2007). Becoming innovators in an era of hyperchange. *American Journal of Occupational Therapy, 61,* 629–637. https://doi.org/10.5014/ajot.61.6.629

Hirsh, J. (with Doherty, B.). (1954). *Saturday, Sunday and everyday: The history of the United Hospital Fund of New York.* United Hospital Fund of New York.

Hollis, L. I. (1979). Eleanor Clarke Slagle Lecture—Remember? *American Journal of Occupational Therapy, 33,* 493–499.

Holm, M. B. (2000). Our mandate for the new millennium: Evidence-based practice. *American Journal of Occupational Therapy, 54,* 575–585. https://doi.org/10.5014/ajot.54.6.575

Hudson, B. B. (1954). What is research? *American Journal of Occupational Therapy, 8,* 140–141, 150.

Hudson, H. (1947). Occupational therapy for the tuberculous. In H. S. Willard & C. S. Spackman (Eds.), *Principles of occupational therapy* (pp. 301–316). Lippincott.

Hudson, H., & Fish, M. (1944). *Occupational therapy in the treatment of the tuberculous patient.* National Tuberculosis Association.

Huss, A. J. (1977). Touch with care or a caring touch? *American Journal of Occupational Therapy, 31,* 11–18.

Individuals With Disabilities Education Act of 1990, Pub. L. 101-476, renamed the Individuals With Disabilities Education Improvement Act, codified at 20 U.S.C. §§ 1400–1482.

Individuals With Disabilities Education Improvement Act of 2004, Pub. L. 108-446, 20 U.S.C. §§ 1400–1482.

Iwama, M. K. (2005). The Kawa (river) model: Nature, life flow, and the power of culturally relevant occupational therapy. In F. Kronenberg, S. Simo Algado, & N. Pollard (Eds.), *Occupational therapy without borders: Learning from the spirit of survivors* (Vol. 1, pp. 213–228). Churchill Livingstone.

Jackson, B. N. (1970). The occupational therapist as consultant to the aged. *American Journal of Occupational Therapy, 24,* 572–575.

Jenkins, F. W. (1923). Occupational therapy: A selected bibliography. *Bulletin of the Russell Sage Foundation Library, 62,* 1–4.

Johnson, J. A. (1973). Occupational therapy: A model for the future. *American Journal of Occupational Therapy, 27,* 1–7.

Johnson, J., & Smith, M. (1966). Changing concepts of occupational therapy in community rehabilitation centers. *American Journal of Occupational Therapy, 20,* 267–273.

Kauffman, N. A. (1978). Occupational therapy theory, assessment, and treatment in educational settings. In H. L. Hopkins & H. D. Smith (Eds.), *Willard & Spackman's occupational therapy* (5th ed., pp. 609–632). Lippincott.

Kielhofner, G. (1980). A model of human occupation, Part 2: Ontogenesis from the perspective of temporal adaptation. *American Journal of Occupational Therapy, 34,* 657–663. https://doi.org/10.5014/ajot.34.10.657

Kielhofner, G., & Burke, J. P. (1980). A model of human occupation, Part 1: Conceptual framework and content. *American Journal of Occupational Therapy, 34,* 572–581. https://doi.org/10.5014/ajot.34.9.572

King, L. J. (1978). Toward a science of adaptive responses. *American Journal of Occupational Therapy, 32,* 429–437.

Kronenberg, F., Simo Algado, S., & Pollard, N. (Eds.). (2005). *Occupational therapy without borders: Volume 1. Learning from the spirit of survivors.* Churchill Livingstone.

Krusen, F. H. (1944). The future of physical medicine. *Journal of the American Medical Association, 125,* 1093–1097. https://doi.org/10.1001/jama.1944.02850340019007

Law, M., Cooper, B., Strong, S., Stewart, D., Rigby, P., & Letts, L. (1996). The Person–Environment–Occupation model: A transactive approach to occupational performance. *Canadian Journal of Occupational Therapy, 63,* 9–23. https://doi.org/10.1177/000841749606300103

Licht, S. (1947). The objectives of occupational therapy. *Occupational Therapy and Rehabilitation, 26*(1), 17–22.

Linker, B. (2011). *War's waste: Rehabilitation in World War I America.* University of Chicago Press.

Llorens, L. A. (1970). Facilitating growth and development: The promise of occupational therapy. *American Journal of Occupational Therapy, 24,* 93–101.

Llorens, L. A. (Ed.). (1973). *Consultation in the community: Occupational therapy in child health.* American Occupational Therapy Association.

Loomis, B. (1992). The Henry B. Favill School of Occupations and Eleanor Clarke Slagle. *American Journal of Occupational Therapy, 46,* 34–37. https://doi.org/10.5014/ajot.46.1.34

Maloney, C. C. (1976). The occupational therapist on a geriatric rehabilitation team. *American Journal of Occupational Therapy, 30,* 300–304.

Mann, W. C. (1976). A quarterway house for adult psychiatric patients. *American Journal of Occupational Therapy, 30,* 646–647.

Mattingly, C. (1994). The search for tacit knowledge. In C. Mattingly & M. H. Fleming (Eds.), *Clinical reasoning: Forms of inquiry in a therapeutic practice.* F. A. Davis.

Mattingly, C., & Fleming, M. H. (1994). *Clinical reasoning: Forms of inquiry in a therapeutic practice.* F. A. Davis.

McDaniel, M. L. (1968). Occupational therapists before World War II (1917–40). In R. S. Anderson, H. S. Lee, & M. L. McDaniel (Eds.), *Army Medical Specialist Corps.* (pp. 69–97). Office of the Surgeon General, Department of the U.S Army. https://achh.army.mil/history/corps-medical-spec-chapteriv

Mellinger, M. A. (1963). Occupational therapy in the treatment of the tuberculous patient. In H. S. Willard & C. S. Spackman (Eds.). *Occupational therapy* (3rd ed., pp. 139–145). Lippincott.

Meyer, A. (1922). Philosophy of occupational therapy. *Archives of Occupational Therapy, 1,* 1–10.

Molke, D., Laliberte-Rudman, D., & Polatajko, H. J. (2004). The promise of occupational science: A developmental assessment of an emerging academic discipline. *Canadian Journal of Occupational Therapy, 7,* 269–280. https://doi.org/10.1177/000841740407100505

Mosey, A. C. (1968). Recapitulation of ontogenesis:a theory for practice of occupational therapy. *American Journal of Occupational Therapy. 22,* 426–432.

Mosey, A. C. (1985). Eleanor Clarke Slagle Lecture: A monistic or a pluralistic approach to professional identity? *American Journal of Occupational Therapy, 39,* 504–509. https://doi.org/10.5014/ajot.39.8.504

Mosey, A. C. (1992). Partition of occupational science and occupational therapy. *American Journal of Occupational Therapy, 46,* 851–853. https://doi.org/10.5014/ajot.46.9.851

Mosey, A. C. (1993). Partition of occupational science and occupational therapy: Sorting out some issues. *American Journal of Occupational Therapy, 47,* 751–754. https://doi.org/10.5014/ajot.47.8.751

Myers, C. (Ed). (1973). *The twenty-five year cumulative index of the American Journal of Occupational Therapy.* American Occupational Therapy Association.

Nelson, D. L. (1997). Eleanor Clarke Slagle Lecture—Why the profession of occupational therapy will flourish in the 21st century. *American Journal of Occupational Therapy, 51,* 11–24. https://doi.org/10.5014/ajot.51.1.11

Nelson, D. L., Peterson, C., Smith, A. A., Boughton, J. A., & Whalen, G. M. (1996). Effects of project versus parallel groups on social interaction and affective responses in senior citizens. *American Journal of Occupational Therapy, 42,* 23–29. https://doi.org/10.5014/ajot.42.1.23

Newton, I. G. (1917). Consolation House. *Trained Nurse and Hospital Review, 59,* 321–326.

Paisley, S. A. (1929). Occupational therapy treatments for a group of spastic cases: Children under 12 years of age. *Occupational Therapy and Rehabilitation, 8,* 83–92.

Peloquin, S. (2005). Embracing our ethos, reclaiming our heart. *American Journal of Occupational Therapy, 59,* 611–625. https://doi.org/10.5014/ajot.59.6.611

Penn Medicine. (n.d.-a). *Dr. Benjamin Rush.* https://www.uphs.upenn.edu/paharc/timeline/1751/tline7.html

Penn Medicine. (n.d.-b). *History of Penn Medicine.* https://www.pennmedicine.org/about/mission-and-history/history-of-penn-medicine#:~:text=Pennsylvania%20Hospital%2C%20part%20of%20Penn,the%20nation%27s%20first%20teaching%20hospital

Peters, C. O. (2011). History of mental health: Perspectives of consumers and practitioners. In C. Brown & V. C. Stoffel (Eds.), *Occupational therapy in mental health: A vision for participation* (pp. 17–30). F. A. Davis.

Proceedings of workshop on graduate education in occupational therapy. (1963). Vocational Rehabilitation Administration and American Occupational Therapy Association.

Ransom, J. E. (1943). The beginnings of hospitals in the United States. *Bulletin of the History of Medicine, 13,* 514–539. http://www.jstor.org/stable/44440813

Reed, K. (1986). Tools of practice: Heritage or baggage? *American Journal of Occupational Therapy, 40,* 597–605. https://doi.org/10.5014/ajot.40.9.597

Rehabilitation Act of 1973, Pub. L. 93-112, 29 U.S.C. §§ 701–796l.

Reilly, M. (1962). Eleanor Clarke Slagle Lecture—Occupational therapy can be one of the great ideas of 20th century medicine. *American Journal of Occupational Therapy, 16*(1), 1–9. https://doi.org/10.1177/000841746303000102

Rood, M. S. (1958). Everyone counts. *American Journal of Occupational Therapy, 12,* 326–329.

Royeen, C. B. (2003). Chaotic occupational therapy: Collective wisdom for a complex profession. *American Journal of Occupational Therapy, 57,* 609–624. https://doi.org/10.5014/ajot.57.6.609

Schkade, J. K., & Schultz, S. (1992). Occupational adaptation: Toward a holistic approach for contemporary practice, Part 1. *American Journal of Occupational Therapy, 46,* 829–837. https://doi.org/10.5014/ajot.46.9.829

Schultz, S., & Schkade, J. K. (1992). Occupational adaptation: Toward a holistic approach for contemporary practice, Part 2. *American Journal of Occupational Therapy, 46,* 917–925. https://doi.org/10.5014/ajot.46.10.917

Schwartz, K. B. (2009). Reclaiming our heritage: Connecting the Founding Vision to the Centennial Vision. *American Journal of Occupational Therapy, 63,* 681–690. https://doi.org/10.5014/ajot.63.6.681

Slagle, E. C. (1914). History of the development of occupation for the insane. *Maryland Psychiatric Quarterly, 4,* 14–20.

Slagle, E. C. (1922). Training aides for mental patients. *Archives of Occupational Therapy, 1,* 11–17.

Slagle, E. C. (1930). Occupational therapy. In F. S. Hall & M. B. Ellis (Eds.), *Social work yearbook* (pp. 298–300). Russell Sage Foundation.

Social Security Act of 1935, Pub. L. 74-271, 42 U.S.C. §§ 301–1397mm.

Social Security Amendments of 1965, Pub. L. 89-97 97, 42 U.S.C. §§ 1395–1395kkk1 (Medicare) and 42 U.S.C. §§ 1396–1396w5 (Medicaid).

Sokolov, J. (1957). Therapist into administrator: Ten inspiring years. *American Journal of Occupational Therapy, 11,* 13–19.

Stattel, F. M. (1956). Equipment designed for occupational therapy. *American Journal of Occupational Therapy, 10,* 194–198.

Townsend, E., & Whiteford, G. (2005). A participatory occupational justice framework: Population-based processes of practice. In F. Kronenberg, S. Simo Algado, & N. Pollard (Eds.), *Occupational therapy without borders: Learning from the spirit of survivors* (Vol. 1, pp. 110–126). Churchill Livingstone.

Townsend, E., & Wilcock, A. A. (2004). Occupational justice and client-centred practice: A dialogue in progress. *Canadian Journal of Occupational Therapy, 71,* 75–87. https://doi.org/10.1177/000841740407100203

Trombly, C. A. (1995). Occupation: Purposefulness and meaningfulness as therapeutic mechanism. *American Journal of Occupational Therapy, 49,* 960–972. https://doi.org/10.5014/ajot.49.10.960

U.S. Federal Board for Vocational Education. (1918). *Training of teachers for occupational therapy for the rehabilitation of disabled soldiers and sailors: Letter from the federal board for vocational education transmitting, in response to a Senate resolution of January 27, report on a study of the federal board entitled "Rehabilitation of disabled soldiers and sailors and teacher training for occupational therapy."* U.S. Government Printing Office.

U.S. War Department. (1944). *Occupational therapy. War Department technical manual, TM8-291.* U.S. Government Printing Office.

Veltri, D. (Producer). (1997). *The power of 504* [Film]. https://www.youtube.com/watch?v=SyWcCuVta7M

Welch, M. B., Watson, C. A., Vanderkooi, F. B., & Matthews, M. (1954). Research in occupational therapy. *American Journal of Occupational Therapy, 8,* 139.

Wemett, L. C. (2017). Celebrating 100 years of occupational therapy. *Life in the Finger Lakes.* https://www.lifeinthefingerlakes.com/celebrating-100-years-occupational-therapy/

West, W. L. (1966). Occupational therapy in neuropsychiatry. In R. S. Anderson, A. J. Glass, & R. J. Bernucci (Eds.), *Neuropsychiatry in World War II: Zone of interior* (Vol. 1, pp. 651–686). Office of the Surgeon General, Department of the Army. https://achh.army.mil/history/book-wwii-neuropsychiatryinwwiivoli-chapter22

West, W. L. (1968). Eleanor Clarke Slagle Lecture—Professional responsibility in times of change. *American Journal of Occupational Therapy, 22,* 9–15.

Wiemer, R. B., & West, W. L. (1970). Occupational therapy in community health care. *American Journal of Occupational Therapy, 24,* 323–328.

Willard, H., & Spackman, C. (Eds.). (1954). *Principles of occupational therapy* (2nd ed.). Lippincott.

Wolfensberger, W. (1975). *The origin and nature of our institutional models.* Human Policy Press.

Yerxa, E. (1967). Eleanor Clarke Slagle Lecture: Authentic occupational therapy. *American Journal of Occupational Therapy, 21,* 1–9.

Yerxa, E., Clarke, F., Frank, G., Jackson, J., Parham, D., Pierce, D., . . . Zemke, R. (1990). An introduction to occupational science: A foundation for occupational therapy in the 21st century. *Occupational Therapy in Healthcare, 6*(41), 1–17. https://doi.org/10.1080/J003v06n04_04

Youngstrom, M. J. (2002). The Occupational Therapy Practice Framework: The evolution of our professional language. *American Journal of Occupational Therapy, 56,* 607–608. https://doi.org/10.5014/ajot.56.6.607

Zemke, R., & Clarke, F. (1996). *Occupational science: The evolving discipline.* F. A. Davis.

3

Occupation and Activity Analysis

KAREN A. BUCKLEY, MA, OT/L;
SALLY E. POOLE, OTD, OT/L, CHT;
AND DIANA CHEN WONG, OTD, OTR/L, CAPS

CHAPTER HIGHLIGHTS

- History of activity analysis
- Occupational therapy's perspectives on activity and occupation analysis
- Occupation/activity analysis process
- Multicomponent activity analysis
- Occupation analysis summary
- Occupation and activity analysis within a frame of reference

KEY TERMS AND CONCEPTS

• acquiring skills • activity analysis • analysis summary • arts and crafts movement • attention • auditory processing • basic learning • basic skills • bilateral integration • body scheme • body strength • categorization • complex skills • concept formation • context • contextual factors • coping skills • copying • crossing the midline • depth perception • endurance • extremity strength • figure–ground perception • fine motor coordination and dexterity • fine motor skill • form constancy • generalization • grasp patterns • gustatory processing • initiation of activity • interpersonal skills • job analysis • kinesthesia • kinetic analysis • knowledge • laterality • learning • level of arousal • memory • mobility • motor control • occupation analysis • occupation-based activity analysis • occupations • ocular–motor control • olfactory processing • oral–motor skill • orientation • position in space • postural alignment • postural control • postural praxis • praxis • prehension/pinch patterns • proprioceptive processing • range of motion • reciprocal patterns • recognition • rehearsing • restricted activity analysis • reverse a sequence • right–left discrimination • routines • self-control • sensory modulation • sensory processing • sequencing • skills • social skills • spatial operations • spatial relations • stereognosis • tactile processing • termination of activity • time management • topographical orientation • vestibular input • visual fixation • visual–motor integration • visual reception • visual tracking

Introduction

This chapter presents a brief historical overview of the importance of activity and occupation in the health and well-being of a person. We begin by reviewing the evolution of activity and occupation analysis. We then provide a systematic approach for occupational therapy practitioners and students to use as a template in the analysis of both an occupation and an activity by means of an outline in the chapter.

Historical Perspective

As early as 2600 BC, historical records document the concept that humans must use both mind and body to maintain health and well-being. The ancient Chinese, Persians, and Greeks understood that a mutually dependent relationship existed between physical and mental health and well-being. Egyptians and Greeks saw diversion and recreation as treatment for the sick. Later, the Romans recommended activity for those with mental illness (Hopkins & Smith, 1978).

Many centuries later in Europe and the United States, the use of activity and occupation was described as a treatment modality for people with mental and physical illness. In 1798, Benjamin Rush, the first American psychiatrist, advocated the use of domestic occupations for their therapeutic value. Weaving, spinning, and sewing were occupations that he considered therapeutic because of their personal interest to the patients of the era and because of their social and cultural relevance (Dunton & Licht, 1957). During the 18th and 19th centuries in the United States, people accepted the use of occupations in the care of patients with mental illness. In 1892, Edward N. Bush, superintendent of a psychiatric hospital in Maryland, wrote, "The benefits of occupation are manifold. Primarily, even the most simple and routine tasks keep the mind occupied, awaken new trains of thought and interests, and divert the patient from the delusions or hallucinations which harass and annoy him" (as cited in Dunton & Licht, 1957, p. 9).

In addition to the use of occupations in psychiatric treatment in the 18th and 19th centuries, early documentation has shown that people used occupations to build muscles and improve joint range. In 1780 in France, Clément-Joseph Tissot, a physician in the French cavalry, described the beneficial use of arts and crafts and recreational activities to mediate the physical effects of chronic illness (Dunton & Licht, 1957). Tissot named "shuttlecock, tennis, football, and dancing" (as cited in Dunton & Licht, 1957, p. 9) as activities to promote range of motion for all joints of the upper and lower extremities. In this early literature about the use of occupations or activities, little description is available about the precise methodology used to select activities that addressed specific problems. Instead, activities appear to have been selected for their cultural, social, recreational, and diversional characteristics and, one assumes, meaningfulness to the person.

In the early 1900s, occupational therapy practitioners embraced the arts and crafts movement that was a backlash against the social ills perceived to have resulted from the Industrial Revolution (Reed, 1986). The ***arts and crafts movement*** promoted a simpler life in which activities were performed at a slower pace than required by factory production, in which the process was as important as the end product, the creative spirit was valued, and manual learning was valued rather than intellectual learning alone (Reed, 1986). In 1928, the American Occupational Therapy Association (AOTA) provided guidelines for analyzing crafts in terms of joint motion and muscle strength (Creighton, 1992). Before World War II, little literature indicated that therapists selected activities on the basis of anything other than intuition (Creighton, 1992; Reed, 1986).

At the end of World War I, two factors had a strong influence on occupational therapy practitioners' use of activities and related occupations. First, the end of the arts and crafts movement in the United States and Europe meant that many activities were not valued in the same way. Second, therapists found themselves treating patients who were exhibiting both physical and psychological trauma. Therapists began selecting activities based on the patient's particular deficits and needs. They first carefully analyzed each patient's deficits and, using a problem-solving approach, determined which specific activity would be appropriate to address the deficit. Therapists used activities because of their characteristics, but no formal analysis was part of the therapist's treatment routine. Therapists and physicians, however, began to look beyond the profession of occupational therapy to gain knowledge about activity analysis.

In this early development of the occupational therapy profession, activity selection and subsequent intervention were influenced by three men outside the profession: (1) Frank Gilbreth, (2) Jules Amar, and (3) L. J. Haas (Creighton, 1992). Gilbreth, an engineer by training, studied jobs to identify the most productive and least fatiguing methods of job performance. His work, which industry accepted, examined the worker, environment, and motion. While visiting European hospitals to study physicians and how they worked, he became acquainted with the research of Amar, a French physiologist. Amar had been commissioned by the French government to study how to prepare wounded soldiers for reentry into the workforce, which he did by measuring the physiological requirements of many jobs. His work influenced Gilbreth by making him aware of the possibilities of applying motion studies to the reeducation of returning wounded veterans. Gilbreth presented his work at the 1917 annual meeting of the National Society for the Promotion of Occupational Therapy, which led to the eventual inclusion of this concept of activity analysis into the field of occupational therapy. L. J. Haas, a psychiatrist, contributed the importance of the social and emotional benefits of crafts as an intervention to address the patient's needs. He also created a system of classification of activities that was embraced by AOTA and reflected in their published documents (Halladay, 1945), Activity analysis was incorporated into occupational therapy textbooks as early as 1919 (Creighton, 1992).

The years between World War I and World War II saw the establishment of AOTA, formerly the National Society for the Promotion of Occupational Therapy, and further development of the profession in general. AOTA encouraged therapists to establish departments and to publish papers to help them do so. In addition, AOTA published papers to assist therapists with the appropriate selection of activities. Crafts were the treatment activities of choice, although *crafts* included both work-related and recreational activities (Creighton, 1992).

World War II propelled women out of the home and into the workforce and moved occupational therapy practitioners into new, real-life circumstances. As a result of improvement in medical and surgical care, veterans were surviving severe physical injuries and living with permanent disability. Practitioners began to specialize in the practice area of physical disabilities. Again, practitioners referred to Gilbreth's work, now being carried on by his wife, Lillian, who proposed that engineers and rehabilitation professionals work together to assist soldiers with disabilities (Creighton, 1992). At the same time, the U.S. Army developed its own manual of therapeutic activities (U.S. Department of War, 1944) that detailed activities to use to improve joint range of motion and the strengthening of all extremities. The military "divided" the body so that occupational therapists worked with the upper body, and physical therapists worked with the lower body (Hinojosa, 1996). Many policies and procedures laid down by the military for occupational therapists are still followed today.

Soon after World War II, Sidney Licht, who, at the time, was president of the American Congress of Rehabilitation Medicine and the editor of the Physical Medicine Library series, published an article in 1947 that advocated the use of a more precise method for analyzing activity for those occupational therapists working in the area of physical disabilities. He believed that craft analysis looked at "psychomotor values, economic factors, tempo, or other inherent characteristics" (Licht, 1947, p. 75). He coined the term ***kinetic analysis,*** however, to refer to when the tools or activities were to be analyzed for the motions involved. Many of Licht's ideas continue to influence practice in the area of physical disabilities. Contemporary practitioners who are concerned about muscle contractions, joint range of motion, precision and accuracy of intervention, ergonomics of body mechanics, and control variants continue to use the criteria for examining motion that Licht originally proposed for kinetic analysis.

Occupational therapy practitioners working in physical medicine appear to have become interested in activity analysis before those working in mental health. In 1948, Gail Fidler (1948) proposed that practitioners working in psychiatric occupational therapy use scientific analysis of activities:

> While the functioning of a personality is certainly not as quantifiable as a muscle, the use of activity for the psychiatric patient should be more scientifically allied with the principles of dynamic psychiatry and treatment objectives than it is at the present. (p. 284)

Fidler also proposed an outline for activity analysis to help practitioners meet the aims of treatment so that occupational therapy in psychiatry could be elevated from a simple diversion to an activity that addressed specific therapeutic goals.

Activity Analysis as a Critical Tool of the Profession

Activity analysis remained rudimentary in occupational therapy and focused almost exclusively on the product rather than the process of analysis. Gradually, the process of analysis has become more important than the end product. For example, Mosey (1981) proposed that activity analysis is the process of closely examining an activity to distinguish its component parts. A careful examination allows a skilled occupational therapy practitioner to select the most therapeutic and appropriate activity from those activities available. A careful examination ensures that the activities selected are relevant and correspond to the individual's needs.

Activity analysis also plays an important part of deductive reasoning in whatever frame of reference or approach the occupational therapy practitioner uses with clients. Mosey (1986) suggested two goals for using an activity analysis that would serve to firmly establish the process as a legitimate tool of the profession. The first purpose enables the student or the practitioner to learn more about the activity's inherent properties and the range of skills the person needs to perform it—in other words, the generic approach. After the has an understanding of the person, their personal goals, and their present performance skills, the needs to select an appropriate frame of reference to initiate intervention. Under these conditions, the practitioner can then perform a restricted activity analysis—that is, focus on the function–dysfunction continuum of the specific frame of reference. This is an alternative purpose for activity analysis. The intent is to identify whether the activity is well suited to be used to promote change in the underlying skills or abilities deemed to be the focus of intervention. This approach to activity analysis is directly related to the postulates regarding change that were identified in the selected frame of reference.

Activity analysis enables occupational therapists to determine an activity's therapeutic properties so that they can make an appropriate match between the individual's interests and abilities and the activity that will meet the person's health needs (Mosey, 1986) and established intervention goals. Activity analysis can be approached from many perspectives, depending on the reason for the analysis and the specific focus of interest. Trombly and Scott (1977) proposed that performance areas be analyzed first. Cynkin and Robinson (1990) proposed that occupational therapists begin an activity analysis with the performance context. In Chapter 6 in the 4th edition of this text, Kramer and Hinojosa (2014) stated that activity analysis assesses the person, activity, and context. For example, a therapist who works in a hand therapy practice would begin with an analysis of the activity-based motor and sensory skills; hence, activities used in the clinic would be selected on the basis of how they address specific deficits. An activity analysis should consider the person's present, past, and future occupations.

Pierce (2001) attempted to clarify the difference between occupation and activity as well as emphasize the importance of analysis for our profession. In her work, Pierce (2001) suggested that "occupation is the experience of a person who is the sole author of the occupation's meaning. Activities are more general, descriptive categories whose meaning are culturally shared rather than originating with the person" (p. 19). Recently, Boyt Shell et al. (2019) suggested that there are two levels or perspectives of activity analysis: (1) occupation analysis and (2) activity analysis. Accordingly, an occupation analysis examines the details of the individual's occupation within their context. An activity analysis investigates the demands of the activity and its context and personal meaning. Activity analysis, not unlike Mosey's (1981) restricted analysis, asks the occupational therapist to determine the therapeutic use of an activity on the basis of practice theory. Crepeau (2003) stated that activity analysis and theory-based activity analysis are done in the abstract. Only ***occupation-based activity analysis*** studies the person "engaging in occupations within [that person's] unique physical, cultural, and social environment" (Crepeau, 2003, p. 192).

We believe that the activity analysis outline, as presented in this chapter, can be used for either the occupation or activity analysis. When all three parts of our activity analysis are completed, one will have a comprehensive understanding of either an occupation or activity analysis.

Occupational Therapy's Perspectives on Occupation and Activity Analysis

Occupational therapy practitioners have an organized conceptual approach to activity analysis. The activity is first viewed as a whole, and then an analysis is done to break it down into its component parts. It is our belief that the practitioner does an activity analysis and then can see how the activity relates to the occupation. In this section, we outline one method of completing both an occupation and activity analysis drawn from various sources within the occupational therapy literature. Many of the ideas presented have become common knowledge within occupational therapy.

Learning how to perform an occupation or activity analysis is an integral part of professional occupational therapy education. Traditionally, students learn to analyze an activity by focusing on performance skills that support the ability of the individual to engage in the activity that underlies their desired occupation. Students are encouraged to consider the context in which the activity is performed—that is, the meaningfulness of the activity to their desired occupations. Performing an activity analysis enables the student and practitioner to explore the demands of the activity beyond the skill that is present. They need to understand to what degree the skill is being used in the context of the activity being performed and its relevance to the individual.

The analysis begins with a description of the activity and each of its fundamental elements as well as the steps necessary for completion. The occupational therapy practitioner describes the activity and how a person would perform it under typical circumstances. What follows is a suggested outline for students to follow when analyzing the component aspects of occupations or activities. We present it in three parts: (1) an introduction and description of the activity, (2) the activity analysis outline itself, and (3) a summary that relates the activity to the individual. Like many other analysis forms, Appendix 3.A, "Occupation and Activity Analysis Form," is based on several documents, including the third and fourth editions of the *Occupational Therapy Practice Framework: Domain and Process* (*OTPF–3* and *OTPF–4,* respectively; AOTA, 2014, 2020), the *International Classification of Functioning, Disability and Health* (*ICF;* World Health Organization [WHO], 2001), and *Uniform Terminology for Occupational Therapy—Third Edition* (AOTA, 1994).

Occupation/Activity Analysis

Historically, occupational therapy practitioners focused only on activity analysis. Today, the emphasis in education and practice is directed toward a more comprehensive occupation analysis. What is the distinction? An ***activity analysis*** is a neutral examination of the activity divided into its component parts. When a practitioner does an activity analysis, they are interested in breaking down the components to understand the decontextualized activity (Crepeau et al., 2014). For example, a practitioner might be interested in knowing what is required to saw a board. The practitioner examines the sensory, physical, cognitive, and social requirements of completing the activity itself. This activity analysis is neutral because it is not specific to a particular person or situation unless they are a carpenter or someone interested in woodworking. Thus, the practitioner will be able to decide if they can use this activity as part of an intervention.

Today, an occupational therapy practitioner is interested in understanding the activity in context of occupation and in the environmental and personal factors affecting the individual. Because this analysis is from the person's unique perspective, it is an ***occupation analysis.*** The practitioner centers the analysis on how a person with their unique experiences and abilities performs the activity in their natural environment. The examination of the activity recognizes that personal attributes, environment, previous experiences, personal beliefs and values, and other factors that influence a person's performance of an activity. This perspective acknowledges that an occupation is supported by several underlying activities meaningful to the person performing them. As an example, an occupational therapy student was assigned the analysis of buying a greeting card. The student decided to purchase a birthday card for her grandfather. She explained the meaning of the activity as part of a role. Her mother always purchased birthday cards for her grandfather, and once the student was older and earning her own money, she took on that responsibility. Snow (2013), the student, indicated that she saw this as a sign of her own "adulthood and independence" (p. 13): "When I buy my grandfather a card, I am fulfilling one of my responsibilities of my role as his granddaughter" (p. 24).

Another student's analysis of the same task was completely different because it had little personal meaning to him. He explained that he does not buy cards but sends personal text messages instead. For this student, this was an activity, not an occupation, because it lacked personal meaning. When the occupational therapy practitioner is interested in an individual's personal performance of activities in context, they conduct an occupation analysis.

As our world evolves, we, as occupational therapy practitioners, must be able to assess, anticipate, and adapt as these changes occur. Thus, the activities performed and analyzed must be considered in relation to the context of the individual. For example, the advent of technology has made significant changes in how we live our lives. Who, for instance, is without a cell phone or iPad™ or other form of hand-held technology? Although these devices have made some aspects of our lives easier—for example, texting has kept us connected (Pottorff, 2020)—the use of this technology has led to varied overuse injuries. The "BlackBerry thumb," for instance, was the tip of the iceberg (O'Sullivan, 2013) as injuries increased even with the advent of advanced technology. The overuse of these items has continued to cause many hand and wrist injuries as well as, unfortunately, more serious injuries, including life-threatening ones, with the careless use of handheld devices (Pottorff, 2020).

Because occupational therapy practitioners have been using activity analysis to understand the interaction between the individual and the task, activity analysis has been used to return individuals to work. Specifically, a ***job analysis*** is a more comprehensive activity analysis performed to identify the demands of a specific job. According to Joss (2007), a job analysis is a "natural extension of the skills that occupational therapists use in activity analysis" (p. 301). The practitioner must be familiar with the demands of the job and what is required of the worker: the specific tasks and how they are performed, materials used, the expected outcomes, and the environment in which the work is performed. Indeed, experienced practitioners may work in industry so that the analysis is done at the individual's actual location. For further information regarding the occupation of work, refer to Chapter 14, "Work Occupations."

According to *OTPF–4* (AOTA, 2020), ***occupations*** are "personalized and meaningful engagement in daily life events by a specific client" as influenced by their context (p. 7). For example, ADLs are considered an occupation; they are subdivided into individual tasks, such as bathing, toileting, and dressing (AOTA, 2020, p. 30). Each self-care task requires different skills and presents different challenges to the individual (e.g., fine motor, cognitive, balance, mobility). It would be impossible to do an activity analysis on an ADL as a whole, but once the component parts are identified, the occupational therapy practitioner can do an analysis on the individual components (e.g., upper-body dressing or toileting), as outlined in this chapter. Therefore, the component or activity is more specific and more succinct in scope.

Occupational therapy practitioners' ability to examine the component parts or various elements of an occupation allows us to identify what may be an obstacle to successful completion of the task or activity. The activity analysis enables the practitioner to direct intervention. This ability to analyze an activity or component of an occupation is a cornerstone of our profession. Once this skill is integrated into our intervention, the practitioner assists the individual to regain their desired skill. In the next section, we describe the activity and the factors that influence the person's ability to perform it, including both internal and external factors.

Description of the occupation, activity, or related activities

After the occupational therapy evaluation, the occupational therapy practitioner considers potential activities based on the patient's performance skills, context, client factors, and occupations. Data collected from the occupational profile allow us to select treatment intervention that will be meaningful to the individual relative to their roles, personal goals, and the context in which they are performed. See Chapter 4, "The Occupational Profile," for a more detailed discussion of the occupational profile.

In this section, we name the activity and describe the sequential steps required to perform it (see Appendix 3.A). Each step is identified in the order in which it is performed to complete the full activity and is described in detail. The following considerations are made concerning the time needed to complete the activity:

- Can the person complete the activity in one session?
- Does the activity naturally divide into segments so that a person can perform it over time?
- Do the steps in the activity require that it be performed over time?

The required objects, materials, tools, equipment, and their properties, along with space and social needs, are considered. In addition, safety precautions and contraindications are identified and included.

Context

According to the *OTPF–4* (AOTA, 2020), ***context*** includes environmental and personal factors that influence engagement in occupations (see Exhibit 3.1). Thus, this section of the occupation analysis form includes demographics and the person's values, beliefs, and spirituality. The occupational therapy practitioner identifies ideas or beliefs that are important to the person.

Determine which of the following features potentially influence the person's participation or engagement in the activity:

- the person's value for the activity/occupation
- the person's perceived purpose of the activity/occupation
- the activity's ability to promote independence or self-efficacy

EXHIBIT 3.1. Context as Present in the *OTPF–4*

Context
Environmental and personal factors that enhance engagement and participation
Environmental factors
Natural environment and human-made changes; products and technology; support and relationships; attitudes; service, systems, and policy
Personal factors
Chronological age; sexual orientation; gender identity; cultural identity and attitudes; habits; past and current behavioral patterns; social background and status; socioeconomic status; life experiences; education, profession, and lifestyle; health conditions; psychological assets; temperament; coping styles

Source. Adapted from AOTA (2020). Used with permission.

Does the activity or occupation provide opportunities for independence, self-expression, or creativity, or all three?

On completion of the occupational therapy evaluation, which includes the occupational profile, the therapist, in collaboration with the individual, identifies the activities that are meaningful and relevant to their roles. The analysis is used to identify whether the activity incorporates skills that can be associated with a desired role. An appraisal of the activity relative to the context is also considered. For example, does the person perform the activity alone or with others? Does their context and client factors (i.e., values, beliefs, spirituality) influence performance?

Activity analysis outline

Activity analysis has multiple components that influence a person's ability to perform the activity. The *ICF* is concerned with people's ability to participate in activities and society. Its taxonomy is divided into two broad categories: (1) functioning and disability and (2) contextual factors. According to the *ICF*, functioning and disability themselves include two components: (1) body function and structures and (2) activities and participation. ***Contextual factors*** include personal factors and environmental factors that influence performance of the activity and the level of participation. There are also components, which are specific descriptors for both personal and environmental factors. The broad categories of required action and performance skills are included in both the *OTPF–4* and the *ICF* (AOTA, 2020; WHO, 2001) and serve as a framework for the analysis presented in this chapter. We do not use the *ICF* taxonomy in its entirety; rather, we limit its use to categories that we determined were most relevant to the process of occupation analysis.

The *ICF* taxonomy (WHO, 2001) provides a broad structure for the analysis and the basis for identifying basic requirements of the activity. The therapist identifies whether a specific skill is necessary during the performance of the activity (yes or no). A *yes* response indicates that the performance skill will need to be focused on in the subsequent sections of the analysis form. Based on the client's performance, the therapist determines the level of influence that each component has on the individual's ability to perform the activity. Eventually, the therapist must understand how impairment affects or challenges the client's performance of the activity. Another reason for analyzing an activity is to identify its potential for providing stimulation or opportunities to use specific skills as part of intervention. A 5-point scale is used to rate the influence of each element:

- *0* = The component has no effect or influence on the ability to do the activity.
- *1* = The component has only a minimal effect or influence on the ability to do the activity. The activity would not substantially stimulate or address the performance component element.
- *2* = The component has a moderate effect or influence on the ability to complete the activity. If an individual has a deficit, compensation may have to be made for them to perform the activity. The activity would present a challenge to the performance component element.
- *3* = The component has a significant effect or influence on the ability to complete the activity. The activity would be extremely difficult to complete if the client has a deficit in this performance component. The activity would present a significant stimulation or opportunity to address the performance component element.
- *4* = The component has a major effect or influence on the completion of the activity. A performance component deficit in this area would seriously influence the person's ability to do the activity. Such a person would very likely be unable to complete the activity. The activity would present a major stimulation or opportunity to address this performance component element.

The observation section is used to describe special circumstances or concerns and provides space to include any other comments a practitioner has relative to performance.

Learning and applying knowledge

In this section, we define each skill and provide several questions that an occupational therapy practitioner or an occupational therapy student would consider when assessing the role skill plays in completing the activity. These questions are not definitive but, rather, a starting point when considering each skill or action. After considering each question, the practitioner rates the skill or action's influence and writes observational notes.

Knowledge and learning. ***Knowledge*** is what is learned. ***Learning*** is based on thinking, solving problems, and making decisions. Learning is also influenced by sensory experiences. Activities are about applying knowledge for a meaningful outcome. The first step to examining this aspect of the activity is to consider what the activity requires the person to do. This screening gives the occupational therapy practitioner guidance about which components need to be analyzed further. Answering the following questions guides practitioners to the next step of the analysis:

- Does the activity require watching—that is, using the sense of seeing intentionally to experience visual stimuli, such as watching a sporting event or children playing? Visual reception is the underlying prerequisite.
- Is intentional hearing required, such as listening for a timer, lecture, or music?
- Does the activity require other intentional sensory experiences? Tactile, proprioceptive, vestibular, olfactory, and gustatory senses may need to be examined.

Occupational therapy practitioners also analyze activities in relation to their sensory-processing demands. A person's central nervous system processes sensory information and integrates this information so that the person can make an adaptive response. Sensory processing may influence their ability to reach a calm state of alertness and thus their ability to engage in and complete the activity. Each activity presents unique sensory-processing requirements. Thus, the ability to organize and integrate multiple sensory processes is necessary for an adaptive response during performance of an activity.

Sensory processing. ***Sensory processing*** is the internal mechanism a person uses to process and respond to sensory input:

- Does the activity require the person to make changes on the basis of sensory input?
- Is the ability to end performance based on sensory processing (e.g., physical discomfort, a problem with the activity)?
- Will a diminished or adverse response influence performance (e.g., defensiveness)?

Visual Reception. ***Visual reception*** involves interpreting stimuli through the eyes, including peripheral vision, acuity, and awareness of color and pattern:

- Does the activity require the person to fixate on a stationary object—that is, the skill of ***visual fixation***?
- Does the activity require slow, smooth movements of the eyes to maintain fixation on a moving object—that is, the skill of ***visual tracking***?
- Does the person need to rapidly change fixation from one object in the visual field to another (near to far)—for example, while driving a car, when crossing a busy street, or when a student is copying from a blackboard?
- Is discrimination of fine detail required to do the activity (e.g., sewing, handwriting)?

Depth perception. ***Depth perception*** is determining the relative distance between objects, figures, or landmarks and the observer and changes in planes and surfaces:

- Does the person have to reach distances to acquire objects or complete the activity?
- Does the person need to place body parts in relation to changing elements of the environment (e.g., step up or down)?

Auditory processing. ***Auditory processing*** involves interpreting and localizing sounds and discriminating among background sounds:

- Does the activity require the person to listen to sounds and interpret their meaning (e.g., musical notes, verbal communication, warning sounds)?
- Are there functional sounds that assist the person with monitoring the environment (e.g., water running, frying, traffic)?
- Does the activity produce loud sounds during its performance (e.g., alarm clock, hammering, power tools)? Could these sounds be stressful to the person?
- Does the environment require the person to discriminate or suppress background sounds (e.g., excessive outside noise while in the classroom)?
- Does sound contribute to or influence safe performance?

Tactile processing. ***Tactile processing*** includes light touch, pressure, temperature, pain, and vibration though skin contact and receptors:

- Does the activity require the person to hold objects gently, or is a degree of pressure important (e.g., a paper cup versus a mug)?
- Are the materials at room temperature or cool/warm/hot to the touch?
- Does the activity require the person to appreciate or tolerate vibration (e.g., electric toothbrush, vacuum cleaner)?
- Does the activity require tactile discrimination (e.g., textures)?
- Are body parts always within the visual field? When must a person rely on tactile input (e.g., putting a necklace)?
- Could the tactile properties be perceived as noxious (e.g., sticky tape, rough surfaces)?

Proprioceptive processing. ***Proprioceptive processing*** involves interpreting stimuli originating in muscles, joints, and other internal tissues that give information about the position of one body part in relation to another:

- Does the activity distract or compress joints and soft tissue?
- Is weight-bearing part of the activity on lower or upper extremities?
- What is the degree of pushing, pulling, or lifting that occurs during the activity?
- Do movements and position of the extremities occur outside the visual field?

Vestibular input. ***Vestibular input*** involves interpreting stimuli from the inner ear receptors regarding head position. It contributes to appropriate righting and equilibrium reactions, automatic postural responses, and maintenance of posture and movement during activity performance:

- Does the activity require quick movements of the head or body?
- Does the activity require postural maintenance or change in relation to gravity or acceleration and deceleration forces (e.g., sit to stand, sudden change in forward movement, vertical or horizontal changes)?
- Does the activity require muscular co-contraction?
- Does the activity require coordinated eye movements?
- Does the activity require postural background movements (e.g., adequate extension; ability to dissociate head, neck, and arm movements)?

Olfactory processing. ***Olfactory processing*** involves interpreting odors:

- Does the activity involve odors that might be interpreted as noxious?
- Does the activity involve odors that might be alerting (e.g., burning toast, smoke) or calming (e.g., fresh baked bread, cookies)?
- How might the scents affect someone who is overresponsive?

Gustatory processing. ***Gustatory processing*** involves interpreting tastes:

- Does the person need to interpret taste to enhance or contribute to performance?
- Does the taste or texture elicit an overresponsive reaction?

Spatial relations. ***Spatial relations*** means determining the position of objects relative to one another:

- Does the activity require the use of spatial concepts (manipulation, take apart, put together)?
- Does the activity require the person to estimate sizes?
- Does the activity require the person to judge distances?
- Does the activity require orientation of shapes, sizes, or designs?
- Does the activity require attention to detail in positioning?

Position in space. ***Position in space*** involves determining the spatial relationship of figures and objects to the self and other forms and objects:

- Does the activity require the person to determine front, back, top, bottom, beside, behind, under, or over (e.g., during dressing)?
- Does the activity require that the person understand the relationship between action and their body (e.g., rolling to the side of the bed before sitting up)?

Sensory modulation. ***Sensory modulation*** is the ability to respond appropriately to incoming stimuli:

- Does the person overrespond to sensory stimuli (e.g., sensory defensiveness, becoming overly stressed by stimuli)?
- Does the person underrespond to sensory stimuli (e.g., does not appear to register stimuli, slow to respond)?
- Does the person seek out or avoid sensory stimuli (e.g., rocking, spinning, or nonparticipation)?

Attention. ***Attention*** refers to the ability to focus on a task over time:

- How long must the person attend?
- Will the person be required to selectively attend (e.g., focus on specific stimuli) or disregard irrelevant stimuli?
- Does the activity demand sustained or divided attention?
- Does the activity require the person to shift attention (e.g., frying eggs, making toast, pouring coffee while cooking)?

Motor control. ***Motor control*** is the use of functional and versatile movement patterns:

- Does the activity require repetition? If so, what kind (e.g., putting a puzzle together, catching a ball)?
- Which specific joints of the body need to be controlled during a complex activity?
- Does the activity require the person to inhibit movements to be more efficient (e.g., using scissors)?
- Does the activity require constant or variable changes in speed, tempo, or rhythm (e.g., dealing cards, dribbling a basketball)?

- Is the pace of the activity externally or internally controlled (e.g., jumping alone or playing double Dutch)?

Praxis. ***Praxis*** involves conceiving and planning a motor act in response to an environmental demand:

- Is the activity new and unusual for the person?
- Does engagement require the person to have a plan when movements are not habitual?
- Does the activity require the person to assume a novel position—that is, ***postural praxis*** (e.g., yoga, martial arts, dance routines for the novice)?
- Does the activity involve the use of new tools?

Basic learning

Basic learning encompasses the skill areas of copying and rehearsing. Answering the following questions guides the occupational therapy practitioner to the next step of the analysis:

- Does the activity require ***copying*** (i.e., imitating or mimicking as a basic component of learning, such as copying a gesture, a sound, or the letters of an alphabet)? Prerequisites to be examined are recognition, form constancy, spatial relations, and position in space.
- Does the activity require ***rehearsing,*** which is repeating a sequence of events or symbols as a basic component of learning (e.g., counting by 10s or practicing the recitation of a poem)? Sequencing is the prerequisite skill.

Recognition. ***Recognition*** means identifying familiar faces, objects, and other previously presented material:

- Does the person have to recognize people, body parts, and objects to engage in the activity?

Form constancy. ***Form constancy*** refers to recognizing forms and objects as being the same in various environments, positions, and sizes:

- Does the activity occur in two or three dimensions?
- Does the activity require the person to respond to changing presentation of objects (e.g., ice melting to water, hanging versus folded laundry)?
- Does the size of the tools, utensils, or letters change?

Sequencing. ***Sequencing*** is the placing of information, concepts, and actions in order:

- Does the activity require the person to arrange items or perform steps in a serial order?
- Does the activity require an understanding of "before" and "after"?
- Does the activity require the person to ***reverse a sequence,*** that is, perform the sequence backward (e.g., put on clothing or take it off, put a toy together or take it apart)?
- Does the activity allow the person to have personal choice in the manner of sequencing (e.g., morning care, dressing, showering)?

Acquiring skills

Acquiring skills means engaging in an activity that creates situations in which people gain skills. ***Skills*** are the sets of actions that a person has learned and is able to apply in given situations. Skills are often divided into basic and complex skills. ***Basic skills*** are elementary and purposeful actions, such as learning to manipulate eating utensils, a pencil, or a simple tool. ***Complex skills*** are integrated sets of actions to follow rules and to sequence and coordinate movements, such as learning to play board games, using a power drill, or engaging in organized sports.

Answering these questions provides guidelines to the occupational therapy practitioner for the next step of the analysis:

- Practitioners must assess a person's cognitive abilities before determining their capacity to learn or apply knowledge. Does the activity require the participant to focus intentionally on specific stimuli, such as filtering out distracting noises? Level of arousal, orientation, and attention span must be considered.
- Does the person have adequate skills to support the efficient completion of the activity? Consider motor control, endurance, praxis, body scheme, fine motor coordination and dexterity, crossing the midline, right–left discrimination, laterality, bilateral integration, and visual–motor integration.
- What thinking processes does the activity require the person to use (formulating and manipulating ideas, concepts, and images whether goal oriented or not, either alone or with others—e.g., creating fiction, providing a theorem, playing with ideas, brainstorming, meditating, pondering, speculating, reflecting)? Consider memory, categorization, spatial operations, generalization, and concept formation.
- Solving problems requires that a person find solutions to concerns about completing the activity. Simple problems involve a single issue or question. Solving complex problems requires the person to consider multiple and interrelated issues. To solve problems, a person must identify the problems, analyze issues, develop and evaluate solutions, and execute the chosen solution. Therefore, learning and memory must be examined.
- Making decisions requires choosing among options, implementing the choice, and evaluating the effects of that choice. Consider memory, concept formation, categorization, and generalization.

Level of arousal. ***Level of arousal*** is demonstrating alertness and responsiveness to environmental stimuli:

- Does the time of day influence the person's arousal level?
- What arousal level is needed to provide an adequate length of time to complete the activity?
- Do fatigue and pain factors affect arousal level and the ability to attend to the task?

Orientation. ***Orientation*** involves identifying person, place, time, and situation.

To identify orientation to person, consider:

- Does the activity relate to the person's lifestyle?
- Is the activity associated with a role that is meaningful to the person?
- Could the activity be influenced by the person's ***routines*** (e.g., cleaning the bathroom on Saturday versus cleaning the bathroom when it needs it)?
- Could the activity be associated with a personal ritual or symbolic action that contributes to the person's identity?

To identify orientation to place, answer this question:

- Does the activity require the person to know where they are?

To identify orientation to time, answer this question:

- Does the person need to know the exact time, date, or time of year to engage in the activity?

To identify orientation to situation, answer these questions:

- What is the relationship between the activity and the person's environment and roles?
- Does the person need to understand the circumstances in which the activity is performed?
- Does the person understand time restrictions or demands placed on performance?

Body scheme. ***Body scheme*** refers to having an internal awareness of the body and the relationship of body parts to each other. This component is closely related to kinesthesia and proprioception because it requires integration of sensation from muscles and joints:

- Does the activity require that the person have an appreciation for their body and be able to sense how the parts work together during movement (e.g., playing sports)?
- Does the activity require the person to have internal awareness of body actions that must happen in a specific sequence (e.g., ballroom dancing)?

Ocular–motor control. ***Ocular–motor control*** involves the ability to move the eyes to focus on and follow objects:

- Does the person need to fixate on a stationary object or track or scan a moving object?

Oral–motor skill. ***Oral–motor skill*** means to use the muscles in and around the mouth:

- Is the person able to coordinate tongue, lips, and jaw for the purposes of clear speech or eating?

Fine motor coordination and dexterity. ***Fine motor coordination and dexterity*** refers to using small muscle groups for controlled movements, particularly in-hand object manipulation:

- What degree of isolated finger use is required?
- Which grasp patterns are used during different functions (e.g., hook, cylindrical, spherical)?
- Which pinch patterns are used (e.g., tripod, lateral pinch, tip-to-tip pinch)?
- Is speed a necessary element of the activity?

Visual–motor integration. ***Visual–motor integration*** is the ability to coordinate the interaction of information from the eyes and body movement:

- What degree of eye–hand or eye–foot coordination is required (e.g., handwriting, tracing, copying, walking on a balance beam, kicking a ball)?

Crossing the midline. ***Crossing the midline*** means moving the limbs and eyes across the midline sagittal plane of the body:

- Does the activity require the person to scan the environment to find required materials to perform the activity? If so, how frequently?
- Does the activity require that the person cross the midline of the body with their arms or legs (e.g., dressing)?

Right–left discrimination. ***Right–left discrimination*** involves differentiating one side from the other.

- Does the person need to be able to use or apply right–left concepts?
- What degree of bilateral coordination is required to do the activity?
- Does the activity require that the person be able to follow verbal or written directions that require actions to the left, right, or both sides of the body?
- Does the activity involve tools that require bilateral coordination, such as the use of one hand as a stabilizer or assist while the other hand operates the tool (e.g., cutting food with a knife and fork)?
- Does the activity require the person to differentiate right and left on another person (e.g., demonstrated instruction as in karate, dancing)?

Laterality. ***Laterality*** involves using a preferred or dominant hand or foot:

- Does the activity require a high degree of skill in which the person needs to use a preferred hand or foot (e.g., handwriting, kicking a ball)?
- Does hand or foot preference influence how smoothly or effortlessly the person performs the activity?

Bilateral integration. ***Bilateral integration*** means coordinating both sides of the body. Bilateral integration is considered a prerequisite for gross and fine motor coordination and affects acquisition of skills:

- How frequently do both sides of the body have to cooperate during the activity?
- Does one side of the body need to stabilize while the other side acts?
- Does the activity require crossing the midline in a rotatory or asymmetrical pattern (e.g., golf swing, baseball swing)?
- Does the activity require that the person use both sides of the body symmetrically (e.g., pushing a shopping cart, playing tug-of-war)?
- Does the activity require ***reciprocal patterns,*** which are corresponding actions with the other extremity (e.g., bike riding, swimming, running)?

Memory. ***Memory*** is the recoding of information after a brief or long period:

- What are the activity's memory requirements—for example, immediate, short term, or long term?
- What information related to personal experience (episodic) is needed?
- What factual knowledge of the world (semantic) is needed?
- What knowledge of the activity or how to do it (procedural) is needed?
- Is the long-term memory sensory specific (visual, auditory, verbal)?

Categorization. ***Categorization*** involves identifying similarities and differences among pieces of environmental information:

- Does the activity require the person to group objects or information according to characteristics (e.g., visual features, tactile features, similarities, differences)?
- Does the activity require mental grouping (e.g., playing cards, different name brands to be purchased, price differences, nutritional contents)?
- Does the activity require construction in which the person must understand how parts relate to a whole or how to break the whole down into its parts?

Concept formation. ***Concept formation*** involves organizing a variety of information to form thoughts and ideas. This component is related to the ability to categorize:

- Does the activity require synthesis of ideas (e.g., formulation of a hypothesis about the how or why)?
- Does the activity require abstract thought processes?
- Does the activity require symbolic thinking?
- Does the activity require the person to question or evaluate their performance?

Spatial operations. ***Spatial operations*** refers to mentally manipulating the position of objects in various relationships:

- Does the activity require the person to mentally visualize different perspectives (e.g., two-dimensional diagrams, three-dimensional objects)?
- Does the activity involve mental visualization of performance?
- Does the activity require that the person visualize how the object or activity should look on completion (e.g., clothing on a hanger or one's body, how a table will be set for a dinner party, how a cake will look after baking)?

Learning. ***Learning*** refers to acquiring new concepts and behaviors:

- Does the activity provide a structured or unstructured learning experience?
- Does the activity provide feedback about performance?
- What type of learning is expected (e.g., motor, verbal, feelings, attitudinal)?

Generalization. ***Generalization*** involves applying previously learned concepts and behaviors to a variety of new situations:

- Can the activity be performed in different contexts (e.g., bathing at bedside, sponge bathing at sink, tub bathing)?
- Does the activity provide opportunities to apply learned skills to a new situation?

General activity demands

Completing an activity requires that people carry out simple or complex and coordinated actions. These actions are related to its mental, physical, and social components. Some actions produce a single simple activity that is clearly defined or time limited, such as initiating or terminating the activity. Single complex tasks need to be carried out in sequence or simultaneously, such as arranging the furniture in one's home or completing an assignment for school. Moreover, activities are influenced by the people who participate in them.

Consideration of the following guides occupational therapy practitioners to the next step of the analysis:

- A person's mental and physical status influence how they carry out simple or complex activities. Prerequisite components to be examined are initiation of activity, time management, termination of activity, coping skills, and self-control.
- Some activities comprise multiple tasks that need to be carried out in sequence or simultaneously, such as preparing a multicourse meal with each course requiring initiation and management of time. Space to prepare a salad, main course, and side dishes must be organized, and several tasks may occur together or sequentially. For example, the salad ingredients and vegetables are washed together, and a sequence of peeling and chopping vegetables and salad ingredients must occur to complete the activity. Prerequisite components to be examined are initiation of activity, time management, termination of activity, coping skills, and self-control.
- Simple, complex, and multiple activities may be carried out independently or within a group setting. When they occur independently, prerequisite components to be examined are initiation of activity, time management, termination of activity, coping skills, and self-control. When tasks occur in a group, the practitioner assesses social conduct and interpersonal skills as well.

Initiation of activity. ***Initiation of activity*** is the starting of a physical or mental activity:

- Does the activity require the person to self-start?
- Does the person have to plan the start (e.g., alarm clock or timer)?
- Is the activity motivated by personal meaning and relevance (e.g., vacuuming as the result of visual feedback of a dirty floor)?
- How would the person's cognitive or mental health status affect the performance of this activity?

Time management. ***Time management*** involves anticipating, planning, and using parcels of time as they relate to completion of activities:

- Is the activity performed in one session or multiple sessions?
- Are there set time constraints for portions of the activity (e.g., bake at 350° for 30 minutes)?
- Is the activity part of a personal routine that has self-imposed time restrictions (e.g., morning care consisting of 10 minutes for shower, 10 minutes for dressing, and 10 minutes for grooming)?
- Does the activity allow for choices about the use of time (e.g., a craft project in which the detailing could require additional time because of increased interest or skill level)?
- Does the activity require organizing and setting realistic priorities to complete it?

Termination of activity. ***Termination of activity*** means stopping an activity at an appropriate time:

- What is the person's control over engaging in and disengaging from the activity?
- Is the activity time limited?
- Is the activity rote or repetitive?

Coping skills. ***Coping skills*** involve identifying and managing stress and related factors:

- Is this activity new for the person, or is it part of an established personal routine?
- Are parts of the activity automatic and therefore less stressful (e.g., habitual)?
- Does the activity environment influence the perceived stress?
- Does the activity provide an appropriate level of challenge without promoting undue stress?
- Does the activity require exactness, or is there a range of acceptable performance?
- Is performance of the activity externally or internally controlled?

Self-control. ***Self-control*** occurs when one modifies their own behavior in response to environmental needs, demands, constraints, personal aspirations, and feedback from others:

- Should mishaps in the activity or environment be expected?
- Does the outcome of the activity lead to attainment of goals?
- Do the activity demands require the person to adapt performance in response to changes in the environment?
- Will the person be required to respond to feedback about performance (e.g., criticism or praise)?
- To what degree does the activity challenge physical, social, or cognitive ability?

Social skills. ***Social skills*** refers to interacting while using manners, personal space, eye contact, gestures, active listening, and self-expression appropriate to one's environment and satisfying to oneself and others:

- In what type of social environment does the activity occur?
- Does the activity require cooperative behavior?
- What are the accepted personal boundaries of the activity (e.g., sports, card game, shopping)?
- Does the social environment present expectations regarding appropriate interaction and communication (e.g., authority figures, or children)?
- Does the activity require the person to initiate or answer questions or make suggestions?

Interpersonal skills. ***Interpersonal skills*** refers to the use of verbal and nonverbal communication to interact in a variety of settings:

- Does the activity require independence, cooperation, or competition?
- What degree of verbal interaction or casual conversation is required?
- Does the activity require active verbal and nonverbal participation?
- Does the activity require expression of emotions?
- Does the activity require specific nonverbal behavior (e.g., appropriate sitting posture, signs of active listening, changes in facial expression, use of appropriate gestures)?
- Does the activity require the person to assume an unfamiliar interaction style?
- Does the activity require the person to recognize and respond to others' nonverbal behavior?

Mobility

Mobility includes changing body positions or location by transferring from one place to another; by carrying, moving, or manipulating objects; by walking, running, or climbing; and by using various forms of transportation. Changing and maintaining body position may occur during performance of the activity. Prerequisite performance components to be examined are postural alignment, muscle tone, postural control, depth perception, and body strength:

- Does the activity require changes in body positioning before, during, and after engagement in the activity?
- Does the activity require moving from one location to another, such as getting up from a chair to lie down on a bed and getting into and out of kneeling or squatting positions?
- Does the activity require the person to transfer from one surface to another, and what degree of control is required?

Postural alignment. ***Postural alignment*** means maintaining the biomechanical integrity among body parts:

- What degree of axial alignment does the activity require?
- Does the pelvic position change during performance of the activity (e.g., taking off shoes)?
- Does the activity require frequent changes in alignment (e.g., texting while seated, playing racquetball)?
- What postures are needed to optimally perform the activity?

Postural control. ***Postural control*** is using righting and equilibrium reactions to maintain balance during functional movements:

- Does the activity have the potential for a sudden displacement of the center of gravity?
- Do changes in the base of support occur while engaging in the activity?
- Does head position change frequently?
- Must the person stabilize against the forces of gravity when engaged in the activity (e.g., lean forward, lean back, lean to the side)?
- Does the activity require the person to anticipate postural adjustments?

Body strength. ***Body strength*** is the degree of muscle strength required to complete the activity:

- How does gravity influence the performance of the activity?
- Does the activity provide resistance to movement of the body?
- Does the activity require concentric, eccentric, or isometric muscle contractions?

Carrying, moving, and handling objects

Many activities require that a person be able to handle, move, and manipulate objects with their upper extremities and hands. Movements may be gross or fine or a combination of both. Sometimes, the actions demand intricate, coordinated finger movements. Other actions require lower-extremity strength and control:

- Are any of the following upper-extremity movements done while performing the activity: pulling, pushing, reaching, throwing, or catching? Prerequisite components to be examined are range of motion, strength, and endurance.

- Must the person move and manipulate objects with their upper extremities? Prerequisite skills for upper-extremity control are range of motion, strength, endurance, stereognosis, kinesthesia, and figure–ground perception.
- Must the person carry or transport objects while walking? Prerequisite skills are range of motion, postural control, strength, endurance, and topographical orientation.

Range of motion. ***Range of motion*** means actively moving body parts through an arc of motion:

- What movements are required of the head, neck, and trunk during the activity?
- What directions and degree of range of motion of the extremities are required and necessary to perform the activity?
- Which joints are positioned statically, and which joints are active?
- Does the activity require the person to control movements at multiple joints?
- What rotational movements (internal or external rotation, pronation or supination) are required to perform the activity?
- Are there any soft-tissue conditions that would affect range of motion (hyper- or hypomobility)?

Extremity strength. ***Extremity strength*** is the grade of muscle strength required in the extremities to complete the activity:

- How does gravity influence the performance of the activity?
- Does the activity require concentric, eccentric, or isometric muscle contraction?
- What muscle grade is required at the extremities to complete the activity?

Endurance. ***Endurance*** refers to sustained cardiac, pulmonary, and musculoskeletal exertion over time:

- What is the duration of the activity (e.g., time needed to complete the activity)?
- How repetitive is the activity?
- Are portions of the activity resistive?
- Does fatigue occur as a result of the activity?

Stereognosis. ***Stereognosis*** is identifying objects through proprioception, cognition, and the sense of touch:

- Does the activity require the hands or feet to identify or manipulate objects without reliance on vision (e.g., reaching into a pocket to find a coin, reaching into a drawer)?
- Do aspects of the activity require vigilance when the person needs to find, manipulate, or reach for objects outside the visual field?

Kinesthesia. ***Kinesthesia*** involves identifying the excursion and direction of movement:

- Does the activity require movements to be coordinated over multiple joints?
- Does the activity require visual attention so that the person must rely on the ability to move their extremities without reliance on vision (e.g., swinging a bat at a baseball, playing tennis, doing ballet)?
- Does the activity require the person to change directions of movements (e.g., fingers during typing, fingers while playing an instrument)?

Grasp patterns. ***Grasp patterns*** refers to the types of coordinated hand movements required to perform the activity:

- What specific grasp patterns are used to complete the activity?
- Does the person demonstrate age-appropriate grasp patterns?

Prehension/pinch patterns. ***Prehension/pinch patterns*** refers to the types of prehension (pinch) required to perform the activity:

- What specific pinch patterns are required to complete the activity?
- Does the person demonstrate an age-appropriate pinch pattern?

Fine motor skill. ***Fine motor skill*** is the ability to use small hand muscles and joints to perform refined actions:

- What kind of fine motor action does the activity require?
- Does the activity require in-hand manipulation of small objects or small tool use?
- Does the activity require small, joint-isolated movements?

Figure–ground perception. ***Figure–ground perception*** involves differentiating between foreground and background forms and objects:

- Does the activity require the person to distinguish an object or image from a complex background (e.g., doing word search games, finding a spoon in a drawer)?
- Does the activity require the person to locate objects from a cluster of objects (e.g., food in a refrigerator, clothes in a closet)?

Topographical orientation. ***Topographical orientation*** is concerned with determining the location of objects and settings and the route to the location:

- Does the activity require the person to follow a familiar route or negotiate new or different surroundings (e.g., shopping in an unfamiliar store)?
- Does the activity require the person to retrace routes from spatial memory?
- Does the activity rely on the person's ability to identify visual landmarks?

Analysis Summary

The ***analysis summary*** included on the analysis form serves as a tool for the occupational therapy student or practitioner to reflect and analyze the information culled from the analysis. This section is particularly useful when the practitioner is using the analysis to determine if the activity is appropriate for intervention (occupation-as-means) strategy.

When the analysis is complete, consider the following in relation to the individual:

- Is the activity relevant to the person?
- It is critical to determine whether the activity will enable the person to be engaged and be a challenge to their present abilities, thus improving their skills during the intervention process. The therapist, in collaboration with the individual, decides if the activity will contribute to the development of competence and mastery of the task in their context.
- Is the occupation part of the individual's habits, routines, roles, or rituals?

An analysis for a particular person does not occur in isolation. An occupational therapy practitioner should give consideration to the process of engaging in the selected activity. Does the activity encompass basic, automatic behaviors (i.e., habits) and routines? Does the sequence provide structure for engagement in occupations? Does the activity support the individual's occupational identity as defined by their personal roles, history, future goals, and essential social and cultural expectations? Has the person assigned symbolic meaning to the activity or portions of the activity?

EXERCISE 3.1. An Example of an Occupation or Activity Analysis

Review the sample activity analysis in Appendix 3.B. Read through this occupational/activity analysis that documents the task of repotting a plant as part of the occupation of gardening. Would you view this activity the same way? How would an occupational therapy practitioner use this information in practice?

EXERCISE 3.2. Analysis of a Daily Life Activity

Consider either the activity of frying an egg for breakfast or folding clothes. Think about the way in which you normally do the task. Follow the process outlined in the form presented in Appendix 3.A.

The purpose of this assignment is to appreciate that everything you do is potentially a therapeutic activity. Through the analysis, you learn the component pieces outside the context of the real-world of activities. In practice, occupational therapy practitioners collaborate with the individual to determine if the activity is important to them within their context.

Occupation and Activity Analysis Within the Context of a Frame of Reference

Activity analysis is a tool that occupational therapy practitioners use to determine an activity's therapeutic potential. As such, activity analyses provide the means for understanding the individual and their ability to perform specific purposeful activities.

Up to this point, activity analysis has been described as a process for examining or analyzing specific activities. When an analysis is used within the context of a frame of reference or a guideline for practice, it is called a ***restricted activity analysis***. The *OTPF–4* (AOTA, 2020) provides the guidelines for the activity analysis. A restricted analysis allows us to select the most relevant areas to analyze. For example, if the occupational therapy practitioner is working with a person with left hemiparesis with motor impairments only, the practitioner will determine the elements to be analyzed from the analysis template.

After assessing the individual, the occupational therapist observes that postural control, sitting and standing balance, and upper-extremity motor function are impaired. Based on this information, the therapist may determine that the neurodevelopmental treatment (NDT) approach is most appropriate to restore performance skills. If the individual wants to be able to dress, the practitioner analyzes the motor skills required for safe and efficient dressing. For example, a button-down shirt versus an overheard garment presents different challenges to an individual's postural control as well as upper-extremity motor control. The practitioner selects the NDT frame of reference to guide the intervention for the dressing task. Once the practitioner has done an activity analysis within the context of a frame of reference, they can then relate the analysis to the broader occupation.

Summary

The ability to analyze an occupation or activity competently is a critical skill for an occupational therapist or occupational therapy assistant's knowledge base. The ability to analyze an activity in the person's context enables both the individual and the occupational therapy practitioner to collaborate on setting goals for intervention. The primary function of this activity analysis form is to guide students in the development of prerequisite skills needed to analyze and interpret the underlying skills of occupations and activities.

This form is designed to direct students to consider the contextual issues that affect each individual, client, or patient during engagement. For occupational therapy practitioners, this form can be used to review and refine basic skills. The form also may benefit practitioners who are transitioning from one practice area to another.

Occupational/activity analysis remains a foundational skill for the practice of occupational therapy. The nature and purpose of an analysis has changed and adapted over time and will continue to evolve based on the emerging needs of the people we serve. Thus, it is our responsibility as occupational therapy practitioners to understand these changes and accommodate accordingly.

References

American Occupational Therapy Association. (1994). Uniform terminology for occupational therapy—Third edition. *American Journal of Occupational Therapy, 48*(11), 1047–1054. https://doi.org/10.5014/ajot.48.11.1047

American Occupational Therapy Association. (2014). Occupational therapy practice framework: Domain and process (3rd ed.). *American Journal of Occupational Therapy, 68*(Suppl. 1), S1–S48. https://doi.org/10.5014/ajot.2014.682006

American Occupational Therapy Association. (2020). Occupational therapy practice framework: Domain and process (4th ed.). *American Journal of Occupational Therapy, 74*(Suppl. 2), 7412410010. https//doi.org/10.5014/ajot.2020.74S2001

Boyt Shell, B. A., Gillen, G., Crepeau, E. B., & Scaffa, M. E. (2019). Analyzing occupations and activities. In B. A. Boyt Shell & G. Gillen (Eds.), *Willard and Spackman's occupational therapy* (13th ed., pp. 320–334). Wolters Kluwer.

Creighton, C. (1992). The origin and evolution of activity analysis. *American Journal of Occupational Therapy, 46*(1), 45–48. https://doi.org/10.5014/ajot.46.1.45

Crepeau, E. B. (2003). Analyzing occupation and activity: A way of thinking about occupational performance. In E. B. Crepeau, E. S. Cohen, & B. A. Boyt Schell (Eds.), *Willard and Spackman's occupational therapy* (10th ed., pp. 189–198). Lippincott Williams & Wilkins.

Crepeau, E. B., Schell, B. A. B., Gillen, G., & Scaffa, M. E. (2014). Analyzing occupations and activity. In B. A. B. Schell, G. Gillen, & M. E. Scaffa (Eds.), *Willard and Spackman's occupational therapy* (12th ed., pp. 234–248). Wolters Kluwer Health/Lippincott Williams & Wilkins.

Cynkin, S., & Robinson, A. M. (1990). *Occupational therapy and activities health: Toward health through activity.* Little, Brown.

Dunton, W. R., & Licht, S. (1957). *Occupational therapy principles and practice.* Charles C Thomas.

Fidler, G. S. (1948). Psychological evaluation of occupational therapy activities. *American Journal of Occupational Therapy, 2,* 284–287.

Halladay, H. S. (1945). Practical occupational therapy for the mentally and nervously ill [Book review]. *American Journal of Nursing, 45*(3), 250.

Hinojosa, J. (1996). Practice makes perfect. *OT Practice, 1*(1), 34–38.

Hopkins, H. L., & Smith, H. D. (1978). *Willard and Spackman's occupational therapy* (5th ed.). Lippincott.

Joss, M. (2007). The importance of job analysis in occupational therapy. *British Journal of Occupational Therapy, 7*(70), 301–303. https://doi.org/10.1177/030802260707000705

Kramer, P., & Hinojosa. (2014). Activity synthesis as a means to structure occupation. In J. Hinojosa, & M. L. B. Blount (Eds.). *The texture of life: Occupations and related activities* (4th ed., pp 121–140). AOTA Press.

Licht, S. (1947). Kinetic analysis of crafts and occupations. *Occupational Therapy and Rehabilitation, 26*(2), 75–78.

Mosey, A. C. (1981). *Occupational therapy: Configuration of a profession.* Raven Press.

Mosey, A. C. (1986). *Psychosocial components of occupational therapy.* Raven Press.

O'Sullivan, B. (2013). Beyond Blackberry thumb. *Canadian Medical Association Journal, 185*(4), E185–186. https://doi.org/10.1503/cmaj.109-4395

Pierce, D. (2001). Untangling occupation and activity. *American Journal of Occupational Therapy, 55*(2), 138–146. https://doi.org/10.5014/ajot.55.2.138

Pottorff, T. (2020, December). Hand-held tech dangers are worse than we thought: Mobile device overuse, misuse can lead to deaths, injuries, health concerns. *ISE Magazine, 52*(12), 42–46.

Reed, K. L. (1986). Tools of practice: Heritage or baggage. *American Journal of Occupational Therapy, 40*(9), 597–605. https://doi.org/10.5014/ajot.40.9.597

Snow, D. (2013). *Activity analysis* [Unpublished manuscript]. New York University.

Trombly, C. A., & Scott, A. D. (1977). *Occupational therapy for physical dysfunction.* Williams & Wilkins.

U.S. Department of War. (1944). *Occupational therapy.* U.S. Government Printing Office.

World Health Organization. (2001). *International classification of functioning, disability and health.*

Appendix 3.A. Occupation and Activity Analysis Form

Part 1. Occupation/Activity Analysis

Description of the activity

Sequence (steps) of the activity. (*Note.* Include as many steps as necessary.)

1.
2.
3.

Time needed to complete the occupation or perform individual steps:

Required objects, materials, tools, equipment, and their properties:

Space demands:

Social demands:

Safety precautions and contraindications:

Context

Environmental and personal factors that influence engagement and participation in the occupation?

Environmental factors:

Natural environment and human-made changes

Products and technology

Support and relationships

Attitudes

Services, systems, and policies

Personal factors:

Age, (chronological and placement in life cycle), sexual orientation, gender identity, cultural identity and attitudes, race, and ethnicity

Social background, social status, and socioeconomic status; upbringing and life experiences; education profession, and professional identity; lifestyle

Psychological assets, temperament traits, coping styles

Other health conditions and fitness status

Part 2. Activity Analysis

Required knowledge, abilities, and skills

Check "yes" or "no" to indicate whether the activity requires watching, listening, or other purposeful sensing. Next, rate each element's influence according to the following scale:

- 0 = *Component has no effect or influence on the ability to do the activity.*
- 1 = *Component has only a minimal effect or influence on the ability to do the activity.*
  The activity would not substantially stimulate or address the performance component element.
- 2 = *Component has a moderate effect or influence on the ability to complete the activity.*
  If a client has a deficit, compensation may have to be made for the client to perform the activity. The activity would present a challenge to the performance component element.
- 3 = *Component has a substantial effect or influence on the ability to complete the activity.*
  The activity would be extremely difficult to complete if the client has a deficit in this performance component. The activity would present a substantial stimulation or opportunity to address the performance component element.
- 4 = *Component has a major effect or influence on the completion of the activity.*
  A performance component deficit in this area would seriously influence the person's ability to do the activity. Such a person would very likely be unable to complete the activity. The activity would present a major stimulation or opportunity to address this performance component element.

Learning and applying knowledge (sensory–perceptual skills)

(*Note.* Categories with gray shaded headings indicate *International Classification of Functioning, Disability and Health* [World Health Organization, 2001] terminology.)

ACTIVITY REQUIRES	YES	NO	FOCUS ON
Watching			Sensory processing, visual reception
Listening			Auditory processing, sensory processing
Other purposeful sensing			Tactile, proprioceptive, olfactory, gustatory, and depth perception, and sensory processing; vestibular input; spatial relations; position in space; sensory modulation; attention; motor control; and praxis

Sensory processing: Internal mechanism used by the person to process and respond to sensory input	
Level of influence: ☐ 0 ☐ 1 ☐ 2 ☐ 3 ☐ 4	Observations:

Visual reception: Decoding stimuli through the eyes, including peripheral vision, acuity, and awareness of color and pattern	
Level of influence: ☐ 0 ☐ 1 ☐ 2 ☐ 3 ☐ 4	Observations:

Depth perception: Determining the relative distance between objects, figures, or landmarks and the observer and changes in planes and surfaces	
Level of influence: ☐ 0 ☐ 1 ☐ 2 ☐ 3 ☐ 4	Observations:

Auditory processing: Interpreting and localizing sounds and discriminating among background sounds	
Level of influence: ☐ 0 ☐ 1 ☐ 2 ☐ 3 ☐ 4	Observations:

Tactile processing: Interpreting light touch, pressure, temperature, pain, and vibration through skin or receptor	
Level of influence: ☐ 0 ☐ 1 ☐ 2 ☐ 3 ☐ 4	Observations:

Proprioceptive processing: Interpreting stimuli originating in muscles, joints, and other internal tissues that give information about the position of one body part in relation to another	
Level of influence: ☐ 0 ☐ 1 ☐ 2 ☐ 3 ☐ 4	Observations:

Vestibular input: Interpreting stimuli from the inner-ear receptor regarding head position	
Level of influence: ☐ 0 ☐ 1 ☐ 2 ☐ 3 ☐ 4	Observations:

Olfactory processing: Interpreting odors	
Level of influence: ☐ 0 ☐ 1 ☐ 2 ☐ 3 ☐ 4	Observations:

Gustatory processing: Interpreting tastes	
Level of influence: ☐ 0 ☐ 1 ☐ 2 ☐ 3 ☐ 4	Observations:

Spatial relations: Determining the position of objects relative to each other	
Level of influence: ☐ 0 ☐ 1 ☐ 2 ☐ 3 ☐ 4	Observations:

Position in space: Determining the spatial relationship of figures and objects to self and other forms and objects	
Level of influence: ☐ 0 ☐ 1 ☐ 2 ☐ 3 ☐ 4	Observations:

Sensory modulation: Ability to generate responses that are appropriately graded in relation to incoming sensory stimuli	
Level of influence: ☐ 0 ☐ 1 ☐ 2 ☐ 3 ☐ 4	Observations:

Attention: Focusing on a task over time	
Level of influence: ☐ 0 ☐ 1 ☐ 2 ☐ 3 ☐ 4	Observations:

Motor control: Use of functional and versatile movement patterns	
Level of influence: ☐ 0 ☐ 1 ☐ 2 ☐ 3 ☐ 4	Observations:

Praxis: Conceiving and planning a new motor act in response to an environmental demand	
Level of influence: ☐ 0 ☐ 1 ☐ 2 ☐ 3 ☐ 4	Observations:

Basic learning

ACTIVITY REQUIRES	YES	NO	FOCUS ON
Copying			Recognition, form constancy
Rehearsing			Sequencing

Recognition: Ability to identify familiar faces, objects, and other previously presented material	
Level of influence: ☐ 0 ☐ 1 ☐ 2 ☐ 3 ☐ 4	Observations:

Form constancy: Recognizing forms and objects as the same in various environments, positions, and places	
Level of influence: ☐ 0 ☐ 1 ☐ 2 ☐ 3 ☐ 4	Observations:

Sequencing: Placing information, concepts, and actions in order	
Level of influence: ☐ 0 ☐ 1 ☐ 2 ☐ 3 ☐ 4	Observations:

Acquiring skills

ACTIVITY REQUIRES	YES	NO	FOCUS ON
Basic skills			Motor control, body scheme, ocular–motor control, oral–motor skill, fine motor coordination and dexterity, visual–motor integration, crossing the midline, right–left discrimination, laterality, bilateral integration
Complex skills			
Applying knowledge			Level of arousal, orientation, attention
Thinking			Memory, categorization, concept formation, spatial operations, learning, generalization
Solving problems—simple			Learning, memory
Solving problems—complex			
Making decisions			Memory, concept formation, categorization, generalization

Level of arousal: Demonstrating alertness and responsiveness to environmental stimuli	
Level of influence: ☐ 0 ☐ 1 ☐ 2 ☐ 3 ☐ 4	Observations:

Orientation: Ability to identify person, place, time, and situation	
Level of influence: ☐ 0 ☐ 1 ☐ 2 ☐ 3 ☐ 4	Observations:

Motor control: Use of functional and versatile movement patterns	
Level of influence: ☐ 0 ☐ 1 ☐ 2 ☐ 3 ☐ 4	Observations:

Body scheme: Internal awareness of the body and the relationship of body parts to each other	
Level of influence: ☐ 0 ☐ 1 ☐ 2 ☐ 3 ☐ 4	Observations:

Ocular–motor control: Ability to move eyes to focus and follow objects	
Level of influence: ☐ 0 ☐ 1 ☐ 2 ☐ 3 ☐ 4	Observations:

Oral–motor skill: Use of muscles in and around the mouth	
Level of influence ☐ 0 ☐ 1 ☐ 2 ☐ 3 ☐ 4	Observations:

Fine motor coordination and dexterity: Using small muscle groups for controlled movements, particularly in-hand object manipulation	
Level of influence: ☐ 0 ☐ 1 ☐ 2 ☐ 3 ☐ 4	Observations:

Visual–motor integration: Coordinating the interaction of information from the eyes and body movement	
Level of influence: ☐ 0 ☐ 1 ☐ 2 ☐ 3 ☐ 4	Observations:

Crossing the midline: Moving the limbs and eyes across the midline sagittal plane of the body	
Level of influence: ☐ 0 ☐ 1 ☐ 2 ☐ 3 ☐ 4	Observations:

Right–left discrimination: Differentiating one side from the other	
Level of influence: ☐ 0 ☐ 1 ☐ 2 ☐ 3 ☐ 4	Observations:

Laterality: Use of a preferred or dominant hand or foot	
Level of influence: ☐ 0 ☐ 1 ☐ 2 ☐ 3 ☐ 4	Observations:

Bilateral integration: Coordinating both sides of the body	
Level of influence: ☐ 0 ☐ 1 ☐ 2 ☐ 3 ☐ 4	Observations:

Memory: Recoding information after a brief or long period	
Level of influence: ☐ 0 ☐ 1 ☐ 2 ☐ 3 ☐ 4	Observations:

Categorization: Identifying similarities and differences among pieces of environmental information	
Level of influence: ☐ 0 ☐ 1 ☐ 2 ☐ 3 ☐ 4	Observations:

Concept formation: Involves organizing a variety of information to form thoughts and ideas	
Level of influence: ☐ 0 ☐ 1 ☐ 2 ☐ 3 ☐ 4	Observations:

Spatial operations: Mentally manipulating the position of objects in various relationships	
Level of influence: ☐ 0 ☐ 1 ☐ 2 ☐ 3 ☐ 4	Observations:

Learning: Acquiring new concepts and behaviors	
Level of influence: ☐ 0 ☐ 1 ☐ 2 ☐ 3 ☐ 4	Observations:

Generalization: Applying previously learned concepts and behaviors to a variety of new situations	
Level of influence: ☐ 0 ☐ 1 ☐ 2 ☐ 3 ☐ 4	Observations:

General activity demands

ACTIVITY REQUIRES	YES	NO	FOCUS ON
Simple task			Initiation of activity, time management, termination of activity, coping skills, self-control
Complex task			
Multiple tasks			
Independent performance			
Group performance			Social skills, interpersonal skills

Initiation of activity: Starting a physical or mental activity	
Level of influence: ☐ 0 ☐ 1 ☐ 2 ☐ 3 ☐ 4	Observations:

Time management: Ability to manage parcels of time as they relate to the performance of tasks or activities	
Level of influence: ☐ 0 ☐ 1 ☐ 2 ☐ 3 ☐ 4	Observations:

Termination of activity: Stopping an activity at an appropriate time	
Level of influence: ☐ 0 ☐ 1 ☐ 2 ☐ 3 ☐ 4	Observations:

Coping skills: Identifying and managing stress-related factors, such as anger, disappointment, or frustration	
Level of influence: ☐ 0 ☐ 1 ☐ 2 ☐ 3 ☐ 4	Observations:

Self-control: Modifying one's own behavior in response to environmental needs, demands, constraints, personal aspirations, and feedback from others	
Level of influence: ☐ 0 ☐ 1 ☐ 2 ☐ 3 ☐ 4	Observations:

Social skills: Interacting by using manners, personal space, eye contact, gestures, active listening, and self-expression appropriate to the situation	
Level of influence: ☐ 0 ☐ 1 ☐ 2 ☐ 3 ☐ 4	Observations:

Interpersonal skills: Using verbal and nonverbal communication skills appropriately	
Level of influence ☐ 0 ☐ 1 ☐ 2 ☐ 3 ☐ 4	Observations:

Mobility

ACTIVITY REQUIRES	YES	NO	FOCUS ON
Changing and maintaining body position			Postural alignment, postural control, body strength, and depth perception
Transferring oneself			

Postural alignment: Maintaining biomechanical integrity among body parts	
Level of influence: ☐ 0 ☐ 1 ☐ 2 ☐ 3 ☐ 4	Observations:

Postural control: Using righting and equilibrium reactions to maintain balance during functional movements	
Level of influence: ☐ 0 ☐ 1 ☐ 2 ☐ 3 ☐ 4	Observations:

Body strength: Degree of gross muscle power when body movement is resisted or is against gravity	
Level of influence: ☐ 0 ☐ 1 ☐ 2 ☐ 3 ☐ 4	Observations:

Carrying, moving, and handling objects

ACTIVITY REQUIRES	YES	NO	FOCUS ON
Lifting			Range of motion, extremity strength, endurance
Carrying			
Fine hand use			Range of motion, extremity strength, endurance, stereognosis, kinesthesia, figure–ground perception, grasp patterns, prehension/pinch patterns, fine motor skill
Hand and arm use			
Moving objects with lower extremities			Range of motion, extremity strength, endurance
Walking and moving			Range of motion, extremity strength, endurance, topographical orientation

Range of motion: Moving body parts through an arc of motion	
Level of influence: ☐ 0 ☐ 1 ☐ 2 ☐ 3 ☐ 4	Observations:

Extremity strength: Grade of muscle strength when body movement is resisted or is against gravity	
Level of influence: ☐ 0 ☐ 1 ☐ 2 ☐ 3 ☐ 4	Observations:

Endurance: Sustained cardiac, pulmonary, and musculoskeletal exertion over time	
Level of influence: ☐ 0 ☐ 1 ☐ 2 ☐ 3 ☐ 4	Observations:

Stereognosis: Identifying objects through proprioception, cognition, and sense of touch	
Level of influence: ☐ 0 ☐ 1 ☐ 2 ☐ 3 ☐ 4	Observations:

Kinesthesia: Identifying the excursion and direction of movement	
Level of influence: ☐ 0 ☐ 1 ☐ 2 ☐ 3 ☐ 4	Observations:

Grasp patterns: Identifying the type(s) of grasp required to perform the activity	
Level of influence: ☐ 0 ☐ 1 ☐ 2 ☐ 3 ☐ 4	Observations:

Prehension/pinch patterns: Identifying the type(s) of pinch required to perform the activity	
Level of influence: ☐ 0 ☐ 1 ☐ 2 ☐ 3 ☐ 4	Observations:

Fine motor skill: Ability to use small hand muscles and joints to perform refined actions	
Level of influence: ☐ 0 ☐ 1 ☐ 2 ☐ 3 ☐ 4	Observations:

Figure–ground perception: Differentiating between foreground and background forms and objects	
Level of influence: ☐ 0 ☐ 1 ☐ 2 ☐ 3 ☐ 4	Observations:

Topographical orientation: Determining the location of objects and settings and the route to the location	
Level of influence: ☐ 0 ☐ 1 ☐ 2 ☐ 3 ☐ 4	Observations:

Part 3. Summary

Once you have completed the analysis, consider the following in relation to the individual:

1. Is the activity relevant to the person?
2. Is the activity/occupation part of the person's habits, routine, roles, or rituals?
3. How does performance of this activity address the individual's goals and their overall well-being and quality of life?

Reference

World Health Organization. (2001). *International classification of functioning, disability and health.*

Note. Adapted from materials by Karen A. Buckley, MA, OT/L; Sally E. Poole, OTD, OT/L, CHT; and Diana Chen Wong, OTD, OTR/L, CAPS. Used with permission.

Appendix 3.B. Occupation and Activity Analysis Form: Repotting a Plant (Student Example)

Part 1. Occupation/Activity Analysis

Introduction

Note. A representative example of portions of a completed activity analysis is presented to inform students and practitioners about the degree of detail needed to identify and understand the many performance skills to successfully complete a task. All areas of the activity analysis are important, but it is recognized that for each individual, some areas may take precedence based on their own personal narrative and presentation.

Four sections of the form are included to demonstrate the degree of analysis and detail needed to identify the sequence (steps) to the activity as well as the observations and subsequent method to rate each element. This section is intended to assist students in developing their ability to observe, analyze, and interpret. Areas include:

1. Description of the activity, sequence (steps) and context (physical environment)
2. Learning and applying knowledge (sensory–perceptual skills)
3. Mobility
4. Carrying, moving, and handling objects

What follows is the student's work.

Description of the activity

I chose to repot a 6-inch jade plant from a small plastic container into a larger plastic container. This activity is personally relevant, allowing me to engage in a meaningful leisure activity and fulfill a valued role as a gardener. This activity is also functionally relevant to promote the growth of the plant. Although I have past experience repotting plants outdoors, I had to make adjustments to perform this activity within the context of a small New York City apartment that has no outdoor space.

Context (environment and space demands)

Repotting a plant can be done indoors or outdoors and requires a surface to set your materials. Given the constraints of my apartment (no outdoor space, no free tabletop surface) and the small size of the plant, I completed this activity inside on the wooden floor of my living room. This space provided adequate room for me to spread out the newspaper, place the materials on top of the paper, and position myself in a side-sitting position directly in front of my workspace. Sitting provided enough vertical height over the plant I chose to repot.

Sequence (steps) of occupation

Assuming I've set up my workspace (jade plant in its current pot, new pot, hand shovel, and cup of water placed on top of a piece of spread-out newspaper; open bag of soil placed on the newspaper on my left-hand side) and seated myself in a comfortable side-sitting position on the floor, I follow these steps (with the time taken included):

1. I visually compare the size of the new pot with its current pot and decide I need to fill my new pot roughly two-thirds full of soil. (3 seconds)
2. I grasp the shovel's handle with my right hand and, crossing my midline, dig into the bag of soil using my left hand to make the opening of the bag as wide as possible. (3 seconds)
3. I bring the shovel full of soil toward the new pot, moving my left hand to grip the side of new pot and stabilize it while I fill it with the soil from my shovel. (4 seconds)
4. I repeat Steps 2 and 3 two more times until I have my new pot roughly two-thirds full. (14 seconds)
5. I put down the shovel and, with my right hand, smooth and pat down the soil. (3 seconds)
6. I reach for and grasp the original pot with my right hand and set it on top of the soil in the new pot to see if I need more soil. The soil level in the current pot is level with the lip of the new pot, so I decide I do not need to add more soil. (4 seconds)
7. I take the jade plant out with my right hand, holding it about 1 foot above the ground, gently pinch the stem with my left thumb and index finger, and squeeze the container a couple times while leaning the plant to the side. (3 seconds)
8. Supporting the stem and some of the attached soil with my left hand, I use my right hand to remove the container completely, and I set it down. (2 seconds)

9. I hold the plant horizontally in my left hand and use my right fingers to pinch and remove about one-third of the soil from the bottom of the plant, being careful not to damage any hanging roots and letting the residual dirt drop into the original pot below. (18 seconds)
10. I place the jade plant into the new pot and then use both hands to center it. (5 seconds)
11. Holding the centered plant with my left hand, I pick up the shovel with my right, reach across my midline, scoop a large amount of soil, bring it back to the new pot, and gently let it slide down and fill in the gaps while I rotate the new pot counter-clockwise. I rotate in this direction and reach for five more scoops of soil until the entire round is full and the plant is standing independently. Some soil spills during this step. (37 seconds)
12. I put the shovel down and use index and middle fingers from both hands to pack the soil down in and around the jade plant. (8 seconds)
13. I pick up the shovel again with my right hand and retrieve one more large scoop of soil. (3 seconds)
14. I turn the container counterclockwise with my left hand and slowly add in the soil until it reaches about a 1/2 inch below the lip of the new pot all the way around. (8 seconds)
15. I use both hands to pack down the soil, making sure the plant is standing upright and that the soil is even across the pot. (10 seconds)
16. To remove any air pockets, I lift the pot with both hands a few inches from the ground and let it thump on the floor. I repeat this two more times. (4 seconds)
17. I use my right hand to reach for and grip the cup of water, bring it close to the new pot, and pour about a 1/2 cup across the entire surface of the soil. I use my left hand to stabilize the pot. (4 seconds)

Part 2. Activity Analysis

Required knowledge, abilities, and skills

Check "yes" or "no" to indicate whether the activity requires watching, listening, or other purposeful sensing. Next, rate each element's influence according to the following scale:

- 0 = *Component has no effect or influence on the ability to do the activity.*
- 1 = *Component has only a minimal effect or influence on the ability to do the activity.*
  The activity would not substantially stimulate or address the performance component element.
- 2 = *Component has a moderate effect or influence on the ability to complete the activity.*
  If a client has a deficit, compensation may have to be made for the client to perform the activity. The activity would present a challenge to the performance component element.
- 3 = *Component has a substantial effect or influence on the ability to complete the activity.*
  The activity would be extremely difficult to complete if the client has a deficit in this performance component. The activity would present a substantial stimulation or opportunity to address the performance component element.
- 4 = *Component has a major effect or influence on the completion of the activity.*
  A performance component deficit in this area would seriously influence the person's ability to do the activity. Such a person would very likely be unable to complete the activity. The activity would present a major stimulation or opportunity to address this performance component element.

Learning and applying knowledge (sensory–perceptual skills)

ACTIVITY REQUIRES	YES	NO	FOCUS ON
Watching	X		Sensory processing, visual reception
Listening		X	Auditory processing, sensory processing

Other purposeful sensing	X		Tactile, proprioceptive, olfactory, gustatory, depth perception, and sensory processing; vestibular input; spatial relations; position in space; sensory modulation; attention; motor control; and praxis

Sensory processing: Internal mechanism used by the person to process and respond to sensory input	
Level of influence: ☐ 0 ☐ 1 ☐ 2 ☐ 3 ☒ 4	Observations: • I need to coordinate the following sensory inputs efficiently to complete this activity: visual, tactile, proprioceptive, and vestibular. • I used visual input to estimate how much soil I needed for my new pot. • I relied on proprioceptive input in lifting and handling the objects appropriately and efficiently. • I used vision, touch, and proprioception carefully to remove the plant from its pot. • I depended on my proprioceptive and tactile input when packing down soil to know whether I needed to pack more or move on to the next step. • If someone has an adverse tactile response to dirt, completion of this activity (without gloves) would be difficult. • Diminished vision would affect the time it took to complete this activity, but one could probably still perform it relying primarily on touch. • Diminished tactile input would affect all grasps, pinches, and the pressure needed to hold objects or pack down soil.

Visual reception: Decoding stimuli through the eyes, including peripheral vision, acuity, and awareness of color and pattern	
Level of influence: ☐ 0 ☐ 1 ☐ 2 ☒ 3 ☐ 4	Observations: • The activity required that I fixate on each of my materials as I used them. • I used visual tracking to follow the shovel into and out of the soil bag and when I emptied the soil into the pot. • I had to quickly scan my workspace when I needed to use my shovel and when I needed to grasp the plant in its original container, the water cup, and so forth. • I needed to be able to discriminate fine details, such as the level of soil in my pot, where I should pinch my plant, the roots of the plant, and the water level in the new pot as I poured. • I needed to visually determine the center of the new pot and stand my plant in an upright supported position. • I did not need to focus from near to far because all the materials I needed were within my reach.

Depth perception: Determining the relative distance between objects, figures, or landmarks, and the observer and changes in planes and surfaces	
Level of influence: ☐ 0 ☐ 1 ☐ 2 ☒ 3 ☐ 4	Observations: • I visually estimated the amount of soil I needed for the new pot, given its dimensions and depth. • I had to understand the depth of the soil bag to retrieve an adequate scoop. • I reached for the objects from the floor in front of me, including the plant, pots, soil, shovel, and water cup. • I had to bring objects close together using both hands separately: watering the newly potted plant, bringing the shovel to the soil bag, and moving the plant into its new pot. • My lower body remained static, but I moved my torso in the sagittal plane and my upper extremities in sagittal, coronal, and transverse planes.

Auditory processing: Interpreting and localizing sounds and discriminating among background sounds	
Level of influence: ☒ 0 ☐ 1 ☐ 2 ☐ 3 ☐ 4	Observations: • I did not need to listen or interpret sounds to complete the activity. • There were only a couple of sounds I produced during the activity, but they had no effect on completing the task. They included rustling of the bag as I retrieved soil and a few thuds when I purposely dropped the plant in its new pot to the ground to remove air pockets. • I did not need to suppress any background sound because it was quiet in my apartment.

<table>
<tr><td colspan="2">Tactile processing: Interpreting light touch, pressure, temperature, pain, and vibration through skin contact or receptor</td></tr>
<tr><td>Level of influence:
☐ 0
☐ 1
☐ 2
☐ 3
☒ 4</td><td>Observations:
• I held different objects with varying degrees of pressure:
◦ gentle when handling the plant itself
◦ some pressure to grasp the empty new pot
◦ greater amount of pressure to grasp the heavier shovel, plant in its pot, and water cup.
• I needed to squeeze the original pot a couple of times to remove it from the plant. It was a small, young plant, so it did not take much pressure to loosen it from the pot.
• I depended on tactile input from my left hand to stabilize and keep the plant upright in its new pot while I retrieved soil with the shovel in my right hand.
• I also relied on tactile input when packing down the soil. Once it was fairly solid, I stopped packing it down.
• I used tactile input to differentiate between soil and roots when I was removing excess soil from the bottom of the plant.
• All materials were room temperature.
• Some might not enjoy this activity if they do not like handling soil or getting their hands dirty.</td></tr>
</table>

<table>
<tr><td colspan="2">Proprioceptive processing: Interpreting stimuli originating in muscles, joints, and other internal tissues that give information about the position of one body part in relation to another</td></tr>
<tr><td>Level of influence:
☐ 0
☐ 1
☐ 2
☐ 3
☒ 4</td><td>Observations:
• I am weight-bearing on my pelvis in my side-seated position.
• The shovel and added soil place weight on my right upper extremity, and when I hold the plant in my hand, it places weight on my left upper extremity.
• The only movement that occurs outside of my visual field is when I reach into the depths of the soil bag, I cannot see the entire way down and must judge by proprioceptive input if I am retrieving enough soil.
• I repeatedly lift the shovel with and without added soil, the plant, and the water cup.
• I compress the joints in my hands and wrist when I apply pressure to pack down the soil in and around the plant.
• I need to be able to coordinate the proprioceptive input to make my movements efficient.</td></tr>
</table>

<table>
<tr><td colspan="2">Vestibular input: Interpreting stimuli from the inner ear receptor regarding head position</td></tr>
<tr><td>Level of influence:
☐ 0
☐ 1
☐ 2
☒ 3
☐ 4</td><td>Observations:
• I found myself making quick and subtle head movements, depending on where my gaze focused—I turned my head to the left whenever I reached for soil—and the action being performed.
• In my side-sitting position, it was important for me to maintain an upright posture to be engaged in the activity and manipulate the objects with my upper extremities.
• When I leaned the plant to the side to remove the pot, I moved my torso, head, and neck simultaneously, almost mimicking the action of the plant.
• There were no sudden movements or changes in movement necessary.
• I needed to coordinate my hand–eye movements the entire time.</td></tr>
</table>

<table>
<tr><td colspan="2">Olfactory processing: Interpreting odors</td></tr>
<tr><td>Level of influence:
☐ 0
☒ 1
☐ 2
☐ 3
☐ 4</td><td>Observations:
• I did not attend to any smells during my activity, although the soil does have some earthy fragrance to it. Neither the soil nor the plant was fragrant enough to warrant a reaction.
• In other circumstances, the plant or soil might be fragrant and have either a desirable (i.e., sweet-smelling flower) or off-putting (i.e., if the soil has rotted components or manure) effect.</td></tr>
</table>

Gustatory processing: Interpreting tastes	
Level of influence: ☒ 0 ☐ 1 ☐ 2 ☐ 3 ☐ 4	Observation: I did not use taste when I performed this activity.

Mobility

ACTIVITY REQUIRES	YES	NO	FOCUS ON
Changing and maintaining body position	X		Postural alignment, postural control, depth perception, body strength
Transferring oneself		X	

Postural alignment: Maintaining biomechanical integrity among body parts	
Level of influence: ☐ 0 ☐ 1 ☒ 2 ☐ 3 ☐ 4	Observations: • I maintained a side-seated posture throughout the duration of the activity. • Once seated, I did not change my pelvic position. • The activity required me to make slight adjustments in alignment when I leaned forward, to the side, twisted my torso, or reached my hands through space. • It would still be possible for someone with postural alignment problems to complete this activity by wearing a brace or positioning the materials at a level that does not require trunk flexion.

Postural control: Using righting and equilibrium reactions to maintain balance during functional movements	
Level of influence: ☐ 0 ☐ 1 ☒ 2 ☐ 3 ☐ 4	Observations: • I maintained a static base of support throughout the activity in a side-sitting position. • I used some slight head righting and equilibrium reactions to maintain my balance when I leaned forward and to the side, but given my large base of support, I did not worry about or anticipate losing my balance. • I stabilized my trunk against gravity when I leaned forward to pack down the soil and water the plant and when I leaned to the side to retrieve soil. • I had to maintain posture to actively use my upper extremities and focus visually.

Body strength: Degree of gross muscle power when body movement is resisted or is against gravity	
Level of influence: ☐ 0 ☐ 1 ☒ 2 ☐ 3 ☐ 4	Observations: • Trunk and neck control allowed me to stay upright and lean over my workspace. • I needed moderate strength in my upper extremity to hold the weight of the objects and move them through space. • Lifting the objects required concentric contraction of upper-extremity muscles, whereas setting them down required eccentric upper-extremity muscle contraction, and holding them in space for a moment or two required isometric upper-extremity muscle contraction.

Carrying, moving, and handling objects

ACTIVITY REQUIRES	YES	NO	FOCUS ON
Lifting	X		Range of motion, extremity strength, endurance
Carrying	X		
Fine hand use	X		Range of motion, extremity strength, endurance, stereognosis, kinesthesia, figure–ground perception, grasp patterns, prehension/pinch patterns, fine motor skill
Hand and arm use	X		
Moving objects with lower extremities		X	Range of motion, extremity strength, endurance
Walking and moving		X	Range of motion, extremity strength, endurance, topographical orientation

Range of motion: Moving body parts through an arc of motion	

Level of influence:
☐ 0
☐ 1
☐ 2
☒ 3
☐ 4
	Observations:
	• I rotated my head and neck slightly to shift my visual focus between the soil bag placed on the left and the plant and pots placed on the floor in front of me.
	• My head stayed in a relatively static, slightly flexed position as I concentrated on the objects on the floor in front of me.
	• I moved between 0° and 45° of trunk flexion, depending on what component I was working on. I found myself in the most trunk flexion when patting down the soil and making sure the plant was centered.
	• Regarding the upper extremity, I needed to be able to move through the following ranges:
	  ○ 0° to 45° shoulder abduction when filling the pot with soil
	  ○ 45° to 90° elbow flexion to reach for and manipulate the objects in space
	  ○ 0° to 45° of scapular plane motion to work with the objects in front of me
	  ○ 0° to 30° wrist extension when grasping and manipulating the pots and water cup
	  ○ 0° to 90° forearm supination and pronation when removing the plant from its original pot
	  ○ 0° to 90° forearm pronation when emptying the soil from my shovel and when patting down the soil in the pot.
	• Other movements of the upper extremity:
	  ○ Some shoulder adduction when reaching across the midline to retrieve soil and when patting down the soil in the pot
	  ○ Scapular protraction to manipulate the objects in front of me
	  ○ Finger flexion to grasp and pinch the objects
	  ○ Finger extension to pat down the soil
	  ○ Thumb flexion to pinch, grasp the shovel and pots, and stabilize the plant.
	• All lower extremity and hip joints remained static and served as my base of support: side-sitting position, hips flexed to 90°; left leg abducted to 30° with left knee flexed to 150° and right leg abducted to 60° with right knee flexed to 150°; feet neutral.
	• Someone with upper-extremity issues, especially any hand, wrist, or elbow mobility or range-of-motion limitations, would have trouble completing the activity.

Extremity strength: Grade of muscle strength when body movement is resisted or is against gravity	
Level of influence: ☐ 0 ☐ 1 ☐ 2 ☒ 3 ☐ 4	Observations: • Most of the actions I used to complete this activity are against gravity and with a small amount of resistance (the weight of the shovel, pots, plants, water cup); thus, a muscle strength grade of 4, or good (perhaps a 3+ because of the low weights of the objects) would be needed to successfully complete this activity. • This activity required that I concentrically contract my upper-extremity muscles when retrieving the soil, lifting the plant pots, and lifting the water. • I used isometric contractions to hold the plant in space for a few seconds while I removed extra soil from the bottom and when I poured the water. • I used eccentric contractions of the upper extremity when lowering the pots, plant, water, and shovel to the floor.

Endurance: Sustained cardiac, pulmonary, and musculoskeletal exertion over time	
Level of influence: ☐ 0 ☐ 1 ☒ 2 ☐ 3 ☐ 4	Observations: • This activity required a minimal level of endurance; however, there were some repetitive actions that could be fatiguing for someone with muscle weakness. • I needed some endurance to retrieve an adequate amount of soil for the new pot. I repeated the action of scooping soil with my shovel a total of seven times. • I needed to be able to lift the shovel by itself and when it was filled with soil, and move it through space. • I did not get fatigued because the activity lasted only a couple of minutes, and the weight of the shovel, plant, pots, and soil is relatively low.

Stereognosis: Identifying objects through proprioception, cognition, and sense of touch	
Level of influence: ☐ 0 ☒ 1 ☐ 2 ☐ 3 ☐ 4	Observations: • I used stereognosis when I stabilized the plant in its new pot with my left hand and focused my visual attention to retrieving more soil with my right hand. • I could not see to the bottom of the soil bag and relied on my proprioceptive and tactile input (specifically weight) when retrieving soil.

Kinesthesia: Identifying the excursion and direction of movement	
Level of influence: ☐ 0 ☐ 1 ☐ 2 ☒ 3 ☐ 4	Observations: • I coordinated my thumb, finger, wrist, radioulnar, elbow, and shoulder joints to manipulate the plant pots, cup of water, shovel, and soil bag. • I coordinated all finger joints when I removed soil from the bottom of the plant, moving between flexion and extension at different rates for each finger. • I chose to position myself in side-sitting position, which initially required me to coordinate all lower body joints into a comfortable and stable position. • I made subtle changes between torso flexion, extension, and rotation throughout the entire activity.

Grasp patterns: Identifying the type(s) of grasp required to perform the activity	
Level of influence: ☐ 0 ☐ 1 ☐ 2 ☐ 3 ☒ 4	Observations: • I used a palmar prehension grasp with both hands when dropping and thumping the new pot on the ground. • I used a power grasp to hold the shovel. • I used a cylindrical grasp to manipulate the circular plant pots and the cup of water.

Prehension/pinch patterns: Identifying the type(s) of pinch required to perform the activity	
Level of influence ☐ 0 ☐ 1 ☒ 2 ☐ 3 ☐ 4	Observations: • I used pad-to-pad pinch to hold the stem of the plant as I removed it from its original pot. • I used the three-jaw chuck to hold the plant (in its original pot) as I judged how much soil I needed in the new pot.

Fine motor skill: Ability to use small hand muscles and joints to perform refined actions	

Level of influence:
☐ 0
☐ 1
☐ 2
☐ 3
☒ 4
	Observations:
	• Given the small size of the pots I was working with and the small size of the plant, I needed to use fine motor skills to do the following actions:
	  ○ manipulate the stem of the plant
	  ○ remove soil from the bottom of the plant
	  ○ center and stabilize the plant in its new pot
	  ○ pack down the soil with my fingers.

Figure–ground perception: Differentiating between foreground and background forms and objects	
Level of influence: ☒ 0 ☐ 1 ☐ 2 ☐ 3 ☐ 4	Observation: I did not need to use figure–ground perception when I repotted my plant because I had five very distinguishable tools and objects placed directly in front of me.

Topographical orientation: Determining the location of objects and settings and the route to the location	
Level of influence: ☒ 0 ☐ 1 ☐ 2 ☐ 3 ☐ 4	Observation: I did not use topographical orientation during this activity because I was seated on the floor of my apartment for the entire duration.

Note. The authors of this chapter thank Sunny M. Dawson, a graduate student at New York University, Class of 2014, for providing the activity analysis of her personal experience of repotting a jade plant.

4

The Occupational Profile

JUDITH WILSON, MA, OTR

CHAPTER HIGHLIGHTS

- Defining the occupational profile
- The occupational profile within different frames of reference
- A top-down view of the occupational profile
- Environmental context: physical, social, and attitudinal
- Temporal context
- Evaluation process
- Goal setting and the occupational profile
- Intervention and the occupational profile
- Groups and populations as the client
- Outcomes and the occupational profile

KEY TERMS AND CONCEPTS

• attitudinal barriers • barriers • client-centered interventions • context • environmental context • ethnographies • frames of reference • health • interview • narrative reasoning • narratives • occupational history • occupational justice • occupational patterns • occupational profile • occupation-based goals • occupation-based interventions • outcomes • participant observation • participation • performance patterns • personal factors • physical barriers • roles • temporal context

Introduction

Occupation is a complex concept, and it is the ***occupational profile*** that seeks to understand that complexity at the level of the individual. The occupational profile includes the person's "occupational history and experiences, patterns of daily living, interests, values, needs and relevant contexts" (American Occupational Therapy Association [AOTA], 2020b, p. 21). In the occupational profile, the occupational therapy practitioner seeks to appreciate how these elements come together to make the person.

This chapter focuses on the occupational profile as a concept and tool applied in practice. I offer a series of reflections from the clinic floor about how people's occupational profiles weave through and shape clinical practices. As an occupational therapist, I remain in awe of the mythical and mundane nature of occupational profiles that express the uniqueness of each client.

What *Is* an Occupational Profile?

The occupational profile identifies the series of occupations that currently define a person. It is a story—but a different one from a traditional description of a person. It is a description of routines—but more. It is what we seek when we ask, What are those "things people need to, want to, and are expected to do?" (World Federation of Occupational Therapists, 2022, para. 2).

Some definitions call the occupational profile an interview—even the current (fourth edition) of the *Occupational Therapy Framework: Domain and Process* (*OTPF–4;* AOTA, 2020b). However, depicting the occupational profile as simply an interview robs it of its full value. An interview is an important tool in evaluating the occupational profile, but it is not the profile. The occupational profile is the substance that we work to understand in our evaluation, target in our interventions, and reimagine in our outcomes. It is the focus of our work as occupational therapy practitioners.

The occupational profile contains elements of narrative. ***Narratives*** are stories or representations that are constructed by the client to describe activities; they are infused with meaning and are used in defining oneself (Riessman, 2008). Mattingly (1998) described the use of narrative in occupational therapy as a means to empower the client in using activities to create change and recovery. Occupational profiles overlap with narratives in that both include the volitional selection of certain elements, have a sequential nature, and have meanings that link to identity. It is important to consider these similarities between narratives and occupational profiles when discussing the occupational profile in interventions.

The first difference between narratives and occupational profiles is that a narrative is a story itself with deliberate word choices and images for a particular representation. An occupational profile, on the other hand, focuses on the actions that populate the story. The occupational profile captures the actions as they are described by the individual, described by those close to them, and acted out by the individual.

Narratives often are biographical and focus on significant events, such as achievements or illness (Frank, 2004; Mattingly, 1998). In contrast, occupational profiles focus on the mundane and the routine. In the occupational profile, the occupational therapy practitioner seeks to uncover specific features of the client's story by looking for descriptions of activities performed, patterns of behavior, and where and with whom activities are performed. What does daily life look like? What do they need to do? What do they choose to do? How and where do they do these activities?

No two people will answer such questions in the same way. The occupational profile needs to capture the unique way each person does each task and the unique way each person structures their day. A person often does not think about these routines because those routines are just that: routine. The occupational profile is found in the details that surround the person's story. They provide meaning and context to their stories. In the words of noted occupational therapist Betty Risteen Hasselkus (2006), "Everyday life is like an anchor in our lives" (p. 628). Occupational profiles bring to view the details as well as the breadth of what a person regularly does, coming together to make the person who they are.

The value of the occupational profile has been argued as being mythical (Kelly & McFarlane, 2007). Occupational therapy practitioners believe "that active engagement in occupation promotes, facilitates, supports, and maintains health and participation" (AOTA, 2020b, p. 5). These concepts cannot be seen, but we believe them to be critically important to the person and to health; hence, they are potentially mythical. Myths have power to move us. They give us understanding, guide us, and lead us to action. Thinking of myth in this narrative, meaning-making sense and in dialogue with science allows us to use the occupational profile as a clinical tool to understand the client and work toward changes they value (Kelly & McFarlane, 2007).

Occupational profiles can most strongly be argued to be ***ethnographies,*** which are the product of a form of qualitative research—most often associated with anthropology—that describe social groups and cultural phenomena. Through the occupational profile, the occupational therapy practitioner shares the anthropologist's aim of *Making the Strange Familiar and the Familiar Strange* (Social Science LibreTexts, 2021). Their probings and observations seek to understand practices in our clients' lives that are foreign to us. At the same time, these probings and observations take tasks familiar to all of us and allow us a moment to step back and look more closely. Simple, everyday tasks like getting dressed may not hold much meaning to some, but to others there is great meaning, such as picking out the perfect outfit and making sure it is just right for that day. Some day-to-day tasks have minimal importance to some but greater importance to others. This is the process of making the familiar strange. Practitioners need this ethnographic perspective to see differences and opportunities in the occupations from which they create an intervention plan.

Ethnography generally studies individuals in relation to a group. Occupational profiles may study groups, such as a family or an organization as a client, but frequently, occupational profiles focus on understanding the individual. The primary difference between ethnographies and occupational profiles is their purpose. Most ethnographers value minimalizing their influence on the research participant during research. In clinical practice, occupational therapy practitioners enter the interaction with the specific intent of creating change.

The unique understanding of the client based on the occupational profile provides the groundwork for client-centered care. The meaning embedded in a person's daily routines is a part of their identity. Centering our clinical approach around each unique occupational profile demands that no two approaches are the same. As occupational therapy practitioners, we tailor our approach to the individuality of the client. Change created by treatment means the occupational profile is changing. The occupational profile cannot change without the person living those changes. Therefore, occupational therapy intervention cannot have an effect without recognizing the client at the center of the change.

Occupational profiles reflect the continually morphing substance of a person's daily routines in all their diversity and details. They capture the acts that form the day-to-day experience of a person's identity (see Figure 4.1). Occupational

FIGURE 4.1. Yardwork is an occupation one is expected to do as a homeowner.

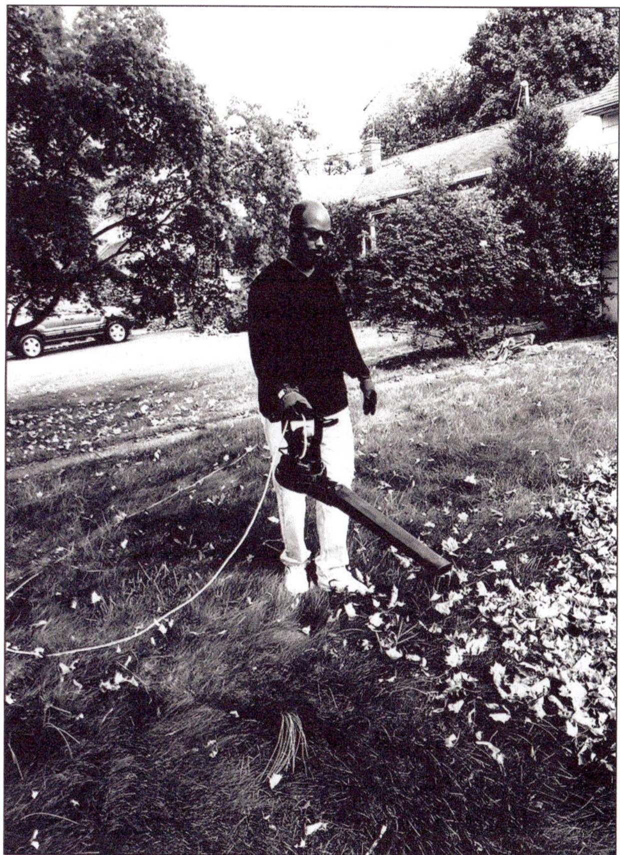

Source. J. Wilson. Used with permission.

profiles are also the first clinical tool we, as occupational therapy practitioners, use to assess our clients. And it is from these profiles that we decide on interventions and outcomes in practice. Appendix 4.A, "AOTA Occupational Profile Template," provides the occupational profile template form developed by AOTA (2020a).

EXERCISE 4.1. Comparing Ordinary Tasks

In Betty Risteen Hasselkus's (2006) Eleanor Clarke Slagle Lecture, "The World of Everyday Occupation: Real People, Real Lives," she reminded us that

> the small behaviors that make up the realm of daily life for each one of us are more than what we have in common with others; they also represent our own exquisite individuality and distinction. We may all brush our teeth every day, perhaps more than once a day, but it's probably fair to assume that we each have our own particular way of doing this tooth brushing. So on one level, we are all doing the same thing, but on another level we are *not* doing the same thing. (p. 628)

For this activity, find a fellow occupational therapy practitioner partner. Compare how you brush your teeth. Create a list of what the differences are.

The Occupational Profile Within Different Frames of Reference

Frames of reference organize our clinical practice using a certain theoretical perspective (Kramer et al., 2020). There are many frames of reference in occupational therapy. The frame of reference you select to use affects what elements the occupational therapy practitioner highlights in the occupational profile. The choice of frame of reference is determined by the type of concerns the client faces, practice standards, and practitioner bias.

When a person seeks or is scheduled to receive occupational therapy, they may have a variety of problems or areas of concern. However, not all of the person's occupations are impaired, changed, or threatened. The frame of reference provides a lens to focus the occupational therapy practitioner's attention on the relevant. The lens shapes the questions asked and the detail to which the practitioner attends. Some of the overarching occupations identified will be the same. However, the details will differ. For example, if a female client has a stroke, the practitioner may choose a neurodevelopmental frame of reference. Part of the occupational profile may describe the client's role as a grandmother. Following the neurodevelopmental frame of reference, the practitioner would focus on the movement patterns used in holding the grandchild or playing games with the child on the floor. The practitioner would watch for the rhythm of the rocking the grandmother uses for her grandchild (Runyan, 2006). In contrast, the practitioner who uses an occupation-as-end model to work with the same client would flesh out the role of grandmother by asking about the range of activities available in the child's home (to seek alternative approaches to the problematic tasks) and may focus more heavily on the meaning of the role to identify where change can be made (Trombly, 2002).

Occupational Profiles: A Top-Down View

Some approaches to intervention start from the bottom up, and others work from the top down. Some start with the details of how someone moves or thinks and then piece these client factors together to see how those factors are used in routines, habits, and roles. Others start with the routines, habits, and roles, and then break them down to find the performance patterns and the client factors, which influence how they are done. An occupation-based perspective generally starts from the top down, and the occupational profile is the view from the top. Even if using a bottom-up approach, the perspective of the occupational profile is a top-down view.

The *OTPF–4* (AOTA, 2020b) includes the following components in the occupational profile: the occupational history, roles and context, the reason for seeking services, successful occupations and barriers, occupational history, the client's values and interests, related performance patterns and

TABLE 4.1. **OCCUPATIONS FROM THE *OTPF–4***

OCCUPATION	DESCRIPTIONS
ADLs: Activities oriented toward taking care of one's own body; these activities are completed on a routine basis	Bathing, showering, toileting, and toilet hygiene; personal hygiene and grooming; dressing; eating and swallowing; feeding; functional mobility; sexual activity
IADLs: Activities to support daily life within the home and community	Care of others (including selection and supervision of caregivers), care of pets and animals, and child rearing; driving and community mobility; financial management; home establishment and management; meal preparation and cleanup; religious and spiritual expression; safety and emergency maintenance; shopping
Health management: Activities related to developing, managing, and maintaining health and wellness routines, including self-management, with the goal of improving or maintaining health to support participation in other occupations	Social and emotional health promotion and maintenance, symptom and condition management, communication with the health care system, medication management, physical activity, nutrition management, personal care device management
Rest and sleep: Activities related to obtaining restorative rest and sleep to support healthy, active engagement in other occupations	Rest, sleep preparation, sleep participation
Education: Activities needed for learning and participating in the educational environment	Formal educational participation, informal personal educational needs or interests exploration (beyond formal education), informal educational participation
Work: Labor or exertion related to the development, production, delivery, or management of objects or services; benefits may be financial or nonfinancial	Employment interests and pursuits, employment seeking and acquisition, job performance and maintenance, retirement preparation and adjustment, volunteer exploration, volunteer participation
Play: Activities that are intrinsically motivated, internally controlled, and freely chosen and that may include suspension of reality, exploration, humor, risk-taking, contests, and celebrations	Play exploration, play participation
Leisure: Nonobligatory activity that is intrinsically motivated and engaged in during discretionary time—that is, time not committed to obligatory occupations, such as work, self-care, or sleep	Leisure exploration, leisure participation
Social participation: Activities that involve social interaction with others, including family, friends, peers, and community members, and that support social interdependence	Community participation, family participation, friendships, intimate partner relationships, peer group participation

Note. Based on the *Occupational Therapy Practice Framework: Domain and Process* (4th ed.; AOTA, 2020b). Used with permission.

client factors, and the client's desired outcomes. These come together for a comprehensive, detailed view of the person as an occupational being.

Overall, occupations are grossly categorized as ADLs, IADLs, health management, rest and sleep, education, work, play, leisure, and social participation (AOTA, 2020b; see Table 4.1). These categories remind occupational therapy practitioners to appreciate the breadth of the occupational profile and not limit our perspective to just one, such as ADLs.

Occupational History

The occupational profile includes an ***occupational history,*** which includes the past occupations, leading up to the moment, that the client values or views as essential. It also includes the current occupations of the client, and their views of their performance.

Roles

The occupational profile helps us to appreciate how occupations combine to identify the roles of the individual. These ***roles*** are sets of behaviors that are defined by context and culture and expected by society (AOTA, 2020b) and are often what make the occupations meaningful to the person. The occupational profile also looks at ***performance patterns***—that is, the manner and sequence in which these occupations are performed to appreciate the person's routines and habits. These patterns are infinitely varied. The job of the occupational therapy practitioner is to discover those unique performance patterns.

FIGURE 4.2. One man's occupational history includes engineering. A current occupation is assembling a telescope with his family.

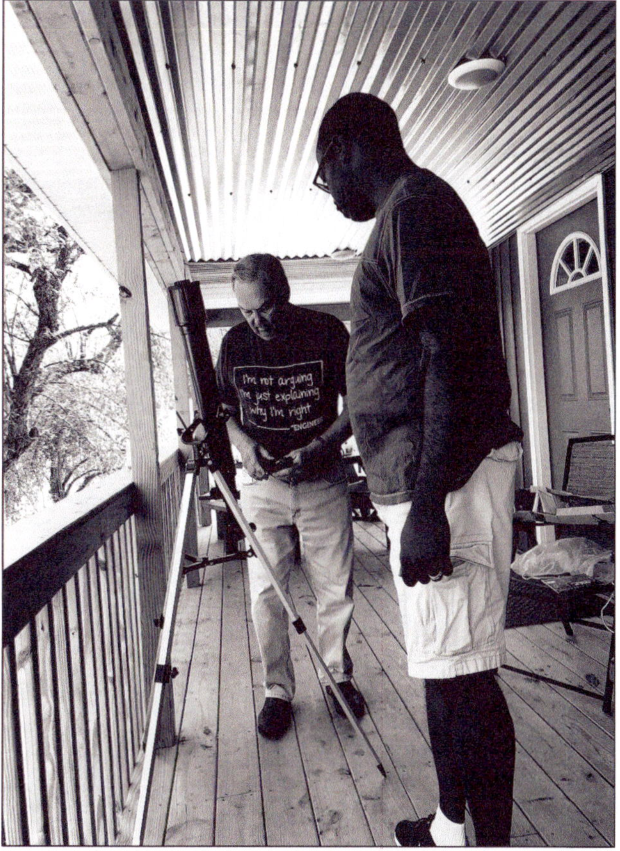

Source. J. Wilson. Used with permission.

Because these unique performance patterns are intrinsic to meaningful roles for the client, it is important to appreciate that meaning as defined by the client. Occupational therapy practitioners must take care not to impose their own values on that meaning. The occupational profile includes the person's values and interests. The values and interests invest meaning in these actions. They shape the choices in occupations and patterns of performance that are incorporated into the occupational profile (see Figure 4.2).

Context

Context, an essential element of the occupational profile, includes the environmental and culture surrounding and inherent to the person and includes the personal factors. Personal factors include individual and social factors that affect how we engage in occupations. These include, but are not limited to, age, sexual orientation, gender identity, race, culture, socioeconomic status, personality, education, professional identity, and lifestyle (AOTA, 2020b). People and their occupational profiles do not exist in a vacuum. Clients are responding to the world, and their occupations are being carried out in relation to a social world. At 25 or 75 years of age, a person experiences toothbrushing, studying, or having tea differently. Common experiences like making dinner or riding a bus are the same whether someone is educated and working as an occupational therapy practitioner or is recently unemployed from a housecleaning job. An appreciation of diversity among people allows us as practitioners to listen better to our clients' individual occupational profiles.

When occupational therapy practitioners explore the occupational profile, they seek to identify what works well and where barriers exist. ***Barriers*** relate directly to why the client is seeking services and to the analysis of healthy engagement in life activities. The barriers are only part of the picture. The practitioner needs to have a more complete view of the client by also discovering which occupations and routines in occupations are currently successful. This is probably most important when the client feels there are no successful occupations. Exploring current, persisting occupations provides a strength focus to empower the therapeutic process that lies ahead.

EXERCISE 4.2. Understanding Personal Daily Routines

Interview a friend or family member (not an occupational therapy practitioner or occupational therapy student). Find out about their daily routines, responsibilities, work, and leisure activities. Learn specifics.

Environmental Context: Physical, Social, and Attitudinal

The ***environmental context*** is what surrounds and situates the performance of an occupation. Without this context, the occupation does not have meaning. Therefore, any occupational performance in the clinic is not truly occupational. The occupation becomes real when it occurs in its real-world context (see Figure 4.3).

Disability rights activists have long argued against medicine's definition of "disability." They point out that the person is not disabled; rather, the environment is disabling (Brown, 2014). The occupation does not exist in isolation; it exists within a certain environmental context. The person and the context interact when a person takes a shower, walks their dog, or a attends a concert. How these occupations are done depends on the context. Possible barriers occur in the client factors, the environment, and, most important, in their interaction.

Context can change the meaning of an occupation. Consider the act of washing a car. One person may work at a car wash. Another may own a car and wash their car regularly, priding themselves on the shine of the hood. Several others might join in washing a car, with the hose and soap flying about, and it becomes play. The setting and the person's view of the occupation changes in each of these examples, so the context of the occupation changes. In each of these examples,

FIGURE 4.3. Currently, this girl's main occupation is basketball. The environmental context is the neighborhood with a long-standing basketball history, which suits her emerging interest in the WNBA.

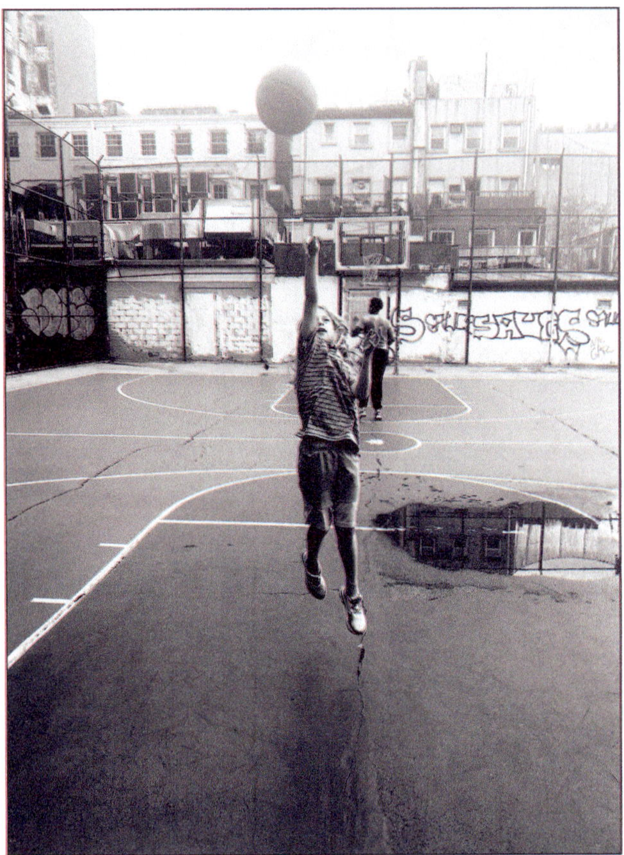

Source. J. Wilson. Used with permission.

the critical differences are in the social context of the task, the institutions related to the task, and the attitudes of the social groups associated with the task.

The occupational profile must view each occupation as an interaction between the activity and the environment. For example, a middle-aged woman steps into the kitchen of a five-star restaurant as a chef. The owner looks at her distrustfully because he is used to having a male chef. She starts to gather the cooking supplies she needs, but they are hung from hooks on high ceilings out of her reach, and she cannot find half the ingredients in the multiple stock shelves. Some sous chefs are present, but they have never worked together. Her meal is a flop. When this same woman goes home, she enters her kitchen with the shelves she has organized, and two young kids cheer when she enters, ask for their favorite dish, and start to get the ingredients out for her. Dinner is magnificent. The activity is the same. The environments are different. At the restaurant environment, she faced discriminatory attitudes, physically inaccessible spaces, and an unfamiliar social environment. At home, she was supported by positive attitudes, space modeled for her, and her team of kids to join in. Could she likely master the occupation of cooking in the restaurant? Yes, but there are barriers she must overcome.

Many health disparities can be best understood by analyzing the environmental aspects of occupations. Variations in who people interact with, the nature of the relationship, and with what social groups they associate create different ***occupational patterns*** (Umberson & Montez, 2010). These occupational patterns may or may not support health. Occupational performance outside the expectations produced in popular media or current power structures places ***attitudinal barriers*** on the individual (Borisoff & Chesebro, 2011). ***Physical barriers***—for example, few dentist's chairs are designed to accommodate wheelchair users (Krahn et al., 2015)—block many people from health maintenance occupations.

Occupational justice seeks environmental changes that support full and diverse occupational opportunities for all. Occupational justice first asks that, as occupational therapy practitioners, we understand ourselves as occupational beings, and as we gather the occupational profile of our client, we are ourselves fulfilling our own occupation and are surrounded by our own history and attitudes. Appreciating our own occupational profile can open us to hearing and seeing our client better. Occupational justice also asks us to recognize the complex barriers our clients may face in their occupations (AOTA, 2020b). Without this complexity, the occupational profile is incomplete.

Environmental context includes ***personal factors,*** which are more personal and individual traits, such as gender, age, education, race, and religion. Personal factors and environmental factors overlap. A person's age affects an occupation in multiple ways, including the roles that are relevant in relation to the life cycle. These stages are defined by their social environment. Is the individual a grandpa, a newly independent young adult, or a toddler? Similarly, how race is defined only has meaning in a social context. However, most people consider their race as a basic piece of who they are (Kramarae, 1996; Wu, 2002).

Learning what personal factors are valued by the individual is an important piece of the occupational profile. The question to answer in relation to the occupational profile is, what elements are a part of the occupational choices that make up the profile? Consider the interplay of these factors to make an occupation meaningful to their identity. For instance, is kneeling for prayers an important part of how a client performs their occupations in relation to their religious identity? Also consider how personal factors may affect how you address their occupations in interventions. For example, if your client has never attended school, you may need to avoid reading in your interventions.

Environmental factors are a defining part of occupational performance. Personal factors often shape how occupations are imbued with meaning. The occupational profile seeks to capture the picture of their complex entwinement with the client's occupations.

EXERCISE 4.3. Self-Reflection on Occupations

Reflect on your own occupational profile. What are the occupations you value the most? Why? What personal factors and environmental context are part of these occupations? How might these occupations influence how you interact with others, including clients?

Time Flows On: Temporal Context

The occupational profile also has a ***temporal context.*** The occupations that make up the profile, how they are done, and what they mean, are constantly evolving. Some changes are small, like starting a new class in school. Some changes are big, like picking up a new hobby or moving to a new city, changing a myriad of routines. Other changes are monumental, such as an accident that places you in the hospital. The occupational profile encompasses the length of the evolution: the past occupations bringing the person to now, the occupations occurring today, and the occupations to which the person aspires.

In placing the occupational profile along the flow of time, we recognize there is a history of occupations that keeps on evolving. For clinical purposes, occupational therapy practitioners focus on the current or recent occupations. These occupations are the ones most relevant to the client's present sense of self and current circumstances. If illness or injury has caused an unfavorable change in occupations, then the occupations performed just before the change are the most critical part of the profile. These recent occupations most accurately reflect the client's values, goals, and aspirations.

A client's current occupations are especially critical to explore when they form a negative sense of self, such as with a drug addiction or a learned helplessness. What are the occupations and the performance patterns that create this occupational dysfunction? Is this dysfunction related to the particular time in their life (i.e., temporal context), or is this a long-term pattern? These are the targets for change in the intervention. For these same clients, we need to explore what positive occupations they have and how we can build on them. Although the occupational profile focuses on the present, some understanding of past and future occupations is also important. Past occupations helped shape the present ones. They are a source of experience from which the client can continue to draw.

Future occupations are the untold story. In collecting the occupational profile, it is important to learn what hopes and goals the person has. Sometimes, by the time someone reaches occupational therapy, they have already revised their vision of future occupations in response to fears and (mis)information. The occupational therapy practitioner needs to delve deeper to encourage the client to share their previous vision of their future as well as their hopes and fears that shape the current vision of those future occupations. This can be a delicate discussion, relying on how the practitioner has built a trusting rapport. There may be changes that make that vision impossible now. However, there are also future possibilities that the client may not have yet started to envision. The outcomes set for the occupational therapy intervention are designed from those future occupations. Those future occupations flow from the occupational history, through the present profile, and into the future. With this outcome in mind, the client and practitioner set goals.

The client seeks change through the occupational therapy process. Occupational profiles are always evolving as part of maturation and in response to life events. A child stops playing with rattles and starts chasing balls. An aunt becomes ill, and a nephew starts to care for her. For the child, the aunt, and the nephew, there are changes in their occupational profiles. At the time of therapy, the occupational profile is set for a change; therapy aims to guide and support that change.

Whether that change is sought because of a sudden event or as a result of long-standing barriers, the occupational therapy practitioner needs to focus on the time frame that will most help them create change. That time frame will be different in different cases. Figuring this out is part of the clinical reasoning for each case. Does the practitioner most want to learn about a time period when the client was successful in their occupations so that they can target that? Does the practitioner most want to understand the activity demands of a new occupation the client is preparing to start? Does the practitioner most want to understand what factors are interacting in the client's current routines to identify what barriers to target?

Using the Occupational Profile in Evaluation

The occupational profile is an essential part of the occupational therapy evaluation. Data collection in assessing the occupational profile is time consuming and extensive. It begins at meeting the client and continues throughout the occupational therapy intervention. The process generally starts with an interview. The client, however, usually does not share much of the most important data with the occupational therapy practitioner until rapport is established, which is accomplished through further interviewing and participant observation. Thus, the intervention plan is refined and adjusted over time as the understanding of the occupational profile emerges.

The pragmatics of an evaluation require the data to be collected within a limited time frame, leaving time for the other pieces of the evaluation. The occupational therapy practitioner must be both thorough and efficient in determining the occupational profile. Looking back at Exercise 4.2, it is reasonable that you may spend 30 minutes to an hour interviewing someone. Hopefully this experience will build your skills so that, in the clinic, you will collect data more quickly, moving efficiently to the most productive questions. Recognizing which time frame is the focus of the occupational profile aids this efficiency. In addition, an important skill is recognizing when to shift from interview to activity, and back. This is partly art and partly recognizing the productivity (or unproductivity) of the interview process.

Interview

The ***interview,*** which entails asking the client or the client's caretakers very detailed questions about their occupations, is usually the first step of data collection. Therefore, good interviewing skills are vital for the occupational therapy practitioner. The key to good interviewing skills lies not in the questions asked but in effective listening. From listening closely to what the client says, the practitioner decides on and adapts their line of questioning. Once a dialogue has been established, the practitioner seeks to clarify details and introduces new topics to expand the discussion. The practitioner probes for clarification and understanding as they listen to what the client says.

People are not accustomed to being asked questions about exactly how they do every task or complete a specific aspect of an activity in their day. When asked what they do in the morning, many people answer that they get up and go to work. The occupational therapy practitioner, however, wants to know when they get up, what kind of bed they slept in, who is in the bed, where they go next, whether they wear slippers, and whether they brush their teeth or drink their coffee first. The practitioner must therefore ask precise and probing questions.

Questions are influenced by the client's particular situation. For example, an occupational therapy practitioner treating a client with a broken finger will ask more about how the client holds the toothbrush and squeezes the toothpaste and less about what kind of slippers they wear. For the client with depression, however, the practitioner will be less concerned about how the client grips the toothbrush but may focus instead on the time or the regularity of the toothbrushing routine. The practitioner uses clinical judgment and knowledge about what brought the client to services to shape the interview.

The occupational therapy practitioner is rarely the first health professional in contact with the client. From previous health care contacts, clients are used to answering questions about their symptoms. They do not expect to be asked about what they enjoy doing in their free time, what community groups they are involved in, and what responsibilities they have at home. It takes extra effort for the practitioner to refocus the conversation, often having to ask questions in multiple ways to find out about the client's activities and occupations.

Sometimes, simply asking the client a question is ineffective. The client may be a young child, be confused, or be unable to communicate. In these cases, the occupational therapy practitioner can usually ask family members for information because the family has much more extensive experience with the person and can flesh out the practitioner's observations. In some cases, the family members may be considered to be clients; therefore, the practitioner may work closely with them to develop intervention priorities. For example, a mother may want to be able to fit her daughter into a car seat to ease transportation to school. In another family, the older son may worry about his elderly mother wandering into the kitchen and turning on the stove. The family is the client, and the practitioner will glean most of the information from the one family member who can communicate.

Sometimes, a client cannot speak for themselves, and no family members or friends are available to provide information. This scenario includes both clients who are unable to communicate and those who are resistive to intervention because of confusion or depression. In these cases, a standard interview will be unproductive. The occupational therapy practitioner must become a puzzle solver, piecing together a hypothesized profile. This profile is constantly updated from the general social data available, from pieces of conversations with the client who can communicate, and from the client's reactions to activities.

Participant Observation

Occupational therapy's tools for assessing the occupational profile are ethnographic tools. The first ethnographic method used to learn about the client and their life is the interview, and the second is ***participant observation,*** a research technique in which the researcher engages in activities with people to learn about them and their lives (Bernard, 2011). In occupational therapy, as rapport is being established and the intervention has begun, the occupational therapy practitioner learns more about the client while engaging in activities with them. Thus, even as the intervention has begun, there is an ongoing loop of continuing assessment of the occupational profile.

The occupational therapy practitioner and the client work together to develop and implement a plan for service delivery. As the practitioner and the client jointly engage in the activities within the intervention, they interact, and rapport continues to build. Even when rapport is difficult to develop, interactions between the practitioner and the client provide information that broadens the practitioner's picture of the client. The practitioner uses activities pertinent to the client, often within their known occupational profile. These interactions are the practitioner's "fieldwork" from which observations are made.

Participant observation provides new details about the client's performance—in an environmental context—that support or contrast with what the occupational therapy practitioner learned in the interview. As the client chats with the practitioner, they share information that triggers new ideas for and questions from the practitioner, leading to an increasingly rich occupational profile. An ethnographer would call this "thick description" (Geertz, 1973, p. 3). As this relationship deepens, the client may reach a point at which they share sensitive personal information, which they had withheld earlier, for the occupational profile.

Participant observation is an intimate and invasive process. We cross into the client's personal spaces and "assess" them (Bernard, 2011; Hasselkus, 2006). Through this invasion, we even seek to change them. The ethical implications of this intimacy and trust are daunting. As occupational therapy practitioners, we need to establish trust with the client and must respect the inherent responsibilities of that trust.

As with all ethnographers, the occupational therapy practitioner brings their own worldview to the process. Of course, the practitioner uses clinical reasoning, understanding of medical and psychological conditions, and a growing understanding of the client to inform their decisions about what to ask in developing the occupational profile. However, the practitioner also brings a more personal and subjective perspective to the process. What questions are asked, what is considered relevant, and what actions are noticed depend on what the practitioner brings to the interaction. The practitioner is influenced by the chosen theories and frames of reference, medical knowledge about the diagnosis and prognosis, their experience with other clients, and their personal experiences and prejudices (Urban, 1998). It is important that practitioners understand their own worldview and consider how it affects the interaction.

The Evaluation Process

The occupational profile is half of the evaluation process. The occupational therapy evaluation is a synthesis of the occupational profile and the analysis of occupational performance (AOTA, 2020a). The process of evaluation is a continuous interplay between these two components. The process is not sequential but rather a back-and-forth and an overlap.

The occupational profile identifies which occupations need to be evaluated for occupational performance. It pinpoints which occupations are priorities for interventions and what configuration of activities currently defines an occupation for the client. The occupational therapy practitioner can then evaluate the client's performance in these activities. As the practitioner analyzes the client's performance of the specified occupations, they observe the individual details of the client's task execution, which further flesh out the profile. Because the client may have difficulty describing their habits and routines and because their behaviors are so ingrained in their lives that they do not think about them anymore, the practitioner sees what and how a client performs a task as they attempt the task in the evaluation.

During this part of the evaluation, the occupational therapy practitioner is both analyzing the occupational performance and conducting participant observation to feed the occupational profile. These observations further clarify the occupational profile and, in turn, refocus the direction of the evaluation of the occupational performance. Likewise, as the practitioner identifies specific skill deficits through the analysis of occupational performance, they are able to anticipate what areas of occupations may be problematic and concentrate the questions on that area. For example, for a client with limited elbow flexion of the nondominant arm, based on activity analysis, the practitioner may delve more deeply into the areas of applying makeup rather than painting fingernails, or golfing rather than reading, depending on the desires of the client.

The synthesis of the evaluation process involves a series of questions the occupational practitioner asks to develop an understanding of the data, create an intervention plan, and determine outcome measures. The analysis must identify barriers and facilitators to the occupational performance of their envisioned future occupational profile. Exhibit 4.1 elaborates this synthesis.

EXHIBIT 4.1. Synthesis of the Evaluation Process

- Determining the client's values and priorities for occupational participation
- Interpreting the assessment data to identify supports and hindrances to occupational performance
- Developing and refining hypotheses about the client's occupational performance strengths and deficits
- Considering existing support systems and contexts as well as their ability to support the intervention process
- Determining desired outcomes of the intervention
- Creating goals in collaboration with the client that address the desired outcomes
- Selecting outcome measures and determining procedures to measure progress toward the goals of intervention, which may include repeating assessments used in the evaluation process

Note. Adapted from AOTA (2020b, p. 23). Used with permission.

With a new injury or illness affecting occupational performance, the occupational therapy evaluation may be the first time clients are attempting some of the tasks important to their occupations. This situation makes the clients vulnerable because what they can and cannot do has changed. As they confront familiar tasks with new difficulties, the priorities and values in their occupational profiles shift. Moreover, this shift is emotionally charged. Clients often struggle down a tumultuous road toward self-perceptions, which are tied directly to their occupational profile. They work to gain a vision of themselves in the future, a vision they use to set their goals and give meaning to the present (Morris, 1994). This metamorphosis spans the evaluation and intervention stages.

Goal Setting and the Occupational Profile

The occupational profile identifies which of the client's occupations are desired, valued, and needed, providing details about the occupations in which the client seeks to participate and commits to engage in more fully. In designing the intervention plan, the occupational therapy practitioner uses the occupational profile to determine which occupation areas to target. These will determine the outcomes sought. ***Occupation-based goals*** pull from the occupational profile. They may be current occupations facing barriers or they may be future occupations that the intervention seeks to develop. Some goals may address client factors or performance skills or patterns. These goals should also link to the occupational profile as steps toward occupational performance (see Figure 4.4 and Case Examples 4.1 and 4.2).

Goal setting should be done in a collaborative discussion with the client in relation to their occupational profile and why they are seeking treatment. Often it is helpful to use a

FIGURE 4.4. Goal setting: In treatment for her arthritis, this woman wanted to walk. More important, she wanted to walk down the church aisle to sing in her church choir.

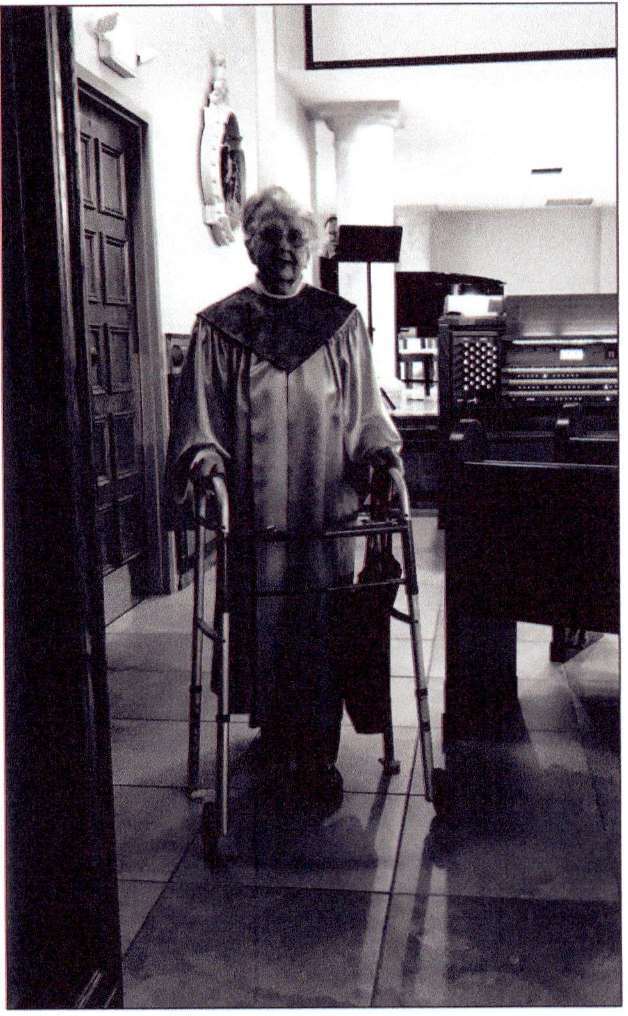

Source. J. Wilson. Used with permission.

formal tool. The Canadian Occupational Performance Measure (COPM; Law et al., 2019) and the Activity Card Sort (Baum & Edwards, 2008) are tools to facilitate a discussion of what occupations the client values and which occupations the client wants to target in treatment.

Frequently, the client's articulated goals are too general to use as intervention goals (e.g., "I want to go home," "I want to be like I used to be," "I want to walk," "I want to get better"). The occupational profile gives the occupational therapy practitioner data with which to interpret these goals and form interventions. For example, in reviewing the client's array of occupations, the practitioner may find answers to questions, such as where the person walked in the past, what activities are necessary to survive at home, and which occupations are presently worse than before.

Through the intervention process, the client and occupational therapy practitioner may become more collaborative in setting goals. The practitioner enters the client's world, whereas the client learns about the perspective and principles of occupational therapy through the shared experience of the intervention. As a client comes to a greater understanding of occupational therapy, they become more self-directed in the process. A client may see themselves successfully completing more activities and may identify which activities they want to work on next in pursuit of valued occupations. The client may bring up an old hobby or a long-held aspiration as they perceive that occupational therapy may be able to help them achieve such goals. For these clients, the occupational therapy process becomes a true partnership.

With clients who do not reach this level of partnership, the occupational therapy practitioner works to interpret the client's responses to activities to expand on the meaningfulness of their goals and interventions. As the practitioner learns about the client's past and present occupations as well as future aspirations, they work with the client to identify occupations that are still attainable or that are especially self-affirming for the client. The practitioner emphasizes the occupations that help the client see their capabilities and encourages the client to actively choose which occupations they wish to set as goals.

Goals can aim to resume impaired occupations, or they can aim to change or redefine the occupations. Activities that are health risks or that are unattainable for the client after a bodily change need to undergo alteration. For example, the intervention plan may target a change in leisure skills for a person with a drug addiction, or it may aim to redefine work for a person after a severe brain injury. Because the profile identifies the client's valued roles, it guides the client and the occupational therapy practitioner in channeling the activity changes to achieve role competence (see Case Example 4.3).

Intervention and the Occupational Profile

Intervention is about creating change. The intervention plan must determine where change is possible and how change can be created. These interventions should be occupation based and client centered. The change occurring through the intervention is ultimately changing the occupational profile.

The evaluation extends into the intervention because there is an ongoing loop of information gathering and modification of the intervention plan. As the process moves into the intervention phase, intervention planning begins to flow more directly from the new data emerging in the profile. The occupational therapist, in collaboration with the occupational therapy assistant, thus uses the occupational profile as an intervention tool. Data collection through participant observation expands the occupational profile, and the occupational therapy practitioner uses the profile to generate intervention ideas.

Occupation-based interventions pull activities from the occupational profile. Treatment settings can make matching

CASE EXAMPLE 4.1. Jorge: Parkinson's Disease

Jorge is a 71-year-old man who has requested occupational therapy services because he wants to regain his ability to be active in his community. Ten years ago, he was diagnosed with Parkinson's disease. Initially, the symptoms were managed with medications, but over the past 5 years, his movements have slowly been declining. He retired as a high school teacher.

Jorge and his wife live in the same two-story home in which they raised their three children. Two years ago, they moved their bedroom to the ground floor. His wife has started to help him with his shower and getting dressed in the morning as well as occasionally assisting with undressing at night. Although he has trouble at times getting out of the car, he has managed to continue driving, although recently, he and his wife discussed her taking over more of the driving responsibilities. In addition, Jorge has had difficulty negotiating getting in and out of the house on the front stoop.

Steps are a bigger problem at their church, so he has had to stop going. He had been a church usher. Some of his friends from church stop by Jorge and his wife's house on Sundays after services. He finds some solace reading the bible. Also, he and his wife used to love to go out to dinner together. The steps, the distances to walk, getting up and down from the chairs, and increasing tremors while eating have resulted in their staying home most nights.

CASE EXAMPLE 4.2. Ling: Carpal Tunnel Syndrome

Ling is a 35-year-old woman. Over the past year, she has had increasing pain in her right hand and was recently diagnosed with carpal tunnel syndrome. The physician referred her for occupational therapy services. Ling works full time as a hairdresser. She is divorced and has three school-aged children who live with her. She is involved in several social and community outreach programs at her temple, including bringing meals to elderly people and teaching Mandarin in the children's program.

EXERCISE 4.4. Applying the Occupational Profile to Case Examples

Review Case Examples 4.1 and 4.2 and answer the following questions for each:

1. What are the contexts (environment and personal factors) in the occupational profile?
2. Which time period would you focus on in the occupational profile?
3. What are occupation-based goals for this client?
4. What do you envision as a possible healthy outcome for this client? (In other words, what would participation in an updated occupational profile look like?)

the environmental context of the occupations difficult. In addition, incorporating the full occupation is often too much. The occupational therapy practitioner may break down the occupations to address components of the occupations. Occupation-based intervention choices use purposeful activities that link to the occupational profile using modifications for both clinical pragmatics and for therapeutic gradations.

Client-centered interventions refer to both the individualizing of treatment in relation to the occupational profile and the inclusion of the client in goal setting. Making interventions occupation based overlaps with making them client centered—with the first focused on the application of the activities themselves and the second focused on the individualization of these selections. The goal-setting discussion between the client and the occupational therapy practitioner empowers the client to make changes for a healthier and richer occupational profile.

The occupational profile also aids the occupational therapy practitioner in choosing a method to approach a goal. Knowing how the client has adapted their occupations at previous stages of life can help in selecting an approach to which the client will be receptive. Where will the client be open to making changes? Would the client rather scale back the performance of an occupation or completely redesign how to fulfill a role? Rather than using the occupational profile as a goal, the occupational profile can be a resource for tools in treatment (see Case Example 4.4).

Narrative reasoning is a form of clinical reasoning in occupational therapy interventions. The occupational therapy practitioner actively engages the client with their occupational profile and directing the path of change the profile follows. The practitioner talks to the client and selects occupation-based activities to encourage "rewriting" their own narrative toward healing and participation in a healthy new occupational profile (Mattingly, 1998). Narrative reasoning uses the evolving nature of the occupational profile as an intervention tool.

The dynamic interplay between assessment and intervention through the occupational profile is where change occurs. During the intervention process, the client's awareness of what they can and cannot do increases and changes. The occupational therapy practitioner exposes the client to new experiences that may open possibilities in the client's eyes. The client travels through different emotional responses to these changes. In addition, the client–practitioner relationship changes from provider–client to guide–partner. Change happens as the client is empowered to change their own occupational profile.

CASE EXAMPLE 4.3. Rosa: Cerebral Palsy

Rosa is age 13 years. She has cerebral palsy. Her family immigrated to the United States 4 years ago, seeking treatment for their daughter. Rosa is bright and responsive in interactions but is very immature. She has had little social contact outside her family. They have been unable to enroll her in school because she does not have a wheelchair that fits; the family has been carrying her. She has multiple contractures from spending most of her time in bed. She has twin brothers who are age 9 years.

CASE EXAMPLE 4.4. Mark's Aspirations

In high school, **Mark** was editor of his yearbook and played the saxophone. He graduated with top grades, and he was the first of his family to attend college. His family was very proud of him and his achievements.

He began college, studying nursing. During his sophomore year, his schoolwork became very disorganized. He began hallucinating, which led to confused behavior, and the school contacted his family. He took a leave of absence and began treatment in a partial-hospitalization program near his parents' home. His family was overwhelmed with this setback. They tried to remain supportive but were also dealing with their own feelings of fear and disappointment. He had one good friend from school who reached out online periodically.

In treatment, Mark stayed focused on returning to school. During his time outside treatment, he was alone in his room, mostly, playing online games.

Three months into treatment, Mark's hallucinations started worsening. He jumped out a window in a suicide attempt. This resulted in his losing his left leg and in a mild head injury. Mark was hospitalized for psychiatric and medical treatment. Mark's family was traumatized by these events. They were very fearful of his returning home and attempting suicide again.

In the hospital, Mark was lethargic and spoke little. He did not respond to texts on his phone, so his family took his phone home. The occupational therapist met him, and he turned his head away, saying, "I can't do anything." Begrudgingly, he eventually sat up and got dressed with help.

The occupational therapist showed him videos online of the Paralympics. He was taken with the swimming when he saw a swimmer with one leg. Afterward, he became animated with plans to become a paralympic swimmer, and his goal was a gold medal. His occupational profile at this point revealed that his primary goal was to become a paralympic swimmer. For several weeks he talked of little else. With some concern, his sister pointed out that he had never been much of a swimmer and, as a child, was afraid of the water.

The occupational therapist continued to use videos in their treatment sessions but mixed in other sports as well as swimming in a more leisurely atmosphere. The therapist used tasks with swimming and with use of the iPad™ for searches.

On discharge home, the family was still nervous. The occupational therapist worked on developing activities they could do together with Mark. Mark continued to want to swim competitively, but his interests were growing. His revised occupational profile revealed a new aspiration: to open a taco stand.

EXERCISE 4.5. Moving From the Occupational Profile to an Intervention Plan

Read Case Example 4.3 and answer the following questions about Rosa (you will have to use your imagination a bit here):

1. What do you think that the occupational profile will tell you about Rosa?
2. What do you see as potential occupations for Rosa?
3. What goals would you set for Rosa?
4. What would be the focus of your intervention plan for Rosa?

EXERCISE 4.6. Using the Occupational Profile for Intervention

Review Case Example 4.4 about Mark and his aspirations, and answer the following questions:

1. As the occupational therapy practitioner at the partial hospitalization program Mark initially was in, how would you handle his occupational profile to set goals? Are there occupations that are dysfunctional? How could you use the occupations in treatment?
2. How did the occupational profile change over time? What triggered the changes?
3. How could the occupational profile be used as a tool for change?
4. How did Mark's environment affect his occupational profile? How could the occupational therapy practitioner address the environment in treatment?
5. On the basis of all the information presented about Mark, what would be the focus of your intervention?

Groups or Populations as Client

It is questionable if an occupational profile is ever about an individual. We are increasingly recognizing that people are social beings. We exist in community. Even "solitary" activities link us with a wider social context. A man knitting alone in his apartment, for example, learned to knit from someone, is likely knitting for someone, and defines this as a meaningful activity in relation to images in society, whether he accepts or rejects those images.

Occupational therapy practice is increasingly recognizing the need to treat the social unit, particularly the family (Stoffel et al., 2017). Family can be both a support and a stressor for a person. Nonetheless, a client must function within the dynamics of the social context (Umberson & Montez, 2010). Therefore, our interventions directed to change how the person carries out their occupational profile must address the social context to be effective. To do this, a truly occupation-based intervention should seek to include the family in their interventions. If the client dons their socks independently in the clinic but lets their spouse do it otherwise, then the intervention is incomplete at best. Guiding a young student to use an adaptive strategy to manage a writing task must include both the classroom and the home environment to be successful.

These occupational profiles, although in a social environment, are still for an individual client. Most of this chapter discusses occupational profiles as if clients were individuals. However, clients can also be a group or a population. They, too, have occupational profiles. These occupational profiles are not a sum of the occupational profiles of the individuals. Rather,

CASE EXAMPLE 4.5. Community Client

Client: a network of Canadian food security programs

Frame of reference: person-occupation-environment

Who is the client (social group associated with a place)? individuals and families who attended food security events and programs; people who worked or volunteered in these programs; schools, businesses, organizations, and coalitions united as clients in supporting and participating in these programs; although the individuals changed, the members agreed that this identified who belonged (and who did not); the places linking them were the sites of the events and programs

Co-occupations (different roles but shared intentionality): gardening, food manufacturing, cooking, political advocacy, high-level communication; examples of the detailing of these occupations include following rotating shift rosters, interactions between leadership and volunteers, interactions between volunteers and those attending events; enjoyment of distributing food together, and creative use of vacant lands

Intervention plan: identification of participant enablement strategies, such as leadership development, leverage outcomes through partnerships and capacity building, facilitation of online participation via social media, and use of multimethod strategies that are socially and culturally diverse

Source. From "Reimagining Occupational Therapy Clients as Communities: Presenting the Community-Centred Practice Framework," by N. Hyett, A. Kenny, & V. Dickson-Swift, *Scandinavian Journal of Occupational Therapy,* Vol. 26, 246–260. Copyright © 2019 by Taylor & Francis. Used with permission.

the occupational profile of a group looks at the resources and dynamics of the group.

Ethnographic methods apply naturally to a group. The occupational therapy practitioner generally interviews a sampling of people, preferably representing different roles in the group. The participant observation is particularly important to learn the dynamics of the group. Once again, there is an interplay between what the clients report in the interview and what is observed in their actions, which moves the collection of data and the analysis forward.

Hyett et al. (2019) presented the community-centered practice framework as a model for occupational therapy practice at the community level, including assessing the community's occupational profile. They delineated the community identity by considering who their community client is. In collecting the occupational profile, they explored what occupations are important to the community as a whole and what actions the community members take together toward shared goals (Hyett et al., 2019; see Case Example 4.5).

EXERCISE 4.7. Applying the Occupational Profile to a Community

Read Case Example 4.5. Design the assessment of the occupational profile of this community. What are the shared goals of this community?

Outcomes and the Occupational Profile

Occupational therapy ***outcomes*** are all tied to the occupational profile, whether by definition of a healthy occupational profile, competence in the roles within the occupational profile, or satisfaction with the occupational profile. The *OTPF–4* (AOTA, 2020b) shares with the World Health Organization's (WHO) *International Classification of Functioning, Disability and Health* (WHO, 2001) the value of participation. ***Participation*** is "involvement in a life situation" (WHO, 2001, p. 123). For occupational therapy practitioners, this is engagement in occupation. The ultimate goal of occupational therapy is participation in a valued and healthy occupational profile (AOTA, 2020a).

The framework also concurs with the WHO definition of ***health:*** "a state of complete physical, mental, and social well-being" (AOTA, 2020b, p. 77). This definition is important in understanding outcomes for occupational therapy. Health is not the opposite of disease. A healthy outcome means the current occupational profile is meaningful and valued by the client. Health must be understood in relation to the person's roles and their environment (see Case Example 4.6).

Occupational measures reflect the decisions made in goal setting. Measures may reassess the occupational profile content to capture change or redefinition in occupations. Measures may assess successful performance of the occupations in the profile. The COPM (Law et al., 2019) and the Activity Card Sort (Baum & Edwards, 2008), used in setting goals, are also outcome measures that capture change.

People describe the experience of participation as fostering a sense of belonging, being meaningful to the person, and allowing self-determination (Häggström & Larsson Lund, 2008; Heinemann et al., 2013). A healthy outcome means the client is able to act to foster their sense of belonging and pur-

EXERCISE 4.8. Applying the Occupational Profile to Intervention With an Infant

Review Case Example 4.6 about Destiny and answer the following questions.

1. Occupational therapist Elsie Vergara (2002) describes infants' primary occupations as play, social interaction, procuring (i.e., getting attention to have needs met), and feeding. In addition, the fourth edition of the *Occupational Therapy Practice Framework: Domain and Process* (AOTA, 2020b) identifies sleep as an occupation. Which aspects of these five occupations will be included in Destiny's intervention plan?
2. What would be the first area of focus for your intervention with Destiny? Why would you choose this first?
3. What outcomes would you hope for with Destiny?

CASE EXAMPLE 4.6. Destiny: Premature Infant

Destiny was born 10 weeks prematurely. After 8 weeks in the neonatal intensive care unit, she was medically stable and feeding by breast and bottle, so she was ready for discharge home. Her family (mom, dad, and a 3-year-old brother) were very excited to welcome her home.

Now, 2 months later, Destiny is referred to occupational therapy because she has dropped below the first percentile in weight for her age. The doctor ruled out metabolic causes and is concerned about her feeding skills. During evaluation, the occupational therapist identified concerns with Destiny's suck–swallow–breathe coordination and endurance while feeding. Destiny eats very small amounts frequently and wakes before getting enough sleep in an inefficient cycle that is exhausting for her and her parents. Her parents describe her as quiet; she has a very weak cry and fusses little. The evaluation also found Destiny's "quiet" behavior included minimal attempts to explore her environment visually or tactilely. Both Destiny and parents would be considered clients in this example.

FIGURE 4.5. Participation: For this parent, attending the high school marching band competition means supporting her daughter and belonging to the band parent community.

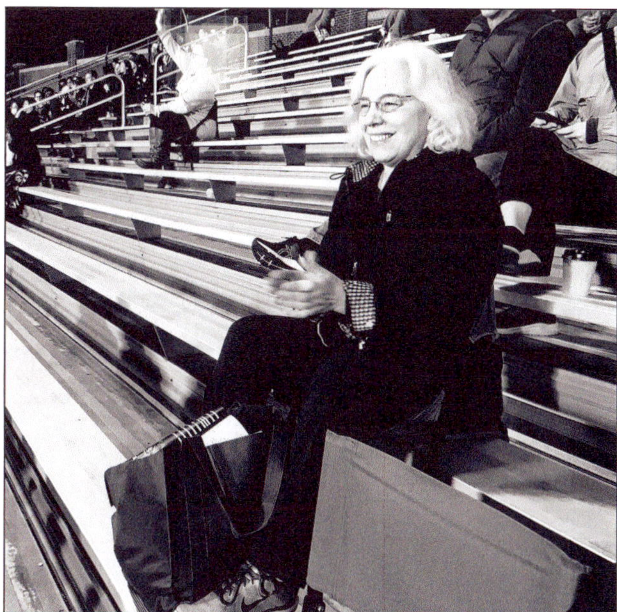

Source. J. Wilson. Used with permission.

pose in their environment. The occupations, embedded in their environment, come together to make the person who they are (Figure 4.5). This is the occupational profile. If the occupational profile is currently fulfilling this role, then the outcome was achieved.

EXERCISE 4.9. Focus on Occupational Outcomes

Review the case examples in the chapter and choose two cases. For these case examples, what do you envision as a possible healthy outcome for each of these clients? In other words, what would participation in an updated occupational profile look like?

Summary

The occupational profile is a morphing narrative of a person's daily routines that forms the day-to-day experience of a person's identity. In the evaluation, the occupational therapy practitioner seeks to identify the occupational profile using the ethnographic tools of interview and participant observation. In practice, the practitioner enters an evolving and engrossing story of the client's occupational profile.

Occupational therapy practitioners are drawn to the intimacy of and the fascination with each client's occupational profile. The discoveries make the strange familiar and the familiar strange. As practitioners, we need an appreciation of health that relies on a fulfilling and balanced occupational profile rather than on a biomedical definition of disease. Understanding the variations in occupational profiles and their fluid nature helps the practitioner to join the client in seeing meaningful outcomes when faced with barriers.

The occupational profile flows through evaluation, treatment planning, intervention, and outcomes. The occupational profile is a dynamic clinical tool that links each part of the occupational therapy process toward the purpose of fostering participation. The occupational therapy practitioner is a witness and guide through these changes in the occupational profile.

Acknowledgments

The author acknowledges the contributions to the discussion and case studies in this chapter by Stephanie Cillo, OTR/L; Mallory Marder, OTR/L; and Charlene Woo, OTR/L.

References

American Occupational Therapy Association. (2020a). *AOTA occupational profile template*. www.aota.org/coding

American Occupational Therapy Association. (2020b). Occupational therapy practice framework: Domain and process (4th ed.). *American Journal of Occupational Therapy 74*(Suppl. 2), 7412410010. https://doi.org/10.5014/ajot.2020.74S2001

Baum, C., & Edwards, D. (2008). *Activity Card Sort* (2nd ed.). AOTA Press.

Bernard, H. R. (2011). *Research methods in anthropology: Qualitative and quantitative approaches* (5th ed.). Altamira Press.

Borisoff, D. J., & Chesebro, J. W. (2011). *Communicating power and gender*. Waveland Press.

Brown, L. (2014). Disability in an ableist world. In C. Wood (Ed.), *Critiques* (pp. 37–45). May Day Publishing.

Frank, A. W. (2004). *The renewal of generosity: Illness, medicine, and how to live*. University of Chicago Press.

Geertz, C. (1973). *The interpretation of cultures*. Basic Books.

Häggström, A., & Larsson Lund, M. (2008). The complexity of participation in daily life: A qualitative study of the experiences of persons with acquired brain injury. *Journal of Rehabilitation Medicine, 40*(2), 89–95. https://doi.org/10.2340/16501977-0138

Hasselkus, B. R. (2006). The world of everyday occupation: Real people, real lives. *American Journal of Occupational Therapy, 60*(5), 627–640. https://doi.org/10.5014/ajot.60.6.627

Heinemann, A. W., Magasi, S., Bode, R. K., Hammel, J., Whiteneck, G. G., Bogner, J., & Corrigan, J. D. (2013). Measuring enfranchisement: Importance of and control over participation by people with disabilities. *Archives of Physical Medicine and Rehabilitation, 94*(11), 2157–2165. https://doi.org/10.1016/j.apmr.2013.05.017

Hyett, N., Kenny, A., & Dickson-Swift, V. (2019). Reimagining occupational therapy clients as communities: Presenting the community-centred practice framework. *Scandinavian Journal of Occupational Therapy, 26*(4), 246–260. https://doi.org/10.1080/11038128.2017.1423374

Kelly, G., & McFarlane, H. (2007). Culture or cult? The mythological nature of occupational therapy. *Occupational Therapy International, 14*(4), 188–202. https://doi.org/10.1002/oti.237

Krahn, G. L., Walker, D. K., & Correa-De-Araujo, R. (2015). Persons with disabilities as an unrecognized health disparity population. *American Journal of Public Health, 105*(52), S198–S206. https://doi.org/10.2105/AJPH.2014.302182

Kramarae, C. (1996). Classified information, race, class, and (always) gender. In J. T. Wood (Ed.), *Gendered relationships* (pp. 20–38). Mayfield Publishing.

Kramer, P., Hinojosa, J., & Howe, T. (2020). *Frames of reference for pediatric occupational therapy* (4th ed.). Wolters Kluwer/Lippincott Williams & Wilkins.

Law, M., Baptiste, S., Carswell, A., McColl, M., Polatajko, H., & Pollock, N. (2019). *Canadian Occupational Performance Measure* (5th ed., rev.). COPM, Inc.

Mattingly, C. (1998). *Healing dramas and clinical plots: The narrative structure of experience*. Cambridge University Press.

Morris, J. (1994). Spinal injury and psychotherapy in treatment philosophy. In G. M. Yarkony (Ed.), *Spinal cord injury: Medical management and rehabilitation* (pp. 223–229). Aspen Publishers.

Riessman, C. K. (2008). *Narrative methods for the human sciences*. SAGE Publications.

Runyan, C. (2006). Neuro-developmental treatment of adult hemiplegia. In H. M. Pendleton & W. Schultz-Krohn (Eds.), *Pedretti's occupational therapy: Practice skills for physical dysfunction* (6th ed., pp. 169–170). Mosby Elsevier.

Social Science LibreTexts. (2021, July 23). *4.2: Making the strange familiar and the familiar strange*. https://socialsci.libretexts.org/@go/page/56388

Stoffel, A., Rhein, J., Khetani, M. A., Pizur-Barnekow, K., James, L. W., & Schefkind, S. (2017). Family centered: Occupational therapy's role in promoting meaningful engagement in early intervention. *OT Practice, 22*(18), 8–13.

Trombly, C. A. (2002). Restoring the role of independent person. In C. A. Trombly & M. V. Radomski (Eds.), *Occupational therapy for physical dysfunction* (5th ed., pp. 629–663). Lippincott Williams & Wilkins.

Umberson, D., & Montez, J. K. (2010). Social relationships and health: A flashpoint for health policy. *Journal of Health and Social Behavior, 51*(Suppl. 1), S54–S66. https://doi.org/10.1177/0022146510383501

Urban, J. (1998, 31 May–5 June). Cultural issues in occupational therapy [Paper presentation]. *12th International Congress of the World Federation of Occupational Therapists*, Montreal, Canada.

Vergara, E. R. (2002). Enhancing occupational performance in infants in the NICU. *OT Practice, 7*(12), 8–13.

World Federation of Occupational Therapists. (2022). *About occupational therapy*. https://www.wfot.org/about/about-occupational-therapy

World Health Organization. (2001). *International classification of functioning, disability and health*.

Wu, F. H. (2002). *Yellow: Race in America: Beyond Black and White*. Basic Books.

Appendix 4.A. AOTA Occupational Profile Template

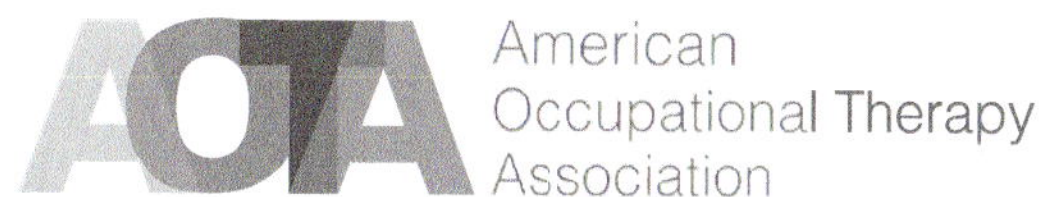

aota.org

AOTA Occupational Profile Template

"The occupational profile is a summary of a client's (person's, group's, or population's) occupational history and experiences, patterns of daily living, interests, values, needs, and relevant contexts" (AOTA, 2020, p. 21). The information is obtained from the client's perspective through both formal and informal interview techniques and conversation.

The information obtained through the occupational profile contributes to a client-focused approach in the evaluation, intervention planning, intervention implementation, and discharge planning stages. Each item below should be addressed to complete the occupational profile. Page numbers are provided to reference the description in the *Occupational Therapy Practice Framework: Domain and Process* (4th ed.; AOTA, 2020).

<table>
<tr><th colspan="4">OCCUPATIONAL PROFILE</th></tr>
<tr><td rowspan="4">Client Report</td><td>Reason the client is seeking service and concerns related to engagement in occupations (p. 16)</td><td colspan="2">Why is the client seeking services, and what are the client's current concerns relative to engaging in occupations and in daily life activities? (This may include the client's general health status.)</td></tr>
<tr><td>Occupations in which the client is successful and barriers impacting success (p. 16)</td><td colspan="2">In what occupations does the client feel successful, and what barriers are affecting their success in desired occupations?</td></tr>
<tr><td>Occupational history (p. 16)</td><td colspan="2">What is the client's occupational history (i.e., life experiences)?</td></tr>
<tr><td>Personal interests and values (p. 16)</td><td colspan="2">What are the client's values and interests?</td></tr>
<tr><td rowspan="3">Contexts</td><td></td><td colspan="2">What aspects of their contexts (environmental and personal factors) does the client see as supporting engagement in desired occupations, and what aspects are inhibiting engagement?</td></tr>
<tr><td>Environment (p. 36)
(e.g., natural environment and human-made changes, products and technology, support and relationships, attitudes, services, systems and policies)</td><td>Supporting Engagement</td><td>Inhibiting Engagement</td></tr>
<tr><td>Personal (p. 40)
(e.g., age, sexual orientation, gender identity, race and ethnicity, cultural identification, social background, upbringing, psychological assets, education, lifestyle)</td><td>Supporting Engagement</td><td>Inhibiting Engagement</td></tr>
</table>

<table>
<tr><td>Performance Patterns</td><td>Performance patterns (p. 41)
(e.g., habits, routines, roles, rituals)</td><td colspan="2">What are the client's patterns of engagement in occupations, and how have they changed over time? What are the client's daily life roles? (Patterns can support or hinder occupational performance.)</td></tr>
<tr><td rowspan="4">Client Factors</td><td></td><td colspan="2">What client factors does the client see as supporting engagement in desired occupations, and what aspects are inhibiting engagement (e.g., pain, active symptoms)?</td></tr>
<tr><td>Values, beliefs, spirituality
(p. 51)</td><td>Supporting Engagement</td><td>Inhibiting Engagement</td></tr>
<tr><td>Body functions (p. 51)
(e.g., mental, sensory, neuro-musculoskeletal and movement-related, cardiovascular functions)</td><td>Supporting Engagement</td><td>Inhibiting Engagement</td></tr>
<tr><td>Body structures (p. 54)
(e.g., structures of the nervous system, eyes and ears, related to movement)</td><td>Supporting Engagement</td><td>Inhibiting Engagement</td></tr>
<tr><td rowspan="9">Client Goals</td><td rowspan="9">Client's priorities and desired targeted outcomes (p. 65)</td><td colspan="2">What are the client's priorities and desired targeted outcomes related to the items below?</td></tr>
<tr><td colspan="2">Occupational Performance</td></tr>
<tr><td colspan="2">Prevention</td></tr>
<tr><td colspan="2">Health and Wellness</td></tr>
<tr><td colspan="2">Quality of Life</td></tr>
<tr><td colspan="2">Participation</td></tr>
<tr><td colspan="2">Role Competence</td></tr>
<tr><td colspan="2">Well-Being</td></tr>
<tr><td colspan="2">Occupational Justice</td></tr>
</table>

For a complete description of each component and examples of each, refer to the *Occupational Therapy Practice Framework: Domain and Process* (4th ed.).

Resources

American Occupational Therapy Association. (2020). Occupational therapy practice framework: Domain and process (4th ed.). *American Journal of Occupational Therapy, 74*(Suppl. 2), 7412410010. https://doi.org/10.5014/ajot.2020.74S2001

The occupational therapy evaluation and reevaluation *CPT*® codes established in 2017 require the inclusion of an occupational profile. For more information, visit https://www.aota.org/coding.

5

Activity Synthesis as a Means to Structure Occupation

PAULA KRAMER, PhD, OTR, FAOTA,
AND WENDY E. WALSH, PhD, OTR/L, FAOTA

CHAPTER HIGHLIGHTS

- Activity synthesis: everyday life
- Occupational synthesis: a critical end product
- Theory
- Activity synthesis and analysis
- Activity synthesis as a precursor to occupational synthesis
- Process of activity synthesis in occupational therapy
- Importance of activity and occupational synthesis to intervention
- Other uses of activity and occupational synthesis in intervention
- Activity and occupational synthesis of health promotion
- Artful practice and synthesis

KEY TERMS AND CONCEPTS

• acquisitional theory • activity modification • activity synthesis • adaptation • artful practice • client-centered approach • clinical reasoning process • frames of reference • grading • guidelines for intervention • layered adaptation • models of practice • occupational synthesis • performance • scaling the activity • theoretical orientations

Introduction

Activity synthesis appears simple to the person viewing it, but it is actually a complex process. In this chapter, we review the complexities of activity synthesis as used by occupational therapy practitioners to effectively engage clients in occupations and meet therapeutic goals. Activity synthesis is often at the heart of what practitioners do with clients. Occupational therapy practitioners engage in activity synthesis directed by a theoretical focus. This theoretical focus determines the process of adapting and grading activities.

After discussing the basic components of activity synthesis, we discuss the complex process of creating new activities through the use of activity synthesis as that process moves toward occupational synthesis. The ways in which practitioners use activities to teach and refine skills are presented, along with the role that activity synthesis can play in health promotion. The chapter ends with a discussion of the importance of artful practice when using activity synthesis, because it is foundational to occupational synthesis, and it takes art for practitioners to create a revised activity that is meaningful to the client. Throughout the chapter, we consider the complexities of this seemingly simple process and explain how practitioners master these complexities.

Activity Synthesis: Everyday Life

It is interesting that the *Occupational Therapy Practice Framework: Domain and Process* (4th ed.; *OTPF–4;* American

Occupational Therapy Association [AOTA], 2020b) does not specifically mention activity or occupational synthesis. The term *synthesis* is used in two areas of the *OTPF–4,* in the analysis of occupational performance and in the synthesis of evaluation process (AOTA, 2020b). In the "Analysis of Occupational Performance" section of Exhibit 2 (AOTA, 2020b, p. 16), synthesis is discussed as one of the processes used by occupational therapists in putting together information from the occupational profile to understand the occupations that are important to the client and the contexts that therapists might need to address in the evaluation. The synthesis of evaluation process (AOTA, 2020b, p. 16) occurs when therapists put together all of the information gathered during the assessment process, along with the client's concerns, personal priorities, and context, to identify the goals of and desired outcomes from the therapy process. Synthesis is not mentioned in either the intervention plan or the outcomes.

However, occupational therapy practitioners frequently use synthesis in a very different manner, as they devise activities that will support engaging clients in occupations. The synthesis of activities can be compared to a magic trick. The magician's sleight of hand is smooth and creates the illusion of reality. The audience watches and is not sure that what they are seeing is real, and they try to reconcile what they know with what they think they are seeing. It seems simple, yet creating the illusion is very complex (Hunt, 1997). In many ways, activity synthesis, which is so integral to practice, mirrors the magician's act. ***Activity synthesis*** is the act of changing or modifying a specific activity so that the person can engage in it successfully. It is a complex task that requires the occupational therapy practitioner's knowledge. Occupational therapy practitioners put much thought and skill into developing and creating activities so that the client's experience with the activities in therapy becomes seamless, much like the misleading simplicity of a magician's illusion.

Activity synthesis occurs in everyday life. People frequently adapt, adjust, and create activities all the time. For example, many young children do not like to have clothes put on over their heads because it occludes their eyes. Parents often turn this task into a game; for example, a parent may say, "Where did Maria go?" while putting a shirt over the child's head so that the child will laugh rather than be frightened. This parent has just synthesized the activity, making it into a game instead of something frightening so that it will lead to a successful outcome. Similarly, if a person becomes tired while performing a task standing up, they might try to find a way to do the same task sitting down or, if too much sitting is causing stress, a standing desk might be an excellent solution. This synthesis could be as simple as moving the activity from a sitting position to a standing position to combat inactivity with sedentary work and reduce repetitive stress on joints (Figure 5.1).

FIGURE 5.1. Adapting an activity from (a) sitting to (b) standing can help with body mechanics and is something that people often do naturally.

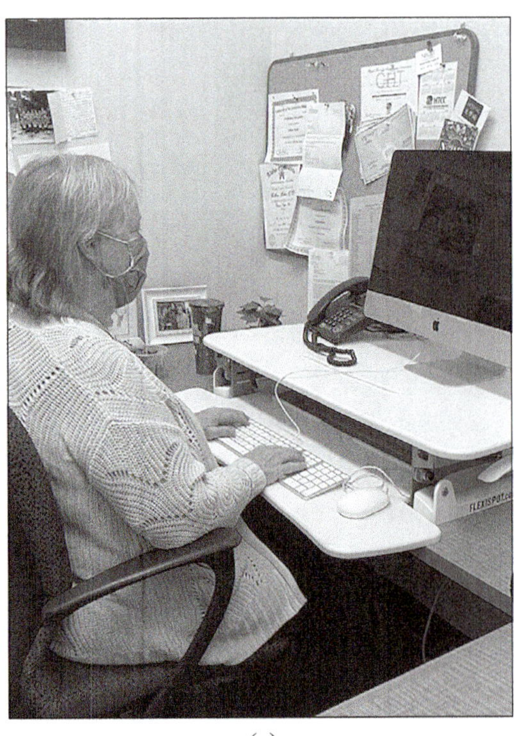

(a)

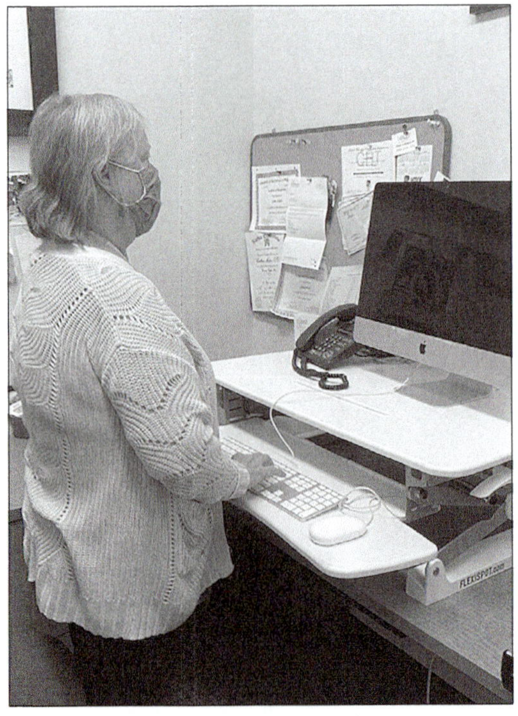

(b)

Source. W. Walsh. Used with permission.

People may think that devising an activity is something that is easy or natural, but it is actually very complex. Because it looks easy and is so common, people generally do not conceptualize the development of activities as synthesis in any special way. Occupational therapy practitioners, however, view activities and their synthesis in a complex and theoretical manner that centers on people's occupational preferences. Because occupational therapy's domain of concern focuses on human occupation, practitioners synthesize activities as a means of advancing a client's ability to participate in meaningful activities and, ultimately, occupations. Despite activity synthesis being central to the art and practice of occupational therapy, very little has been written specifically about this aspect of intervention. In this chapter, we delve into the myriad concerns and reasoning processes involved in activity synthesis in occupational therapy.

Synthesizing activities is something people take for granted—they often modify, adapt, or alter activities seemingly without even thinking. However, even though many people view activity synthesis as part of a natural process, it requires either some conscious thought or an intuitive sense of what changes need to be made to the activity for a successful outcome to occur. In other words, it requires a deeper understanding on some level of why a task is not working the way it was originally supposed to and why it is important to make modifications to successfully complete the task. It must also be centered around occupations that are meaningful to the client.

Occupational Synthesis: A Critical End Product

Occupational synthesis is critical to the practice of occupational therapy. But what is occupational synthesis? ***Occupational synthesis*** is a process that takes place internally (and sometimes unconsciously) within the client, in which the client internalizes the activity synthesis that has been performed by the occupational therapy practitioner as a result of the therapeutic process. At the initiation of occupational therapy services, the client (or their family or significant others) conveys to the practitioner the client's meaningful occupations, the things they do that are important to them. It is important that the occupational therapist incorporate these occupations into their synthesis of the evaluation data. The practitioner uses this knowledge in the intervention process for activity synthesis. Once the client is involved in the occupational therapy process, they can work with the practitioner to begin engaging in tasks and activities that improve functional performance. At this point, the client either has already developed an understanding of which of those activities contribute to personally meaningful occupations or will develop that understanding through the therapy process.

The identified meaningful occupations are critical to the client. In other words, they are occupations that the client truly wants to continue to do once occupational therapy is completed. For the client, these occupations are essential to the maintenance of functional performance. For example, a client who injured her shoulder has been working on range of motion of the shoulder during occupational therapy, but the therapy is about to end. To help her maintain the gains she made during therapy, she and her occupational therapy practitioner decide to rearrange her closet and put some of her favorite sweaters on a higher shelf. This rearrangement forces her to reach up, thereby maintaining the range of motion in her shoulder and becoming part of her occupational synthesis. The ongoing use of the activity, and its adoption into the client's routine, signal that it has been incorporated into her daily life and occupations, which is essential for occupational synthesis to be effective.

Occupational therapy practitioners facilitate occupational synthesis by determining the occupations that are meaningful to the client and working toward synthesizing appropriate therapeutic activities so the client can perform their desired occupations. In addition, to successfully carry out this synthesis process, practitioners must gain an understanding of the client as a person. They need to examine all the available data to develop interventions that will meet the client's occupational needs. This process requires a ***client-centered approach,*** in which a practitioner explores the value of the occupation to the client and the client's personal choices in terms of occupations. It is not up to the practitioner to determine what is important to the client; it is up to the client and their family or significant others to identify those meaningful occupations.

When occupational therapy practitioners are unable to obtain useful information from the client about their occupational needs or desires, they must find other sources of information. They can talk with the client's caregivers, partners, parents, and significant others; review evaluation data; and consider the client's occupational profile in terms of contextual factors, including both environmental and personal factors as well as temporal needs. Practitioners must then use trial and error, by presenting various tasks, activities, and approaches to discover what motivates the client. It is important that practitioners not make assumptions about a client's motivation, nor should they just choose occupations for the client. When a client values an occupation, they are more likely to engage in the activities related to the occupation. When a client is not motivated, however, practitioners must use their clinical judgment to explore the situation. Is the client unmotivated because of the tasks and activities being presented, or does the client lack motivation in general? If nothing seems to spark the client's engagement and motivation after trial and error with various tasks, another approach needs to be considered. Practitioners should select a theoretical perspective that addresses motivation to guide the intervention. Such perspectives might include the Model of Human Occupation (Forsyth & Kielhofner, 2003; Kielhofner, 2008; O'Brien, 2017), the Canadian Model of Occupational Performance (Law, 2002; Law et al., 2019; Polatajko et al., 2007), the Person–Environment–Occupation–Performance

Model (Baum et al., 2015), and the Cognitive Orientation to daily Occupational Performance approach (Polatajko, 2017).

To effectively use occupational synthesis with clients who can articulate their occupational needs and goals, occupational therapy practitioners should consider the following questions:

- Why is this activity important to the client?
- How does this activity relate to the client's occupations?
- What role does this occupation play in the client's life?
- How does this occupation need to be synthesized to fit into the client's life?
- How will this occupational synthesis fit into the context of the client's life?
- How will the synthesized activity help the client engage in meaningful occupations overall?

Determining the answers to these questions will allow practitioners to understand the activity and its relationship to the client's occupations.

Occupational therapy practitioners should also consider context when the synthesis of activities is related to intervention, because the ultimate goal is for the client to be able to perform the activity in the real world, not just in the simulated environment of the occupational therapy practice setting. Therefore, context is critically important to consider in any intervention plan. In the *OTPF–4*, the description of context is greatly expanded and includes environmental factors and personal factors (AOTA, 2020b). Context determines the demands on the person in many ways, so it is critical for practitioners to choose tasks and activities with the person's contextual factors in mind. Understanding the person's contexts is also part of the evaluation process and needs to be taken into account throughout the planning of therapy sessions, before occupational synthesis is even considered. Clearly, context is vital to developing meaningful occupational synthesis for the client. Context is discussed extensively in Chapter 9, "Occupations and Contexts."

Theory

In this section, we discuss the relationship between occupational therapy and theory related to activity analysis. Although people naturally modify activities in a relatively unconscious manner, they do not generally adapt them in an organized fashion. No theoretical rationale exists for the adaptation of an activity; people rely instead on what appears to be common sense. In doing so, people tend to look for a simple change in the activity that will bring about success rather than looking critically at the activity as a whole. Occupational therapy practitioners, however, use activity synthesis in an organized manner, determined by the frame of reference or theoretical perspective they are using to guide their intervention.

Returning to the metaphor of the magician, the magician creates the illusion by using principles of physics, visual misdirection, and knowledge of how people may perceive various situations. Thus, the magician uses the distraction of attractive people or lots of movement on the stage so that the viewer will not focus on the specific actions the magician does as part of the act. Occupational therapy practitioners do not use distraction but theory as the basis for what they do to allow the client to focus on changing an activity to meet their goals. The client is then able to complete their desired activity in a way that is easier for them and allows for success.

Occupational therapy practitioners are guided by theory to plan the synthesis of an activity to meet therapeutic goals. For example, a practitioner may use an ***acquisitional theory*** based on teaching and rewarding the learned behavior, such as Piaget's (1963) theory of cognitive development, to synthesize activities because they understand that the children innately actively seek knowledge and desire rewards. The practitioner presents activities consistent with the child's stage of development and is sensitive to the child's cognitive level. For example, for a child younger than age 2 years, the practitioner would synthesize an activity based on its sensorimotor aspects at an age-appropriate cognitive level. This could involve using larger blocks or building a small tower rather than a more complicated building-block activity that is at a much higher physical and cognitive level. The practitioner might start with a synthesized task that is at a lower level than the child's to promote a feeling of success and very gradually make the activity more difficult, to develop higher-level skills. Thus, the theory provides the practitioner with an understanding of how to synthesize the activities in a therapy session and an understanding of what is expected to happen in a therapeutic way (Figure 5.2).

Occupational therapy interventions should always be based on theoretical perspectives. These perspectives include ***models of practice,*** in which one or more theories are used to devise a method for translating theory into practice (Hinojosa et al., 2010); ***theoretical orientations,*** in which a theory underlies a model of practice, frame of reference, or particular theoretical perspective; ***guidelines for intervention,*** which provide specific information about putting theoretical information into practice; or ***frames of reference,*** which describe the theory or theories used with specific methods of evaluation and how to use theory to guide the intervention.

Many occupational therapy practitioners synthesize activities using established theoretical perspectives, paradigms, or frames of reference. Some more well-known examples are the Model of Human Occupation (MOHO; Kielhofner, 2008; O'Brien, 2017), Ecological Model of Occupation (Dunn, 2017; Dunn et al., 2003), Person–Environment–Occupation–Performance model (PEOP; Bass et al., 2017; Baum et al., 2015), Cognitive Orientation to daily Occupational Performance approach (Missiuna et al., 2001; Polatajko, 2017), Bobath or neurodevelopmental treatment approach (Barthel, 2020; Gellert & Pulaski, 2021), and Ayres Sensory Integration® (Schaaf et al., 2010; Smith-Roley et al., 2020).

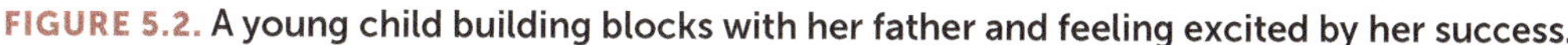

FIGURE 5.2. A young child building blocks with her father and feeling excited by her success.

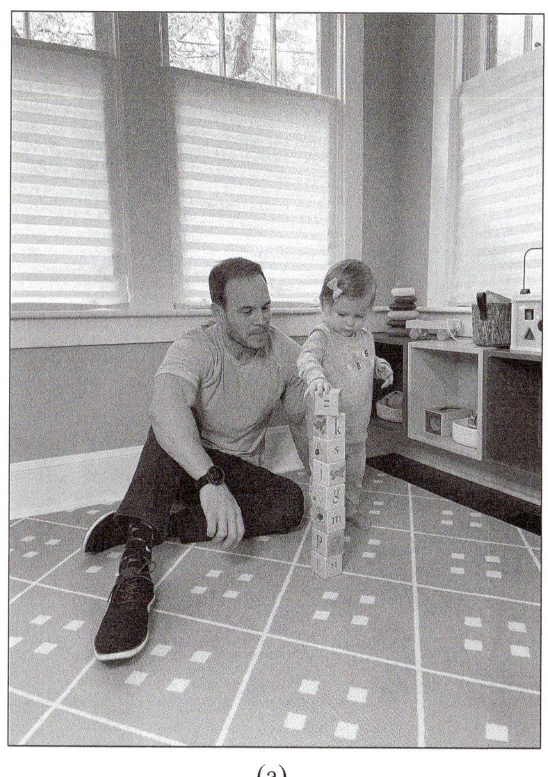

(a)

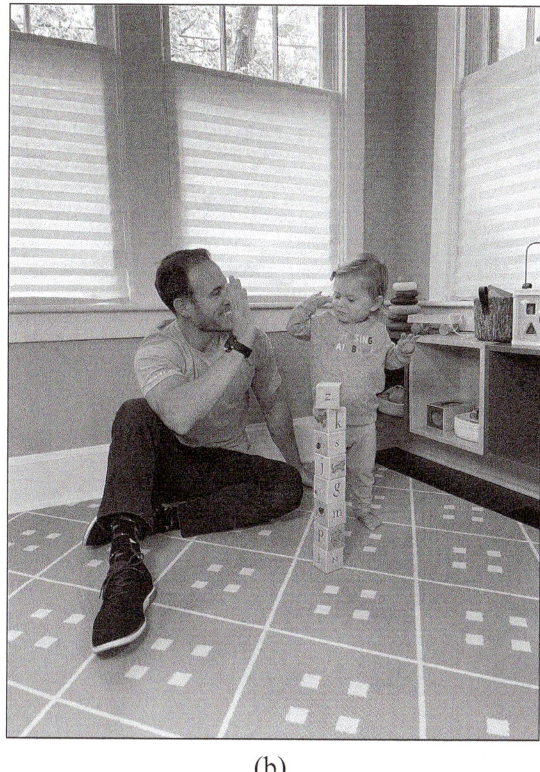

(b)

Source. G. K. Antinore. Used with permission.

The theoretical perspective directs practitioners on how to modify the specific activity during the intervention. Thus, activity synthesis takes place within a theoretical framework that guides the intervention. Then, using the creative process within a theoretical framework, practitioners devise or synthesize activities that will meet the client's needs. If the client has no interest in the activity or does not see it as meaningful to their life, they will probably go through the actions with no personal investment or possibly refuse to engage in the activity. The client may not be self-motivated to participate in the activity at all, and then it has no significant therapeutic value. Moreover, this client may have a negative view of occupational therapy because they do not see it as meeting their personal needs.

Whenever possible, occupational therapy practitioners should use a client-centered approach (AOTA, 2020b) to ensure that the therapeutic activities are meaningful to and elicit a positive response from the client. For the intervention to be successful, the synthesis of activities must always take the client's needs and wants into account. Some theoretical perspectives, such as the MOHO (Kielhofner, 2008) and the Life Style Performance Model (Fidler, 1996; Fidler & Velde, 2002), explicitly address the client's personal motivation; most others, such as the Ecological Model of Human Occupation (Dunn, 2017; Dunn et al., 1994) and the PEOP model (Bass et al., 2017; Baum et al., 2015) address the meaningfulness of the activity to the client, which is also being client centered. Practitioners should select a theoretical perspective that meets the client's needs and incorporates the client's personal interests and choice.

In those models that focus on the importance of the activity to the client, the occupational therapy practitioner provides activities and presents options for the client as a means of intervention. The client then incorporates some of these activities into personally meaningful occupations. The occupational synthesis begins as a collaboration between the practitioner and the client and then ultimately takes place within the client as they choose which occupations to continue as part of their everyday life. We believe that practitioners work with the client to develop an activity synthesis, whereas occupational synthesis ultimately occurs within the client as they choose to include meaningful occupations in their everyday lives. Note that the perspective we propose is not consistent with that proposed by Nelson and Jepson-Thomas (2003). They defined *occupational synthesis* as what the practitioner does; they did not use the term *activity* at all.

Activity Synthesis and Analysis

Activity synthesis is based on the occupational therapy practitioner's comprehensive understanding of the activity and occupation. The initial understanding of the activity and occupation is based on the activity analysis. Activity analysis has been a basic competency for all practitioners since the 1940s (Creighton, 1992; Fidler, 1948; Mosey, 1981). As discussed in detail in Chapter 3, "Occupation and Activity Analysis," activity analysis provides the practitioner with an understanding of the activity and its components. Activity synthesis uses this knowledge of the component elements to reconstruct or design a therapeutic activity. Although activity analysis and synthesis are usually discussed as two separate but associated processes that are used together, they provide the practitioner with the means to understand and successfully use purposeful activities for the client's benefit.

In occupational therapy professional education, much time is spent on activity analysis and, interestingly, very little time is spent on activity synthesis. Therefore, students and practitioners often get the impression that activity analysis is more important to the intervention process than activity synthesis. However, if one observes children on a playground for a short period of time, one can see that adaptation and synthesis occur continuously in play (Figures 5.3 and 5.4). This points to the need for greater emphasis on synthesis in professional education.

The assumption in the focus on activity analysis is that once the practitioner understands the step or stage of a task that is problematic to the client, intervention can take place, and the client will then work toward the successful completion of the task. The notion, however, that synthesis is not as important as analysis is not accurate; in fact, a constant interplay exists between analysis and synthesis. Nelson (1997) characterized *occupational analysis* as "what occupational therapists do" (p. 15), thus noting the importance of synthesis being interconnected with analysis rather than separate from it. Synthesis is thought to be an intellectual process and part of the clinical reasoning and decision-making aspects of practice (Mosey, 1996; Nelson & Jepson-Thomas, 2003). It is not an automatic process on the part of the practitioner, but one that requires careful thought and an understanding of the theoretical perspectives being used.

FIGURE 5.3. Adapting activities is part of synthesis: Playing on an outdoor playset requires adaptation of movements; the older child can adapt her movements on her own, but the younger child is being assisted by her mother.

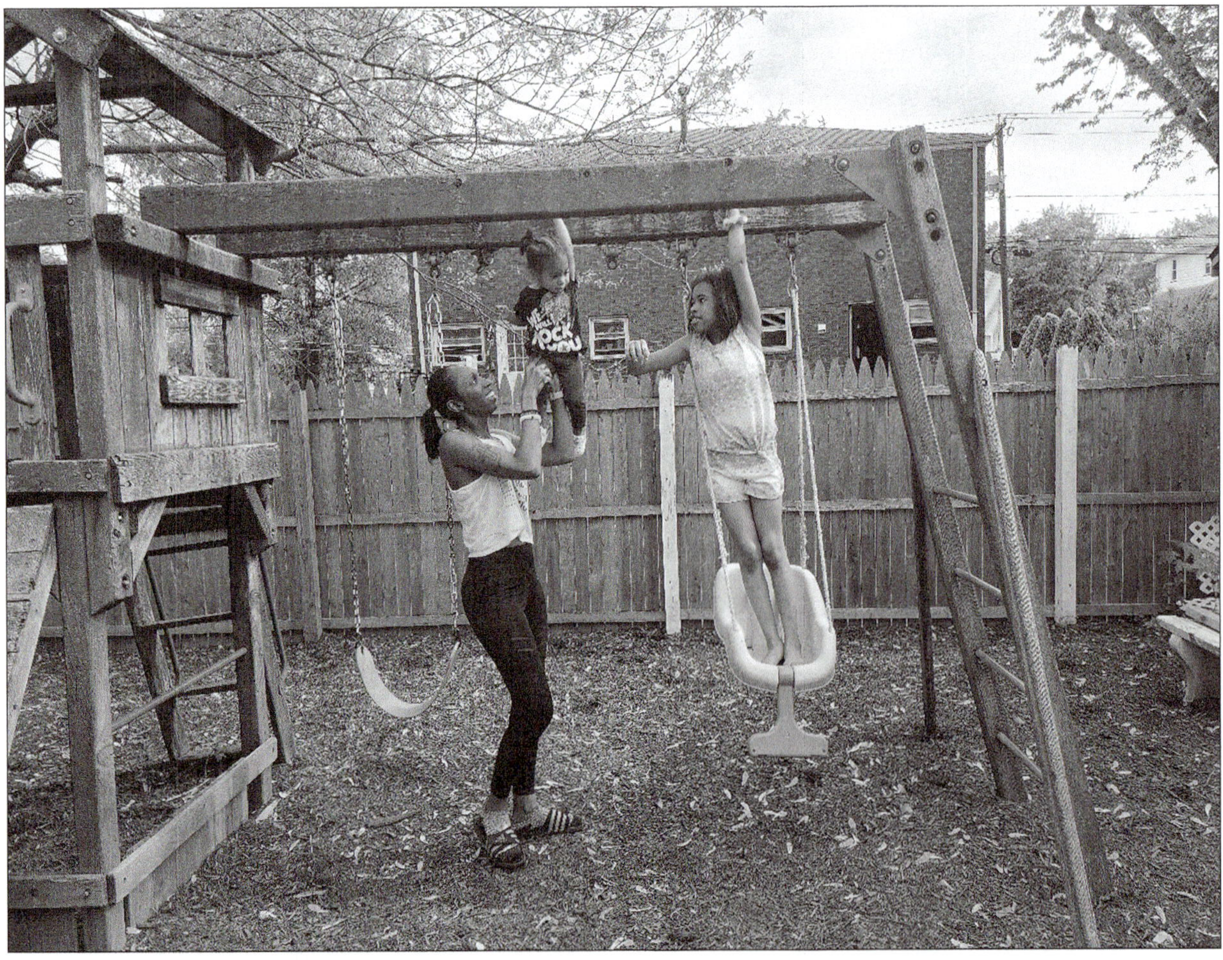

Source. J. Wilson. Used with permission.

FIGURE 5.4. Sometimes trying a new activity can be a little scary, but this little boy is still moving forward.

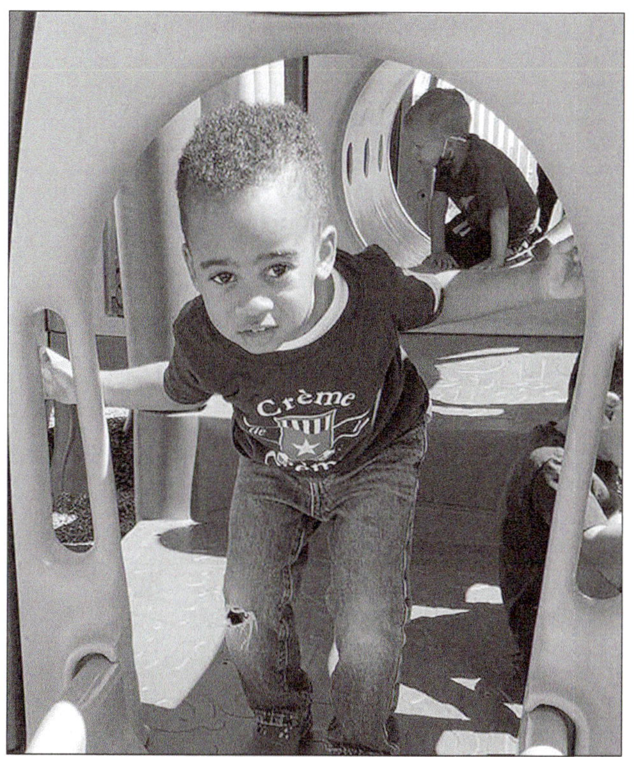

Source. B. DeVeaux. Used with permission.

Activity Synthesis as a Precursor to Occupational Synthesis

Generally, activity synthesis takes place before occupational synthesis and sets the stage for the client to be able to achieve occupational synthesis. How do occupational therapy practitioners use activity synthesis as part of their intervention? Where does activity synthesis fit into the overall intervention process? As presented in this chapter, activity synthesis involves and encompasses a complex reasoning process guided by theory that directs practitioners in the therapeutic use of activities. From a practitioner's perspective, activity synthesis begins with conceptualizing the activities that the client wants or needs to perform. Responsibility rests with the client and the practitioner to determine the importance of these actions, to think them through carefully, and to use this knowledge as the foundation for activity synthesis. This activity analysis ensures that the practitioner understands the components of the activity in the context of the client's performance of that activity.

Before analysis or synthesis can take place, the practitioner needs to understand the client and the client's life situation, which involves understanding their personal goals, desires, interests, capacities, and limitations. Personal goals and desires may depend on context, and in some cases, they may be those of the family (such as with a child) or society (when something is considered socially appropriate) and may depend on certain life circumstances. Much of this information can

FIGURE 5.5. Synthesizing the occupation of gardening by sitting instead of standing or kneeling and using a raised planter.

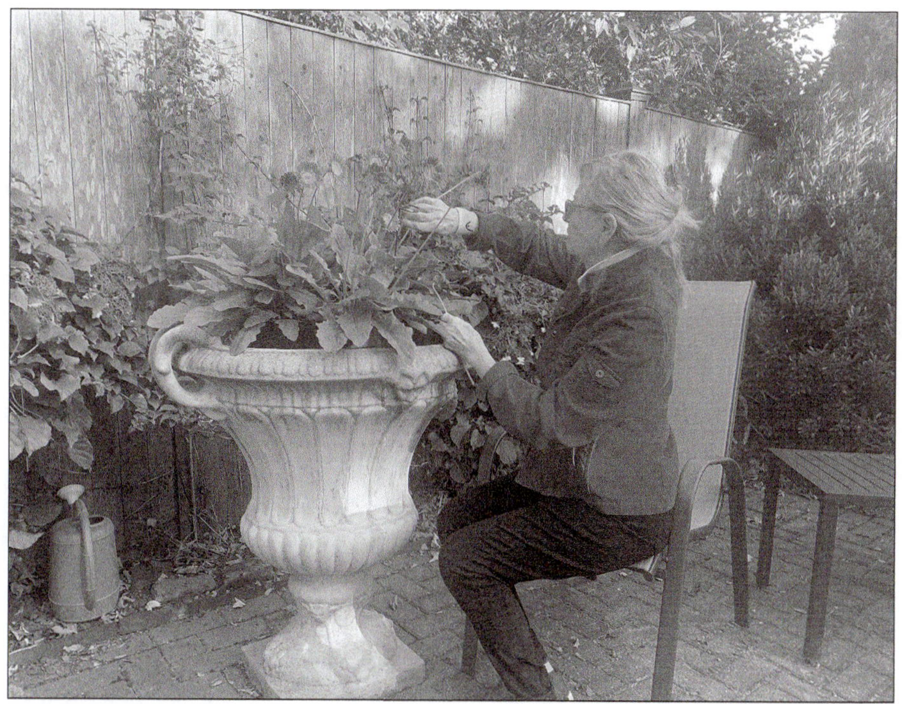

Source. P. Kramer. Used with permission.

be obtained from the occupational profile. Goals, interests, and desires then need to be explored within the context of capacities and limitations. Although one may have the desire to achieve something, the capacity for that achievement may not be present. Activities can be synthesized effectively only when the practitioner has a clear understanding of the client, the client's life, and all the contextual factors that affect the client (Figure 5.5).

Once the occupational therapy practitioner has selected the appropriate activity, they complete an activity analysis, taking into consideration the client's strengths and areas of concern. With experience, this process becomes fairly automatic. The activity analysis gives the practitioner a rudimentary understanding of the tasks that might need to be adapted or changed. With this information, the practitioner can begin to create modifications to the activity that meet the client's needs. The practitioner synthesizes an activity that is consistent with the theoretical perspective, model, or frame of reference that has been selected to guide their interventions with the client. The theoretical perspective determines how and in what ways an activity is synthesized in the therapeutic situation. By putting together the practitioner's professional knowledge, the expected outcomes of the therapeutic process, and the client's (or family's) mutually agreed-on goals, synthesis begins.

Identifying and defining potential goals for the intervention require collaboration and sometimes negotiation between the client and the occupational therapy practitioner. This process goes two ways, and each person involved brings their own perspective. The practitioner brings a clinical understanding of the client's condition from a medical and a psychosocial perspective and an understanding of the potential sequelae of the disease, and the client brings their unique sense of self and an understanding of their own aspirations, along with the drive to achieve the goal. Together, the practitioner and client develop goals that define the course of treatment and outcomes of the intervention. Ideally, the goals should relate to the occupations that the client currently wants to carry out or will engage in at some point in the future, and they should be oriented to the ability to participate in life and society. If the activities that are synthesized are meaningful to the client, the client will be more likely to incorporate them into daily life as part of an occupational synthesis.

Process of Activity Synthesis in Occupational Therapy

In occupational therapy, once the activity analysis is complete and the theoretical perspective has been considered, the activity synthesis begins. This process starts with defining the key elements of the activity because an activity can only be adapted so much until it becomes a different activity. For example, is it still cooking if no stove or heat is involved? Is it still football if a round ball is used and there is no running on a field? When key elements are no longer present, the activity is not the same. Once the activities are created and presented to the client, the occupational therapy practitioner observes the client's performance and continually reanalyzes it to adapt and resynthesize the activity to meet the client's changing needs and to move toward the end goal. The process is ongoing and dynamic.

Sometimes the activity needs to be reconstructed or synthesized in a different way to allow the client to be successful. The dynamic nature of this process confirms that analyzing the activity is not enough; understanding how one can construct or synthesize an activity is equally as important. It is important to remember that synthesis involves more than just the activity itself; it involves the personal meaning of the activity. As discussed earlier, occupational therapy practitioners view synthesis in the context of the person as an occupational being. They should ask the following questions:

- Who is the person involved in the intervention process?
- What occupations are important to this person?
- How do specific purposeful activities relate to these occupations?
- Does the accomplishment of an important activity build on or allow this person to engage in meaningful occupations at their current stage of life or in the future?

The creative process of synthesis requires a thorough understanding of the activity, as well as a visualization of the goal and the desired end product for the client.

All activities used by occupational therapy practitioners are viewed within the context of the occupations that are critical to the client. Practitioners use an organized conceptual approach to activity synthesis, based on the understanding of the occupation and its component activities. They view each activity as a whole, and the activity analysis is done to break it into its component parts. The final step in the process is to synthesize or re-create the activity with changes, modifications, or adaptations to allow the client to achieve success in the task.

Traditional activity synthesis requires that the chosen activity be reconstructed, incorporating the client's therapeutic goals, areas of strength and limitations, and the therapeutic relationship. The activity is reconfigured in ways that allow the client to approach it with minimal fear of failure and with greater potential for success. At this point, the activity synthesis can be used for two purposes: (1) as an evaluative tool to see how the client responds to the modifications or (2) as part of the intervention process. More specifically, activity synthesis can be used to evaluate occupational performance within a context, teach a new skill, refine a skill, or maintain a client's functional status or performance ability. These applications of activity synthesis are discussed later in this chapter.

Activity synthesis is based on the occupational therapy practitioner's skills and abilities and an understanding of the theoretically based guidelines (e.g., models of practice, theoretical orientations, guidelines for intervention, or frames of reference) that the practitioner has determined to be the most appropriate for the client, the client's needs, and the context in which the activity will occur. Throughout the process of activity synthesis, the practitioner is guided by the theoretical framework. Thus, activities are used, adapted, modified, or created within the parameters of the chosen theoretically based guidelines (see Case Example 5.1). Activity synthesis involves complex processes of adapting and grading activities, modifying activities, and creating new activities that are based on theory. These processes are discussed in the following sections. Although we address each process individually as though it were distinct from the others, in practice, one or more processes may be used in combination; they may overlap and are not mutually exclusive. As with learning any process, it is important that each component be appreciated and understood in relation to the others. By understanding the components of activity synthesis, one can attain a distinct knowledge of the whole process of synthesis (Case Example 5.1).

Adapting and Grading Activities

Adapting and grading activities are critical to activity synthesis. ***Adaptation*** involves a change to the environment or the

CASE EXAMPLE 5.1. Mustafa: Two Frames of Reference to Address Difficulties With Fine Motor Coordination

Mustafa, age 6 years, is referred to occupational therapy for a fine motor coordination problem. After a comprehensive evaluation, the occupational therapist assigns Mustafa to an occupational therapy assistant to implement a program to develop hand and fine motor coordination by working with manipulative tools that strengthen muscles. Thus, a sensorimotor frame of reference is chosen. The therapist selects this frame of reference because she has determined that Mustafa has poor muscle strength and limited experience with fine motor activities. The intervention is carried out within the context of Mustafa's classroom because that is his natural context at school.

After meeting Mustafa, reviewing the recommendations, and discussing the frame of reference with the therapist, the occupational therapy assistant uses activity analysis and synthesis to develop activities for Mustafa. These activities involve Mustafa using an adapted pencil for writing and paper with raised lines that will give him increased sensory feedback. Another activity is spending playtime using interlocking building blocks. In addition, the assistant observes the computer-based activities used in the classroom. After careful analysis of these computer-based activities, the assistant decides to replace Mustafa's keyboard with one that provides more resistance. The keyboard is also raised so that Mustafa must use more shoulder motion while working on the computer.

If a different frame of reference is chosen—for example, one based on play (thus, the context is outside the classroom)—and theories of psychosocial development are chosen to address Mustafa's fine motor problems, a very different approach would be used. The focus would be on Mustafa's personal choice of toys or play activities, his personal interests, an analysis of purposeful activities, and synthesis of activities in response.

For instance, the occupational therapy assistant observes that Mustafa enjoys the game Connect 4™. The objective of the game is to pick up small disks and put them into a vertical form to line up four in a row. An understanding of theories of psychosocial development suggests that a 6-year-old boy can relate to others in a cooperative manner. Therefore, the occupational therapy assistant involves Mustafa in creating a way to play Connect 4 while working on his fine motor skills.

After adapting the game to address some of Mustafa's fine motor needs, the assistant plays the game with Mustafa. Together, they then decide to place the disks under various heavy objects around the room, forcing Mustafa to develop his strength by lifting the objects. Mustafa might also be positioned prone over a bolster, using his nondominant hand to balance and support his weight and his dominant hand to place the disks into the vertical form. Guided by the psychosocial development frame of reference, the assistant has synthesized an activity to engage Mustafa in terms of his developmental stage and to be therapeutically valuable for his particular motor needs.

After this initial activity helps Mustafa develop more strength, the assistant uses cooperative play again to work on another, more demanding fine motor task, such as constructing with interlocking building blocks. The assistant then engages another child in cooperative play with Mustafa to develop both his psychosocial and fine motor skills while the children work together on a building project.

activity, not a change to the person. Adaptation of activities, therefore, involves changing the environment in which the activity occurs or the activity itself rather than working to bring about change in the person doing the activity. When a client is having difficulty with a task or activity, the activity is adapted for the client.

Adaptation begins with an activity analysis that considers the capabilities of the client, the activity, and the context in which it will be done. After analyzing the activity or completing the activity analysis, the occupational therapy practitioner uses the theoretical perspective to decide how the activity should be adapted or changed to meet the client's abilities, allowing the client to perform the activity in a specific context.

For instance, using a simple rehabilitation frame of reference, the occupational therapy practitioner might modify the activity by having the client grip an implement (e.g., spoon with a built-up handle), changing the client's position when engaging in the task, or having the client sit down during the activity for energy conservation. If the therapist selects a different theoretical perspective, a different adaptation would be involved, which might involve a more complicated process in which the defining features of the activity are changed. An example is using the Ecological Model of Human Development, in which the environment of the task is significantly changed or the utensils used in the task are changed completely. Theoretical perspectives thus guide the adaptation and modification process.

Grading is a common way to adapt an activity. Although it is a basic principle in learning theory, occupational therapy practitioners almost universally use grading. For this reason, it is critical to think about grading and how it is used in the context of specific theories that guide intervention. ***Grading*** can involve simplifying the activity, making the activity more complex, modifying the sequence or physical nature of the activity, or modifying the amount of time taken to complete the activity. Simplifying the activity (also known as *grading the activity down*) entails making the activity easier for the client in some way, whereas *grading the activity up* entails making it more difficult or more complex (Figure 5.6).

For example, for a child who is learning how to undress themself (using an acquisitional frame of reference, which is a theory-based intervention based on teaching and learning), grading might involve having the parent roll down the sock from the heel and then having the child pull it off or opening the child's pants fastenings and then having the child remove the pants. In this case, the parent does part of the task and allows the child to do the remainder. Once the child has accomplished a certain segment of the task, the task can be made slightly more difficult, thus grading the activity up. Another way of grading a dressing task down while still using an acquisitional frame of reference is to buy the child pants with an elastic waist rather than those with a fastening at the waist or to use pullover shirts rather than ones with buttons. Grading a task down allows the client to feel successful and gain confidence so that they are willing to try more difficult tasks, develop skills, or build on a previously acquired level of skill.

FIGURE 5.6. Grading an activity up: Once a child can climb on stable surface, she adapts her skills to walk across a rope ladder, a less predictable surface.

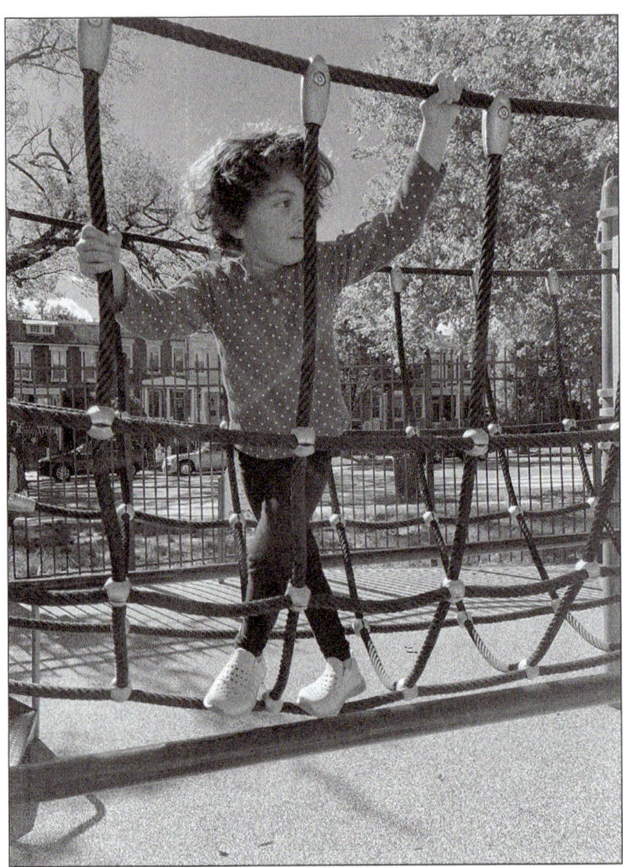

Source. D. Joseph. Used with permission.

Whether adapting or grading an activity, theoretical perspectives often require that the physical nature of an activity be changed by modifying the materials used in a task. From a developmental perspective, this usually involves changing

EXERCISE 5.1. Adaptation

Think about an activity that you adapted to make your life easier. Reflect on the adaptation and the answers to the following questions:

- How did you deduce an appropriate adaptation?
- How did knowing your capabilities and having a goal in mind influence the way you approached the adaptation?
- Did your first attempt at adaptation yield a successful outcome?
- What theoretical orientation did you use? (You may not have consciously been thinking of a theory, but whatever made you change the activity in the way you did is probably a theoretical orientation.)
- Can you make a different adaptation to the same activity using a different theoretical orientation?
- Did the adaptation of the activity affect the overall occupation? How?

EXERCISE 5.2. Adapting an Activity From a Biomechanical Perspective

Observe children playing on a playground or in a schoolyard. Select one activity in which they are engaged and answer the following questions:

- What is the overall occupation in which the child is engaged?
- What are three activities that are component activities of this occupation?
- Using a biomechanical perspective (i.e., increasing strength, endurance, and range of motion), how could you adapt one of these activities so that a child in a wheelchair could participate?
- What supports are needed? What barriers, if any, are present?

EXERCISE 5.3. Adapting an Activity Using a Sensory Integration Frame of Reference

Observe a child in a therapy session in which the occupational therapy practitioner is using a sensory integration frame of reference.

- What is the overall occupation in which the child is engaged?
- What are three activities that are component activities of this occupation?
- Using a sensory integration frame of reference, how could you adapt a playground activity for a child with tactile defensiveness?
- What supports might be needed? What barriers, if any, might be present?

EXERCISE 5.4. Grading an Activity

Select an activity at which you are very competent but that one of your classmates cannot perform. For example, if you are good at playing chess or the piano or at baking, then select a student who does not know the rules of chess, how to play the piano, or how to bake. Develop and carry out one teaching session with your classmate that involves grading in some way.

- How did you grade the activity so that the other person would have a positive learning experience?
- How difficult was this to do?
- How would you have graded the activity for a different person?

an activity so that it is easier for the client to complete it successfully. For example, if a child has difficulty building with wooden blocks because they are hard to grasp and lift, then smaller foam blocks can be provided that are lighter and easier to handle. This adaptation is grading the activity down so that the child can participate in block building despite having limited strength and grasping ability.

Modifying Activities

Activity modification involves not changing the activity, but rather changing the way the activity is done. It can be seen as a specific type of grading that focuses on the activity itself. The purpose and goal of the activity remain the same, but the sequence or time requirements of the tasks encompassed in the activity may be altered. Modifying the sequence of tasks involves changing the order in which tasks are done so that the person can engage in the task more successfully. This approach is frequently used for energy conservation.

For example, to avoid energy depletion caused by repeatedly walking up and down stairs or back and forth across a room, the client can change the order in which they perform ADL tasks to minimize the walking involved in the task. Modifying the activity may also mean moving the venue of the activity—for example, from the kitchen counter, where the client has to stand to complete the activity, to the kitchen table, where the client can complete the task while sitting down (see Figure 5.1). Another type of activity modification may involve ***scaling the activity*** (i.e., breaking the activity into smaller parts that are required to complete the activity as a whole), such as finishing part of a puzzle (e.g., the outer edges of the puzzle or one section) rather than the whole puzzle or completing the puzzle in smaller sections.

Performance (i.e., the actual doing) of tasks involves a time factor. To be functional, tasks have to be done either within a specified amount of time or at a certain time of the day or year. For example, spending a half hour putting on a shirt would not be considered functional. In the therapeutic environment, the timing of a task can be modified or the time requirements of a task or activity can be changed; initially, a client can take longer to complete a task without repercussions, or dressing can be done in the middle of the day rather than earlier in the morning. Once a client has mastered an activity within an extended timeframe, the time allotted can be decreased.

For example, when working with a child who is learning to put on a pullover shirt, the child might at first be allowed to take as much time as they need. Slowly, a time requirement would be added. After the child has mastered putting on the pullover shirt in a reasonable amount of time, they might be asked to put on a shirt with buttons in the same amount of time, even though this shirt is more difficult to put on. In this way, the task of putting on a shirt is made more challenging using ***layered adaptation,*** which involves placing increasing

EXERCISE 5.5. Altering the Sequence of Tasks

Think about the way in which you accomplish the self-care occupation of getting ready for work or school in the morning. List the tasks that you do to accomplish each activity (e.g., personal hygiene, selecting clothes, dressing). Select one activity. Consider how you would change the sequence of the task if you had to get ready in a shorter period of time one morning. What would be different? Would you leave out some tasks? Would you shorten certain task components (i.e., forgo ironing a shirt, not drying your hair, donning slip-on shoes vs. lace-up boots)?

EXERCISE 5.6. Altering the Timing of Tasks

Select an activity at which you are very skilled. Determine how much time it takes you to do the activity from beginning to end. Divide the time in half and do the activity. How is your performance affected? Now, double the time it takes to do the activity. How is your performance affected?

How long does it take you to shower or bathe? In the clinic, clients will often vastly underestimate the time necessary to properly complete a showering activity after injury. They only think of time physically in the bathtub or shower area, forgetting all of the preparatory steps before and necessary steps after cleansing the body to bring the activity to completion so that they can go about their day dressed and ready. List the tasks necessary from start (dressed in night clothes and completely dry) to finish (bathed and redressed), and compare the list with your initial response to the question.

demands in the activity as the client attains greater skill to improve performance. Each successive task is more complex than the previous one, with time becoming a more important component of the task at each stage.

Creating New Activities

The most complex type of activity synthesis is creating new activities. This synthesis occurs after the occupational therapy practitioner evaluates a client and determines the areas that require intervention. In response to the evaluation, the practitioner creates an activity specifically for the client. Two types of activity can be created: (1) one that arises from the practitioner's responsibility to present a specific level of challenge to the client and thus promote growth and (2) one based on the client's occupational needs and desires to move to a certain level of performance. Note that creating an activity is different from adapting and grading or modifying an existing activity because an entirely new activity emerges from the process.

Some theoretical perspectives and frames of reference, such as neurodevelopmental treatment and sensory integration, require the occupational therapy practitioner to be the creator of the majority of activities during the intervention, placing responsibility for defining the activities on the practitioner. The role of the practitioner is based on the client's therapeutic needs and interests, and the goal of the frame of reference is to promote future growth and skills. From these perspectives, client collaboration is secondary to client need and is derived from engagement in the task. If the client does not engage, the practitioner must create new activities to entice them into the activity. Therefore, the practitioner's understanding of the client is critically important, and their ability to create activities that engage the client is paramount to the success of these perspectives.

In other theoretical perspectives and frames of reference, such as occupational adaptation and occupational performance, the creation of activities comes from the client and is based on the client's perceived occupational needs rather than their therapeutic needs. This synthesis requires the practitioner to have skill, creativity, and an in-depth understanding of the client. The resultant activity is based on an understanding of the client's interest, problem areas, and goals. It is not based on activity analysis but is very much client centered and has a just-right fit, perfectly related to the client's needs and abilities.

In this type of synthesis, the nonhuman environment plays a very important role. The occupational therapy practitioner, therefore, must gain an understanding of both the human environment (i.e., the people in the environment who are important to the client) and the nonhuman environment (i.e., important things surrounding the person that are not live human beings) of the client's occupations to create activities that will engage the client. The *OTPF–4* describes different aspects of the environment that should be considered when

EXERCISE 5.7. Creating a New Activity

Identify a skill, such as playing catch with another person. How would you create an activity to teach someone to play catch? Determine what your goal would be for a client in this situation, such as "the client will be able to catch the ball three times in a row." You can choose any new activity and devise how you will use an activity to teach the skill and identify goals for the client in that situation. This involves both activity synthesis and activity analysis (see Chapter 3, "Occupation and Activity Analysis").

EXERCISE 5.8. Creating New Activities With Defined Developmental Goals

You have been hired to work in a new occupational therapy practice with limited space and materials. All you have in the treatment environment are two chairs and one small table. In the supply closet, you have access to masking tape, a box of different colored 1-inch blocks, and two boxes of 12 (unsharpened) pencils. You have two children scheduled for the day: Alex, a 21-month-old boy with developmental delays who functions at about a 9-month developmental level, and Maria, a 3-year-old girl with cerebral palsy, athetoid type. Outline one to two goals for an individual treatment session with Alex and then with Maria. Develop an activity (or activities) for each child using only the materials, supplies, and environment as described.

EXERCISE 5.9. Creating New Activities Based on the Client's Needs

Tanisha is a 10-year-old girl who wants to go to her local school's dance program. She has attention deficit hyperactivity disorder. Identify the skills required to attend dance classes and what abilities would be necessary to interact appropriately with peers and instructors. Identify the theoretical perspective that you are using. Create several activities that will help Tanisha develop the skills and control she needs to attend a dance class.

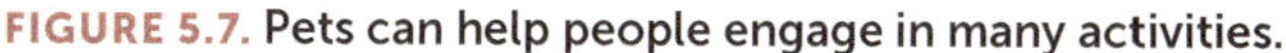

FIGURE 5.7. Pets can help people engage in many activities.

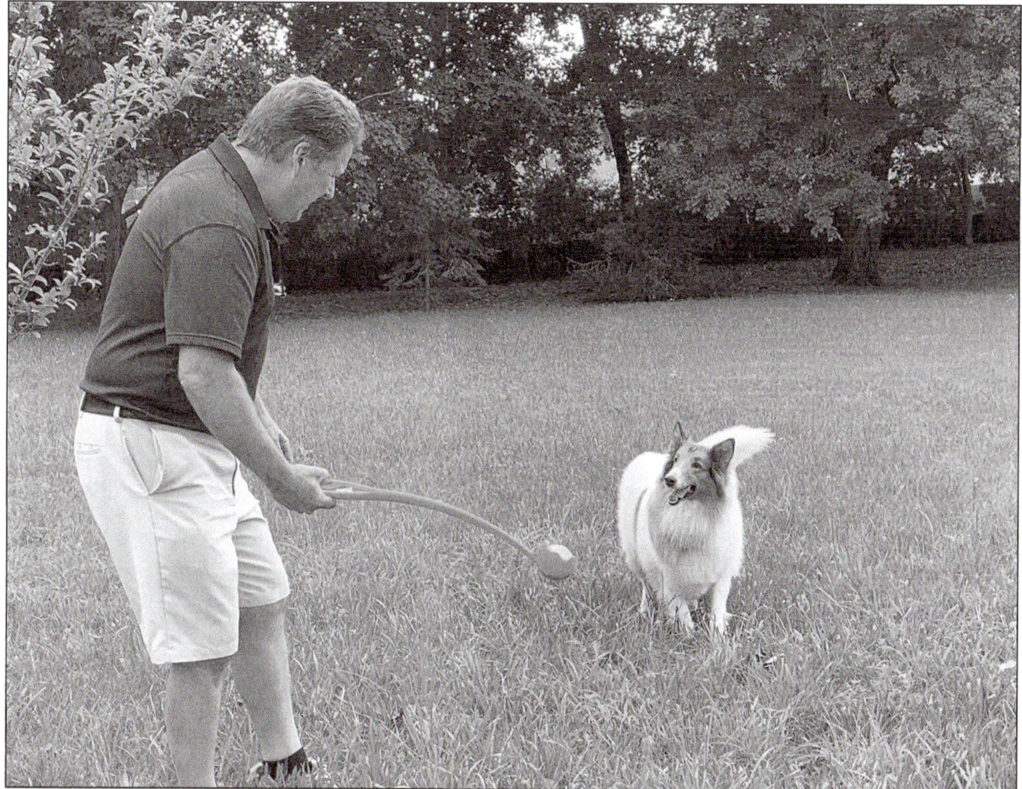

Source. P. Kramer. Used with permission.

CASE EXAMPLE 5.2. Carol: Multiple Sclerosis

Carol, age 62 years, has advanced multiple sclerosis, uses a wheelchair, and has resided in a long-term-care facility for the past 4 years. Before she came to the facility, she raised several dogs who were very important to her and to whom she referred as family members. The facility has a pet therapy dog, and the occupational therapist found that Carol was much more likely to come to group activities when the therapy dog was present. This understanding of Carol's interest in pets allowed the therapist to design appropriate and meaningful activities for her to engage in.

synthesizing treatment activities. One example might be if the client has a special pet. The practitioner can involve the care of that pet in an aspect of the intervention, and the client will then be more likely to engage in the intervention (see Figure 5.7 and Case Example 5.2).

Importance of Activity and Occupational Synthesis to Intervention

Both activity synthesis and occupational synthesis are critical to the intervention process. People sometimes automatically adapt the way they do a task with little problem. For example, if a person is accustomed to preparing a meal standing at the kitchen counter and then develops limited standing tolerance, they can move meal preparation to the kitchen table and complete the task sitting down. This modification is likely to be acceptable. However, it is often difficult for people to modify the way they do particular tasks, especially when they have done those tasks in a particular way for many years. Even if completing the task in the usual manner becomes very difficult, change may still be hard to accept because the modification alters the value of or enjoyment they derive from the original task.

CASE EXAMPLE 5.3. Francesca: Adapting an Activity

Francesca, age 78 years, had collected porcelain figurines over the years, and she liked to clean them periodically. These objects, however, were displayed on high shelves and could be reached only by standing on a ladder. Francesca conducted her own analysis of the task: As a senior citizen, she was aware that climbing on a ladder was no longer an acceptable option because she risked falling and injuring herself. She considered hiring someone to do the task for her, but her collection was personally valuable to her, and she did not like the thought of other people handling the objects, fearing that they might break them. Francesca eventually decided to hire someone to help her, but she was very clear in defining this person's role in the task. The helper was to climb the ladder to retrieve the objects from the shelf, and Francesca would then clean them and direct how they were to be put back in place. This modification of the activity allowed Francesca to have control over the task and to handle the things that were precious to her while avoiding the aspects of the activity that were difficult and potentially dangerous. Francesca synthesized the revised activity in a way that was both acceptable to her and safe.

For example, when cleaning the home becomes too difficult, some obvious options include accepting assistance from others, cleaning one room each day until all the rooms are done, or doing minimal cleaning. Some of these options may be more acceptable than others. For some people, getting assistance with cleaning is perfectly acceptable, whereas for others it is not a suitable alternative because cleaning has been one of their life's occupations and a source of enjoyment and pride. For others, doing minimal cleaning may not be acceptable because of their personal beliefs or their desired standard of living. Case Example 5.3 illustrates how a client successfully adapted an activity to make it easier in a way that retained the value of the occupation.

Other Uses of Activity and Occupational Synthesis in Intervention

Up to this point, we have discussed activity synthesis as an intervention process used to bring about change in the client and how it relates to occupational synthesis. We have stressed the use of theoretical grounding in this process. Indeed, occupational therapy practitioners typically think about activity synthesis as a tool for treating a client. It is generally a medium that is used to improve function once a deficit has been identified.

Activity synthesis can, however, be used creatively in many more ways. As discussed previously, it can be used as a tool with which to evaluate client performance. We also noted earlier in the chapter that activity synthesis may be used to teach a new skill, refine a skill, or maintain functional status or performance abilities. In the next sections, we present the use of activity synthesis for these various purposes. Note that occupational synthesis is an end product and does not occur at this point in the process.

Evaluating Performance

Activity synthesis can assist the therapist in evaluating a client's performance in a certain context. For example, the therapist may first see whether a child can zip a zipper on a doll or on an ADL board, a piece of equipment used for practicing specific tasks related to ADL skills that includes things such as buttons, zippers, and ties. The therapist may then observe the child's ability to close a zipper on their own coat. It may be easy for a child to close a zipper on an ADL board or on a doll, but it is critical for the child to be able to also close a zipper on their own coat, generalizing this skill to real-life contexts.

The therapist uses the synthesized activity to evaluate the child's performance in two different contexts and by doing so can determine whether intervention is necessary and how to proceed with it. Even if the child can zip a zipper on an ADL board, if the child is unable to zip a zipper on their own coat, intervention would be warranted, because this skill is required in daily life (see Case Example 5.4).

Teaching New Skills

Using learning theories, an occupational therapy practitioner can use synthesis to teach new skills. This type of intervention is what an occupational therapy practitioner typically thinks of as activity synthesis. How does one devise a meaningful activity that will assist the client in developing new skills? Expanding on a previous example, when teaching a child to fasten clothes, a practitioner may first work on the skill in isolation with a doll and then make it more complex by applying the skill to the child's own clothes. In this situation, the practitioner is identifying the skills that need to be developed and creating activities that will promote the development of that new skill (see Case Example 5.5).

Refining Skills

The occupational therapy practitioner can use activity synthesis to refine a skill, again using learning theories. Once the client has attained a basic skill level, the practitioner can enhance and modify the activity to make the required skill level more complex. For example, when working on the development of communication skills with a client with psychosocial dysfunction,

CASE EXAMPLE 5.4. Dipesh: Developing Social Skills

An occupational therapist works with **Dipesh,** age 12 years, on developing social skills. In a group, Dipesh role-plays purchasing a shirt in a department store. During the role-play, the therapist observes how Dipesh handles himself, whether his verbalizations are appropriate, and his ability to count out money to pay for the item. On the basis of Dipesh's ability to perform well in the role-playing situation, the therapist takes Dipesh into an actual store and observes his abilities in a real context rather than in a simulated situation. The therapist uses these observations to give feedback to Dipesh and develop a plan for intervention. The therapist can also point out to Dipesh the differences between his performance in the simulated situation and in the real-life activity to help set mutually acceptable goals for performance.

CASE EXAMPLE 5.5. Tasha: Money Management

Tasha has difficulties with money management skills. She does not watch how much money she gives the store clerk and does not count her change. The occupational therapist uses an acquisitional frame of reference and sets up a simulated store. Tasha must pay for everything she wants from the store, and the therapist works with her on money management within this context. Periodically, the therapist takes on the role of consumer and has Tasha take on the role of the cashier. Through this activity, the therapist can begin to teach Tasha the basic skills necessary to develop the ability to manage her money.

CASE EXAMPLE 5.6. Jose: Developing Social Skills

Jose is developing social skills through role-playing in a group. He then tries the skills he has acquired in a real situation. The occupational therapist works with Jose on refining his behavior in the real-world environment. Is he dressed appropriately to go out shopping? Does he appear well groomed? Does he make eye contact with store personnel? Can he ask questions appropriately if he needs to find an item? Can he handle money responsibly? What are some additional areas to explore in terms of his development of social skills?

the practitioner might first work on having the client say "good morning" to others in a protected environment, such as a therapy group. They may then work on asking people how they are and finally move on to conducting an entire conversation. Although the activity synthesis might begin in a protected environment, eventually the skills would need to be tested in the real world to determine their viability (see Case Example 5.6).

As skills increase, the occupational therapy practitioner continually resynthesizes the activity to increase the demands on the client and refine the skills necessary for application in a real-life situation. In essence, by grading up the task, the practitioner is synthesizing the activity to meet new goals.

Maintaining Functional Status or Performance Abilities

Synthesis can be used to maintain a person's functional status or performance ability. For example, if a client has been working on strengthening her hands and has achieved an acceptable level of strength, then it would be incumbent on the occupational therapy practitioner to work with her to synthesize activities that would maintain that level of strength after completion of the intervention. The practitioner would first need to understand the client's meaningful occupations and then, with this understanding, synthesize activities that would be of sufficient interest to her so that she would want to continue doing them to maintain her hand strength (see Case Example 5.7).

If the activities devised by the occupational therapy practitioner hold no interest for the client, the client will have little incentive to do them. Therefore, synthesized activities should incorporate purposeful and meaningful occupations for the client to maximize their success. For example, squeezing therapy putty may not be a meaningful occupation for one particular person, but molding clay into animals that could be given as gifts might be more purposeful, enjoyable, and rewarding. In

CASE EXAMPLE 5.7. Alicia: Maintaining Functional Status

Alicia had difficulty with range of motion in her shoulder from a fall. She received an inpatient occupational therapy intervention and was very responsive to treatment. At discharge from the hospital, she was able to raise her arm to 180° of shoulder flexion. During a subsequent home visit, the occupational therapist observed that Alicia's range of motion had decreased slightly from the measurements noted on the hospital discharge paperwork. The therapist suggested that, to work on improving shoulder motion, Alicia place the dishes that she uses most often on the second shelf of her cabinets so that she will have to reach for them. Alicia agreed to the embedded exercise in daily activities because this occupational approach was more meaningful to her. Thus, the maintenance of her shoulder range became a part of her everyday life (Figure 5.8).

FIGURE 5.8. Woman placing objects on a higher shelf to maintain shoulder motion.

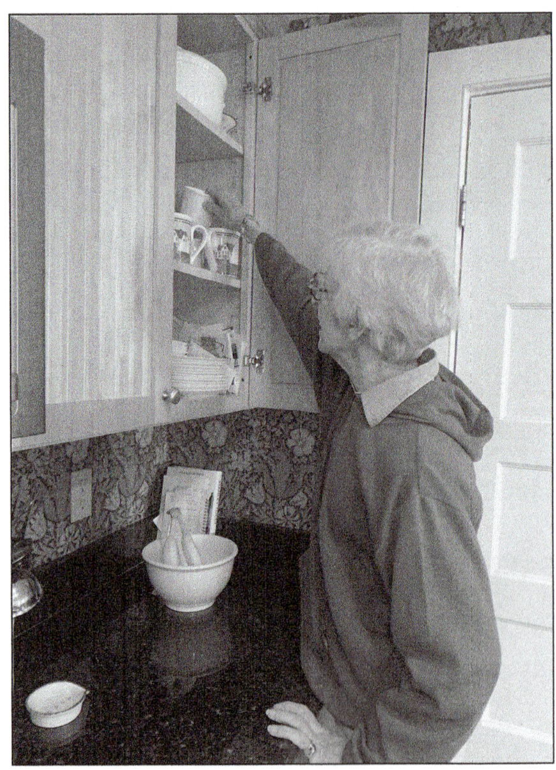

Source. P. Kramer. Used with permission

this case, activity synthesis is based on a fundamental assumption of the profession—that is, engagement in occupations keeps people healthy—rather than basing activities purely on a theoretical perspective.

Another fundamental assumption of occupational therapy is that people are more likely to engage in activities that are meaningful to them; in other words, these activities are important to the individual. Therefore, the primary goals of the occupational therapy process are not only to assist people in finding meaningful occupations but also to help them maintain and restore function so that they can use the activity synthesis process to continue to engage in meaningful occupations. When people can explore how they can continue to engage in their chosen occupations, occupational synthesis can occur. Knowing the client and what the client enjoys are critical to synthesizing an activity that will be successful for the client and result in occupational synthesis.

Activity and Occupational Synthesis for Health Promotion

Occupational therapy practitioners have a responsibility that goes beyond intervention, to promote health in the client

EXERCISE 5.10. Synthesizing Activities Using a Frame of Reference

You have just been assigned to a new client, Luis. He has right hemiplegia secondary to a cerebrovascular hemorrhage. Before this trauma, Luis was an engineer in the U.S. Air Force. He had a very high-level position designing logistics equipment for aircrafts. His hobbies included building things for his family and home, using multiple means (e.g., woodworking tools, electrical and mechanical devices). Choose a frame of reference or a theoretical perspective, and synthesize several therapeutic activities for Luis using your chosen perspective and incorporating his personal interests and preferred occupations. Describe the activities and how they reflect both Luis's interests and the theoretical perspective you have chosen.

EXERCISE 5.11. Activity Synthesis in a Clinical Environment

Observe an intervention with a client. Identify the activities that have been synthesized for that client. Try to identify the theoretical perspective or perspectives that provide the foundation for this intervention.

- Have the activities been synthesized specifically for this particular client?
- Can you determine the client's investment in the intervention?
- Are you observing artful practice?
- Is the intervention client centered?
- How could the intervention better touch on the concepts of artful practice and client-centered practice?
- How can this activity can become part of the client's occupational synthesis?

through activity and occupational synthesis. Activity synthesis is an important tool in this process; the practitioner takes an active role with the client, collaborating on the development of activities to promote health. Synthesis may be necessary to develop activities that will assist the client in meeting goals and optimizing their lifestyle. With the knowledge the practitioner has gained about the client's desires and abilities, the practitioner can assist in the development of specific activities that maintain physical, mental, and social health. For example, through activity synthesis, the practitioner can customize activities that promote continued engagement in social activities that reinforce participation. Synthesis may take many forms. For example, the practitioner may encourage the client to participate in a community center or may customize a home exercise program to address specific needs and abilities. Successful activity synthesis is necessary for successful occupational synthesis to occur.

Artful Practice and Synthesis

In the synthesis of activities with the intent to move toward occupational synthesis, practitioners need to be artful in developing or choosing an activity that suits the client's needs from both a functional perspective and a personal perspective (Case Example 5.8). If both needs and interests are not met, the activity will not be successful in achieving its goal (Case Example 5.9). Occupational therapy practitioners should first take time to learn about the client, focusing on who they are as a person and their strengths and limitations. The use of the occupational

CASE EXAMPLE 5.8. LinMae: Hand Weakness

LinMae has weakness in her hands from peripheral neuropathy. When first synthesizing activities for LinMae, the occupational therapy practitioner considered using modeling clay as a therapeutic intervention, but LinMae showed no interest in working with clay. She enjoys baking and has expressed an interest in learning to bake bread. Baking bread requires kneading the dough, which will strengthen LinMae's hands. Thus, not only does baking bread have therapeutic value, but it is a meaningful and pleasurable activity for LinMae. The successful merging of therapeutic and personal needs specific to LinMae and her situation will lead to a more successful intervention.

CASE EXAMPLE 5.9. Morris: Mild Fine Motor Problems and Endurance Issues

Morris is a 62-year-old man who was a naval engineer and enjoyed designing and making mechanical objects. He has emphysema and is experiencing some mild fine motor problems. He needs to increase his standing tolerance, so his occupational therapist has had him putting together nuts and bolts while standing. The therapist devised the activity without discussion with Morris. Morris was very upset, finding the activity demeaning and way below what he was used to creating. He told that therapist that he did not see the purpose of occupational therapy and did not want to continue.

- The therapist thought they were considering Morris's background, but what else should the therapist have considered?
- What do you think the therapist should do now?

Read Case Example 5.8 and this case and discuss the differences in the way the cases were handled.

profile (AOTA, 2020a; see Chapter 4, "The Occupational Profile") can be very helpful in achieving this level of understanding of the client. Then it is possible for the practitioner and the client together to identify goals for the intervention.

This step may involve analyzing the client's performance in particular activities and identifying performance components that interfere with successful completion of the task. It may also involve some aspect of client education to increase the client's awareness of how performance can be improved or how performance in a particular area is affecting overall functioning. It is critically important, however, that this step be as collaborative as possible so that the intervention can be truly client centered. Activities are then synthesized with the client so that they are meaningful and beneficial to them. Unless the activity is viewed as meaningful to the client, it will not result in occupational synthesis.

Remember that synthesis is not concrete: It does not follow a step-by-step process and may instead be undertaken in many different ways. Several elements, however, should be present for synthesis to be successful: developing an understanding of the client, including what is important to this person and their meaningful occupations; analyzing activities to determine how deficits interfere with performance; and selecting a theoretically based guideline for intervention. In addition, together with the client, the practitioner must be creative in identifying or devising activities that will help the client overcome their deficits or develop the skills necessary for successful task performance.

Development of Artful Practice

Activity and occupational synthesis require artful practice on the part of the occupational therapy practitioner. ***Artful practice*** is the skill with which the practitioner engages the client in occupations and activities, so that the therapeutic intervention is meaningful and enjoyable to the client. It is not something that can be easily taught. It is, in part, the product of experience because one does not start out as an artist. One must learn how to use and play with materials, study techniques, develop skill with the materials, and, finally, develop a personal style. It also involves an element of creativity. Some people are by nature more creative than others. These factors are the prerequisites to becoming an artist. Once a person possesses the basic skills, they may be able to develop into a creative artist, but it will take time, practice, and experience.

The same is true of occupational therapy practitioners. Initially, practitioners start out as novices with a technical or procedural understanding of what is going on with the client. They develop into experts with time and experience. They learn how to get to know the client quickly, how to collaborate easily with the client, and, ultimately, how to use this information to synthesize meaningful occupations for the client. This takes time and practice. Some practitioners develop this skill more quickly; others take more time to be able to effectively use synthesis.

The ***clinical reasoning process***—or the way in which the practitioner makes decisions on the basis of understanding theory, disabilities or functional deficits, and the client and their particular needs—is part of the art of practice. The practitioner develops reasoning skills in different areas and at various stages of professional development. Some aspects of clinical reasoning include scientific reasoning, professional reasoning, narrative reasoning, pragmatic reasoning, and ethical reasoning (Schell & Schell, 2017). The various types of reasoning are presented in depth in Chapter 6, "Professional Reasoning and Reflective Practice." Clinical reasoning skills develop as practitioners mature and reflect on their cumulative experiences. Engaging in the practice of synthesis, however, involves more than just reasoning; it involves understanding the client, their life, and oneself as a practitioner.

Experience contributes to one's ability to be an artful occupational therapy practitioner, enhancing knowledge of different approaches, a range of techniques and responses, and greater interaction skills. Having a multitude of experiences with clients with various disabilities and cultures, in various settings, expands one's repertoire. The knowledge gathered from experience provides the practitioner with options for both intervention and interaction. Such knowledge is not necessarily an expansion of theoretical knowledge but an expansion of practical knowledge and a greater understanding of the self and the human condition—all elements essential to successful and appropriate occupational synthesis. Practitioners need to be reflective (Cohn et al., 2010; Robertson, 2012; Schell & Schell, 2017; Schell & Gillen, 2018; Schön, 1983) and have a clearer understanding of the role of activity and occupation in the client's life. They are then able to creatively match the intervention with the client's needs. The art thus comes from within the practitioner, not from a greater understanding of theory (Schell & Schell, 2017). It is a personal and professional development, not exclusively an intellectual development.

Although the art of practice does not come from an understanding of theory, it does occur within a theoretical context. Occupational therapy practitioners should choose a theoretical framework or frame of reference that will fit the setting, the client's needs, and their own knowledge base. The choice of a theoretical approach and, therefore, the synthesis of activities requires consideration of all these things and should not be based on one area alone. Understanding one's personal and organizational context and the client's context is critical to effective practice.

Artful occupational therapy practitioners create the circumstances in which occupational synthesis can take place within the client. Practitioners use their knowledge of human occupation integrated with theoretically based guidelines for intervention to provide activities and opportunities that the client then uses for occupational synthesis. The definitive goal of occupational therapy is to provide interventions that will produce the desired changes so that service recipients can participate in occupations that are personally meaningful to them (Hinojosa et al., 2003, 2017, 2020). The practitioner facilitates opportunities for occupational synthesis to occur by providing interventions that are relevant and creative. Again, this synthesis requires a successful interaction between the practitioner and the client so that the practitioner can gain an understanding of activities that are meaningful to the client, and the client can give feedback to the practitioner on the effectiveness of specific activity syntheses.

Artful practice requires that occupational therapy practitioners experience the treatment with the client, using their own life experience as an active agent of change to design and implement treatments (Weinstein, 1998). As proposed by Schön (1983), the art of professional practice is built on a professional's reflection in action. Practitioners reflect on what is happening during treatment to continually modify, adapt, or change the intervention process or activity. Beyond the theoretical perspective, practitioners experience what is happening and are prepared to change strategies spontaneously. This skill does not occur automatically, but a seasoned practitioner may make it look like it does; it is based on both reflection and experience. In some cases, modifying the activity, the environment, or the interaction will help to make the intervention more effective for the client. In other situations, when the predicted changes do not occur, practitioners decide to change the intervention. In these cases, the artful practitioner proposes new hypotheses and implements the revised intervention. These modifications ensure that occupational synthesis takes place and that interventions are also related to the client's future occupations.

When interventions are relevant, the client can easily transpose the tasks or activities into their real-life occupations. Relevant interventions are judged by two criteria. First, are they appropriate for addressing the client's deficits? Second, are they pertinent to the client's life situation (e.g., goals, values, culture, lifestyle) as defined by the client?

Occupational synthesis is more likely to take place when the occupational therapy program is client centered. The practitioner begins this process by considering the following four questions to ensure that the client's life situation is being addressed:

1. Do I understand the client's occupations?
2. Do I respect the client's occupations and personal choices?
3. Do I understand the client's activity patterns, particularly in relation to their cultural background, and do I respond to them appropriately?
4. How do my client's occupations influence other people in their daily lives?

Hinojosa (2003) identified five additional questions that an occupational therapy practitioner might ask after reflecting on this first set of questions, to assess the relevance of their interventions as it relates to the concept of occupation:

1. Are my interventions reflecting an understanding of the client's life situations and their culture?
2. Have I developed an understanding of my client's occupations through discussions with them?
3. Have I considered clear ethical reasoning when developing my interventions within the context of the client's goals, priorities, and capacities?
4. Are my interventions based on an understanding of how the client defines their own personal occupations?
5. Do my interventions result in enabling the client to engage in occupations and increase their life satisfaction?

Developing meaningful intervention using synthesis is a complex process. The occupational therapy practitioner usually starts by developing an understanding of activity synthesis. At the same time, the practitioner is developing sound clinical reasoning skills and, over time, gaining experience to develop the art of practice. With experience, the practitioner comes to understand the client's critical role and their unique situation. This process is not necessarily linear, but it is one that takes time and experience to develop. Once this development has occurred, occupational synthesis can be facilitated, and intervention becomes truly meaningful. The ultimate demonstration and most valuable outcome of occupational synthesis can be observed when the client engages in their chosen occupations in real life rather than in an artificial clinical situation.

Summary

Activity synthesis is a common phenomenon that occurs in everyday life. People have many occupations and activities that are meaningful to them, and they modify and change activities so that they can perform them successfully. Activity synthesis appears simple precisely because it is so commonplace, yet most people do not synthesize activities in an organized and systematic manner, in the way that occupational therapy practitioners approach this task. True activity synthesis is a complex skill, but very little has been specifically written about it.

Occupational therapy practitioners approach activity synthesis from an organized theoretical perspective that requires an understanding of activity analysis, the underlying components, the context, and the client. Moreover, activity synthesis is strongly influenced by the frame of reference chosen for intervention and the artfulness of the practitioner. Activity synthesis is a critical function of the practitioner and is used frequently in day-to-day interventions. If used successfully in the intervention process, activity synthesis should result in occupational synthesis within the client.

In this chapter, we proposed that occupational therapy practitioners need to understand the importance of activity synthesis and how to approach it in an organized and systematic manner. Through effective activity synthesis and an understanding of the client, practitioners will be able to help the client develop true occupational synthesis to enhance the client's everyday life. Then, through ongoing development, reflection, and experience, practitioners become both skillful and artful in developing interventions that are meaningful for the client.

References

American Occupational Therapy Association. (2020a). *AOTA Occupational Profile Template*. https://www.aota.org/~/media/Corporate/Files/Practice/Manage/Documentation/AOTA-Occupational-Profile-Template.pdf

American Occupational Therapy Association. (2020b). Occupational therapy practice framework: Domain and process (4th ed.). *American Journal of Occupational Therapy, 74*(Suppl. 2), 7412410010. https://doi.org/10.5014/ajot.2020.74S2001

Barthel, K. A. (2020). A frame of reference for neuro-developmental treatment. In P. Kramer, J. Hinojosa & T. Howe (Eds.), *Frames of reference for pediatric occupational therapy* (4th ed., pp. 205–246). Wolters Kluwer.

Bass, J., Baum, C. M., & Christiansen, C. H. (2017). Person–Environment–Occupation–Performance Model. In J. Hinojosa, P. Kramer, & C. Royeen (Eds.), *Perspectives on human occupation: Theories underlying practice* (2nd ed., pp. 161–182). F. A. Davis.

Baum, C. M., Christiansen, C., & Bass, J. (2015). The Person–Environment–Occupation–Performance (PEOP) Model. In C. Christiansen, C. M. Baum, and J. Bass (Eds), *Occupational Therapy: Performance, participation, and well-being* (4th ed., pp. 49–55). Slack.

Cohn, E. S., Schell, B. A. B., & Crepeau, E. B. (2010). Occupational therapy as a reflective practice. In N. Lyons (Ed.), *Handbook of reflective inquiry* (pp. 131–157). Springer.

Creighton, C. (1992). The origin and evolution of activity analysis. *American Journal of Occupational Therapy, 46,* 45–48. https://doi.org/10.5014/ajot.46.1.45

Dunn, W. (2017). The Ecological Model of Occupation. In P. Kramer, J. Hinojosa, & C. Royeen (Eds.), *Perspectives on human occupation: Theories underlying practice* (2nd ed., pp. 207–236). F. A. Davis.

Dunn, W., Brown, C., & McGuigan, A. (1994). The ecology of human performance: A framework for considering the effect of context. *American Journal of Occupational Therapy, 48,* 595–607. https://doi.org/10.5014/ajot.48.7.595

Dunn, W., Brown, C., & Youngstrom, M. J. (2003). Ecological model of occupation. In P. Kramer, J. Hinojosa, & C. Royeen (Eds.), *Perspectives in human occupation: Participation in life* (pp. 222–263). Lippincott Williams & Wilkins.

Fidler, G. S. (1948). Psychological evaluation of occupational therapy activities. *American Journal of Occupational Therapy, 2,* 284–287.

Fidler, G. S. (1996). Life-style performance: From profile to conceptual model. *American Journal of Occupational Therapy, 50,* 139–147. https://doi.org/10.5014/ajot.50.2.139

Fidler, G. S., & Velde, B. (2002). *Lifestyle performance: A model for engaging the power of occupation*. Slack.

Forsyth, K., & Kielhofner, G. (2003). Model of Human Occupation. In P. Kramer & J. Hinojosa (Eds.), *Perspectives in human occupation: Participation in life* (pp. 45–86). Lippincott Williams & Wilkins.

Gellert, K. M., & Pulaski, K. H. (2021). Functional uses of neurological approaches: Rood, Brunnstrom, proprioceptive neuromuscular facilitation, and neuro-developmental treatment. In D. P. Dirette & S. A. Gutman (Eds.), *Occupational therapy for physical dysfunction* (8th ed., pp. 717–734). Wolters Kluwer.

Hinojosa, J. (2003). Occupation and continuing competence: Part II. *OT Practice, 8,* 11–12.

Hinojosa, J., Kramer, P., & Howe, T.-H. (2020). The structure of the frame of reference: Moving from theory to practice. In P. Kramer & J. Hinojosa (Eds.), *Frames of reference for pediatric occupational therapy* (4th ed., pp. 3–19). Wolters Kluwer.

Hinojosa, J., Kramer, P., & Luebben, A. J. (2010). The structure of a frame of reference. In P. Kramer & J. Hinojosa (Eds.), *Frames of reference for pediatric occupational therapy* (3rd ed., pp. 3–22). Lippincott Williams & Wilkins.

Hinojosa, J., Kramer, P., Royeen, C. B., & Luebben, A. (2003). The core concept of occupation. In P. Kramer, J. Hinojosa, & C. B. Royeen (Eds.), *Perspectives in human occupation: Participation in life* (pp. 1–17). Lippincott Williams & Wilkins.

Hinojosa, J., Kramer, P., Royeen, C. B., & Luebben, A. (2017). The core concept of occupation. In P. Kramer, J. Hinojosa, & C. Royeen (Eds.), *Perspectives on human occupation: Theories underlying practice* (2nd ed., pp. 23–38). F. A. Davis.

Hunt, D. (1997). *The magician's tale*. Putnam.

Kielhofner, G. (2008). *Model of Human Occupation: Theory and application* (4th ed.). Lippincott Williams & Wilkins.

Law, M. (2002). Participation in the occupations of everyday life. *American Journal of Occupational Therapy, 56,* 640–649. https://doi.org/10.5014.ajot.56.6.640

Law, M., Baptiste, S., Carswell, A., McColl, M. A., Polatajko, H., & Pollock, N. (2019). *The Canadian Occupational Performance Measure* (5th ed., rev.). CAOT Inc.

Missiuna, C., Mandich, A. D., Polatajko, H. J., & Malloy-Miller, T. (2001). Cognitive Orientation to daily Occupational Performance (CO–OP): Part I—Theoretical foundations. *Physical and Occupational Therapy in Pediatrics, 20,* 69–81.

Mosey, A. C. (1981). *Occupational therapy: Configuration of a profession*. Raven Press.

Mosey, A. C. (1996). *Applied scientific inquiry in the health professions: An epistemological orientation* (2nd ed.). American Occupational Therapy Association.

Nelson, D. L. (1997). Eleanor Clarke Slagle Lecture—Why the profession of occupational therapy will flourish in the 21st century. *American Journal of Occupational Therapy, 51,* 11–24. https://doi.org/10.5014/ajot.51.1.11

Nelson, D. L., & Jepson-Thomas, J. (2003). Occupational form, occupational performance, and a conceptual framework for therapeutic occupation. In P. Kramer, J. Hinojosa, & C. B. Royeen (Eds.), *Perspectives on human occupation* (pp. 87–155). Lippincott Williams & Wilkins.

O'Brien, J. C. (2017). Model of human occupation. In P. Kramer, J. Hinojosa, & C. Royeen (Eds.), *Perspectives on human occupation: Theories underlying practice* (2nd ed., pp. 93–136). F. A. Davis.

Piaget, J. (1963). *Psychology of intelligence*. Littlefield, Adams.

Polatajko, H. J. (2007). Canadian Model of Occupational Performance and Engagement (CMOP–E). In E. A. Townsend & H. J. Polatajko (Eds.), *Enabling occupation II: Advancing an occupational therapy vision for health, well-being, and justice through occupation* (pp. 22–36). CAOT Publications.

Polatajko, H. J. (2017). Cognitive Orientation to daily Occupational Performance approach. In P. Kramer, J. Hinojosa, & C. Royeen (Eds.), *Perspectives on human occupation: Theories underlying practice* (2nd ed., pp. 183–206). F. A. Davis.

Robertson, L. (2012). *Clinical reasoning in occupational therapy: Controversies in practice*. Wiley-Blackwell.

Schaaf, R. C., Schoen, S. A., Smith-Roley, S., Lane, S. J., Koomar, J., & May-Benson, T. A. (2010). Frame of reference for sensory integration. In P. Kramer & J. Hinojosa (Eds.), *Frames of reference for pediatric occupational therapy* (3rd ed., pp. 99–186). Lippincott Williams & Wilkins.

Schell, B. A. B., & Gillen, G. (2018). Professional reasoning in practice. In B. A. B. Schell & G. Gillen (Eds.), *Willard & Spackman's occupational therapy* (13th ed., pp. 482–497). Wolters Kluwer.

Schell, B. A. B., & Schell, J. W. (2017). *Clinical and professional reasoning in occupational therapy* (2nd ed.). Wolters Kluwer

Schön, D. A. (1983). *The reflective practitioner: How professionals think in action*. Basic Books.

Smith-Roley, S., Schaaf, R. C., & Balthzar-Mori, A. (2020). Ayres Sensory Integration® frame of reference. In P. Kramer, J. Hinojosa, & T.-H. Howe (Eds.), *Frames of reference for pediatric occupational therapy* (4th ed., pp. 87–158). Wolters Kluwer.

Weinstein, E. (1998). *The nature of artful practice in psychosocial occupational therapy* (Unpublished doctoral dissertation). School of Education, New York University.

6

Professional Reasoning and Reflective Practice

CAROLYN A. UNSWORTH, PHD, BAppSci(OccTher), GCTE, OTR, MRCOT, FOTARA

CHAPTER HIGHLIGHTS

- Decision making and reasoning
- Professional and clinical reasoning and reflective practice
- Experience and expertise
- Tacit knowledge and what we can say
- Professional reasoning, experience, and expertise
- Professional reasoning in occupation-focused practice

KEY TERMS AND CONCEPTS

• advanced beginners • chart talk • clinical reasoning • competent therapists • conditional reasoning • decision making • embodied knowledge • expertise • expert therapists • generalization reasoning • Gibbs' Reflective Cycle • Hierarchical Model of Clinical Reasoning • interactive reasoning • intuition • language • narrative reasoning • nonpropositional knowledge • novices • personal knowledge • pragmatic reasoning • procedural reasoning • professional craft knowledge • professional reasoning • proficient therapists • propositional knowledge • reflection • reflection-in-action • therapist with the three-track mind • two-bodied practice • worldview

Introduction

While meeting with Carol, her Level II fieldwork supervisor, Anya, who is studying occupational therapy, starts to explain the outcome scores she gave her client, 82-year-old Nathan. Anya's supervisor interrupts her, saying, "And tell me your reasoning, Anya." Anya freezes, and her mind goes blank: "What is she thinking, and why?"

This chapter examines the concept of *professional reasoning*. Using the case study of Anya, Nathan, and Carol (see Case Example 6.1), the chapter provides examples of how occupational therapy practitioners can confidently talk through their own reasoning. Specifically, it explores what professional reasoning is and differentiates this type of thinking from decision making. Briefly outlined are the history and development of clinical and professional reasoning in occupational therapy, followed by details on the different modes or "tracks" of reasoning. Concepts that relate closely to professional reasoning in occupational therapy, such as embodied knowledge, intuition, and worldview are explored. The chapter ends with a presentation of information on how professional reasoning grows as a student progresses from novice to expert as well as a description of a model to enhance reflective practice to promote professional reasoning.

Clinical and Professional Decision Making and Reasoning

As a profession, occupational therapy practitioners share certain patterns of thinking and ways of viewing the world that

CASE EXAMPLE 6.1. Introduction to Anya (Occupational Therapy Student), Nathan (Client), and Carol (Supervisor)

Anya is an occupational therapy student undertaking a Level II fieldwork at a local acute care facility. She has been at the facility for 2 weeks, and her supervisor, **Carol,** has asked her to assess a new client, **Nathan,** and then score his baseline status using the Australian Therapy Outcome Measures for Occupational Therapy (AusTOMs–OT; Perry et al., 2004) outcome measure.

Anya learned about the AusTOMs–OT at school and knows it is an evidence-based global outcome measure used internationally, with more than 25 publications supporting its use (Perry et al., 2004; Unsworth & Duncombe, 2014; Unsworth et al., 2009, 2015, 2018). She downloaded the scales and manual for free (see https://austoms.com/) and knows that she will score Nathan on admission to the service and at discharge by choosing a small number of scales from the 12 available that reflect the goals she and Nathan set.

The 12 scales are "Learning and Applying Knowledge," "Functional Walking and Mobility," "Upper Limb Use," "Carrying Out Daily Life Tasks and Routines," "Transfers," "Using Transport," "Self-Care," "Domestic Life—Home," "Domestic Life—Managing Resources," "Interpersonal Interactions and Relationships," "Work, Employment, and Education," and "Community Life, Recreation, Leisure, and Play." For each scale selected, Anya will make four ratings, which is one for each health domain of impairment, activity limitation, participation restriction, and distress/well-being. The ratings are made on an 6-point scale—from 0 (most severe impairment/does not perform/unable to fulfil roles/high concern) to 5 (no impairment/no limitations in performing/no restriction in fulfilling roles/able to cope) with half points—with lower values suggesting poorer outcomes (Unsworth & Duncombe, 2014).

Carol, Anya's supervisor, is an expert occupational therapist with more than 20 years of experience working in acute care, rehabilitation, and community-based occupational therapy. This morning, Carol asked Anya to conduct the typical initial interview and score Nathan on the FIM™ (Functional Independence Measure; Uniform Data Set for Medical Rehabilitation, 1997). In the afternoon session just completed, Anya and Nathan set goals together, and Anya and Carol are meeting so that Anya can score Nathan on the AusTOMs–OT as well as provide her professional reasoning to support her scoring. Anya had previously used the AusTOM–OT at another fieldwork experience, so she has knowledge of using and rating the scales.

set them apart from other health professionals. Many aspects of this thinking are shared with specialists from other disciplines, but it is the way the thinking is constructed and how this reasoning enables our theories of human occupation to be practiced that are unique to our profession. The *Oxford Dictionary* defines *reasoning* as "the intellectual faculty by which conclusions are drawn from premises . . . [and] to reach conclusions by connected thought" (Thompson, 1995, p. 1144). But this definition does not do justice to professional reasoning in occupational therapy and what it means in practice. ***Professional reasoning*** is the reflexive thinking associated with engaging in a client-centered professional practice. This includes the thinking associated with planning to be with the client (and their caregivers and other health professionals); when the practitioner is with the client; and afterward, when reflecting on time with the client. Professional reasoning occurs in the context of a practitioner's empathy, intuition, judgment, and common sense. As professionals, our reasoning is constantly evolving in response to a multitude of both concealed and explicit influences and contextual factors. Professional reasoning unfolds in the practitioner's mind in narratives and images.

When occupational therapy practitioners began to write about the thinking processes of therapists in the 1980s and 1990s (see, e.g., Cohn, 1989; Fleming, 1991; Rogers & Masagatani, 1982), the clinical focus of occupational therapy at the time shone through, and the term ***clinical reasoning,*** which refers to how practitioners think through and understand a clinical problem, was widely adopted. However, occupational therapy practice is conducted in a wide range of environments, such as schools, prisons, and community settings, and with individuals and groups of clients who may be experiencing social or politically related occupational disruption or deprivation. Hence, "clinical" reasoning may not always provide the best description of how practitioners think because the environments in which they practice are not always clinical. Furthermore, clients do not always present with clinical problems. Consequently, Schell (Schell & Schell, 2018) and others (Unsworth & Baker, 2016) have begun to use the term "professional" reasoning, which has been formally adopted in the American Occupational Therapy Association's (2020) *Occupational Therapy Practice Framework: Domain and Process* (4th ed.) and is the term adopted in this chapter.

In other clinical fields, such as medicine, thinking processes have also been widely studied but often with a different focus. For example, in medicine, the focus on accessing physicians' thinking processes is firmly on decision making and, more specifically, on diagnostic decision making. Unlike the "thinking" process that underpins reasoning, ***decision making*** is concerned with weighing up options to arrive at a choice. Although a treating physician may make diagnostic decisions, treatment decisions are increasingly being made by the medical team, client, and their family using a shared decision-making model (Hoffmann et al., 2016). Although occupational therapy practitioners also make many decisions, such as the choice of an upper-limb splint or a licensing recommendation following a driver assessment (Harries et al., 2018), and work collaboratively with clients on care-related decisions, such as goal setting and housing decisions on discharge, the focus of this chapter is on the reasoning processes that are constantly in use and that underpin every aspect of therapy. To gain a full appreciation of this area of the literature, see the seminal tests on decision making—for example, those by Dowie and Elstein (1988) or more recent works by Sox et al. (2013).

Professional Reasoning: History and Theory Development

Clinical reasoning—the original term in occupational therapy—was formally born through the publication of a special issue on the topic in the *American Journal of Occupational Therapy* in November 1991 and the subsequent book by Cheryl Mattingly and Maureen Hayes Fleming (1994) called *Clinical Reasoning: Forms of Inquiry in a Therapeutic Practice*. However, this important area of inquiry had been developed over many years. Rogers and Masagatani published the first study on professional reasoning in occupational therapy in 1982 that examined the reasoning process of 10 occupational therapists undertaking client evaluations. The following year, Rogers (1983) delivered an Eleanor Clarke Slagle lecture that focused

FIGURE 6.1. Hierarchical Model of Clinical Reasoning in occupational therapy.

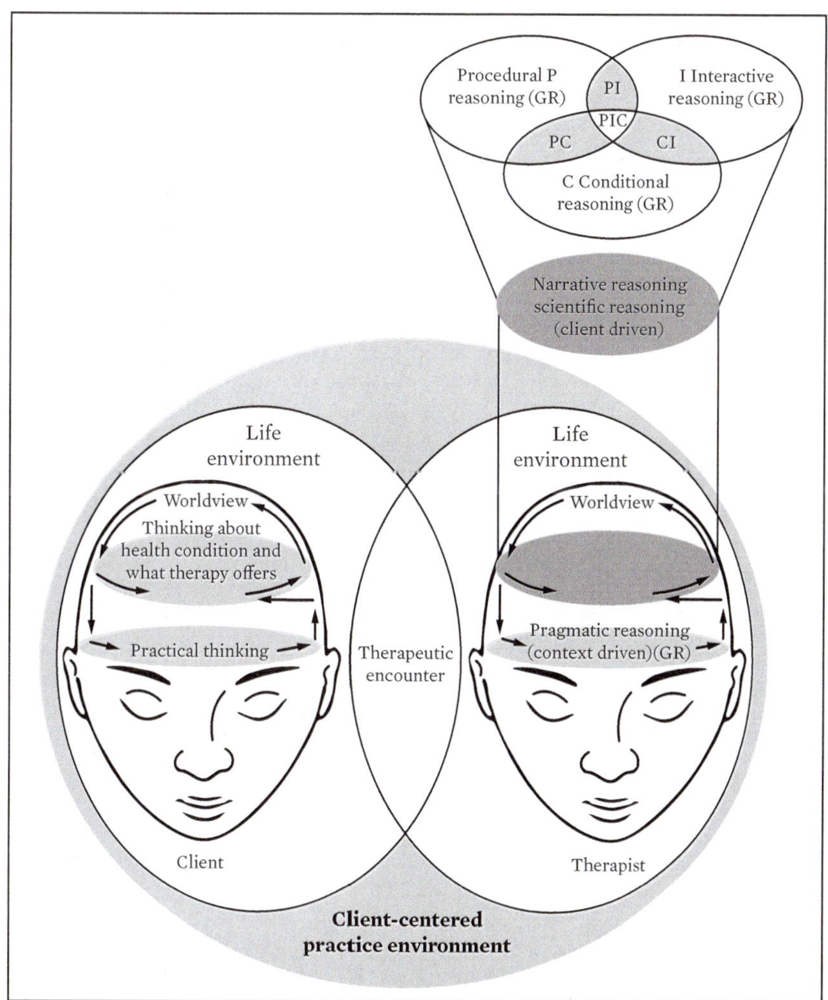

Source. Unsworth (2004, 2017). Copyright (2017) by Elsevier. Used with permission.

EXHIBIT 6.1. Modes of Thinking in the Hierarchical Model of Clinical Reasoning

Worldview

This is a global outlook on the world and underlying assumptions about life and reality. Worldview is not a type of reasoning but influences all professional reasoning and, therefore, is at the top of the Hierarchical Model. Worldview encompasses an occupational therapy practitioner's ethics, values, beliefs, faith, and spirituality.

Ethical Reasoning

This is the thinking that accompanies an analysis of a moral dilemma, whereby one moral conviction or action conflicts with another, and then generating possible solutions and selecting action to be taken.

Scientific Reasoning	Narrative Reasoning
This draws on a biomedical approach. When reasoning scientifically, practitioners use the language of chart talk. The process of hypothesis generation and testing generally is referred to as "hypothetico-deductive reasoning."	This draws on a phenomenological approach to understanding the person and involves storytelling and story creation. The emphasis is on understanding the meaning of the person's illness and illness experience.

Diagnostic Reasoning	Procedural Reasoning	Interactive Reasoning	Conditional Reasoning
This is used to identify underlying impairments or occupational performance issues, define desired outcomes, set goals, and develop interventions or solutions. It provides a basis for procedural reasoning.	These are the reasoning processes associated with the evaluations and interventions to be used with a person. This reasoning refers to all the "procedures" of therapy. Procedural reasoning includes systematic data collection, hypothesis formation and testing, and the reasoning that underpins interventions.	This is used when communicating, both verbally and nonverbally. Interactive reasoning is used to engage the person in therapy; consider the best approach to communicate with the person; understand who the person is and the problems from the person's point of view; individualize therapy; convey a sense of acceptance, or trust, or hope; break tension through the use of humor; build a shared language of actions and meanings; and monitor how the treatment session is going. It is referred to as the "underground practice" because practitioners often describe what they do with the person but generally not their interactions.	This is one of the more complex models to understand and has several components. A practitioner is reasoning conditionally when thinking about the person's condition and how change is conditional on participation in the therapeutic process. The therapist is reasoning conditionally when thinking temporally about the person's past, present, and future to understand what the person's life was like before the therapy encounter, what it is like now, and what it could be in the future. Hence, this type of reasoning is used when trying to understand what is meaningful to the person in their social and cultural world.

Pragmatic Reasoning

This is reasoning related to personal, organizational, political, and economic contexts. Hence, this thinking is about how therapy can operate given resource and financial considerations, such as who is funding therapy. Personal context includes the reasoning surrounding the therapist's own motivation, negotiation skills, repertoire of therapy skills, and life knowledge and assumptions.

Source. Adapted from Unsworth (2021).

on this topic. Rogers argued that therapists should be able to describe why they had undertaken the therapy delivered, but they were not skilled in doing so. However, the value and importance of being able to articulate how and why occupational therapy is conducted and the goal to achieve its outcome were universally recognized by the profession, and since the mid-1990s, almost every occupational therapy program (if not all programs) across the globe teach professional reasoning to students, and more than 140 studies have since been reported across the literature (Unsworth & Baker, 2016).

Although several developing theories of professional reasoning are described in Schell and Schell's (2018) book on the topic, relatively few empirical studies have been conducted to test and advance the field. This chapter draws on Unsworth's ***Hierarchical Model of Clinical Reasoning,*** (2004, 2021), which is grounded in empirical research (Chaffey et al., 2012; Mitchell & Unsworth, 2005; Unsworth, 2001, 2004, 2005) and reflects contemporary thinking in occupational therapy. The model is presented in Figure 6.1, and key terms from the model are further explored in Exhibit 6.1.

This model explores how the occupational therapy practitioner and client interact in a client-centered practice environment to promote optimal occupational engagement. The client has their own worldview, which sits at the top of their hierarchy and affects (often unrecognized) their thinking about their health condition and what therapy can offer them. The client's thinking also occurs in the context of the base-level practical thinking around what can be achieved given real-world constraints, such as their time and budget. Similarly, the professional reasoning processes of the practitioner are influenced and colored, often without insight, by worldview and overarching ethical reasoning. The middle layer of the hierarchy is where occupational therapy practitioners use their skilled reasoning processes, which are driven by both scientific and narrative reasoning. The Venn diagram (see Figure 6.1) shows the overlapping relationship between the key modes of reasoning, which are discussed in a later section in this chapter: procedural, interactive, and conditional reasoning with generalization reasoning imbedded in each. Practitioners also reason pragmatically concerning how they can achieve therapy goals with the client within the context of the service, environment, funding models, and the personal contexts of the client and the clinician (Unsworth, 2013, 2021).

A Framework and Language for Professional Reasoning in Occupational Therapy

To explicate the often tacit (i.e., knowing more than we can say) professional reasoning process of occupational therapy practitioners, a language is required. ***Language*** enables phenomena to be shared, examined, promoted, and also learned by students and novices as explored later in this chapter. In this section, language is given to foundational concepts in professional reasoning, including a simple way of how we "know things," the two-bodied practice, and the therapist with the three-track mind. Furthermore, the two main modes of communication used by practitioners—narrative reasoning and chart talk—are described.

To set the scene, first we need to consider that the "knowledge" we have in occupational therapy (and, of course, all knowledge) takes two main forms: (1) ***propositional knowledge,*** or knowing "that;" and (2) ***nonpropositional knowledge,*** which is also called *procedural knowledge,* or knowing "how" (Burgin, 2016; Stanley & Williamson, 2001). Propositional knowledge is derived through research and scholarship and is published in texts through which the knowledge is shared. This knowledge has been peer reviewed and ratified by the field. In contrast, nonpropositional knowledge is derived through practice and incorporates ***professional craft knowledge,*** which is the practical knowledge gained through "doing" therapy, and ***personal knowledge,*** which is knowledge tied to an individual's reality or experience. Nonpropositional knowledge enables us to "do" the practice of occupational therapy and, in many cases, expert occupational therapy practitioners simply "do," which makes it is difficult for students and novices to access this knowledge and therefore learn. This is because much of this knowledge is tacit. Hence, providing a language and framework for professional reasoning helps students to use but, importantly, to move beyond propositional knowledge to embrace, understand, and use nonpropositional knowledge.

Two-Bodied Practice

As part of the foundation study of clinical reasoning in occupational therapy, Mattingly (1994) noted that, as a profession, occupational therapy sits comfortably between two practice spheres: a (1) biomedical sphere in which the body is viewed as a machine and (2) phenomenological sphere in which the client's experience of their health and circumstance is examined, and the focus is on the lived body. In occupational therapy, it makes perfect sense for these two spheres to coexist because of occupational therapy's holistic view of a person managing their occupations in the context of a health-related or sociopolitical context. In Mattingly and Fleming's (1994) text, this phenomenon is described as the ***two-bodied practice.***

Narrative Reasoning and Chart Talk

When communicating with other health professionals, occupational therapy practitioners use a shared language described as ***chart talk,*** whereby they present client information orally in team meetings; chart talk also occurs when the practitioner writes notes in a client medical history or case summary. Factually focused, chart talk succinctly presents core information about the client that is required across multiple professions. In contrast, telling the "story" of the client necessitates ***narrative reasoning*** (Mattingly & Fleming, 1994), which involves storytelling and story creation and has an emphasis on understanding the meaning of the person's health experience. The occupational practitioner describes the client as a person with the rich tapestry of life woven into the discussion. This includes who the client is as a person, their lived experience of both health and illness, and the person's motivations. Practitioners, as mentioned earlier, seem to thrive in a two-bodied practice. What Mattingly and Fleming (1994) also delineated, which is now widely understood in occupational therapy, is that practitioners tend to use chart talk when considering the person in their biomedical sphere and narrative reasoning when taking a more phenomenological view of the whole person.

Therapist With the Three-Track Mind

Although the modes of clinical reasoning have been enhanced and expanded since the 1990s (Schell & Schell, 2018; Unsworth & Baker, 2016), Mattingly and Fleming (1994) coined the term ***therapist with the three-track mind*** to describe three main modes of clinical reasoning in occupational therapy: (1) procedural, (2) interactive, and (3) conditional (described later in this chapter). What was unique in the original conceptualization of the three-track mind was the notion that occupational therapy practitioners can reason in one, two, or all three tracks simultaneously, and examples of this are provided in Case Example 6.1. This is particularly important for novice practitioners to consider because the tendency for new practitioners is to reason sequentially (Robertson et al., 2015; Unsworth, 2001).

Modes of Professional Reasoning in Occupation-Focused Practice

Within the Hierarchical Model of Clinical Reasoning (Unsworth, 2004, 2021), several tracks or modes or types of reasoning have been identified. Although Mattingly and Fleming (1994) described the therapist with the three-track mind, these forms of reasoning have been teased out to now include procedural reasoning, interactive reasoning, conditional reasoning, pragmatic reasoning, and generalization reasoning, as

EXHIBIT 6.2. Case Notes, Scoring, and Professional Reasoning From Anya

INTRODUCTION TO NATHAN (CHART TALK)	ANYA'S NARRATIVE REASONING (IN THE FIRST PERSON)
Nathan is an 82-year-old man who lives alone in a small retirement community. He has congestive cardiac failure, diabetes, and a pressure injury on his left foot. He was admitted to acute care with a severe bladder infection and developed pneumonia. Medically stable, he is ready for intensive therapy to get home. Previously independent in personal care (with a nurse dressing his pressure injury) with adaptive equipment. Uses his mobility scooter to visit the local shops and church and to get around the retirement community. Nathan has main meals at the dining room, could make hot drinks and simple snacks, did his own laundry, and put the trash cans out. Nathan usually spent afternoons visiting neighbors or going to the social group at the leisure area. Went to church 1x per week and a nearby friend's house 1x per week for "cards, football, and beer." Goals are to return home and go to the card game, social group, and visit neighbors once again. Has conceded to have his pressure injury dressed and PADL help from the visiting nurse but wants to be able to prepare simple snacks and get to the central dining hall for meals.	I'm getting to know Nathan through the initial interview, and I followed the occupational therapy checklist using procedural reasoning to cover all questions. I then undertook a PADL (showering, dressing, and grooming) and MoCA cognitive screen in the morning and used this to score all the FIM items. Throughout it all, I found Nathan to be in good humor and have a sharp wit. Carol [Anya's supervisor] reminded me about using my interactive reasoning to get to know my client better, and I really spent some time in the interview trying to get to know Nathan as a person. For example, I shared a story about my grandpa and his love of using his scooter to get to the local Powerball lotto outlet, and how important scooter use is for both of them. Using my pragmatic reasoning, Carol and I have discussed how Nathan is likely to be in the facility only for a few days, and I may need to refer Nathan to outpatient services and increase the nursing care to include assistance with showering and dressing in the morning and getting into bed for a few weeks after discharge. His pressure injury means he is at risk of repeated infections, and it's possible that he will be hospitalized again for care or possible surgery. I haven't seen his pressure injury to know how bad it is but will ask the nurses if I can observe the dressing change and, using my embodied reasoning, I can observe for pain and also ask Nathan directly about this. Reasoning conditionally, I'm thinking about what Nathan's life was like before this admission and how to help him reach his goals to get back home again and enjoy the things he likes to do. Given his goals to return home and go to the social group and visit his neighbors, procedurally, I will choose the AusTOMs–OT, Scale 8: Domestic Life—Home and Scale 12: Community Life, Recreation, Leisure, and Play, to score and work on as priorities over this admission. Pragmatically, I'm also thinking about fitting everything in today, as well as getting to my part-time job tonight, doing a shift, and planning everything for fieldwork tomorrow. I sure am tired!

(Continued)

EXHIBIT 6.2. Case Notes, Scoring, and Professional Reasoning From Anya *(Cont.)*

ANYA'S ADMISSION SCORES FOR NATHAN ON THE AUSTOMS–OT: SCALES 8 AND 12	SCORE	ANYA'S REASONING UNDERPINNING THE SCORES AWARDED
Scale 8: Domestic Life and Home (Inside House: Impairment) Scale 12: Community Life, Recreation, Leisure and Play: Impairment	3 3	For both scales, Nathan has several physical/sensory impairments but no cognitive impairments. His pressure injury is responding to treatment but is moderate to severe, he has difficulty with walking more than a few steps because of overall weakness, and his upper limbs have mild to moderate weakness as well.
Scale 8: Domestic Life and Home (Inside House): Activity Limitation Scale 12: Community Life, Recreation, Leisure and Play: Activity Limitation	0 3	On admission, Nathan was unable to tolerate standing for more than a few minutes in the kitchen area and could not make a hot drink and toast or carry out any of the domestic activities he described that he usually does at home. Can't manage any laundry. Nathan needs to be taken in a wheelchair to the dayroom to socialize with the other patients for short periods (about an hour before fatiguing). He was also able to go in a wheelchair (with an attendant pushing) to the chapel area in the facility on the weekend for a simple service.
Both Scales 8 and 12: Participation Restriction	2	Using interactive and conditional reasoning, I think Nathan currently has very limited social integration compared to his usual routines but, with assistance, can get to the dayroom. He is otherwise restricted in fulfilling his roles as a homemaker and neighbor, so a 2 is the best fit. I hope that we can get Nathan back to his home routines as soon as possible, but the deconditioning associated with being bedbound while he recovered from the pneumonia and his general weekend stats as evidenced by the pressure injury have left him weak.
Both Scales 8 and 12: Distress/Well-Being	3	Generally, Nathan seems to be doing fine and is in good humor but just wants to go home. He is accepting that he will need extra help when he returns home, although the pressure injury isn't healing and could lead to an infection again. However, I think Nathan's good humor could easily turn if he can't get back to his routines soon. Using generalization reasoning, I have been told by Carol that this is a common pattern and that clients are often fine and manage their situation well if they are going home. But things can rapidly change if the client has doubts about this or there are suggestions of transfer to an SNF, and it's important to watch for change in mood and depression, if this is a possibility.

Note. This exhibit presents Anya's written notes using chart talk (column 1) and her narrative reasoning (column 2). The different forms of professional reasoning are identified. PADL = personal activities of daily living; MoCA = Montreal Cognitive Assessment (Nasreddine et al., 2005); FIM = Functional Independence Measure (Uniform Data Set for Medical Rehabilitation. 1997); AusTOMs–OT = Australian Therapy Outcome Measures for Occupational Therapy (Perry et al., 2004); SNF = skilled nursing facility.

described shortly. Furthermore, as illustrated in the Venn diagram in the central portion of the hierarchy (see Figure 6.1), several of these forms of reasoning overlap and can be seen occurring together. Illustrations of this are provided in Exhibit 6.2: Anya and her supervisor, Carol, are discussing scoring Nathan on the AusTOMs–OT outcome measure. Exhibit 6.1 also provides a summary of these different modes of reasoning in the same "hierarchy" configuration, which are presented next.

EXERCISE 6.1. Alternative Reasoning

Once you explore Anya's reasoning with Nathan, can you think of any different reasoning you might have with this case? Consider what you might have done differently and how that might change the intervention process.

Procedural Reasoning

Rooted in scientific reasoning, ***procedural reasoning*** dominates when occupational therapy practitioners think about what theoretical orientation to apply, the therapy process from admission through to discharge, the specific evaluations and interventions to use with a client, and the outcomes attained to determine what comes next. Research evidence suggests that novice practitioners usually have good rule-based procedural reasoning, but this form of thinking often is dominant, and they rarely use other forms of reasoning (Unsworth, 2001).

Interactive Reasoning and the Intentional Relationship

Occupational therapy involves close collaboration—interaction—between the client and the occupational therapy practitioner. However, ***interactive reasoning*** goes well beyond this and is concerned with the practitioner's understanding who the client is as a person. A practitioner engages the client in therapy using a variety of intentional interactive strategies designed to motivate the client to achieve what the person wants, needs, or has to do, and to their level of satisfaction. Using interactive reasoning, the practitioner collaborates, advocates, encourages, empathizes, educates, and problem solves with the client to achieve therapy goals (Taylor et al., 2011).

Conditional Reasoning

The most elusive mode of professional reasoning is ***conditional reasoning.*** In part, this may be related to the multiple descriptions of this mode of reasoning presented by Mattingly and Fleming (1994). Simplistically, the client's progress is conditional on participation in occupational therapy. But at a deeper level, the occupational therapy practitioner needs to create a shared temporal vision of what the client's life was like before the therapeutic encounter, what the client's life is now, and what the client's life could be in the future. Conditional reasoning is more frequently used by experts than novices (Unsworth, 2001) when trying to understand what is meaningful to the client in their social and cultural world (Mattingly & Fleming, 1994).

Pragmatic Reasoning

Pragmatic reasoning occurs when an occupational therapy practitioner's reasoning centers around what can be achieved given the client's context; family circumstances; physical environment; funding/insurance circumstances; availability of equipment and other resources; and temporal issues, such as client length of stay, time available for therapy, and pressure of clients waiting to be seen. Pragmatic reasoning was identified by Schell and Cervero (1993) and further elaborated and refined by Unsworth (2004) through a qualitative study with 13 experienced occupational therapists.

Generalization Reasoning

Within each of the modes of procedural, interactive, conditional, and pragmatic reasoning, occupational therapy practitioners use ***generalization reasoning*** when drawing on past experience or knowledge to assist in making sense of a current situation or client circumstance. The practitioner thinks about the client, then reflects on general experiences or knowledge, and relates this back to the current situation, refocusing on the client (Unsworth, 2005). For example, when working with Nathan, Anya reflected to another older deconditioned client she had worked with the previous year, and combining procedural and generalization reasoning, Anya reasoned that using AusTOMs-OT would again be a successful way of measuring client outcomes.

Knowing More Than We Can Say: Hidden Reasoning and Influences on Reasoning

Although Unsworth's (2004, 2021) Hierarchical Model of Clinical Reasoning (see Figure 6.1) positions worldview as a major influence on professional reasoning, two other significant factors affect the professional reasoning of occupational therapy practitioners that are not directly portrayed in the model. They are (1) embodied knowledge and (2) intuition.

Worldview

Worldview was defined by Wolters (1989) as a person's global outlook on life and the world. Worldview incorporates an occupational therapy practitioner's values and beliefs, ethics, faith and spirituality; personal style; ability to read the practice culture; repertoire of therapy skills; and motivation for practice. Some occupational therapy scholars draw out ethical reasoning as a distinct form of reasoning, as shown in Exhibit 6.1. Ethical reasoning is described as the thinking that accompanies analysis of a moral dilemma where one moral conviction or action conflicts with another, and then generating possible solutions and selecting action to be taken. However, ethical reasoning is closely aligned with worldview, and it is not a simple task to articulate one's reasoning associated with these constructs.

Worldview was first explored in occupational therapy by Hooper (1997) through the thinking of an expert clinician, but little exploration of the topic has occurred since. The only other study examining this construct revealed that although worldview affects professional reasoning, it is not a form of reasoning itself (Unsworth, 2004). This research also revealed that worldview is distinct from pragmatic reasoning, which contrasts with the original idea of pragmatic reasoning proposed by Schell and Cervero (1993), who posited that pragmatic reasoning incorporates both the practical as well as personal views of the occupational therapy practitioner. In contrast, Unsworth's (2004) research separated out the elements of values, beliefs, and ethics as "worldview" and referred only to the elements' day-to-day reasoning that practitioners use when considering the practice context, resources, and temporal issues as being concerned with pragmatic reasoning.

Embodied Knowledge

Embodied knowledge describes the way occupational therapy practitioners use their whole body to gather or sense information. When interacting with their clients, practitioners gather information not only from what the person says through aural reception but from all their other senses as well (Kinsella, 2018).

When interacting with their clients, occupational therapy practitioners gather information, not only from what the person says through aural reception, but from all their other senses as well (Kinsella, 2018). For example, information may be gathered through smell (signifying wound healing or deterioration), sight (monitoring a client's face and posture for pain) and touch (palpating for muscle contraction). In addition, as noted by Noe (2004), knowledge is not only revealed to our minds but also through our actions in the world. As we interact with a client, a practitioner needs to use their body and therapeutic touch to work effectively, reflecting our knowledge. For example, a practitioner working on a burn unit needs to feel the features of a scar as well as detect the temperature of the client's skin to understand how healing is progressing. Professional reasoning may therefore be described as "embodied" because we reason with our whole bodies. Although practitioners may actively gather embodied knowledge, they may also arrive at information intuitively, as discussed in the next section.

Intuition

Professional reasoning is a complex process that occupational therapy practitioners can have difficulty articulating. Part of why clinicians may have difficulty putting language to practice is that there is undoubtedly an intuitive element to therapy, and intuition is inherently difficult to articulate (Chaffey et al., 2012). ***Intuition*** is the opposite of overt analysis and has been described as subconsciously knowing something: It is "knowledge of a fact or truth, as a whole; immediate possession of knowledge; and knowledge independent of the linear reasoning process" (Rew, 1986, p. 23). Intuition is also described as having a gut feeling or instinct. Occupational therapy practitioners' thinking and reasoning are grounded in evidence-based analysis but also their subconscious intuition.

These constructs of worldview, embodied knowledge, and intuition can be illustrated through the case study of Anya. We know that through Anya's home life and upbringing, her spiritual, moral, and ethical views were largely formed and influence all her reasoning unconsciously. However, she is slowly learning how to listen to herself, her knowledge base, and her intuition to understand her clients and what is happening to them. Carol has been supervising Anya to consider embodied knowledge when an opportunity presents itself. Carol has also been suggesting to Anya that she develop and listen to her intuition, although this is harder to coach and nurture. Anya has had a feeling that Nathan is very lonely and that the time in hospital has provided much-needed company. Anya learned that Nathan had always had a dog until about 10 years ago. Anya is really interested to explore pet therapy and intuitively feels that having a dog around could provide much-needed company for Nathan. Carol suggested that Anya follow up with a phone call and visit to Nathan's nearby retirement community to determine whether a therapy dog could become a shared pet for the community. Over time, occupational therapy practitioners become more tuned into and comfortable with having a worldview and using embodied knowledge and intuition to inform their professional reasoning.

Professional Reasoning, Experience, and Expertise

One of the most widely used descriptions of the development of ***expertise*** among professionals was provided by Dreyfus and Dreyfus (1980) through the examples of chess players and airline pilots. The authors' descriptions of stages in the development of expertise have been translated across multiple sectors, including health, where it was adapted by nursing academics (Benner, 1984). Professional reasoning and the development of expertise are often described together because research has consistently revealed that experts think and reason differently from novices. Although experts use their nonpropositional and tacit knowledge to know "how" to practice, novices need to rely on their propositional or factual book knowledge to know "what" to practice (Dreyfus & Dreyfus, 1980).

Although there are more than 17 studies on the development of expertise among occupational therapy practitioners (Unsworth & Baker, 2016), most were conducted between 1991 and 2001. Furthermore, few studies have been able to tease out the stages of expertise attained by clinicians empirically, with most only able to view the dichotomy of novice and experts (Gibson et al., 2000; Mitchell & Unsworth, 2005). Many studies have focused solely on expert practice so that the professional reasoning of these practitioners can be better understood and disseminated to contribute to the learning of other practitioners. For example, a recent study successfully used grounded theory to examine how practitioners hone expertise and develop skills in home modifications (DuBroc & Pickens, 2015). The next section explores five stages of expertise commonly described in the literature.

Stages in the Development of Expertise

As delineated by Dreyfus and Dreyfus (1980) and nuanced by Benner (1984), the five stages an occupational therapy practitioner passes through on the continuum from novice to expert are

1. novice,
2. advanced beginner,
3. competent,
4. proficient, and
5. expert.

As depicted in Figure 6.2, an occupational therapy practitioner often commences as a novice and takes a journey across these five stages. However, the journey is not necessarily linear. Increasing years of experience do not always equate with

FIGURE 6.2. Stages and key concepts on the journey from novice to expert.

Novice
No practice experience in the situation and dependent on theory. Factual and rule driven. Cannot grasp whole situation.

Advanced Beginner
Incorporates contextual information into rule-based thinking. Uses pattern recognition.

Competent
Planning is deliberate, efficient, and responsive to practice and other contextual issues.

Proficient
Perceives situation as a whole. Intuitive behavior begins to replace reasoned responses.

Expert
Has an intuitive grasp of the whole situation. Professional reasoning is internalized, fast, and focused.

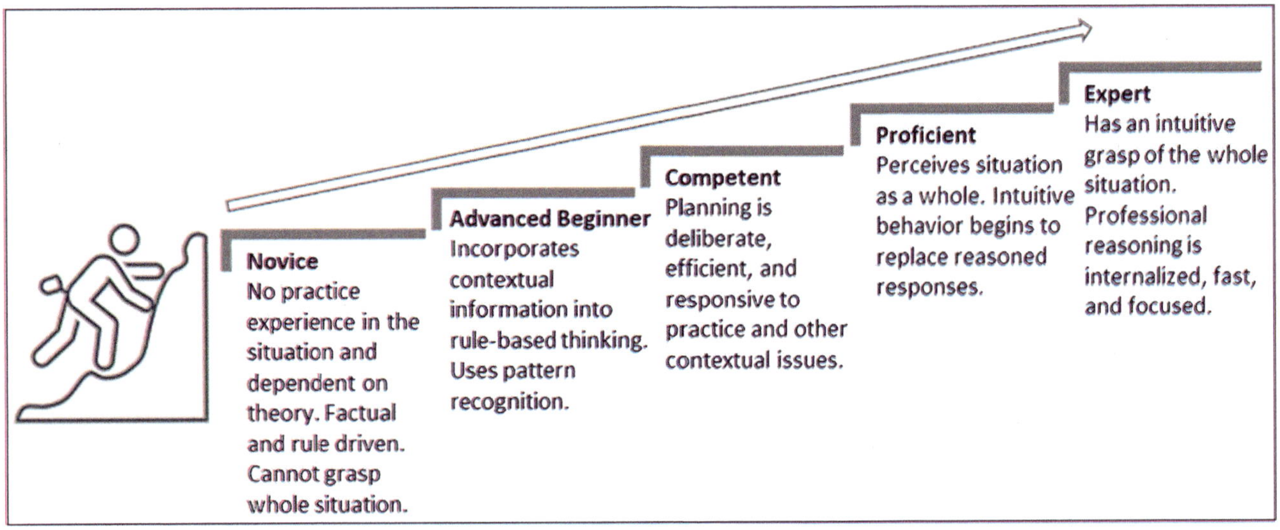

increasing expertise. Some practitioners graduate and rise quickly to expert status, whereas others can remain stuck in the advanced beginner, competent, or the proficient stage for years. Therefore, it is helpful for novices to consider strategies to build their skills and development toward expert practice, as described next.

As ***novices,*** newly graduated occupational therapy practitioners have knowledge of theories, principles, and specific disabilities, but they are usually rigid in their application of this knowledge. Novices do not have experience of the clinical situations they will be involved in. ***Advanced beginners*** can start to modify rules, principles, and theories so that they are adapted to the specific situation. However, because practitioners at this stage have to concentrate on remembering rules, principles, and theories, they are less flexible in their application. Advanced beginners have sufficient clinical experience to identify recurring themes and the information on which reasoning is based. However, they may have difficulty determining a course of action when circumstances differ or do not present as expected.

Competent therapists have typically worked for several years and are able to adjust the therapy to the specific needs of the client and the situation, but they lack the speed and flexibility of the proficient clinician. ***Proficient therapists*** are flexible and able to alter an occupational therapy intervention plan as needed, have a clear understanding of the client's whole situation, and have a perception of the situation based on experience rather than deliberation. These therapists are highly skilled but are not quite at the level of experts.

The final stage of becoming an expert is not attained by all occupational therapy practitioners. ***Expert therapists*** approach therapy from client-generated cues rather than preconceived therapeutic plans. Experts quickly anticipate and recognize client strengths and weaknesses based on their experience of other clients. An expert clinician does not need to rely on rules to take appropriate action; rather, they have an intuitive grasp of the situation. Based on the research of King et al. (2008), experts can often be recognized as possessing the following six attributes:

1. They achieve superior outcomes to their peers.
2. They use a range of technical, interpersonal, self-regulation, cognitive, and metacognitive skills.
3. They are knowledgeable about content (propositional/factual knowledge) and how to do things (nonpropositional knowledge), and they possess self-knowledge (insight to own knowledge).
4. Their personal attributes and qualities, such as values and traits, are respected by others.
5. They have practiced in the field for some time.
6. They have a reputation as an expert among their peers.

Novice clinicians often find it difficult to understand how an expert is working unless the expert can translate their tacit and intuitive processes into language.

Boosting Therapists on Their Journey From Novice to Expert

Occupational therapy education programs strive to graduate students with the skills, tools, behaviors, attitudes, and professional reasoning abilities needed to boost them on their journey toward expert status. Therefore, educators actively seek ways to help students and novices gain insights into expert thinking so they may hasten their journey on this continuum. A Canadian research team working in medical education identified a taxonomy of clinical reasoning difficulties (Audétat et al., 2013) as well as strategies for supervisors to manage (Audétat et al., 2017a) and remediate such difficulties (Audétat et al., 2017b). Although this research is not of direct relevance to occupational therapy practice because the focus is on diagnostic reasoning, the idea of being able to identify and assist students to manage professional reasoning difficulties is of great importance to occupational therapy and deserves research attention in the future.

For occupational therapy students and novices, practical strategies can enhance professional reasoning and propel their journey toward expert status. These strategies include seeking feedback from an expert who observes the novice in a therapy session (either in-person or through video); actively participating in regular continuing professional development activities from in-services and journal clubs through to enrollment in formal courses; and asking supervisors and mentors for dedicated time to ask questions and reflect on practice using the structure of our shared professional reasoning language. This technique of using reflection to enhance and promote professional reasoning is explored in more detail in the next section.

The Reflective Practitioner: Enhancing Professional Reasoning and Practice

Schön (1983) wrote extensively about ***reflection,*** which is the process of turning experiences into learning. He proffered the idea that reflection is a cyclical process in which occupational therapy practitioners engage when looking forward or anticipating an encounter—while they are in action and also after an encounter when they engage in reflection on their action—and that reflection promoted reasoning. In occupational therapy, reflection-for-action and reflection-in-action require complex thinking processes that demand the practitioner to plan for, monitor, and then adjust the ever-changing and sometimes extremely subtle shifts in client performance. ***Reflection-in-action*** refers to contemplative reflection after the therapeutic encounter. However, as Harries and Gilhooly (2010) noted, reflection does not automatically result in improved self-insight and concomitant improvements in practice. Rather, many practitioners, and particularly novices, need structure to assist them in reflection and allow them to grow their insight and understanding of practice and reasoning to improve it and ultimately reach expert status.

Reflective activities designed to enhance professional reasoning can be undertaken alone, with a reflective partner as an informal sharing activity, or formally through supervision. Reflective activities include storytelling, prebriefing and debriefing, reflective questions after working with a client, reflective journal writing, a review of critical incidents with a mentor, participation in discussion groups, and videotaping and viewing sessions with clients (McKay, 2009; Schell & Schell, 2018; Wong et al., 2016). These processes all require occupational therapy practitioners to translate what is going on into language that can then be shared, examined, and critiqued orally or through prose. ***Gibbs' Reflective Cycle*** (Gibbs, 1988) presents an excellent model for students to use to guide and develop their reflective practices. Developed in 1988, Gibbs' Reflective Cycle provides a structured framework for examining experiences as depicted in Figure 6.3 (Buman & Schultz, 2013). Novices can follow the six steps in the cycle related to the experience: (1) description, (2) thoughts and feelings, (3) evaluation, (4) analysis, (5) conclusion, and (6) action plan. The structure of this model assists practitioners in developing their reflective skills in an organized way.

FIGURE 6.3. Gibbs' Reflective Cycle to support reflective practice.

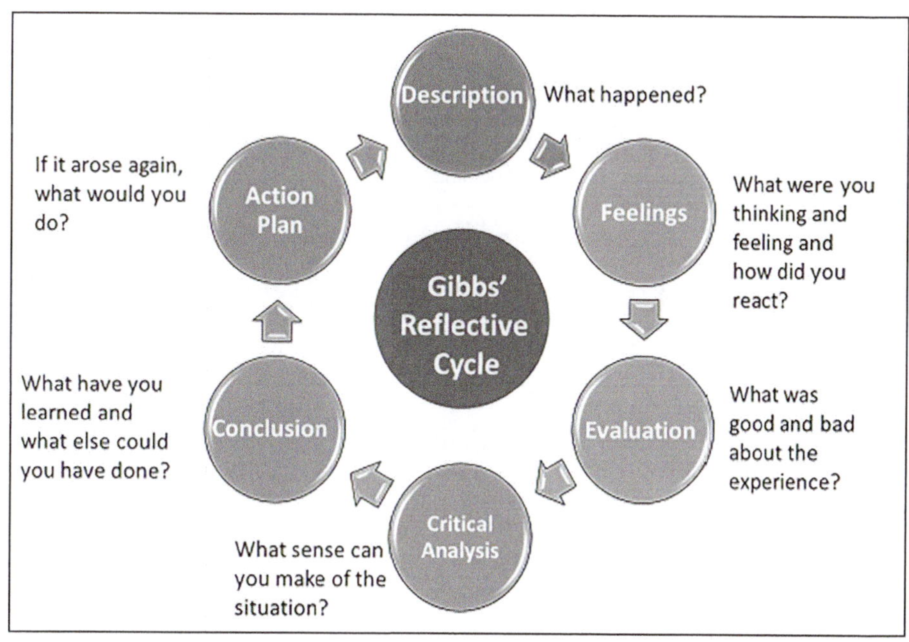

Source. Buman & Schultz (2013).

EXHIBIT 6.3. Example of Anya's Using Gibbs' Reflective Cycle in Occupational Therapy Practice

CYCLE STAGE	ANYA'S REFLECTIONS ON AN INCIDENT WITH NATHAN AFTER HIS THERAPY
Description: What happened? This part is descriptive—**not** analytical—and describes an experience. 	I took Nathan to the dayroom after his therapy session to socialize with the other patients. I knew Nathan was tired, but he wanted to go, and I said I would come back after my next client in an hour and take him back to the room—but to call for an orderly if he wanted to go back sooner. Then when I got to the dayroom, I was a bit late, and Nathan looked grey, tired, and upset. All the other patients had left, and he was alone. Nathan was cross with me for being late and said he was disappointed it had taken me so long to come to get him and that he was exhausted and needed to go lie down. I apologized to Nathan for being late and agreed that it had been a long session and then a lot to manage to be in the dayroom as well. I took Nathan back to his room in silence.
Feelings: What were you thinking and feeling, and how did you react? This part is also **not** analytical and describes personal feelings and thoughts and actions or reactions. 	When I took Nathan to the dayroom, I didn't think too much about it, and actually, I was a bit distracted, thinking about my next client and whether I was keeping up with everything Carol [Anya's supervisor] was asking of me. But when I got to the dayroom about 70 minutes later, and I saw how tired and grey Nathan looked, I felt really bad and actually a bit guilty. I was unhappy with my actions as I should have known how tired he already was after his therapy session and that it would be too much to go to the dayroom.
Evaluation: What was good and bad about the experience? This part is also **not** analytical but requires positive or negative thoughts about an experience. 	When I think back on the day, I think it was a good therapy session with Nathan, and he was able to build his physical tolerance while making a cup of coffee and crackers with spread. I know I was a bit distracted thinking about my next client and worrying I was getting everything done, and it was too much for Nathan to be in the dayroom after therapy. I guess I took it at face value that Nathan wanted to go to the dayroom to meet some of the other patients, and I didn't really stop to think about it.
Critical analysis: What sense can you make of the situation? This part **is** analytical and requires explanation of the causes and consequences of the things that happened. Questions like "Why?" and "So what?" and "What if?" are asked. 	Nathan had a day that was too long, and this led to him being overtired, and this will possibly slow down his recovery. It's possible that he will need additional rest tomorrow. Given his limited number of days at the facility, this is a problem. I contributed to this situation negatively and should have used my interactive reasoning to suggest an alternative plan for Nathan's afternoon. There wasn't really anyone else present in this situation as Carol had left me to finish up the session and take Nathan back. I haven't had this kind of experience before.
Conclusion: What else could you have done? In this step, you sum up what you have learned from the experience. 	I think I really could have done things differently. I should have been thinking about Nathan, and his session ending, and what was next for him rather than my next patient. I could have recommended he go back to his room after therapy and have a rest first and then socialize with some of the other patients at dinner or before dinner if he felt up to it. I guess my inexperience meant I didn't pick up the cues that Nathan had done enough at that time and needed to rest, and I wasn't aware that I even needed to check in with Nathan or look at nonverbal cues to see that he was already tired when I took him to the dayroom. Maybe when I have seen more clients, I will have a better feel for fatigue levels and be better able to gauge when clients have had enough.

(Continued)

EXHIBIT 6.3. Example of Anya's Using Gibbs' Reflective Cycle in Occupational Therapy Practice *(Cont.)*

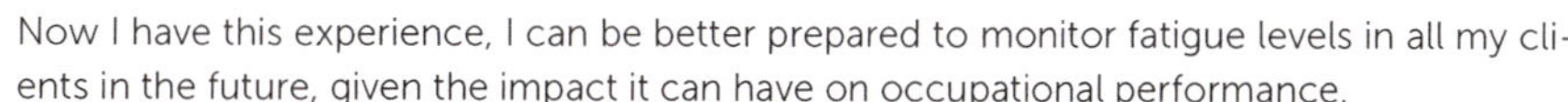

CYCLE STAGE	ANYA'S REFLECTIONS ON AN INCIDENT WITH NATHAN AFTER HIS THERAPY
Action plan: If it arose again what would you do? In this step, state actions designed to improve knowledge, ability, experience, and so on. Include what you plan to do and why. Be specific.  And cycle back to the start for the next experience. . . . 	Now I have this experience, I can be better prepared to monitor fatigue levels in all my clients in the future, given the impact it can have on occupational performance. When working with older deconditioned clients I can also use generalization reasoning to really think and talk with clients about when they have done enough and when it's time to rest. Next time, I can use my interactive reasoning to pitch the rationale for rest to the client at the just-right level that is engaging and persuasive for that particular client. I think I have to be better prepared when I'm seeing clients so I can juggle the changeover between clients more smoothly. I think I need to make sure I am really attending to my client for the whole time and not get distracted by what's next. I need to have all my plans for the next client ready to go, so I don't need to think about this in the changeover time.

Note. Cycle stages from Gibbs (1988).

On the third day that Anya went to meet and work with Nathan, she found him upset and unwilling to join in the plans they had made the previous day. Anya used Gibbs' Reflective Cycle to structure her reasoning and promote her understanding of the situation after a discussion with Carol. Anya's reflections are noted in Exhibit 6.3.

EXERCISE 6.2. Applying Professional Reasoning to Your Own Case

Think about a case that you have seen in class or during fieldwork. Review the case and describe what your reasoning process was and what types of reasoning you used you decide on your intervention process.

Summary

Professional reasoning can be a difficult concept for occupational therapy students and practitioners to fully understand. It is helpful to view it as a bridge that links theory and classroom-based propositional knowledge to everyday practice; when observing and then practicing occupational therapy during fieldwork, the concept of professional reasoning falls quickly into place. This chapter provided an overview of how professional reasoning is the thinking that guides occupational therapy practitioners to plan, direct, undertake, and reflect on client care.

Professional reasoning is informed by and sits alongside our worldview and intuition in an embodied practice. Occupational therapy practitioners have developed a language to describe the often-tacit fund of knowledge held by the profession, and through using the terms *procedural, interactive, conditional, scientific, narrative, ethical,* and *generalization reasoning*, novices can help shape and organize their own thinking, and more readily converse with experts to gain insight into their practice as well. Reflection was presented as a vital element supporting the development of professional reasoning. Therefore, this chapter concluded by describing reflection as an active process that students and novices can use to help grow their reasoning skills and ultimately achieve the best possible outcomes with clients.

Dedication

This chapter is dedicated to former colleague Maureen Hayes Fleming (1940–2019) whose collaborative research into clinical reasoning in occupational therapy laid important foundation stones in the bridge spanning theory to practice.

References

American Occupational Therapy Association. (2020). Occupational therapy practice framework: Domain and process (4th ed.). *American Journal of Occupational Therapy, 74*(Suppl. 2), 7412410010. https://doi.org/10.5014/ajot.2020.74S2001

Audétat, M.-C., Laurin, S., Dory, V., Charlin, B., & Nendaz, M. R. (2017a). Diagnosis and management of clinical reasoning difficulties: Part I. Clinical reasoning supervision and educational diagnosis. *Medical Teacher, 39*(8), 792–796. https://doi.org/10.1080/0142159X.2017.1331033

Audétat, M.-C., Laurin, S., Dory, V., Charlin, B., & Nendaz, M. R. (2017b). Diagnosis and management of clinical reasoning difficulties: Part II. Clinical reasoning difficulties: Management and remediation strategies. *Medical Teacher, 39*(8), 797–801. https://doi.org/10.1080/0142159X.2017.1331034

Audétat, M.-C., Laurin, S., Sanche, G., Béïque, C., Caire Fon, N., Blais, J.-G., & Charlin, B. (2013). Clinical reasoning difficulties: A taxonomy for clinical teachers. *Medical Teacher, 35*(3), e984–e989. https://doi.org/10.3109/0142159X.2012.733041

Benner, P. (1984). *From novice to expert. Excellence and power in clinical nursing practice.* Addison–Wesley.

Buman, C., & Schultz, S. (2013). *Reflective practice in nursing.* Wiley-Blackwell.

Burgin, M. (2016). *Theory of knowledge: Structures and processes.* World Scientific.

Chaffey, L., Unsworth, C. A., & Fossey, E. (2012). Relationship between intuition and emotional intelligence in occupational therapists in mental health practice. *American Journal of Occupational Therapy, 66*(1), 88–96. https://doi.org/10.5014/ajot.2012.001693

Cohn, E. S. (1989). Fieldwork education: Shaping a foundation for clinical reasoning. *American Journal of Occupational Therapy, 43*(4), 240–244. https://doi.org/10.5014/ajot.43.4.240

Dowie, J., & Elstein, A. (1988). *Professional judgment: A reader in clinical decision making*. Cambridge University Press.

Dreyfus, S. E., & Dreyfus, H. L. (1980). *A five-stage model of the mental activities involved in directed skill acquisition* (Unpublished report, Air Force Office of Scientific Research, United States Air Force Contract No. F49620-79-C-0063). University of California at Berkeley.

DuBroc, W., & Pickens, N. D. (2015). Becoming "at home" in home modifications: Professional reasoning across the expertise continuum. *Occupational Therapy in Health Care, 29*(3), 316–329. https://doi.org/10.3109/07380577.2015.1010129

Fleming, M. H. (1991). Clinical reasoning in medicine compared with clinical reasoning in occupational therapy. *American Journal of Occupational Therapy, 45*(11), 988–996, https://doi.org/10.5014/ajot.45.11.988

Gibbs, G. (1988). *Learning by doing: A guide to teaching and learning methods*. Oxford Polytechnic.

Gibson, D., Velde, B., Hoff, T., Kvashay, D., Manross, P. L., & Moreau, V. (2000). Clinical reasoning of a novice versus an experienced occupational therapist: A qualitative study. *Occupational Therapy in Healthcare, 12*(4), 15–31. https://doi.org/10.1080/J003v12n04_02

Harries, P. A., & Gilhooly, K. J. (2010). Occupational therapists' self-insight into their referral prioritisation policies for clients with mental health needs, *Australian Occupational Therapy Journal, 57*(6), 417–424. https://doi.org/10.1111/j.1440-1630.2010.00881.x

Harries, P. A., Unsworth, C. A., Gokalp, H., Davies, M., Tomlinson, C., & Harries, L. (2018). A randomised controlled trial to test the effectiveness of decision training on assessors' ability to determine optimal fitness-to-drive recommendations for older or disabled drivers. *BMC Medical Education, 18*, Article 27. https://doi.org/10.1186/s12909-018-1131-4

Hoffmann, T. C., Légaré, F., Simmons, M. B., McNamara, K., McCaffery, K., Trevena, L. J., . . . Del Mar, C. B. (2016). Shared decision making: What do clinicians need to know and why should they bother? *Medical Journal of Australia, 201*(1), 35–39. https://doi.org/10.5694/mja14.00002

Hooper, B. (1997). The relationship between pretheoretical assumptions and clinical reasoning. *American Journal of Occupational Therapy, 51*(5), 328–338. https://doi.org/10.5014/ajot.51.5.328

King, G., Currie, M., Bartlett, D. J., Strachan, E., Tucker, M. A., & Willoughby, C. (2008). The development of expertise in paediatric rehabilitation therapists: The roles of motivation, openness to experience, and types of caseload experience. *Australian Occupational Therapy Journal, 55*(2), 108–122. https://doi.org/10.1111/j.1440-1630.2007.00681.x

Kinsella, E. A. (2018). Embodied reasoning in professional practice. In B. A. Schell & J. W. Schell (Eds.), *Clinical and professional reasoning in occupational therapy* (2nd ed., pp. 105–121). Wolters Kluwer.

Mattingly, C. (1994). Occupational therapy as a two-body practice: The body as machine. In C. Mattingly & M. H. Fleming (Eds.), *Clinical reasoning: Forms of inquiry in a therapeutic practice* (pp. 37–63). F.A. Davis.

Mattingly, C., & Fleming, M. H. (Eds.). (1994). *Clinical reasoning: Forms of inquiry in a therapeutic practice*. F.A. Davis.

McKay, E. A. (2009). Reflective practice: Doing, being and becoming a reflective practitioner. In E. A. S. Duncan (Ed.), *Skills for practice in occupational therapy* (pp. 55–72). Churchill Livingstone.

Mitchell, R., & Unsworth, C. A. (2005). Clinical reasoning during community health home visits: Expert and novice differences. *British Journal of Occupational Therapy, 68*(5), 215–223. https://doi.org/10.1177/030802260506800505

Nasreddine, Z., Phillips, N. A., Bédirian, V., Charbonneau, S., Whitehead, V., Collin, I., . . . Chertkow, H. (2005). The Montreal Cognitive Assessment (MoCA): A brief screening tool for mild cognitive impairment. *Journal of the American Geriatrics Society, 53*, 695–699. https://doi.org/10.1111/j.1532-5415.2005.53221.x

Noe, A. (2004). *Action in perception*. MIT Press.

Perry, A., Morris, M., Unsworth, C., Duckett, S., Skeat, J., Dodd, K., . . . Riley, K. (2004). Therapy outcome measures for allied health practitioners in Australia: The AusTOMs. *International Journal for Quality in Health Care, 16*, 285–291. https://doi.org/10.1093/intqhc/mzh059

Rew, L. (1986). Intuition: Concept analysis of a group phenomenon. *Advances in Nursing Science, 8*(2), 21–28. https://doi.org/10.1097/00012272-198601000-00006

Robertson, D., Warrender, F., & Barnard, S. (2015). The critical occupational therapy practitioner: How to define expertise? *Australian Occupational Therapy Journal, 62*(1), 68–71. https://doi.org/10.1111/1440-1630.12157

Rogers, J. C. (1983). Eleanor Clarke Slagle Lectureship—1983; Clinical reasoning: The ethics, science, and art. *American Journal of Occupational Therapy, 37*(9), 601–616. https://doi.org/10.5014/ajot.37.9.601

Rogers, J. C., & Masagatani, G. (1982). Clinical reasoning of occupational therapists during the initial assessment of physically disabled patients. *Occupational Therapy Journal of Research, 2*(4), 195–219. https://doi.org/10.1177/153944928200200401

Schell, B. A., & Cervero, R. M. (1993). Clinical reasoning in occupational therapy: An integrative review. *American Journal of Occupational Therapy, 47*(7), 605–610. https://doi.org/10.5014/ajot.47.7.605

Schell, B. A. B., & Schell, J. (2018). *Clinical and professional reasoning in occupational therapy* (2nd ed.). Wolters Kluwer.

Schön, D. A. (1983). *The reflective practitioner: How professionals think in action*. Basic Books.

Sox, H. C., Higgins, M. C., & Owens, D. K. (2013). *Medical decision making* (2nd ed.). Wiley-Blackwell.

Stanley, J., & Williamson, T. (2001). Knowing how. *Journal of Philosophy, 98*(8), 411–444. https://doi.org/10.2307/2678403

Taylor, R., Lee, S. W., & Kielhofner, G. (2011). Practitioners' use of interpersonal modes within the therapeutic relationship: Results from a nationwide study. *OTJR: Occupation, Participation and Health, 31*(1), 6–14. https://doi.org/10.3928/15394492-20100521-02

Thompson, D. (1995). *Concise Oxford dictionary* (9th ed.). Oxford Clarendon.

Uniform Data Set for Medical Rehabilitation. (1997). *FIM clinical guide, version 5.01*. State University of New York at Buffalo.

Unsworth, C. A. (2001). The clinical reasoning of novice and expert occupational therapists. *Scandinavian Journal of Occupational Therapy, 8*(4), 163–173. https://doi.org/10.1080/110381201317166522

Unsworth, C. A. (2004). Clinical reasoning: How do pragmatic reasoning, worldview and client-centredness fit? *British Journal of Occupational Therapy, 67*(1), 10–19. https://doi.org/10.1177/030802260406700103

Unsworth, C. A. (2005). Using a head-mounted video camera to explore current conceptualizations of clinical reasoning in occupational therapy. *American Journal of Occupational Therapy, 59*(1), 31–40. https://doi.org/10.5014/ajot.59.1.31

Unsworth, C. A. (2013). The evolving theory of clinical reasoning. In E.A.S. Duncan (Ed.), *Foundations for practice in occupational therapy* (5th ed., pp. 209–231). Elsevier.

Unsworth, C. A. (2021). The evolving theory of clinical reasoning. In E. A. S. Duncan (Ed.), *Foundations for practice in occupational therapy* (6th ed., pp. 178–197). Elsevier.

Unsworth, C. A., & Baker, A. (2016). A systematic review of professional reasoning literature in occupational therapy. *British Journal of Occupational Therapy, 79(1)*, 5–16. https://doi.org/10.1177/0308022615599994

Unsworth, C. A., Bearup, A., & Rickard, K. (2009). Benchmark comparison of outcomes for clients with upper-limb dysfunction following stroke using the Australian Therapy Outcome Measures for Occupational Therapy (AusTOMs-OT). *American Journal of Occupational Therapy, 63*(6), 732–743. https://doi.org/10.5014/ajot.63.6.732

Unsworth, C. A., Coulson, M., Swinton, L., Cole, H., & Sarigiannis, M. (2015). Determination of the minimal clinically important difference on the Australian Therapy Outcome Measures for Occupational Therapy (AusTOMs–OT). *Disability and Rehabilitation, 37*(11), 997–1003. https://doi.org/10.3109/09638288.2014.952450

Unsworth, C., & Duncombe, D. (2014). *AusTOMS for occupational therapy [Arabic translation]: Therapy outcome measures for use internationally.* CQUniversity.

Unsworth, C. A., Timmer, A., & Wales, K. (2018). Reliability of the Australian Therapy Outcome Measures for Occupational Therapy (AusTOMs–OT). *Australian Occupational Therapy Journal, 65*(5), 375–386. https://doi.org/10.1111/1440-1630.12476

Wolters, A. M. (1989). On the idea of worldview and its relationship to philosophy. In P. A. Marshall, S. Griffioen, & R. Mouw (Eds.), *Stained glass: Worldviews and social science* (pp. 14–26). University Press of America.

Wong, K. Y., Whitcombe, S. W., & Boniface, G. (2016). Teaching and learning the esoteric: An insight into how reflection may be internalised with reference to the occupational therapy profession. *Reflective Practice, 17*(4), 472–482. https://doi.org/10.1080/14623943.2016.1175341

7

Enhancing and Facilitating Occupational Performance

VIKRAM PAGPATAN, OTR/L, ATP, BCP, CLA,
AND WESLEY BLOUNT, SHRM-CP

CHAPTER HIGHLIGHTS

- Facilitating occupational performance
- Using activities to elicit greater effort, repetition, or duration than traditional exercise
- Using activities to provide graded challenges
- Using activities to develop effective strategies for performance skills

KEY TERMS AND CONCEPTS

• caregivers • client factors • cognitive strategies • compensatory strategies • graded challenges • instructed plan • interpersonal strategies • just-right challenge • motor strategies • nonregulatory conditions • occupation-as-means • performance skills • regulatory conditions • self-developed plan • sensory strategies • strategies

Introduction

Occupational therapy practitioners continuously assess which areas of occupation are meaningful and essential in people's daily lives and which have become difficult for them to perform. Sometimes, the client enjoys an occupation they can no longer do, such as playing piano with an injured hand. That is, the client's injury limits function. Once the hand heals, however, function may return. At that point, the client may need therapy to address not the restoration of function but some sort of restoration of occupational performance. Facilitating, and enhancing, occupational performance focuses on working with a client to find activities to enhance performance, adjustments that may facilitate or enhance performance, or interventions that can facilitate renewed performance.

Improved occupational outcomes, engagement in meaningful activities, and participation in all facets of society are some of the therapeutic goals for which focusing on performance can make a difference. Interventions addressing occupational performance include developing adaptive strategies, introducing compensatory techniques, selecting and modifying assistive devices and technologies, implementing contextual modifications, and implementing guided therapeutic practice of essential and meaningful tasks.

We begin this chapter by describing the use of activities as a means by which occupational therapy practitioners incorporate therapeutic approaches in addressing specific challenges in people's performance skills and patterns and integrate structured challenges to address specific deficits in client factors. We identify four ways to use occupations and their related activities to improve clients' internal factors: (1) foster interest, (2) sustain interest, (3) challenge performance level, and (4) develop effective cognitive strategies, motor strategies, or both.

In the next section, we describe the integration of both regulatory and nonregulatory conditions to facilitate occupational performance and incorporate therapeutically constructed challenges into the rehabilitative process. Examples include physical activities for adult clients and the use of play-based sessions for pediatric clients. Moreover, we highlight in detail the clinical consideration of different factors that affect activity performance, the importance of ongoing goal identification, the variation of structured versus unstructured tasks, the impact of the context or contexts, and the practitioner's therapeutic use of self. In the "Using Activities to Promote Effective Strategies for Performance Skills" section, we discuss how to use activities to promote the development of effective motor, cognitive, interpersonal, and sensory strategies to enhance performance skills. In each section, the focus is on the use of occupations and their related components as effective therapeutic processes that address the central needs of every person in the occupational therapy process.

Each approach is discussed separately, integrating evidence-based practice and principles of diversity, equity, and inclusion in professional practice; implementing culturally sensitive and competent clinical reasoning skills; and addressing care holistically through a life course continuum. Ultimately, by looking at enhancing and facilitating improved occupational performance, we show how, beyond simply restoring function, therapeutic interventions make a difference in the client's restoration of occupational health.

Facilitating Occupational Performance

Occupational therapy practitioners facilitate and enhance occupational performance through a mix of interventions that maximize the potential to improve ***performance skills,*** which are "observable, goal-directed actions and consist of motor skills, process skills, and social interaction skills" (AOTA, 2020b, p. 13), and ***client factors,*** which are "specific capacities, characteristics, or beliefs that reside within the person, group, or population and influence performance in occupations" (American Occupational Therapy Association [AOTA], 2020b, p. 15; see Figure 7.1).

Performance Skills

Examples of performance skills include the breaking down of performance into motor, process, and social interaction skills. An example of breaking down a new occupation might be determining the skills involved in donning a prosthetic device after an amputation. In this case, the occupational therapy practitioner should already have considered the healing of the wound and care for the body before use of the device. Once the client is ready, the therapist can work on breaking down the performance skills needed.

A process skill for donning a prosthetic device, for example, involves organizing the material, problem solving and sequencing the steps, and adapting the steps to account for time. The motor skills involved in learning those steps then follow and may require additional adaptation as limitations arise. Last, social interaction skills can include how to integrate the prosthetic device into a social engagement, such as pointing to or verbally describing the device to someone else during a conversation, easing understanding and acceptance.

Client Factors

Using the example of the prosthetic device, the occupational therapy practitioner can look at related client factors, which "influence the clients' performance in occupations" (AOTA,

FIGURE 7.1. **Clinical reasoning skills require occupational therapy practitioners to balance internally and externally directed interventions to address a client's goals, performance in various areas of occupation in changing contexts, and their overall role fulfillment.**

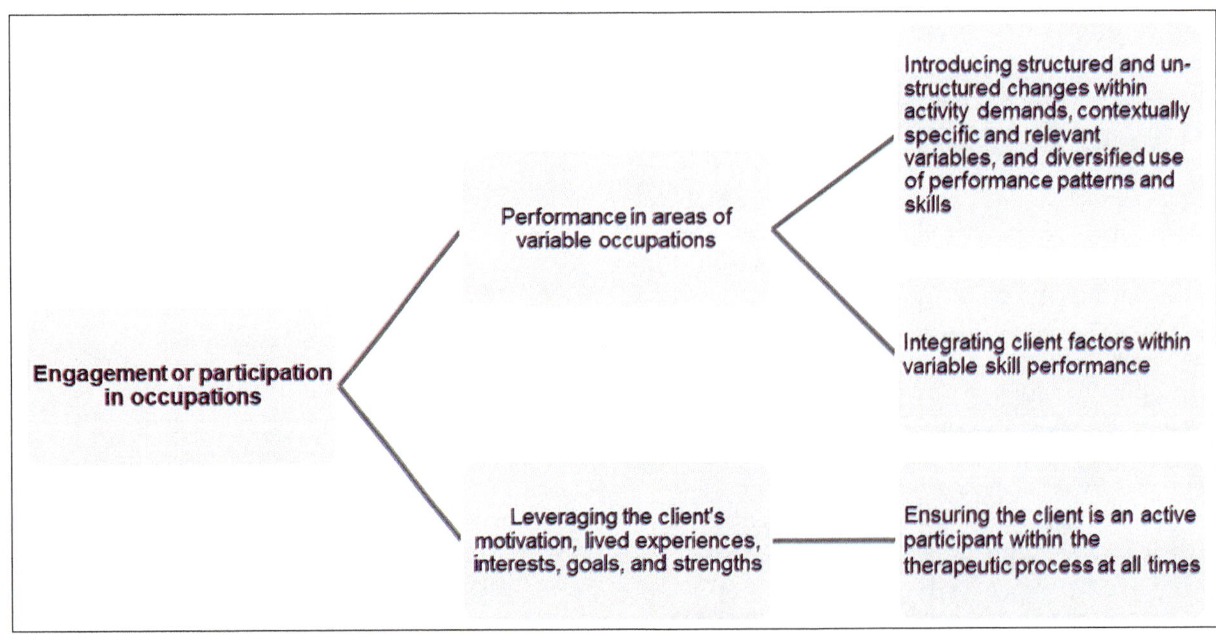

Source. V. Pagpatan. Used with permission.

2020b, p. 51). These factors could include, for example, the muscle tone and endurance of the residual limb, the emotional aspects related to recovering from an amputation, and feelings of pain or discomfort. Addressing these client factors (and others) while improving performance is the goal of the therapeutic intervention.

Occupational therapy practitioners also seek to minimize activity limitation through ***compensatory strategies,*** which are interventions that modify the environment or teach the client adapted procedures to substitute for loss of function. An example of a compensatory strategy is the inclusion of assistive technologies for clients who have difficulty taking notes in a classroom. Adaptive pencil grips, tablets, digital documents, or speech-to-text software (external factors) can be integrated with clients' drive, motivation, and strengths (internal factors) to enable occupational therapy practitioners to promote performance of occupations that will enhance clients' participation in meaningful and essential tasks. Thus, improving occupational performance can also include improving performance as it relates to the functional interventions.

Improvements in internal factors are critical to the occupational therapy process because they enable clients to perform occupations using a variety of methods and with contextual variations. Such improvements also facilitate the development of confidence, motivation, drive, and self-empowerment as clients discover new variations and strategies within occupational performance and role development. Occupational therapy practitioners who work with clients who have had a cerebrovascular accident (CVA) often use neuromuscular techniques as a means to facilitate and encourage the development of more mature performance skills (internal factors). Practitioners constantly incorporate and remove variables in the occupational therapy process to present the client with the ***just-right challenge***—one that is neither so far beyond the client's present abilities that it is frustrating or may compromise the therapeutic process nor so far beneath them that new learning or progress does not occur.

Importance of Occupation as Means

Occupation-as-means refers to an intervention in which the occupational therapy practitioner selects therapeutic activities on the basis of the client's occupational interests and needs. The occupation itself is the means of therapy. In the therapeutic process, practitioners promote improvements in a client's internal factors by analyzing and selecting components of related activities in four major ways:

1. Practitioners present an activity to promote interest, motivation, and drive, which enables a client to exert more effort and follow an activity to completion, allows for performance in multiple contexts, and sustains performance for a longer duration.
2. Practitioners manipulate a selected activity and environmental conditions to present graded challenges to specific skills.
3. Practitioners select activities that will present variables during activity performance that require a client to assess, develop, and implement effective cognitive or motor strategies (responses) that can be generalized to a variety of future situations (generalization of skills).
4. Practitioners educate clients on how components of an occupation (whether partial or whole performance) can be used throughout the rehabilitative process to collaboratively discuss, establish, and work toward goal attainment.

The combination or adaptation of variables can occur in practice, whereby occupational therapy practitioners incorporate variations of occupation-as-means and related activities into various areas of practice. A critical component of using a client's occupation as a form of intervention is ensuring that the intervention is also centered on the client's values, beliefs, and spirituality. Incorporating these features of a client's identity into the treatment process can also affect the client's motivation and be a holistic factor of providing client-centered and inherently meaningful services.

The incorporation of a client's cultural identity begins at the point of evaluation and often continues as a dynamic process along the therapeutic continuum of care. Occupational therapy practitioners must also note that values, beliefs, and spirituality are not exclusive of other determinants of occupational performance such as client factors or performance skills. The generalization of skills is also a critical component of measuring the effectiveness of occupational performance in the intervention process. When a client demonstrates the potential to improve underlying factors or performance skills, the practitioner can include activities that enable the client to work toward the restoration, promotion, modification, or the promotion of desired goals and outcomes in the therapeutic process.

Using Occupation-Based Activities to Enhance Occupational Performance

The incorporation of activities as a form of therapy to address client factors and performance skills dates to occupational therapy's conception (Taylor, 1929). Baldwin (1919) suggested that therapeutic occupations must be aligned with the client's choice if the occupation is to be effective in meeting the therapeutic goals. Compared with traditional rote exercises, the performance of activities elicits improved outcomes within client factors and performance skills (Che Daud et al., 2016a; Hoppe et al., 2008; Powell et al., 2016).

Rote learning is based on repetition and memorization; learning is reinforced through sheer repetition and then stored in a person's long-term memory through a form of automatism (Bergson, 1991; James, 1890/1950). Examples of rote exercises (excluding purposeful motions or occupations) can include jumping in place at a predetermined pace or stretching a resistance band for a set number of repetitions. Although these kinetic motions may be beneficial when increased joint extension or endurance are treatment goals, the movements alone are not a form of occupation-based treatment, because the components themselves cannot be classified as forms of occupation in a variety of contexts. Occupational therapy practitioners can clinically manipulate the motor, cognitive, psychosocial, and social interactional characteristics of therapeutic activities to a greater extent than traditional repetitive exercises, which offer clients less variability or intrinsic meaning.

Activities that elicit a client's interest also promote a greater degree of repetition and prolonged duration of physical output than the performance of a routine exercise program (Lohse et al., 2013; Morton et al., 1992; Omar et al., 2012). With the steady advancements in and access to an array of interactive gaming technologies, occupational therapy practitioners are mainstreaming the use of interactive simulations and gaming systems as a part of virtual rehabilitation in various practice settings as a means of facilitating therapeutic engagement and targeting client-centered interest (Avcil et al., 2020).

For example, in a randomized controlled study, Rand et al. (2014) analyzed purposeful and nonpurposeful repetitions of upper-extremity movements of people with a history of chronic CVA while they interacted with video games or participated in traditional rote exercise programs. In the rote exercise program, participants were instructed to perform isolated movements of the affected upper-extremity through either passive or active range of motion and for a specific number of repetitions and duration. In the video game group, participants engaged in purposeful upper-extremity movements based on visual and audio feedback from the movement-focused, activity-based interactive features of the virtual simulations. Both groups were supervised by occupational therapists, who attempted to minimize compensatory movements and provided verbal encouragement as needed.

The results revealed that among people with chronic CVA, video game simulations elicited more purposeful upper-extremity repetitions and higher acceleration of movement than traditional rote therapy. The researchers also noted that the participants in the video gaming group had a higher degree of activity tolerance and sustained interest than those in the rote exercise program.

Tate et al. (2020) produced similar findings in a qualitative study examining the effectiveness of goal-directed intervention in increasing nonvocational activities for seven people with traumatic brain injury (TBI) and a substantial degree of disability that resulted in an inability to rejoin the workforce. The researchers focused on meaningful activities, leisure performance and satisfaction, and social and cognitive activities that centralized the carryover of skills to a variety of contexts. The results revealed that participants had higher functional outcomes with activities that focused on occupation-based strategies. They reported a higher degree of enjoyment in these activities than in activities that focused only on their diminished capacities. Motivation and interest were essential in this study because participants valued meaningful activities in the context of cognitive, emotional, and physical symptoms of TBI, which also directly improved community reintegration and mental wellness (Tate et al., 2020).

Unique occupation-based activities can be used to treat both acute and chronic conditions, especially when symptoms of these conditions affect meaningful occupational roles and when traditional forms of rehabilitation such as rote exercises produce minimal to no symptom relief. In a qualitative study conducted by Earley and Shannon (2006), a longitudinal case analysis of a 53-year-old woman with primary shoulder adhesive capsulitis focused on meaningful occupations in natural contexts and revealed a heightened degree of client-initiated pain management, decreased negative effects of learned disuse, and fear avoidance. Researchers centralized the application of compensatory occupational techniques and purposeful activities and included therapeutic education focused on occupational role fulfillment.

Compared with the benefits of rote exercises, engagement in everyday activities can be physically and cognitively challenging and rewarding for people with deficits in performance skills and client factors as a result of a disability. For example, Wensley and Slade (2012) qualitatively examined six avid walkers and asked them to describe the benefits of daily walking for their overall health and well-being. Participants described walking as a meaningful activity in which the challenge, wellness, social connectedness, and connection to nature in this daily and routine-based activity engagement were motivating factors. The researchers also determined that people's subjective value and perceptions of occupations are powerful tools in assessing how to incorporate interest-based forms of intervention in practice as a means of promoting health and wellness. The results of Earley and Shannon (2006) and Wensley and Slade (2012) highlight the importance and efficacy of varying the types of therapeutic approach in the intervention process for both acute and chronic conditions, along with an essential component of ensuring that clients find meaning in the practitioner's treatment approaches and clinical reasoning processes.

Is the incorporation of occupation-based treatment more practical and effective in meeting client-centered goals than rote forms of therapeutic exercise and treatment regimens? The answer depends on multiple variables. Occupational therapy practitioners have reported logistical issues such as limited access to space and resources, time, and equipment as factors that limit the use of occupation-based forms of treatment in practice, such as in hand therapy (Che Daud et al., 2016b; Colaianni & Provident, 2010). Practitioners have also attributed the need to further evaluate client experiences, perspectives, expectations, and perceptions as a form of individualized treatment planning that, if discounted, can decrease the incorporation of occupation-based treatment modalities in practice (Kristensen et al., 2016).

Occupational therapy practitioners must account for practical constraints in practice when attempting to incorporate meaningful forms of therapeutic intervention, but they must also be cognizant of the principles of holistic practice that value the person's unique experiences, cultural background, spirituality, and current capacities. In addition, prioritizing client preferences in service delivery can also enhance clients' quality of life in the continuum of practice settings. Occupation-based interventions may produce more favorable outcomes than traditional rote therapeutic programs.

In a qualitative study examining occupational therapy practitioners' perspectives and occupation-based interventions with people after hip fracture, Wong et al. (2018) were able to identify various major themes that contributed to and hindered the integration of occupation-based forms of intervention in treatment delivery. The themes identified were conducting an occupational profile, integrating occupation-based interventions in the facility, and identifying goals for occupational engagement after discharge. Occupational therapy practitioners identified barriers such as partial or unsubstantiated forms of documentation that made it difficult for practitioners to document true occupation-based forms of intervention and limited resources, such as space and equipment. Highlighting occupational therapy's contributions through outcome measures that assess, document, substantiate, and quantify interventions conveys the profession's unique value to the wider health care system (Wong et al., 2018).

Using Client-Relevant and Culturally Relevant Occupations in Practice

Using mock simulations to address ADLs can alleviate the lack of contextual resources in occupation-based interventions. Skills such as planning the steps of preparing a meal from scratch can be learned through tabletop activities as well as through readily available clinic resources. Occupational therapy practitioners can also document the components of performance skills that were addressed through treatment as opposed to the occupation that drove the intervention.

For example, an occupational therapy practitioner can document the kinematics involved in performing laundry-based tasks, such as crossing midline, dynamic standing balance, bilateral manual skills, shifting center of gravity, and visual–motor coordination (occupation as a means), as opposed to describing a client folding and sorting clothes from a dryer as an occupation-based activity (occupation as an end). Moreover, practitioners can also incorporate the sense of enjoy-

CASE EXAMPLE 7.1. Muhammad: Multiple Sclerosis

Muhammad is a 51-year-old Pakistani American man who has a diagnosis of primary progressive multiple sclerosis and is receiving occupational therapy services in an inpatient rehabilitation unit after a fall in his kitchen. Muhammad resides with his wife and daughter in a two-bedroom basement apartment, which requires walking down 10 steps. In the medical center, the collaborative rehabilitative goals were to increase Muhammad's visual attention and awareness of peripheral fields, to improve his bimanual motor control despite the presence of bilateral intention tremors in the upper extremities, and to address overall dynamic standing balance and tolerance.

From an occupational profile and information obtained through a semistructured interview, the occupational therapy practitioner learned that Muhammad values reading his holy scripture; praying throughout the day, which involves kneeling and bowing; and cooking traditional dishes passed down over generations for his family and friends. Muhammad was able to stand for less than 5 minutes when not being distracted by stimuli in the clinic. He also exhibited delayed reaction and termination responses during activities requiring fine motor control, such as manipulating objects, and responding to basic auditory cues when presented through his peripheral line of sight.

The occupational therapist used a culturally sensitive approach to treatment because Muhammad responded less than favorably to bottom-up–based approaches to treatment. In the treatment regimen, the therapist used the motivation of Muhammad's favorite dish, which required Muhammad to stand for a tabletop activity while manipulating the components of the dish as sourced by a family member. While sitting, Muhammad also integrated adaptive strategies to produce controlled trunk flexion and compensatory bilateral movements as alternative forms of movements related to praying while listening to an audio file of his holy scripture as sourced by Muhammad himself. Muhammad was able to stand independently and maintain his standing balance for 10 to 12 minutes before being prompted to take a break because he was eagerly engaged and focused on the task. He reported feeling fulfilled and motivated by his performance, and his bimanual movements also improved as a result of carefully integrated compensatory strategies when engaged in simulated tabletop activities of cooking and alternative postural strategies for praying, which he acknowledged deeply motivated him to resume his meaningful activities.

ment, challenge, and completion of the therapeutic process into treatment planning or implementation if clients find some form of meaning and perceived value (or spiritual satisfaction; see Chapter 16, "Spirituality and Occupation"). A client who enjoys the experience, who finds the treatment to be challenging yet rewarding, and who can reap benefits outside of the intended outcomes (such as enhanced mindfulness) is more likely to comply with therapeutic instruction and carry over skills to other areas of performance of daily tasks (Krpalek et al., 2017; see Case Example 7.1).

Other researchers have found that after sustaining a stroke, adults showed extensively improved motor performance and neurophysiological changes when the treatment context resembled their natural and meaningful space (Guidetti et al., 2009; Skubik-Peplaski et al., 2012). The incorporation of a meaningful client space when using occupation-based forms of treatment is a vital step in addressing interest, motivation, and use of internal factors to successfully attain goals and desired outcomes. As in Case Example 7.1, occupational therapy practitioners can create simulated natural contexts or performance patterns that mirror a client's natural context to address client factors and performance skills through an individualized approach to service delivery.

In pediatric intervention, the integration of occupation-based forms of intervention is often critical in addressing the developmental, cognitive, psychosocial, and adaptive needs of clients in an array of pediatric settings (see Figure 7.2). The use of occupations and how they are incorporated into pediatric practice also depends on the occupational therapy practitioner's ability to support and advocate for caregiver buy-in and inclusion, caregiver confidence and competency, and environmentally focused strategies to incorporate naturalistic contexts in service delivery. The practitioner-driven facilitation of active participation in occupational forms of intervention within the treatment setting should also address how pediatric clients and their caregivers transfer those learned experiences to the home context as a part of holistic, client-centered service delivery (Gurga et al., 2019). Family-centered practice supports the integration of occupation as a viable form of treatment, sometimes as a means and sometimes as an end, across the pediatric practice continuum in which home care, school-based, and clinic-based settings incorporate varying forms of family-centered principles of intervention (Fingerhut et al., 2013).

For example, a school-based occupational therapy practitioner can document their daily notes for a pediatric client and also schedule a weekly meeting with a parent who has a busy work schedule. Along with the parent, the practitioner can then request the assistance of a school district–based interpreter if English is not the primary language, so they can review the child's progress and discuss any sensitive matters in the parent's preferred language and as the parent's weekly availability allows.

FIGURE 7.2. Client engaged in an age-appropriate play-based activity through the use of occupation as an end, incorporating a strengths-based approach to address bimanual integration, dynamic sitting balance, and short-term memory recall.

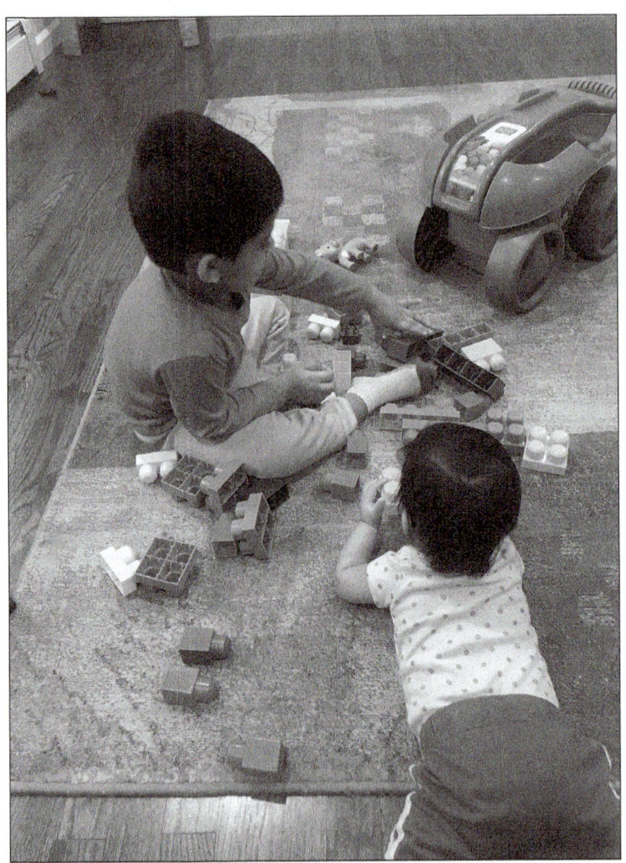

Source. P. Kaur. Used with permission.

Within pediatric and adult practice, the term ***caregivers*** can mean a client's partner; parent; or any other recognized, acknowledged, or legally appointed member of a client's micro or macro form of support. In following this culturally sensitive approach to the diverse and multilayered aspect of the caregiver role, occupational therapy practitioners must learn as much as possible about each client's experiences, strengths, limitations, and motivating variables that can support the therapeutic process and goal attainment. The balance between a client's intrinsic capacity and their understanding of how practitioners use treatment modalities to facilitate goal development must be carefully monitored to integrate a consistent client-focused approach to services into the client's rehabilitative journey.

Providing culturally competent services within occupational therapy is a vital factor for serving the needs of increasingly diverse communities within varying practice contexts and a pivotal factor in supporting the occupational needs of individuals through a truly holistic and client-centered model of care (Govere & Govere, 2016). An occupational therapy practitioner can ask, "Could you tell me something about your cultural or ethnic background that you find meaningful?" "What language do you prefer or feel comfortable with?" or "Are there any physical, cultural, or spiritual restrictions or sensitivities you feel comfortable disclosing to me or to a member of the team so that we can provide services respectfully?" Depending on the practice area and situation, as well as the intrinsic and extrinsic variables of the therapeutic process at hand, practitioners must tread carefully, ethically, and professionally and use a culturally sensitive approach when gathering potentially sensitive information. Transparency and fostering a truly collaborative therapeutic relationship with clients can encourage a greater degree of goal development and attainment. A practitioner's knowledge of a client's meaningful experiences can be used as a tool in occupation-centered practice—for example, working with a child who understands that practicing legible handwriting can be an effective form of self-expression in making new friends and communicating interests or using a client's favorite song as a cue in addressing time management and impulse control. Culturally sensitive communication demonstrates an understanding of and inherent respect for individuals and promotes client and caregiver satisfaction (Claramita et al., 2016; Douglas et al., 2011).

Occupational therapy practitioners can demonstrate verbal and nonverbal forms of culturally sensitive communication practices. Using a culturally sensitive approach to discussing a client's occupation relies heavily on practitioners' ability to critically evaluate their own values, beliefs, preferences, and culture, as is an ongoing understanding of how individuals' and communities' traditions, perspectives, experiences, and practices are a powerful part of a therapeutic approach to holistic care.

In a systematic review, Brooks et al. (2019) explored the concept of culturally sensitive communication and identified clinical practice implications and knowledge gaps related to culturally sensitive communication in health care practice. They found that the health care practitioners' use of open and sensitive communication, understanding of their own culture, and use of culturally sensitive communication that highlights the client's values and beliefs were major themes in the body of research reviewed and were effective strategies to integrate cultural sensitivity into communication approaches with clients and caregivers.

Integrating Both Regulatory and Nonregulatory Conditions Into Activity Performance and Design

Each person is different and performs activities with unique and distinct variations that are symbolic of their roles, experiences, values, and cultural identities. For example, a person who is preparing a meal alone in their home can perform that exact same activity with a noticeable degree of variation while talking to a friend on the phone. Although the basic activity is the same (preparing a meal) and is performed in the familiar context, the extrinsic variable of talking to a friend embedded in the performance of that activity directly affects and alters the performance skills, performance patterns, and client factors used in the performance of this specific occupation. In the latter variation of the activity, the person must now account for differences in range of motion, strength, balance, coordination, cognitive demands, and social skills. A practitioner can use these differences in designing a treatment approach through a continuum of ***graded challenges,*** which can encompass an increase or decrease in the perceived level of difficulty or goal attainment. A component of an activity that can be graded allows the clinician to add or reduce the level of complexity and challenge during activity performance by the client, in turn allowing for controlled variability. Treatment sessions must incorporate activities that provide incremental increases in appropriate demands; the practitioner uses their clinical reasoning skills to identify a specific therapeutic continuum of when and how these gradations are introduced.

Practice, repetition, and variable task performance will not promote improvement in all client factors and performance skills. For example, if a client's goal is to improve their wheelchair propulsion in the context of the workplace, the occupational therapy practitioner must decide whether they should encourage the client to propel for longer distances without taking breaks in the workplace or to propel their wheelchair on the various surfaces of the workplace (e.g., hardwood floors, carpeted and tiled areas). Because activity tolerance is not the focus of the client's goal, the ability to propel themselves within the workplace and its associated contexts requires the practitioner to methodically introduce a series of graded challenges along a client-centered continuum that encourages the client to perform an activity with a variation in the activity demands, leading to an improved therapeutic outcome specific to the client's personal goals.

Gentile's (1972) two-stage model emphasizes the goal of the learner and the influence of task and environmental characteristics on obtaining that goal. A person must conceptualize the pattern or plan of movement as well as be able to discriminate the regulatory and nonregulatory conditions that will affect activity performance. ***Regulatory conditions*** refer to environmental features that directly influence the specific way a person performs an activity or task. ***Nonregulatory conditions*** include factors that are not inherently related to performing a specific activity or task. When designing activities to present a graded challenge, occupational therapy practitioners determine which features in the environment and activity performance are regulatory to the skills and capacities they seek to challenge in the therapeutic process (Jarus, 1994). Practitioners can incorporate a greater awareness of both regulatory and nonregulatory conditions when designing therapeutic tasks that challenge a client's ability to discriminate between both conditions to refine and diversify their own performance capacities for enhanced outcomes. For example, when learning to tie a tie, a client may require time to get accustomed to the material and length of the tie as well as the form and style they are attempting when manipulating the tie (regulatory

FIGURE 7.3. Regulatory conditions that can be graded to challenge activity performance requirements for making a simple sandwich.

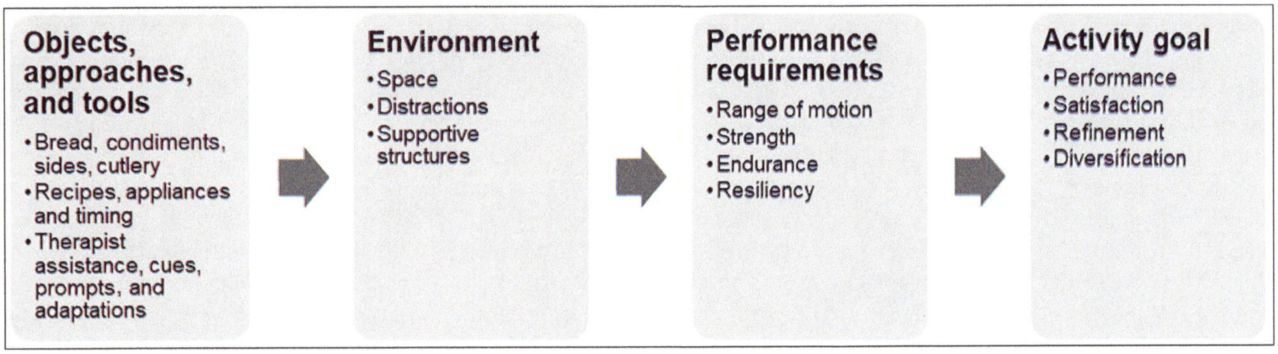

Objects, approaches, and tools		Environment		Performance requirements		Activity goal
• Bread, condiments, sides, cutlery • Recipes, appliances and timing • Therapist assistance, cues, prompts, and adaptations	→	• Space • Distractions • Supportive structures	→	• Range of motion • Strength • Endurance • Resiliency	→	• Performance • Satisfaction • Refinement • Diversification

Source. V. Pagpatan. Used with permission.

conditions). The client may also need to ignore contextual distractors and features such as the pattern or design of the tie that do not affect the movements required to reach their goal (nonregulatory; see Figure 7.3).

Objects, Approaches, and Tools

People can use objects, approaches (i.e., strategies), and tools in a variety of ways to optimize their task performance outcomes. Objects and tools can be manipulated, adapted, customized, simplified, built up, and modified, which will influence how people plan and execute their own movements for task performance. Approaches can also influence goal attainment because the person is always accounting for and reacting to variations in motor planning; kinematics; and available cognitive, sensory, and motor capacities to carry out their desired task performance. Object variations, such as the size and weight of a ball (baseball vs. basketball), or tool variations (using a hammer instead of a nail gun) can influence the outcome of the task performance. Occupational therapy practitioners can manipulate these regulatory conditions in treatment sessions to facilitate both the practice and the mastery of task performance.

Environmental Considerations

Contextual variations and features are forms of both regulatory and nonregulatory conditions that can affect task performance. Auditory distractions, such as residents conversing loudly in a hallway during a treatment session with a client, which requires sustained attention, or intentional obstacles in the path of a client practicing motorized wheelchair maneuvers are variable features that can be used in therapeutic intervention to provide a graded challenge.

Practitioner as a Regulatory Factor

The occupational therapy practitioner may also be a regulatory factor that influences the client's performance requirements. A practitioner can introduce varying forms of therapeutic instruction, education, feedback, and guidance to support, assist, or adapt a client's own task performance strategy. Such assistance can be graded down incrementally to provide clients with the opportunity to develop increasingly refined and diverse abilities to independently and efficiently engage in task performance (see Figure 7.4).

FIGURE 7.4. Client with hemiparesis to her dominant side and occasional inattention after a stroke performing meal preparation by practicing a strategy of therapist-prompted bimanual coordination.

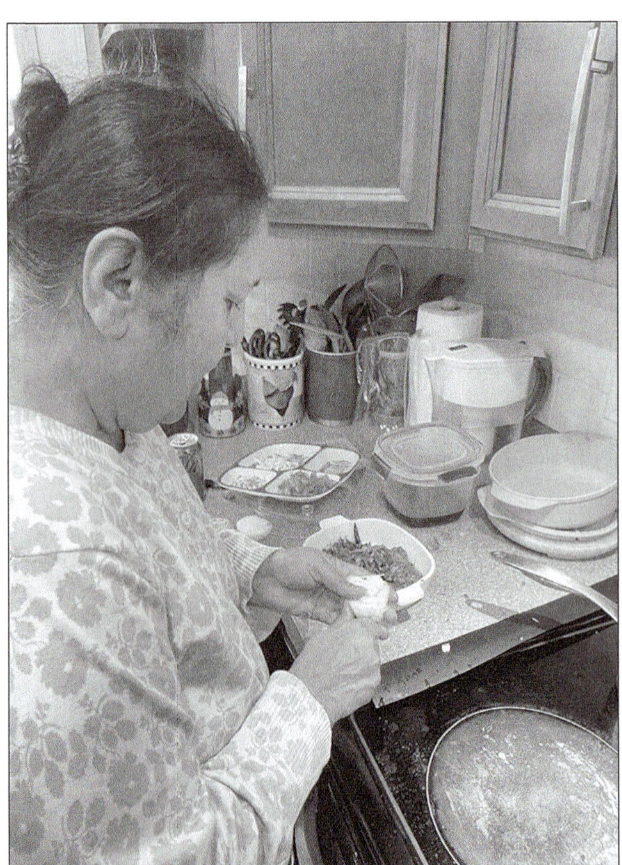

Source. V. Pagpatan. Used with permission.

Leveraging Graded Challenges in Occupational Performance

When incorporating graded challenges in the treatment process, occupational therapy practitioners should critically consider the impact of precautionary measures on the effectiveness and quality of outcomes produced through occupational performance. Precautions can be clearly outlined from referral sources, by members of the interdisciplinary team, or by the occupational therapy practitioner in the evaluation and treatment process. It is vital that a practitioner take precautionary steps when introducing graded challenges with clients to reduce the likelihood of injury and to avoid hindering motivation and confidence or minimizing levels of competence.

In any activity requiring movement, the occupational therapy practitioner must ensure that the client is initiating movement with either an ***instructed plan*** (i.e., visual instructions, an understanding of expectations, modeled behavior, explanation of the intent of the activity, verbal instructions) or a ***self-developed plan*** (i.e., motor praxis) of movement, starting from a position of optimal body alignment and with an understanding of the expectations and outcomes of the therapeutic activity. With an activity centered around cognitive training, the practitioner must ensure that the components of the activity that can be graded are in alignment with the client's current skill level and potential; understand the client's ability to manage and adapt to alterations to activity demands; and account for the client's emotional, mental, and behavioral states when integrating a series of graded challenges (see Case Example 7.2).

Simply providing increasingly difficult challenges does not always result in improved functional outcomes. Before selecting a treatment regimen for graded activity performance, the occupational therapy practitioner must determine whether

CASE EXAMPLE 7.2. Oluwayomi (Ou-lu-y-omi): Activity Grading

Oluwayomi (Ou-lu-y-omi) is coordinating an IADL skills group with a group of veterans in a community Veterans Health Administration outpatient setting. The theme of the group is to analyze and discuss IADL challenges for veterans with posttraumatic stress disorder (PTSD) and strategies to improve their functional performance in meaningful community-based tasks. The group has eight members, and each member has a significant past medical history of orthopedic, psychological, and mobility impairments. Group members are ages 27 to 33 years and are eager to reintegrate into their meaningful occupational roles. Group members exhibit difficulty committing themselves to new styles of communication and social behaviors and to stigmatizing themselves as dependent within society. Oluwayomi will grade the group's activities along a continuum of increasing self-awareness, confidence, and teamwork and will use clients' strengths and interests to maintain drive and attention.

At the first session, group members are required to introduce themselves by nonverbally sharing something positive about their upbringing and cultural experiences through an art-based activity, such as through music, abstract expression, and creative forms of art. At subsequent sessions, clients delve into their perceptions of community-based barriers and supports that drive and influence the day-to-day activities that are meaningful to them. They discuss and explore areas of home-making tasks, shopping, financial management, taking care of their family members, and community mobility (driving and public transportation). They discuss their experiences through a mediated and semistructured discussion with Oluwayomi, who constantly monitors changes in behavior, attitude, and mental state and responds accordingly using a facilitatory approach.

Gradually, Oluwayomi introduces and facilitates self-expression, self-awareness, and insight- and judgment-based activities and discussions on community-based scenarios and situations that may trigger or exacerbate group members' PTSD symptoms. Through active observation, documentation, and monitoring, Oluwayomi monitors the group's performance and how increasingly difficult or complex activities affect each group member's overall level of functioning. Oluwayomi demonstrates compensatory strategies that are centered around mitigating feelings of anxiety, depression, and emotional fluctuations and encouraging forms of coping and wellness-based adaptive responses.

Oluwayomi's long-term goal is for group members to develop adaptive coping mechanisms that can be used in an array of occupational activities. Through a carefully implemented clinical approach, Oluwayomi introduces graded challenges that allow group members to compound the skills they have learned and apply them in various contexts and situations. She remains vigilant for any areas of decline and strives to incorporate meaningful pieces of information that allow for a safe space and a truly client-centered approach in facilitating therapeutic group activities and discussions.

the client has the baseline and potential capacities to benefit from this type of intervention. In many cases, the use of graded challenges requires a deeper understanding of the client's social, medical, and cognitive capacities. This understanding can be gained from a collaborative approach among team members, client, and support systems, as well as the practitioner's knowledge and competencies (i.e., continuing education and training).

Indeed, an occupational therapy practitioner can do unintentional harm to a client and the client's progress if graded challenges hinder, deter, or misguide the client regarding their performance and progress. For example, a practitioner introduces a series of strategically placed obstacles in the path of a pediatric client's wheelchair with the intention of measuring the client's reaction time, spatial awareness, and safety awareness when using their manual wheelchair in the hallway of their school. The practitioner incorporates physical obstacles and environmental auditory distractions and fluctuates the distance of the wheelchair path. However, the client becomes frustrated, says, "I can't do this," and retreats. Rather than, say, increasing obstacles or setting high expectations, this can be a moment to appreciate the progress made and focus on what has been accomplished, and not a new, perhaps unattainable goal. Frustration and setbacks are part of the learning process, but the practitioner needs to integrate the graded challenges after carefully assessing the client's current level of performance, medical status, and documented precautions as well as tips, hints, and recommendations from other team members.

The *AOTA 2020 Occupational Therapy Code of Ethics* (AOTA, 2020a) requires that occupational therapy practitioners ensure that they take care to avoid undue harm or hardship to their clients that may diminish their trust or tarnish the therapeutic rapport established in the process of occupational therapy. Professional errors are unavoidable and have been thoroughly examined in various health care fields. In the field of occupational therapy, practitioners consider the potential not only for physical harm to clients but also psychosocial concerns (Scheirton et al., 2003). For example, consider a 7-year-old client who is struggling to achieve optimal postural

CASE EXAMPLE 7.3. Mr. Singh: Developing Alternative Strategies

Mr. Singh is a 47-year-old Indian American man who has been referred to occupational therapy services in an inpatient setting secondary to a left hip fracture and right humeral fracture after a motor vehicle accident. Mr. Singh has a past medical history of diabetes, hypertension, and chronic renal failure. His occupations are father, husband, brother, and owner of an interior design company. Although proficient in basic social exchanges, Mr. Singh has identified English as his second and nonpreferred language, with Punjabi and Hindi being his primary languages. Mr. Singh must also wear a head covering or head garment (i.e., turban) at all times because of his religious and spiritual beliefs. Mr. Singh is working with Leila, the occupational therapist, and Alexander, the occupational therapy assistant, to address a series of ADL skills and barriers to occupational performance before his scheduled discharge to home.

Mr. Singh exhibits difficulty in upper- and lower-body dressing skills and functional transferring skills (e.g., toilet transfer), as well as an overall lack of activity tolerance secondary to his deconditioned state. Because of length-of-stay restrictions, the rehabilitation team can only partially address these areas of concern with an emphasis on safety and independence. The occupational therapy practitioners work collaboratively to address Mr. Singh's needs through an occupation-as-means approach by targeting his most important tasks first, which he has reported as getting dressed independently.

Using adapted motor strategies, the occupational therapy team educates and instructs Mr. Singh on various kinematic strategies that could enable him to don and remove his upper- and lower-body garments while adhering to his medical precautions. The practitioners use weight shifting, pelvic movement, and adapted one-handed dressing techniques to facilitate the use of alternative motor patterns to allow Mr. Singh to perform his meaningful activity. The team also incorporates a series of sensorimotor strategies focused on using specific types of clothing material that can allow for increased manipulation during donning and removing sequences and interpersonal techniques to help Mr. Singh ask for assistance to apply his religious head garment every day, a meaningful activity that he says provides him with the motivation to continue with his treatment. The team uses conceptual demonstrations and visually guided strategies to allow Mr. Singh to practice in various situations and to challenge and gradually improve his activity tolerance and overall stamina. With a language interpreter on standby, the occupational therapy team also educates Mr. Singh and his family members on potential home adaptation strategies that can better enable his functional performance of other ADLs upon discharge to a subacute facility.

control for notetaking when sitting for a prolonged period of time in a classroom. The practitioner introduces fun and engaging activities that, unexpectedly, force the client to sit for an extended time, past their threshold. The client attempts to find a comfortable position through weight shifting to no avail. In the attempt to upgrade the activity by introducing a graded challenge, the well-meaning practitioner may have had a negative effect on the client's confidence and introduced variables that increase the complexity of the task beyond the client's current capacity, that is, the client's performance skills and client factors.

Using Activities to Promote Effective Strategies for Performance Skills

Skill acquisition and generalization of effective strategies that can be used in the performance of daily tasks is an essential goal for many forms of occupational therapy practice. ***Strategies*** are organized plans or sets of rules that guide action in a variety of situations (Sabari, 2011). People develop strategies in a variety of ways that serve as templates or guides and as foundational blueprints for effective participation in daily activities. Various strategies have been so well learned that they seem to be automatic, such as driving a car or riding a bicycle. The loss of these foundational skills can challenge clients' performance of daily occupations and may also affect many clients' quality of life (see Case Example 7.3).

Children learn strategies through trial and error, exploration of contexts, manipulation of objects, and demonstration of performance skills that result in desired outcomes, such as rewards. Children can also learn and make new associations through environmental forms of reinforcement, such as positive praise from a parent or feedback from a teacher. Such forms of reinforcement can be associated with positive results, thus transforming learning from a primitive to a more client-driven or purposeful action. For example, an occupational therapy practitioner is working with a child to develop core strength for improved static and dynamic sitting balance during play-based activities. The client is provided with a prompt to find their favorite animal. The client supports their trunk independently using their nondominant hand despite numerous failed attempts. Through trial and error, adapting their kinematic strategy, and an overall sense of interest and intrigue, the client is successful (see Figure 7.5). This play-based activity uses the client's strengths and interests in teaching them, a strategy for optimal weight shifting and weight bearing during movements that require dynamic sitting balance or a shift in their center of gravity.

FIGURE 7.5. Client exploring different ways to prop himself up to find and point to his favorite animal in a treatment session focusing on self-expression and postural coordination.

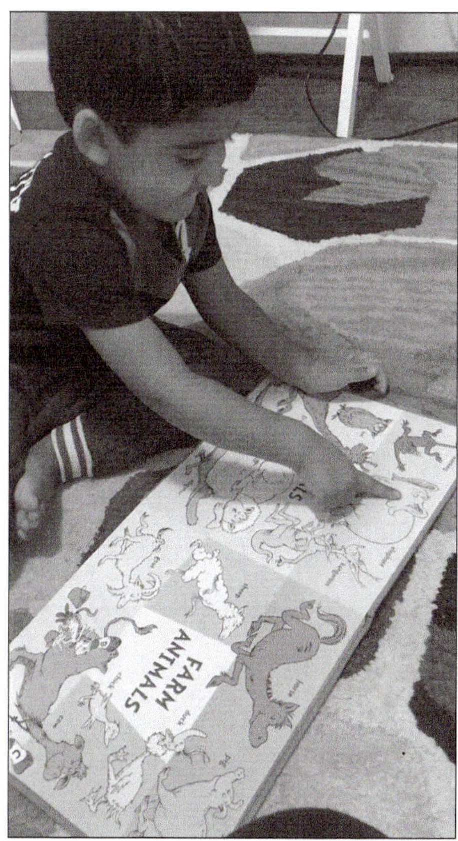

Source. K. Lata. Used with permission.

Motor Strategies

Motor strategies are volitional kinematic movements that underpin the performance of skilled and efficient fine and gross motor performance of everyday tasks. Fine and gross motor disorders can have a negative impact on people's occupational performance across the life course. Among pediatric clients, neurodevelopmental disorders such as cerebral palsy, developmental coordination disorder, and developmental delays can affect underlying performance of daily activities and hinder the ability to generalize the kinematic strategies that underlie efficient and purposeful movement (see Figure 7.6).

Task-oriented interventions that target the development and refinement of motor strategies are effective if practitioners

EXERCISE 7.1. Putting a Phone Case on a New Phone

Think about the task of putting a phone case on a new phone.

1. What strategies would you use to accomplish the task while supporting joint alignment and reducing the likelihood of injury?
2. Would your past experience assist you in the initiation and sequencing of this multistep task?
3. Now consider the onset of a disability that affects fine motor skills and visual–motor coordination. What motor strategy changes would you need to implement to accomplish this task, given the changes to your kinematics and praxis?

FIGURE 7.6. Client using the sink and bimanual strategies to support himself when engaged in self-care.

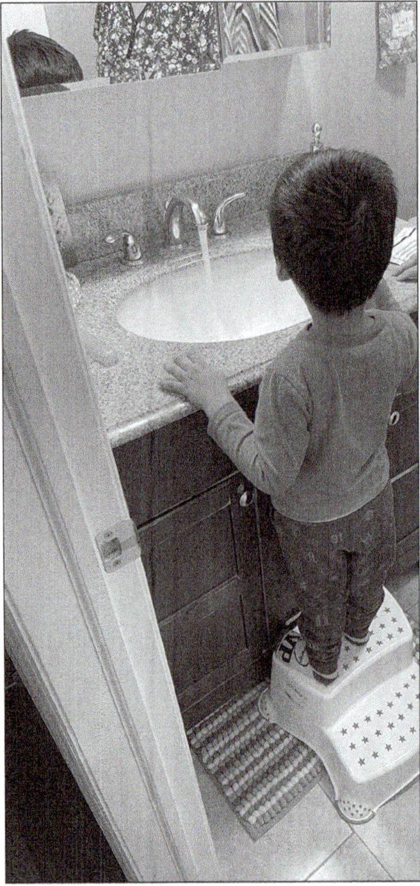

Source. P. Kaur. Used with permission.

couple a cognitive component with the activity demands. The incorporation of cognitive skills such as planning and problem solving has been found to be effective in generalizing motor strategies for daily performance (Lucas et al., 2016; Preissner, 2010; Weinstock-Zlotnick & Mehta, 2019).

Cognitive Strategies

Cognitive strategies include the mental processing of various forms of internal and external stimuli through strategies that involve processing, storage, retrieval, manipulation, application, and generalization of information and experiences. Cognitive strategies are individualized to a person and are often invisible to the provider in the therapeutic process. Such strategies influence all areas of ADL and IADL skills and tasks and are in a constant state of reorganization, refinement, and evolution. As people process new information and experiences, their cognitive strategies are being adapted, simplified, updated, or reinforced through the stimuli they experience in task performance and in different contexts.

Consider what cognitive strategies you have found useful in transitioning from academic to clinical learning experiences, such as fieldwork. Organizing your class notes to create a practice-specific reference guide may be an effective cognitive strategy to be able to quickly locate, reference, and source information used for clinical learning experiences. You may also find that creating a form with abbreviations for nonclinical skills such as documentation saves you much-needed time during stressful on-the-move situations. Categorizing and formulating visual models of reference for retrieving and applying principles of practice may also be helpful in recalling and applying specific forms of clinical information.

The use of cognitive strategies by people with disabilities that affect memory recall, problem solving, sequencing, and judgment may make it possible for them to achieve independence and autonomy in daily life tasks. The use of assistive technologies that enable function and independence for people with cognitive deficits is increasingly becoming a mainstream aspect of today's technology-driven society. For example, the use of software applications that can assist in developing, organizing, and recalling a grocery list can serve as a helpful guide for people with cognitive impairments as a result of TBI or a progressive condition such as Alzheimer's disease (Ienca et al., 2017). Moreover, multidevice cloud integration that allows people to access shared and stored information from any Internet-capable area or device can also serve to support cognitive strategies when a person's occupational deficits may lie in their ability to recall or retrieve stored pieces of information (Evans et al., 2015).

Interpersonal Strategies

Interpersonal strategies are innate templates of social interaction skills that enable people to engage, interact, reciprocate, and react in varying social situations. Every context has its own normative practices of social engagement that are also influenced by sociocultural factors. Interpersonal strategies are developed from childhood into adulthood through a series of diverse engagements and contextual variations. For example, a person would converse with their peers in a breakroom differently than with their Board of Directors in a conference room. The context, individuals, situation, and cultural normative factors all influence the types of interpersonal strategies and social etiquette people use throughout their daily lives.

Interpersonal strategies and their integration as a form of coping mechanism are important factors in adapting to various social situations in daily occupational performance. When engaged in social situations in the community, people with autism spectrum disorder incorporate coping mechanisms into their interpersonal strategies to account for nonverbal forms of social exchange and improve their expressive and comprehension abilities (Wu et al., 2014). When occupational therapy practitioners are following a holistic model of care that is truly client centered, their integration of interpersonal strategies into the therapeutic process can also address clients' ability to self-reflect, express themselves, and advocate for their goals and objectives.

Sensory Strategies

Sensory strategies include the strategies people integrate into their daily lives to regulate and modulate the input and output of sensory stimuli (i.e., auditory, visual, vestibular, olfactory, tactile, oculomotor, gustatory). The modulation of sensory inputs allows them to understand their environments and to regulate their behaviors or actions accordingly (see Figure 7.7). Contextual information generally affects the way people react to stimuli. For example, a student in a classroom who hears a distant noise in the hallway will divide their attention between multiple stimuli for a period of time instead of directing their sustained attention to the primary context of occupational performance (i.e., classroom). Occupational therapy practitioners must identify sensory deficits by methodically selecting and implementing sensory screens that are appropriate to the population, setting, and practice area. Practitioners must also take the time to thoroughly implement a form of sensory screening for vulnerable individuals or client populations who require an alternative assessment of their basic sensory capacities secondary to practical barriers, such as time allotted for evaluations or the progressive nature of their conditions (Wittich et al., 2018).

FIGURE 7.7. Client practicing incorporating her weaker upper extremity in a self-feeding task by verbally prompting herself to hold onto her jacket zipper, a self-produced sensory strategy.

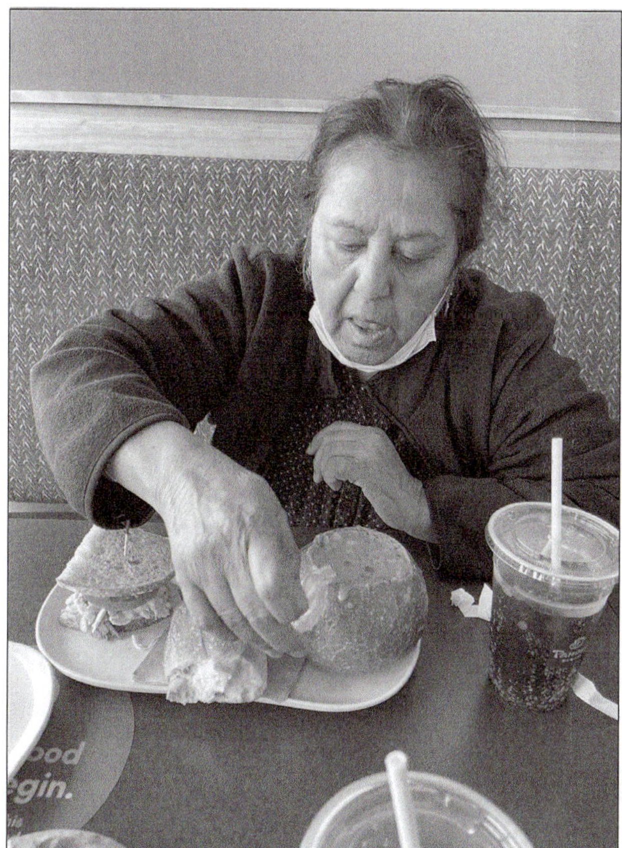

Source. V. Pagpatan. Used with permission

Summary

The use of activities as interventions to enhance client factors or to address performance skills after a disability or illness is a critical component of occupational therapy treatment. Regardless of professional practice setting, the occupational therapy practitioner must address the client's goals through a treatment regimen focused on occupation as an end or as a means to ensure improved performance remains a central theme of the intervention. Critical steps must be taken to assess whether a client meets the necessary requirements to engage in any areas of the occupational therapy process.

First, the client must demonstrate the minimum cognitive, physical, or emotional factors required to engage in the occupational therapy process at a level that can be deemed necessary to remediate, restore, adapt, educate, or compensate for a loss of function, either directly or indirectly. Second, the activity must be individualized for each client and centralized to their occupational identities and goals and to improve their overall status. The provision of occupational therapy services must also incorporate a client's understanding and willingness to receive services and to be a central part of service design and delivery. Finally, improving client factors or performance skills should always incorporate meaningful areas of activities and roles that are critical in adhering to the profession's distinctive scope of delivering services uniquely focused to facilitate a meaningful life.

Ultimately, therapeutic intervention can prove beneficial in many ways, and although some interventions restore or revive performance, others offer the opportunity to facilitate and improve it. Understanding how to introduce and encourage improved performance, bearing in mind the client's individual needs and goals, is essential to the role of the well-rounded occupational therapy practitioner. In many cases, the opportunities to overcome challenges—enhancing performance in what may seem the smallest of ways or facilitating the most meaningful of occupational outcomes—can provide the client with the knowledge and skills to face even greater challenges.

References

American Occupational Therapy Association. (2020a). AOTA 2020 occupational therapy code of ethics. *American Journal of Occupational Therapy, 74*(Suppl. 3), 7413410005. https://doi.org/10.5014/ajot.2020.74S3006

American Occupational Therapy Association. (2020b). Occupational therapy practice framework: Domain and process (4th ed.). *American Journal of Occupational Therapy, 74*(Suppl. 2), 7412410010. https://doi.org/10.5014/ajot.2020.74S2001

Avcil, E., Tarakci, D., Arman, N., & Tarakci, E. (2020). Upper extremity rehabilitation using video games in cerebral palsy: A randomized clinical trial. *Acta Neurologica Belgica, 121,* 1053–1060. https://doi.org/10.1007/s13760-020-01400-8

Baldwin, B. T. (1919). *Occupational therapy applied to restoration of movement.* Walter Reed General Hospital

Bergson, H. (1991). *Matter and memory* (N. M. Paul & W. S. Palmer, Trans.). Zone. (Original work published 1896)

Brooks, L. A., Manias, E., & Bloomer, M. J. (2019). Culturally sensitive communication in healthcare: A concept analysis. *Collegian, 26,* 383–391. https://doi.org/10.1016/j.colegn.2018.09.007

Che Daud, A. Z., Yau, M. K., Barnett, F., Judd, J., Jones, R. E., & Nawawi, R. F. M. (2016a). Integration of occupation based intervention in hand injury rehabilitation: A randomized controlled trial. *Journal of Hand Therapy, 29,* 30-40. https://doi.org/10.1016/j.jht.2015.09.004

Che Daud, A. Z., Yau, M. K., Barnett, F., & Judd, J. (2016b). Occupation-based intervention in hand injury rehabilitation: Experiences of occupational therapists in Malaysia. *Scandinavian Journal of Occupational Therapy, 23,* 57–66. https://doi.org/10.3109/11038128.2015.1062047

Claramita, M., Tuah, R., Riskione, P., Prabandari, Y. S., & Effendy, C. (2016). Comparison of communication skills between trained and untrained students using a culturally sensitive nurse–client communication guideline in Indonesia. *Nurse Education Today, 36,* 236–241. https://doi.org/10.1016/j.nedt.2015.10.022

Colaianni, D., & Provident, I. (2010). The benefits of and challenges to the use of occupation in hand therapy. *Occupational Therapy in Health Care, 24,* 130–146. https://doi.org/10.3109/07380570903349378

Douglas, M. K., Pierce, J. U., Rosenkoetter, M., Pacquiao, D., Callister, L. C., Hattar-Pollara, M., . . . Purnell, L. (2011). Standards of practice for culturally competent nursing care: 2011 update. *Journal of Transcultural Nursing, 22*(4), 317–333. https://doi.org/10.1177/1043659611412965

Earley, D., & Shannon, M. (2006). The use of occupation-based treatment with a person who has shoulder adhesive capsulitis: A case report. *American Journal of Occupational Therapy, 60,* 397–403. https://doi.org/10.5014/ajot.60.4.397

Evans, J., Brown, M., Coughlan, T., Lawson, G., & Craven, M. P. (2015). A systematic review of dementia focused assistive technology. In M. Kurosu (Ed.), *Human–Computer Interaction: Interaction technologies* (pp. 406–417). Springer. https://doi.org/10.1007/978-3-319-20916-6_38

Fingerhut, P. E., Piro, J., Sutton, A., Campbell, R., Lewis, C., Lawji, D., & Martinez, N. (2013). Family-centered principles implemented in home-based, clinic-based, and school-based pediatric settings. *American Journal of Occupational Therapy, 67,* 228–235. https://doi.org/10.5014/ajot.2013.006957

Gentile, M. (1972). A working model of skill acquisition with application to teaching. *Quest, 17,* 3–23. https://doi.org/10.1080/00336297.1972.10519717

Govere, L., & Govere, E. M. (2016). How effective is cultural competence training of healthcare providers on improving patient satisfaction of minority groups? A systematic review of literature. *Worldviews on Evidence-Based Nursing, 13*(6), 402–410. https://doi.org/10.1111/wvn.12176

Guidetti, S., Asaba, E., & Tham, K. (2009). Meaning of context in recapturing self-care after stroke or spinal cord injury. *American Journal of Occupational Therapy, 63,* 323–332. https://doi.org/10.5014/ajot.63.3.323

Gurga, A., Jarvis, J., Khetani, M., & Choong, K. (2019). Caregiver strategy use to promote their child's participation in home-based occupations following pediatric critical illness. *American Journal of Occupational Therapy, 73*(4, Suppl. 1), 7311505178. https://doi.org/10.5014/ajot.2019.73S1-PO7018

Hoppe, K. A., Miller, B. K., & Rice, M. S. (2008). Occupationally embedded exercise versus rote exercise and psychosocial response in college-aged females. *Occupational Therapy in Mental Health, 24,* 176–191. https://doi.org/10.1080/01642120802055317

Ienca, M., Fabrice, J., Elger, B., Caon, M., Scoccia Pappagallo, A., Kressig, R. W., & Wangmo, T. (2017). Intelligent assistive technology for Alzheimer's disease and other dementias: A systematic review. *Journal of Alzheimer's Disease, 56,* 1301–1340. https://doi.org/10.3233/JAD-161037

James, W. (1950). *The principles of psychology* (Vol. 2). Dower. (Original work published 1890)

Jarus, T. (1994). Motor learning and occupational therapy: The organization of practice. *American Journal of Occupational Therapy, 48,* 810–816. https://doi.org/10.5014/ajot.48.9.810

Kristensen, H. K., Ytterberg, C., Jones, D. L., & Lund, H. (2016). Research-based evidence in stroke rehabilitation: An investigation of its implementation by physiotherapists and occupational therapists. *Disability Rehabilitation, 38,* 2564–2574. https://doi.org/10.3109/09638288.2016.1138550

Krpalek, D., Hyun, A., Kim, J., Lee, A., Lee, J., Moningka, D., . . . Pendleton, K. (2017). Exploring the effectiveness of an occupation-based intervention: An experimental study with calligraphy. *American Journal of Occupational Therapy, 71*(4, Suppl. 1), 7111505118. https://doi.org/10.5014/ajot.2017.71S1-PO3151

Lohse, K., Shirzad, N., Verster, A., Hodges, N., & Van der Loos, H. F. M. (2013). Video games and rehabilitation: Using design principles to enhance engagement in physical therapy. *Journal of Neurologic Physical Therapy, 37,* 166–175. https://doi.org/10.1097/NPT.0000000000000017

Lucas, B. R., Elliott, E. J., Coggan, S., Pinto, R. Z., Jirikowic, T., McCoy, S. W., & Latimer, J. (2016). Interventions to improve gross motor performance in children with neurodevelopmental disorders: A meta-analysis. *BMC Pediatric, 16,* 193. https://doi.org/10.1186/s12887-016-0731-6

Morton, G. G., Barnett, D. W., & Hale, L. S. (1992). A comparison of performance measures of an added-purpose task versus a single-purpose task for upper extremities. *American Journal of Occupational Therapy, 46,* 128–133. https://doi.org/10.5014/ajot.46.2.128

Omar, M. T., Hegazy, F. A., & Mokashi, S. P. (2012). Influences of purposeful activity versus rote exercise on improving pain and hand function in pediatric burn. *Burns, 38,* 261–268. https://doi.org/10.1016/j.burns.2011.08.004

Powell, J. M., Rich, T. J., & Wise, E. K. (2016). Effectiveness of occupation- and activity-based interventions to improve everyday activities and social participation for people with traumatic brain injury: A systematic review. *American Journal of Occupational Therapy, 70,* 7003180040. https://doi.org/10.5014/ajot.2016.020909

Preissner, K. (2010). Use of the occupational therapy task-oriented approach to optimize the motor performance of a client with cognitive limitations. *American Journal of Occupational Therapy, 64,* 727–734. https://doi.org/10.5014/ajot.2010.08026

Rand, D., Givon, N., Weingarden, H., Nota, A., & Zeilig, G. (2014). Eliciting upper extremity purposeful movements using video games: A comparison with traditional therapy for stroke rehabilitation. *Neurorehabilitation and Neural Repair, 28,* 733–739. https://doi.org/10.1177/1545968314521008

Scheirton, L., Mu, K., & Lohman, H. (2003). Occupational therapists' responses to practice errors in physical rehabilitation settings. *American Journal of Occupational Therapy, 57,* 307–314. https://doi.org/10.5014/ajot.57.3.307

Skubik-Peplaski, C., Carrico, C., Nichols, L., Chelette, K., & Sawaki, L. (2012). Behavioral, neurophysiological, and descriptive changes after occupation-based intervention. *American Journal of Occupational Therapy, 66,* e107–e113. https://doi.org/10.5014/ajot.2012.003590

Tate, R. L., Wakim, D., Sigmundsdottir, L., & Longley, W. (2020). Evaluating an intervention to increase meaningful activity after severe traumatic brain injury: A single-case experimental design with direct inter-subject and systematic replications. *Neuropsychological Rehabilitation, 30,* 641–672. https://doi.org/10.1080/09602011.2018.1488746

Taylor, M. (1929). Occupational therapy in industrial inquiries. *American Journal of Physical Medicine and Rehabilitation, 8,* 335–338.

Weinstock-Zlotnick, G., & Mehta, S. P. (2019). A systematic review of the benefits of occupation-based intervention for patients with upper extremity musculoskeletal disorders. *SI: Evidence Updates, 32,* 141–152. https://doi.org/10.1016/j.jht.2018.04.001

Wensley, R., & Slade, A. (2012). Walking as a meaningful leisure occupation: The implications for occupational therapy. *British Journal of Occupational Therapy, 75,* 85–92. https://doi.org/10.4276/030802212X13286281651117

Wittich, W., Höbler, F., Jarry, J., & McGilton, K. S. (2018). Recommendations for successful sensory screening in older adults with dementia in long-term care: A qualitative environmental scan of Canadian specialists. *BMJ Open, 8,* e019451. https://doi.org//10.1136/bmjopen-2017-019451

Wong, C., Fagan, B., & Leland, N. E. (2018). Occupational therapy practitioners' perspectives on occupation-based interventions for clients with hip fracture. *American Journal of Occupational Therapy, 72,* 7204205050. https://doi.org/10.5014/ajot.2018.026492

Wu, C. L., Tseng, L. P., An, C. P., Chen, H. C., Chan, Y. C., Shih, C. I., & Zhuo, S. L. (2014). Do individuals with autism lack a sense of humor? A study of humor comprehension, appreciation, and styles among high school students with autism. *Research in Autism Spectrum Disorders, 8,* 1386–1393. https://doi.org/10.1016/j.rasd.2014.07.006

8

Groups, Populations, and Communities in the Context of Occupation

SHERI WADLER, MS, OTR/L,
AND HEIDI MacALPINE, OTD, MED, OTR/L

CHAPTER HIGHLIGHTS

- Yalom's therapeutic factors
- Groups in occupational therapy
- Planning process for groups, communities, and populations
- Profiling and assessment
- Building groups
- Group considerations
- Tracking progress
- Innovative group approaches
- Essential group concepts to consider

KEY TERMS AND CONCEPTS

• active listening • altruism • associative groups • brainstorming • capacity building • catharsis • clients • closed groups • COAST and SMART goals • communities • community development • community profiling • content • cooperative groups • corrective recapitulation of the primary family group • cultural sensitivity • development of socializing techniques • evidence-based practice • existential factors • experiential learning • explicit norms • formal groups • group cohesiveness • group decision making • group development • group norms • group protocol • group stages • groups • health promotion • heterogeneous groups • homogeneous groups • imitative behavior • imparting information • implicit norms • individual roles • informal groups • interpersonal learning • instillation of hope • just-right challenge • long-term goals • mature groups • needs assessment • *Occupational Therapy Practice Framework: Domain and Process* • open groups • parallel groups • person • personal or social roles • population • PRECEDE–PROCEED Model • process • roles • self-disclosure • short-term goals • social determinants of health • Social Profile • task roles • telehealth • therapeutic change • therapeutic factors • therapeutic group • therapeutic norms • therapeutic use of self • third ear • universality

I had no idea how valuable group process courses would be as those classes prepared me to work in groups (which is much of one's professional life) and understand how group dynamics impact productivity. . . . I utilize the principles of task analysis on a daily basis, which has been a cornerstone of my success.
—Anonymous Student, 2021

Introduction

By their very nature, people function within groups from birth and throughout their lives. "From the beginning of time people have congregated in groups to ensure their survival, development and evolution. The knowledge that there was safety in numbers was a motivating factor in the earliest gatherings of people" (Posthuma, 2002, p. 1). Moreover, groups often involve engagement in activities, the "building blocks of occupations, and because people are social animals, they naturally form groups to engage in these activities" (Tomlinson & White, 2014, p. 212). Belonging to groups helps people define themselves and provides them with a sense of identity.

So, what is a group? Simply defined, a ***group*** is three or more people gathered together for a common purpose. A ***therapeutic group*** is one that is conducted in a treatment environment and designed for a defined therapeutic purpose for a specific population of participants. The aim of therapeutic groups is to promote change and growth. In this chapter, we refer to therapeutic groups that are relatively small in size. Leaders are professionals or paraprofessionals, are of differing disciplines, and may work independently or as part of a larger treatment team.

Groups form to meet human needs in particular environmental contexts. They can be formal or informal (Tomlinson & White, 2014). ***Formal groups*** are more structured, such as families, academic classes, sports teams, special interest clubs, volunteer groups, and work teams. Also considered formal in nature are larger social groups, such as religious organizations and political action organizations. ***Informal groups,*** in contrast, occur spontaneously in settings such as the workplace or on the playground. In many cases, groups form in person, but today an increasing number of groups develop over great distances through the Internet. World events, popular culture, and performance contexts all influence and are critical to the creation and maintenance of groups throughout people's lives.

This chapter covers the use of groups in occupational therapy practice, the importance of making a group therapeutic, and working with communities and populations. The chapter also discusses the development of group protocols, planning and implementation of groups, and goal setting.

EXERCISE 8.1. Group Experience

Think of a favorite group in which you are or were a member. Briefly describe the group, its purpose, the leader, and members. Why was it a positive experience? Be specific with examples of what occurred and what circumstances contributed to the group's success.

Yalom's Therapeutic Factors

What are the ingredients of an extraordinary group? Group leaders and members have pondered this question for as long as there have been groups. When planning a new group, following a prescribed, tested method is a good way to start. Thorough planning alone, however, might not account for the group's life-changing outcome.

In retrospect, it is often difficult to pinpoint a single event, discussion, or activity that produced big changes in the participants. Sometimes, members will verbalize intense feelings of gratitude to the leader or members. "Before joining this group, I never thought I could do all that!" or "That was a wonderful group! It gave me a whole new perspective!" What might explain these reactions? ***Therapeutic change*** is "an enormously complex process that occurs through the interplay of human experiences [referred to as ***therapeutic factors***]" (Yalom & Leszcz, 2020, p. 10) that occurs while people are actively involved in a group setting with a therapist leading the group. The 11 factors, which Yalom (1970) first termed and then updated (Yalom & Leszcz, 2020), include the following:

- ***instillation of hope:*** the belief that group membership will produce positive, even curative results
- ***universality:*** the notion that one's problems are not unique and are shared by many (i.e., "we're all in the same boat")
- ***imparting information:*** didactic instruction or direct advice that can teach a helpful skill or explain the nature of an illness or condition
- ***altruism:*** the ability all people have to reach out and help those in distress
- ***corrective recapitulation of the primary family group:*** the tendency of a group to resemble a family and, through interaction, for members' original family conflicts to be relived correctly
- ***development of socializing techniques:*** the learning of adaptive social skills
- ***imitative behavior:*** the learning of new skills by watching and approximating the behaviors of the leader, peers, or both
- ***interpersonal learning:*** the group as a social microcosm, providing opportunities for members to learn about themselves through interacting with others
- ***group cohesiveness:*** the strong and positive bond felt by group members
- ***catharsis:*** the expression of and working through feelings and emotions arising from earlier or current experiences with the group
- ***existential factors:*** the identification of core life issues and beliefs that have the most important meaning and relevance.

These factors are not usually seen in isolation; rather, they occur in conjunction with each other. In all groups, and specifically in occupational therapy groups, the membership, overall purpose, activities, and approach will determine which factors will most likely apply. Schwartzberg et al. (2008) described an additional factor, particularly relevant to occupational therapy treatment, called ***experiential learning.*** Here, the development of a new skill occurs through doing it, as opposed to reading or hearing about it (Tomlinson & White, 2014). Examples include a work simulation activity for survivors of traumatic brain injury, a cooking group for young adults with mental health issues, the organization of a schoolwork area for a group of children, and a fall prevention exercise activity for a group of older adults. Occupational therapy practitioners are trained to look holistically at those with whom they work. Through task analysis, they can create life-changing, hands-on experiences in groups.

EXERCISE 8.2. Looking Through the Lens of Therapeutic Factors

For the group you described in Exercise 8.1, did you identify any of the therapeutic factors noted? How? If you identified an additional factor, comment on this as well.

Groups in Occupational Therapy

A Brief History of Groups in Occupational Therapy

From their earliest days as professionals, occupational therapy practitioners have been running therapeutic groups. Howe and Schwartzberg (2001) have written extensively about occupational therapy's use of group treatment, first recognized in the 1920s and continuing into the modern era.

Throughout the history of the profession, clinicians recognized the value of group work in developing and enhancing social skills. Over time, the recognition of the reparative, creative, and curative aspects of group activities resulted in the use of groups in a greater variety of settings. Today, massive changes have occurred in the way people communicate, use technology, and view culture. In addition, people define their roles on a more macro level (i.e., communities and populations). Despite these changes, elements of occupational therapy's earliest days are still present in the services occupational therapy practitioners provide today, which explains the number of older citations in this chapter, some from the field of occupational therapy and some from other disciplines.

Current Practice With Groups

More recently, innovative and nontraditional approaches have reflected the integration of old and new. Higgins et al. (2015) conducted a national survey to look at group practice in occupational therapy. They found that 50% of practitioners use groups as part of their practice with mental health, physical disabilities, and school-based settings. In addition, there are a greater number of groups in community settings, senior centers, nursing homes and assisted living facilities, and private practices. In these contexts, occupational therapy practitioners may be intervening with communities rather than with just specific groups. Today, groups are conducted face to face and through ***telehealth*** over the Internet. In short, groups are an integral part of the ever-growing practice of occupational therapy.

Occupational Therapy Practice Framework

The evolution of group work, along with related theory, neuroscience, and research methods, is reflected in the recent fourth edition of the ***Occupational Therapy Practice Framework: Domain and Process*** (*OTPF–4;* American Occupational Therapy Association [AOTA], 2020b). This evolution has included new areas such as health management, social participation, and sleep and rest identified as new distinct domains of occupation for practitioners. The *OTPF–4* provides a clear definition of occupational therapy's primary goal—the distinct perspective that engagement in occupation is critically important to health and well-being. Further, it emphasizes the importance of groups and populations (AOTA, 2020a).

Communities and Populations

The Accreditation Council for Occupational Therapy Education (2018) has set standards that require students to learn about ways to grade and adapt processes and environments, consult, and manage care for communities and populations. These standards outline how occupational therapy focuses on persons, groups, and populations as they perform occupations and activities. Moreover, they explain the profession's role as science driven and evidence based "as it relates to the importance of balancing areas of occupation; the role of occupation in the promotion of health; and the prevention of disease, illness, and dysfunction for persons, groups, and populations" (p. 41). The use of groups is critical as we begin to focus our treatment on communities and populations.

Communities are defined as a collection of populations that may be diverse and varied, including people, networks, and organizations. Authors vary in how they define and perceive the word *community,* based on their experience and profession. Scaffa et al. (2014) mentioned a broader definition of *community* to be "non-institutional aggregations of people linked together for common goals or other purposes" (p. 5). The *OTPF–4* further explains the relationships among the individual, community, and population (Table 8.1).

AOTA (2020b) describes ***clients*** in terms of persons, groups, and populations. ***Person*** refers to an individual. ***Groups*** are a collection of individuals with shared characteristics. ***Population*** has been more specifically defined to mean an "aggregate of people with common attributes" (p. 75). Examples of populations include caregivers advocating for their children with special needs who are approaching adulthood and require housing, or vulnerable populations affected by natural disasters and extreme weather.

Through recent occupational therapy research and updates to the *OTPF* and educational accreditation standards, occupational therapy practitioners are becoming more familiar with approaches to practicing within communities to address health disparities and population health (AOTA, 2020a).

TABLE 8.1. **EXAMPLES OF THE OCCUPATIONAL THERAPY PROCESS FOR INDIVIDUAL, COMMUNITY, AND POPULATION**

INDIVIDUAL	COMMUNITY	POPULATION
	Community mobility	
Person with stroke who wants to return to driving	Stroke support group talking with elected leaders about developing community mobility resources	Stroke survivors advocating for increased access to community mobility options for all people living with mobility limitations
	Social participation	
Young adult with IDD interested in increasing social participation	Young adult with IDD in a transition program that sponsors leisure activities through which all may participate in valued social relationships	Young adult with IDD educating their community about their need for inclusion in community-based social and leisure activities
	Home establishment and management	
Person living with SMI interested in developing skills for independent living	Support group for people living with SMI developing resources to foster independent living	People living with SMI in a region advocating for increased housing options for independent living
	Work participation	
Older worker with difficulty performing some work tasks	Group of older workers in a factory advocating for modification of equipment to address discomfort when operating the same set of machines, possibly requiring repetitive motions	Older workers in a national corporation advocating for company-wide wellness support programs

Source. AOTA (2020b). Adapted with permission.
Note. IDD = intellectual or developmental disability; SMI = serious mental illness.

Advocacy for policy or systems change for social justice—for example, mental health initiatives such as professional alliances with larger organizations such as the National Association for Mental Illness (NAMI) and Autism Speaks—is one example of occupational therapy practitioners' work with local and national organizations (e.g., New York State Occupational Therapy Association, AOTA) to address population needs.

Definitions of *community* can also relate to capacity building and community development, both of which help people learn to help themselves in their community. ***Capacity building*** is "the development of systems, processes, and strategies aimed at developing sustainable outcomes for improving health practices" (Touchinsky, 2019, p. 133). ***Community development*** involves clients in developing a level of commitment, gaining a sense of togetherness, being able to solve problems, and accessing resources. Occupational therapy practitioners can provide occupation-based activities by identifying and analyzing the problem and then facilitating knowledge, tools, and resources to help clients gain the necessary skills to engage in familiar or new occupations through community development and capacity building.

Fazio (2017) pointed out the importance of defining the community of a specific group of clients when collaborating with other professionals, so that the goals and objectives are clear and aligned with all stakeholders (invested members) and do not interfere with the outcome (objectives). These community-based settings and practices have become service-learning opportunities for occupational therapy students to better understand, design, and implement occupational therapy programs under the guidance and supervision of a university professor. For example, there are drop-in centers for the homeless where people can get meal or supplies and that have no professional services, but they are very willing to welcome occupational therapy students under faculty supervision.

Global and national organizations, such as the World Health Organization (WHO) and the U.S. Department of Health and Human Services (DHHS), conceptualize groups and populations as clients and promote ***evidence-based practice*** to create awareness and support, and provide resources to groups, communities, and populations. Moreover, this conceptualization of groups and populations expands the occupational therapy practitioner's role to promote health and enable people to have increased control over their health and well-being, thus improving their quality of life. ***Health promotion*** is described by WHO (1986) as reaching a state of complete physical, mental, and social well-being with the ability to identify and realize aspirations, satisfy needs, and change or cope with the environment, which goes beyond a healthy lifestyle to well-being. Health and well-being can be improved by participation in groups in clients' natural settings. Government entities such as DHHS (2020), with its 2030 objectives, align with the mission of occupational therapy and can assist practitioners by recognizing the importance of supporting groups of people with their set data-driven national objectives that measure and focus on the determinants of health and the health and well-being of populations into the next decade. DHHS describes well-being as overall life satisfaction.

Continued emphasis on these alliances has affected occupational therapy's perspective on treatment and group interventions. "If we carefully structure the things we do, review lifestyle choices, and address barriers to participation, engagement in occupation can improve people's health and well-being" (Hocking, 2011, p. 53).

Planning Process for Groups, Communities, and Populations

Profiling and Assessment

Careful research of a population is an important step in planning an effective group. Whether starting a new program or adding a group to an existing one, it is important to look at the population's met and unmet needs. Sometimes, the occupational therapy practitioner conducts a ***needs assessment,*** a procedure that can greatly help in providing ideas for a new group. It is a "formalized approach to collecting data in order to identify the needs of a group of individuals" (Price et al., 2017, p. 85), and it can be conducted in smaller institutions such as schools, worksites, and nonprofit organizations, as well as in larger geographical communities.

Community profiling is a planning model for assessing the needs of a community; it includes social, epidemiological, educational and ecological, and administrative and policy assessments to identify ***social determinants of health.*** It instructs the practitioner on the overall concerns of the targeted population, which theory to use, and how it can be applied to support activity groups. One community profile planning model that is considered a road map and has a step-by-step guide is the ***PRECEDE–PROCEED Model*** (Crosby & Noar, 2011; Grim & Hortz, 2017). This nine-stage model is described in detail as one way to be helpful when working with different populations, such as those in assisted living facilities, senior centers, camps, mental health facilities, and other community programs. PRECEDE is the portion that leads to, or comes before, an intervention, and it stands for Predisposing, Reinforcing, and Enabling Constructs in Educational/Environmental Diagnosis and Evaluation. PROCEED explains how to move forward with an intervention, and it stands for Policy, Regulatory, and Organizational Constructs in Educational and Environmental Development. For more detailed information on the PRECEDE–PROCEED Model, explore the Community Tool Box website (https://ctb.ku.edu).

The occupational profile (AOTA, 2020a, 2020b, 2021b) should be part of the evaluation process and helps to determine the appropriate group placement for specific clients. The practitioner uses the occupational profile to perform an informal assessment with a client-centered approach, using interview and observation to determine the needs, interests, values, and priorities of and barriers faced by the targeted individuals. In addition, formal assessments can be used to assess occupational performance and thus provide important information in planning a group for targeted outcomes. The occupational profile and specific assessments can be used in an ongoing manner throughout the treatment process to ensure that each client's individual needs are met.

Group Membership

A person's ability to benefit from a specific group format is always an important consideration. A member's expressed interest, attention span, or ability to self-regulate their emotions might make one group a better choice than another.

The leader will decide whether the new group is to be open or closed. ***Open groups*** allow members to join at any point. A member may even come to a single session or just part of a session. Open groups may work well on hospital units with short lengths of stay, for members who are reluctant to join, or for those who cannot yet sustain a full group commitment. Open groups are helpful when trying to promote an "everybody's welcome" feeling in a therapeutic or nontraditional health promotion setting. ***Closed groups*** have set membership. Members are expected to attend, which allows for a more focused format to build specific skills and promote a greater sense of cohesion. Naturally, the group's overall purpose and goals help in determining whether it should have open or closed membership.

Clinicians also need to consider the composition of the group (Posthuma, 2002). Relevant qualities may include gender, sexual orientation, age, education, cultural identification, medical conditions, common treatment problems, common strengths or talents, level of experience in a specific occupation, and overall level of functioning. ***Homogeneous groups*** are those in which members share certain of these relevant qualities; for example, a handwriting group for second graders or a group of female breast cancer survivors who are going back to work and have at-home challenges. ***Heterogeneous groups*** are those in which these qualities are substantially different. Here, for example, the therapist may invite all patients in a hospital unit for a community meeting or organize a cooking activity for a culturally diverse group of younger, middle-aged, and older adults.

Both homogeneous and heterogeneous groups have advantages and disadvantages. In a more homogeneous group, members may be better able to identify with each other and quickly develop group cohesion so that group tasks are more readily accomplished. Conversely, a more heterogeneous group will bring a variety of knowledge, experiences, and unique contributions. Practitioners may use these differences to stimulate the group and encourage openness to new ideas and problem solving. Some of the most creatively devised groups will combine aspects of homogeneous and heterogeneous qualities to provide a rich and meaningful growth experience for their members.

A final consideration is group size. For many groups, especially those in which open discussion is encouraged, six to eight members may be ideal. In educational groups, in which there is a teaching–learning approach, a larger number may work successfully. For many school-based groups for young children, in which tasks are narrowly focused, very small groups may work better. In all cases, practitioners should take into consideration safety, setting, available equipment, how much assistance members will need to complete tasks, and the nature of the activity itself to best determine the optimal group size.

Group Models and Theories

Planning groups requires occupational therapy practitioners to have a broad perspective on occupational performance and the needs of specific groups. When assessing and planning groups, specific models are chosen to support a holistic approach. Models are broad and explain the interrelationship of the person, environment, and occupation within a system (Cole, 2012). Several models, such as the Model of Human Occupation (MOHO; Kielhofner et al., 2003), Health Promotion Model (Scaffa et al., 2014), and universal design for learning (AOTA, 2015), may be used to explain and apply concepts to the same performance problems for different outcomes. These theories guide the process of planning, implementing, and evaluating programs and groups and address how changes occur (Grim & Hortz, 2017).

Two examples of broad models are MOHO and the Health Belief Model (Fertman & Allensworth, 2017), a health promotion program model. MOHO is an occupation-based model that views the entire spectrum of health and illness and the connections among person, environment, and occupation (Cole, 2012). MOHO can be used to examine a group's characteristics, change, and the environment that support or hinder the members' roles (Kielhofner et al., 2003). The theories that underlie the Health Belief Model describe, explain, and predict behavior at the interpersonal, intrapersonal, and population levels (Fertman & Allensworth, 2017).

Occupational therapy is a multi-theory profession, so practitioners can use more than one theory and apply it. MOHO examines a group's characteristics, its change, and the environment that supports or hinders the members' roles (Kielhofner et al., 2003). MOHO theory may also be used to address daily living habits. Social cognitive theory (Bandura, 1977, 2004) and Theory of Planned Behavior (Fertman & Allensworth, 2017) could be used to address health maintenance. Practitioners use different theories to predict functional outcomes and design interventions to achieve these outcomes.

The application of models and theories can be seen in the example of a group of older adults ages 65 or older with mild dementia and arthritis who are experiencing upper- and lower-extremity weakness and limited range of motion at the shoulders, hands, hips, and knees. A health promotion model, such as The Health Belief Model (Fertman & Allensworth, 2017), can be used to address these clients' level of motivation and self-efficacy when planning a program of functional exercises and education. The Theory of Planned Behavior (Fertman & Allensworth, 2017) postulates that change occurs when attitudes, norms, and control of behavior are taken into consideration. This group will prepare clients for increased participation in leisure activities, such as gardening and mindful movement groups focused on fall prevention and community engagement.

Building Groups

Protocols

Reflecting the needs of the community and population, a ***group protocol*** (plan) is formulated by the practitioner and guides them in planning the group. According to Cole (2012), a group protocol or plan will include the title of the group; its overall purpose; a description of activity, supplies, and equipment; goals; questions for discussion, including processing, generalizing, and application; and, last, points of summary. It will include both long- and short-term goals. Exhibit 8.1 describes the example of a 6-week gardening group protocol researched, planned, and implemented by an occupational therapy student for older adults at an assisted living facility using Cole's (2012) group format (see Figures 8.1. and 8.2).

Goal Setting

The selection of activities is guided by the members' therapeutic goals and the theories chosen to support the strategies used for the group or program. Relative mastery of an occupation is based on one's sense of effectiveness, efficiency, and satisfaction with self and others (Grajo & Boisselle, 2019). It is important to identify goals that lead to client-centered interventions for the improvement of relative mastery of occupation (Grajo & Boisselle, 2019). The significance of the group to its members is closely related to the development of appropriate goals and to members seeing themselves as agents of change.

The overall purpose and goals of the group are written in the protocol or treatment plan after the initial evaluations. ***Long-term goals*** or outcomes are required for each problem identified in the initial evaluation and provide a clear direction and intention for the intervention. ***Short-term goals*** focus on more immediate change and lead to the achievement of the long-term goals. Occupational performance can be reexamined at the deadline or date stated in the goal. For examples of specific goals, refer to the discussion of group protocols in the preceding section.

The ***SMART*** (Sheu et al., 2017) and ***COAST*** (Gately & Borcherding, 2017) methods are two forms of goal writing that are client centered and work well in occupational therapy settings. Depending on the source, the acronym SMART may stand for differing components; one explanation is **S**pecific,

EXHIBIT 8.1. Group Protocol Example

1. Group title: "Can You Dig It?"
2. Purpose: Engage clients in a group gardening activity to build community and involve people in a positive experience. A 2017 meta-analysis showed that gardening had a significant positive effect on health outcomes, including increased life satisfaction and sense of community and decreased depression and anxiety (Soga et al., 2017).
3. Brief description of activity: 6-week gardening group activity in the courtyard with six to eight members and two co-leaders.
4. Supplies and equipment needed: sun protection (e.g., sun visors), water bottles, sanitized wipes, whiteboard and writing utensils, full buckets of water, and adapted equipment (small 3-D soil scoops and mini watering cans), 11 in. x 17 in. blank transplanting schedule templates, soil, and speech recognition devices, if necessary.
5. Goals:

Example of long-term goal: By Week 6, members will be able to demonstrate the ability to use adapted gardening tools to complete sequenced gardening tasks while interacting with other participants.

Examples of short-term goals: (1) By Week 3, group members will have worked together to make decisions and assign tasks, using an independent, democratic approach, with each member making at least two verbal contributions; (2) each week, each member will choose and successfully use an adapted gardening tool to complete the weekly assigned task; and (3) each week, the members will be able to independently follow the steps of the task, using an enlarged printed sheet with pictures, and complete the daily task.

6. Questions for processing (students should think through the questions, generalize the information, and then move to application):
   - How did the members feel about the activity?
   - How might this activity relate to future leisure endeavors?
   - What has been learned? How does it apply to the member's life?
7. Points for summary: Explain group success, aligning it with short- and long-term goals.

FIGURE 8.1. As part of this health management and leisure group, students modified and adapted a garden activity at an assisted living facility.

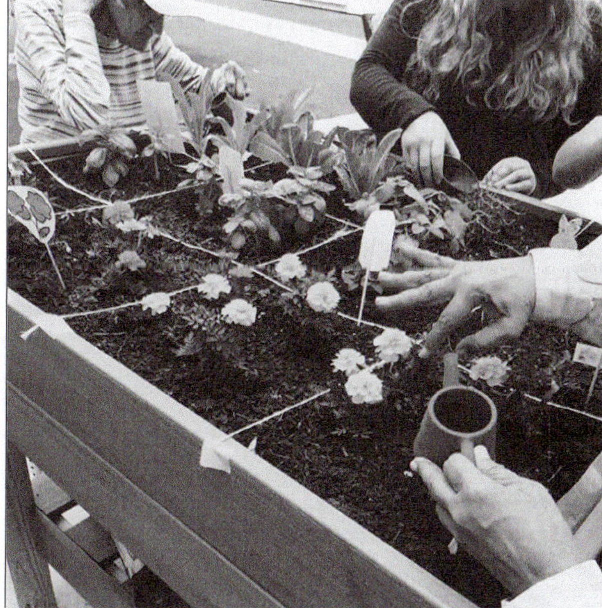

Source. H. MacAlpine. Used with permission.

FIGURE 8.2. A 3-D printer was used to create adapted gardening tools for older adults with cognitive and physical deficits.

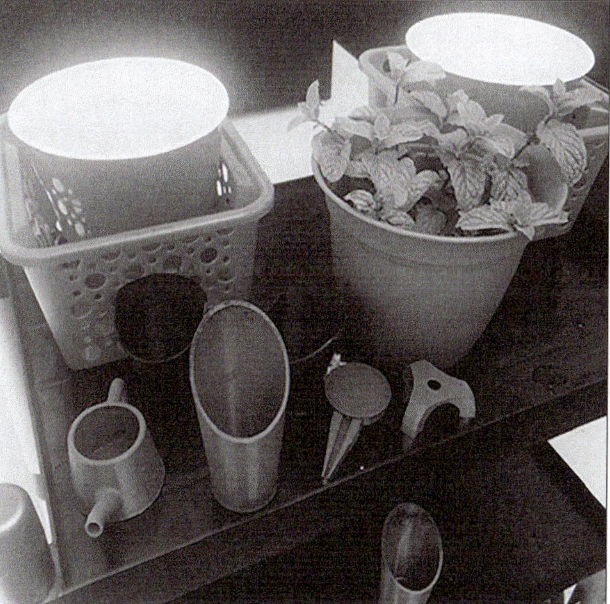

Measurable, **A**ttainable, **R**ealistic (Relatable) and **T**ime specific. SMART goals are used to direct, motivate, and invest clients in attaining specific goals that have value and meaning to them.

The COAST method has been used to communicate occupational therapy's distinct value and focus on occupational performance to third-party payers. The COAST elements are identified as follows: *C* refers to the client and should be written in terms of what the client is expected to do; *O* to the occupation the practitioner wants the client to engage in; *A* to the specific assistance level; S to the specification of any other conditions under which the practitioner expects the client to perform the desired action (e.g., adapted equipment); and *T* to the timeline in which the client is expected to accomplish this goal.

These goals work with populations and communities and align with the *OTPF-4*. The DHHS website, *Healthy People 2030* (http://www.healthypeople.gov), has some good references and resources for understanding objectives, and it provides evidence-based resources and objectives that relate to different topics and health conditions. Sheu et al. (2017) provided details, not only on objectives for programs, but also for each specific SMART goal area. They referred to the "four *W*s" rule when formulating questions to assist in writing specific SMART goals (p. 116):

1. **Who** or what is expected to change or happen?
2. **What** or how much change is expected?
3. **Where** will the change occur?
4. **When** will the change occur?

The seven-step format outlined in Exhibit 8.2 fosters a positive client–therapist relationship that works to support and engage groups in shared tasks, activities, and occupations and allows the occupational therapist to reflect on the potential meaning for each member of the group (Cole, 2012). Although this format is formulated to maximize learning for higher-level groups, it can be adapted to meet the needs of members with lower cognitive levels. The belief in members' ability to self-direct is a catalyst for group confidence and cohesiveness and enables the group to attain its goals. Cole's seven steps are a holistic and dynamic way to plan and implement group interventions that are client centered, strengthen social relationships, and support the use of adaptable and evidence-based protocols for intervention planning.

Selection of Activities

In occupational therapy groups, the primary focus is often on a set of activities. Ideally, sustained engagement in relevant, meaningful activities will improve functioning in particular settings and contexts. The selection of activities is based on the various techniques that are used in a client-centered approach. During the planning process, the choice of activities should reflect at least three steps. The first step is the careful process of reviewing both members' challenges and assets. Therapists are often very aware of the challenges faced by group members. It is easy to overlook members' strengths. For example, groups may have members with artistic talent (e.g., art, music, dance), intelligence, life experiences, and specific work or leisure skills. Acknowledging and incorporating these strengths can greatly enhance the chance for a successful group outcome. The second step involves attention to the group's SMART goals, as described earlier. The third step is the actual selection of appropriate activities. Essentially, the process is the following: Problems and assets → goals → methods (approaches and activities).

Because of their unique training, occupational therapy practitioners are task analysis experts. Through careful task analysis, practitioners plan how an activity will be carried out, adapt it, and grade it up or down (i.e., making it easier or more complex) to meet the group's needs. Occupational therapy practitioners aim to choose activities with the ***just-right challenge***, those activities that will be at the right level for clients. Throughout the activity selection process, practitioners consider how the activity will generalize to future settings in which the members are likely to be after the group concludes.

Activities can take many forms, including task- and discussion-based interventions. Discussions following a task can help to clarify purpose, challenges, and goals achieved. Games (traditional or from popular culture), paper-and-pencil exercises, work and home management simulations, movement, leisure pursuits (often with an emphasis on the task), wellness experiences, sensory activities, and social participation role-playing are just a few of the possibilities. Supplies do not necessarily have to be high tech or expensive. If the activities are safe, purposeful, related to member goals, and attractive enough to hold members' interest and have a reasonable chance for completion and success, then the possibilities are endless.

Occupational therapy practitioners should keep a few additional things in mind. First, in a group, one activity can fulfill several goals. For example, a group of older adults engage in a three-step movement activity. They are encouraged to jointly select music from a given list. Their goals include working on balance, cognitive sequencing, and social participation.

Second, one activity might be used in multiple groups that have completely different goals. For example, a cooking activity can meet daily living goals to teach basic cooking skills, or it can serve as a vocational activity to train members to become short-order cooks. For a group of adolescents, the activity could teach decision making and executive function skills, and for a group of people who already know how to cook, the same activity could focus on interpersonal interaction and communication and exploration of life roles as members plan menus and create sophisticated meals.

For any group activity, it is important for practitioners to consider the approach to use with each activity. For example, how much and what kind of support or encouragement will members need for the activity? Will they need verbal cues? Will they need special supplies or adaptive equipment? Will the members be encouraged to add comments or provide input? Some approaches are devised as the activity progresses in real time, but thinking about helpful approaches in the

EXHIBIT 8.2. Planning a Group Session

Cole's (2012) Seven-Step Group Format is one way to use a client-centered approach to create a single group session. An example, using the "Can You Dig It?" group, follows.

1. Introduction/warm-up

- Reintroduce leader and new members.
- Briefly outline the session and connect it to the previous session.
- Introduce the practitioner's role and relate it to occupation.
- Perform warm-up: relaxation and simple hand exercises.
- Review homework (tending to garden and following the written instructions).
- Summarize the preceding week's activity and identify outside fall hazards for safety reasons.
- Introduce activity, task, and goals.
- Discuss and implement safety precautions as follows:
    - If balance or lower-extremity strength is a concern, residents will remain seated during the entire activity to minimize fall risk.
    - Residents should apply sunscreen and be provided with hats to protect them from the sun.
    - SARS-CoV-2 virus (COVID-19) protocols will be followed (if necessary).
    - Group leader and assistants will monitor residents during standing activity for any evidence of postural instability or impaired balance.

2. Activity

Introduce a new watering can, purpose of watering, and how to water the garden. Consider

- strengths and limitations,
- long- and short-term goals,
- activity analysis,
- therapeutic use of self, and
- adaptations of activity, self, and environment (e.g., adaptive watering containers).

What are the needs of the garden?

- What do plants need (sun, light, water, nutrients, space)?
- What has to be done to meet the plants' needs?
- How have the modified tools helped to increase members' ability to participate in the gardening activity?
- In what ways can falls be prevented in a new environment (carryover of knowledge)?

3. Sharing

After the activity, members are asked to discuss their projects. Members will point to the areas they watered.

4. Processing

Allow members to share their work and experience with using the adaptive watering cans. How satisfied are they with their level of performance in gardening?

5. Generalizing

Discuss future gardening interactions with members and potential new members.

6. Application

Ask members what they learned about their fellow members, the activity, and their own capabilities.

7. Wrap-up, summary, and thanking the group

- Mentally review the group and the activity and help members to connect their experience to the group's goals and objectives.
- Prepare for next week and preview the new gardening tool.
- Thank members for participating in the group.

Note. Steps from Cole (2012).

planning stage can greatly enhance the possibility of a successful group outcome. It is through the professional and clinical reasoning process that activity demands are assessed and the client's strengths and challenges are factored into the equation (see Chapter 6, "Professional Reasoning and Reflective Practice"). The members' needs are considered to support occupational engagement, and goal attainment includes carryover of the occupation to relevant contexts.

Group Considerations

Leadership Roles for Occupational Therapy Practitioners

As far back as 1969, Gail Fidler stated that the overall role of the group leader, specifically the occupational therapy practitioner, is not simply that of a treatment giver but rather that of an agent in maximizing group members' learning potential.

As seen earlier, a leader selects group members, secures a safe environment in which to conduct the group, establishes goals and norms for the group, plans appropriate activities, obtains necessary supplies, and conducts the group in an established time frame. The group's purpose must be clearly stated in language the members can understand. Leaders help the group mark progress on the task and reflect on how this progress was accomplished. Thus, the leader serves many functions, but the specifics of these functions will vary from group to group. In many groups, especially those using a behavioral or learning approach, the leader serves as a technical expert, demonstrating behaviors appropriate to the situation. In a home management group, for example, the therapist might show members how to use the washer and dryer safely, or the therapist might facilitate group members to do the modeling themselves: "Who can show the group how to load the washer?"

For a group leader in any discipline, ***active listening*** is one of the most important skills to be mastered. Here, the leader pays active attention to the member speaking, signaling this attention with appropriate body language (e.g., eye contact, nodding). The occupational therapy practitioner then restates, clarifies, and reflects on the information presented. The goal here is to demonstrate the practitioner's empathy and overall understanding of the members and their situation. Reik (1948) described this ability to empathize and understand the meaning of member feelings as listening to others with the ***third ear.*** Relatedly, it is with this ***therapeutic use of self*** that practitioners use personal understanding to develop and enhance helpful relationships with group members that empower both themselves and the group participants (Bitel, 1999). Active listening and empathy, if mastered by the practitioner, can then be taught to the members to use among themselves. By helping the group to clarify and reflect on what is said, the leader can address communication and intrapsychic and interpersonal goals: "Can anyone explain what Sasha is trying to say?" "I was wondering if anyone else felt uncomfortable when ...?" or "What do you think about what Pedro just shared?"

Many additional skills, techniques, or attributes contribute to strong group leadership. Among them are reliability, enthusiasm, warmth, flexibility, self-confidence, creativity, sense of humor, and—of critical importance—the ability to separate out the leader's needs from those of the group members.

It is important to note that there is no one way to be a great leader—there are a multitude of ways. Although many of the qualities discussed here may come naturally to some, others will develop these qualities over time, with practice and clinical supervision. Each leader must find their own style to meet the needs of both the group as a whole and every individual in the group.

Content and Process

An important job for the occupational therapy practitioner is to be aware of both the content and the process of the group. ***Content*** is the task of the group. It refers to the activity itself (e.g., exercise, game, handwriting, fundraiser, memory activity). ***Process*** refers to the ways in which the activity is completed. It includes the mood of the group, member compliance, cooperation or resistance to the activity, and communication patterns among members or with the leader. "Process needs to be balanced with content or a group will fail to attain its objectives. . . . The manner in which process and content issues are addressed has an impact on how participants view the success of a meeting" (Hulse-Killacky et al., 1999, p. 114).

For many groups run by occupational therapy practitioners, the content dominates. The idea is to complete the task. The group will bake cookies, complete the movement activity, or write two pages in a handwriting journal and share the results. However, what if the group resists the activity, moves slowly, rushes, or seems sad? What if a single member bullies another or threatens to walk out of the group? The leader, who might or might not know the members and group dynamics well at this point, needs to be able to address the situation. "Everyone seems to be working so slowly today. . . . what's going on?" "Sara, you look sad today. Are you okay?" By examining the process, the leader can deal with difficult issues with group dynamics as they arise. These issues include dependency, apathy, monopolization, and resistance. That said, it should be noted that processing does not always address negative dynamics observed in the group. It can also address positive dynamics, for example, "Wow! You all cooperated and compromised so easily. We got this done in no time!" Again, as with the other leadership skills described, any two therapists might handle a situation differently. For guidance, the skilled practitioner will reflect on the group's overall purpose and the participants' treatment goals to help guide the intervention. Understanding the balance between content and process, their link to each other, and how to guide a specific group is often a skill developed over time, and it can have a great impact on the outcome of the group.

Group Norms

All groups are governed by norms; that is, the standards by which people judge behavior as acceptable or unacceptable. Many describe ***group norms*** as the "rules of the game." Some norms are common to many of the groups an occupational therapy practitioner might run, whereas others are specific to a particular group and environment. Many norms are culturally bound by their own uniqueness. They define the way the group interacts and gets things accomplished. Practitioners become aware of the group's norms and the group's acceptance of these norms in relation to its attitudes, biases, and standards of behavior, thus helping the members to become part of the group. Leaders need to become aware of the members' beliefs and values. Norms can, in general, make communities, populations, and the world seem a bit more predictable and, thus, safe to inhabit. In occupational therapy groups, the practitioner gives the client or clients a safe and positive space to share and facilitate change. By becoming culturally sensitive to the group's needs, respecting the confidentiality and diversity of its members, maintaining productive norms can have a great impact on group participation and members' positive outcomes.

Norms can be either implicit or explicit. ***Implicit norms*** are those that are cumulative in nature. They are generally learned over the years, starting when people are young and incorporated into their everyday behaviors. Saying "please" and "thank you" are examples of implicit norms. ***Explicit norms*** are clearly stated in the group, often in the first session: "There is no smoking in this group," "To allow everyone to be able to speak freely, everything said here in group is to be kept here in the group," or "All wellness participants will bring a mat and towel to each session." In general, the older the group member is, the more implicit norms are expected to be displayed (i.e., the norm of saying "please" would be implicit for a 21-year-old adult but not for a 2-year-old child). It is important that practitioners not blindly assume that a person holds an implicit norm. Implicit norms might be closely tied to one's upbringing or culture (e.g., food choices, family interactions, work habits). To clarify, the therapist might ask group members about the origin of the norm. In group, this can lead to a lively discussion, reinforcing similarities and respecting differences among group members.

Yalom and Leszcz (2020) spoke of ***therapeutic norms*** and how they shape the group. Therapeutic norms govern aspects such as ***self-disclosure*** (i.e., what members are willing to reveal about themselves or their challenges), how important the group becomes to the members, how members become "agents of help," and how group members confront each other. In groups generally, and certainly in occupational therapy groups, reviewing explicit norms is often integrated with the description of the overall purpose of the group. For example, a therapist might put together an after-school club for a group of adolescents with social skills challenges. The therapist might start the group by stating,

> Today is the first meeting of our club. The idea here is to get to know each other, to work together to select some fun activities that we will carry out over the next 8 weeks. Some ground rules: Everyone is to be here at 3:00 pm sharp. To work well together as we make decisions, it is important that each of you be respectful, and speak one at a time. This will give everyone an opportunity to be heard.

Establishing the norms early helps members to know what is expected of them.

Finally, norms can have a positive or negative effect on groups. Some group norms can put enormous pressure on members to conform. This can add stress. If left unchecked, antisocial norms (e.g., some gang behaviors) can challenge any group. Conversely, norms can also bring about strong cohesion. Experienced group leaders encourage members to discuss their values, respect individual ideas, and then find agreement where possible, leading to the acceptance of a functional and adaptive set of norms. When this is accomplished, the therapist might ask after some sessions, "Why do you think this group is working so well?" A member might reply, "Because we listen well, and care about each other!" This is an example of positive norms at work.

Group Culture

The uniqueness of each group's culture is influenced by its leader and its members and the emergence of norms and roles established by the leader in the beginning of each session (Cole, 2012). The AOTA Strategic Framework (AOTA, 2021a) states that professional development should focus on cultural sensitivity and strategies to incorporate family perspectives into evaluations, assessments, and interventions. Resources such as the Centers for Disease Control and Prevention's (2021) *Learn the Signs: Act Early Campaign* can provide practitioners, the community, and populations with handouts in multiple languages that review developmental milestones and early signs of autism. This material can be directly distributed to groups (e.g., parent groups). Practitioners are creating blogs and forums on a global level (e.g., CommunOT) to support and share ideas on the development of effective population-based occupational therapy interventions to promote professional growth.

Cultural sensitivity is critical to practice, and it is strongly suggested that occupational therapy practitioners develop skills to integrate culture throughout the occupational process, including the practice of self-reflection, to the degree possible, for both the client and the practitioner. The practitioner–client relationship assists the practitioner in understanding the relevance of the activity and its meaning within a given culture.

In addition, occupational therapy practitioners can provide interventions or develop programs that implement evidence-based and culturally sensitive interventions to address public health concerns with larger populations. Community health organizations (e.g., Alzheimer's Association, Healthy Hearts Program, AOTA) provide materials and education that are culturally inclusive. Such materials and educational programs may include those with careful attention to providing health literacy that is education matched to the reading abilities, interests, and values of the targeted audience. Sometimes it includes looking for materials that make use of universal approaches (e.g., music, exercise, art that crosses cultural lines and considers the physical and cultural barriers that may hinder performance and participation; see Figure 8.3).

AOTA (2017) has formulated a strategy that aligns with *Vision 2025* "as an inclusive profession, occupational therapy maximizes health, well-being, and quality of life for all people, populations, and communities through effective solutions that facilitate participation in everyday living." This mission and vision include advocating for our members, profession, and the public with a plan guided by strategic principles. These principles expand, transform, advocate, support, and educate occupational therapy practitioners to be more diverse, equitable, and inclusive (e.g., with respect to lesbian, gay, bisexual, questioning/queer people, religion, and race).

Group Member Roles

In groups, members will assume different ***roles,*** that is, patterns of behavior that are a result of their character, their

FIGURE 8.3. **Fall prevention and senior movement groups assisted older adults with health maintenance in an assisted living facility. This program provided culturally relevant music and visual aids (on the wall monitor) to increase participation and interest.**

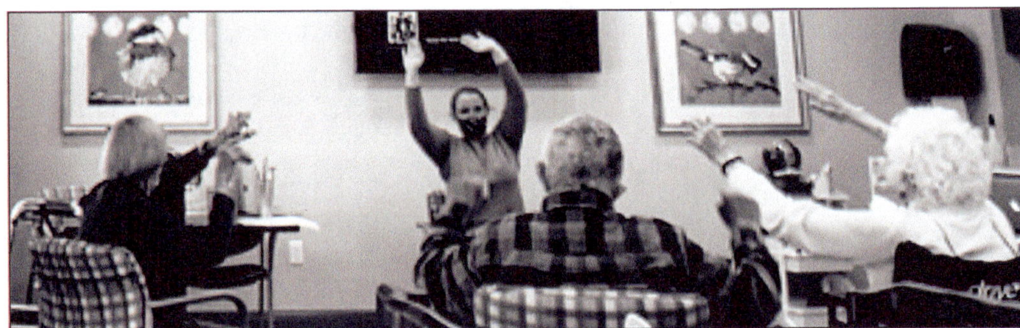

Source. H. MacAlpine. Used with permission.

needs, or pressure experienced within the group. Members may or may not be aware of the roles they occupy. Benne and Sheats (1948) set forth a long list of the roles that frequently occur in groups. A brief overview follows.

Task roles help the group complete its work:

- initiator or contributor—proposes original or new ways of approaching group problems
- information seeker—requests clarification that information is reliable, in terms of its factual adequacy; determines what information is missing; and seeks expert information
- information giver—provides factual information to the group; is seen as an authority on the subject and relates their own experience when relevant
- opinion seeker—asks for clarification of members' values, attitudes, and opinions
- opinion giver—expresses relevant opinions, beliefs, or values
- elaborator—builds on or explains initial ideas with relevant examples and data
- coordinator—pulls together a few different ideas or plans and makes them cohesive
- orienter—summarizes accomplishments; keeps the group organized and on course
- evaluator or critic—judges and evaluates the logic or practicality of proposals
- energizer—challenges and stimulates the group to make decisions or take further action
- procedural technician—attends to practical matters (e.g., meeting location, supplies)
- recorder—records minutes, writes down ideas, and remembers what occurs in group.

Personal or social roles (group building and maintenance roles) describe member relationships and how they contribute to the group's positive functioning.

- encourager—affirms, supports, and praises the efforts of fellow group members
- harmonizer—reduces tension; reconciles disagreement through discussion or humor
- compromiser—offers to change a position or meet halfway for the group's benefit
- gatekeeper or expediter—regulates communication; limits dominators and encourages quieter people to speak
- observer or commentator—provides feedback; helps the group to reset group processes
- follower—passively accepts others' decisions; more of a listener than a contributor.

Individual (dysfunctional) roles also describe member relationships, but these roles interfere with the group's work. They focus on meeting an individual's, not the group's, needs:

- aggressor—attacks others by using belittling and insulting comments
- blocker—opposes group ideas without suggestions; is an obstacle to the group's progress
- recognition seeker—draws personal attention to themselves; may brag or pull stunts
- self-confessor—discloses inappropriate or irrelevant personal feelings and issues
- disrupter or jokester—distracts other people by telling jokes and playing pranks
- dominator—monopolizes conversation; tries to control conversation and members

- help seeker—actively looks for sympathy by expressing feelings of inadequacy
- special interest pleader—makes suggestions based on what others would think or feel; avoids revealing their own biases or opinions.

Members may take on more than one role within the group. For example, an individual could be an information giver (task role), a harmonizer (person or social role), and occasionally a self-confessor (individual role). They might also take on different roles outside the group, in other settings. Identifying member roles has many advantages. Doing so can help members become more self-aware and, thus, identify roles that help or interfere with healthy functioning. The occupational therapy practitioner can also help the group understand the roles played within the group and how these roles get the task done or interfere with the process.

EXERCISE 8.3. What Roles Relate to You?

Study the roles by Benne and Sheats (1948) and your class as a group. What role or roles, as a group member, do you occupy in this group? Are they different from the roles you might play with your family or in other groups? Select one role that you would like to develop in the future. Be specific.

Problem Solving and Decision Making

Practicing problem solving in occupational therapy groups can help members develop essential skills necessary to function well in daily activities found in all performance areas—at home, at school, at work, socially, and in the pursuit of leisure activities. The problems presented can relate to the completion of tasks, or to relationships between those in the group, or between members and individuals outside the group. The leader might teach a specific step-by-step method for problem solving, such as

- identifying the problem,
- proposing solutions for the problem,
- assessing the different suggested solutions,
- selecting a solution,
- implementing the solution, and
- assessing the results.

A commonly used method for proposing solutions is ***brainstorming,*** in which members are encouraged to throw out suggestions with no initial judgment from the group. Naturally, this method might be graded down (the leader might more closely guide the group toward possible solutions) if the group is very young or low functioning. Assessing the possible solutions might involve the group imagining the results and consequences of particular actions. Selecting a solution follows. The implementation of the solution might take place in the group session (if the problem is one concerning a group task or in-group interpersonal interaction), or it might take place at a future time outside the group. In this latter situation, the last step, assessing the results, would be adjusted to a later date as well. Solving problems as a group can have many benefits, reflecting the adage "Two heads are better than one." Relatedly, emphasizing the creative aspects of problem solving can reduce stress, and introducing the idea that there are often several ways to approach a challenging situation can lead to very positive results.

How are group decisions made? That is, how is the group itself managed? Initially, it is the leader who, in planning the group, makes decisions concerning the overall purpose, projected outcomes (goals), methods (approaches and activities), time, place, materials, and so forth. In a very high-functioning group, some initial decisions can be delegated to the group as a whole. After the group is up and running, however, the way in which it makes decisions can be an important part of the therapeutic process. These decisions might be about activity choice, the way in which an activity will be completed, or how leadership is delegated. Providing opportunities for decision making can lead to members' personal growth. Johnson and Johnson (2013) described seven approaches to ***group decision making:***

- decision by authority without discussion
- decision by expert member
- average of members' opinions
- decision by authority after discussion
- minority control
- majority control
- consensus.

There are times when certain approaches to group decision making are preferable. Factors such as the group's purpose and the members' age and level of functioning must all be considered. When it comes to safety issues, these decisions must be made by the leader—the authority—without discussion; for example, "All sharp instruments, must be placed back in the box when you are finished with them," even though an explanation might be furnished to clarify the issue. For a work simulation activity, the occupational therapy practitioner may serve as a boss. In some jobs, many decisions are made by the boss and simply must be followed. However, when all decisions are made by the leader, power issues sometimes arise and will have to be addressed.

It is well known that members' involvement in decision making improves participation and overall motivation. It seems logical that this process might lead to better occupational performance. Also, as members participate in the decision-making process, they feel more a part of the group. For the group, decision making can result in a greater sense of cohesion. Even with small children, providing a choice of activities can be handled democratically, or even through facilitated consensus. In general, decision by consensus is often considered the gold standard. Here, members reach a decision together through discussion, compromise, and final agreement. Consensus can help develop higher level interpersonal skills but tends to take longer. When time is a big factor, a democratic vote is more efficient. For members who are less dominant and have consistently been outvoted, a decision by the minority might be empowering, for example, "Let's hear from you, Joe—you haven't chosen an activity yet." Certainly, group decision making is a complex process, but it is well worth taking the time to integrate it into planning and executing a group.

Levels of Group Interaction

To lead the most effective groups, occupational therapy practitioners carefully study and help build interpersonal relationships within the group, noting how they affect the completion of everyday tasks. Donohue (2011b) expanded on the original work of Mosey (1996) and Parten (1932) to identify five levels, on a developmental continuum, that describe how group members interact with each other. This model can be useful in planning, understanding, and revising the way in which groups are led. The five group levels from simplest to most complex are

1. parallel,
2. associative,
3. basic cooperative,
4. supportive cooperative, and
5. mature.

In ***parallel groups,*** interaction is minimal, and conversation might be rare. Tasks are completed individually within the group, and the therapist is intensely involved in supervising, teaching, and facilitating some interaction. An example is a handwriting group for young children in which there is a focus on concentration, attention to task, and fine motor skills. In ***associative groups,*** brief interaction and cooperation are noted. The therapist sets up the activity to promote social interaction and task sharing. An example is a large monthly calendar made by group members with developmental challenges. The supplies are shared, prompting members to interact.

In ***basic cooperative groups,*** members begin to engage in joint decision making and interact with more social awareness. The leader can facilitate greater problem solving. An example of this, for a group of older adults with mild cognitive challenges, is a game of "Family Feud" (like the TV show) in which members form two teams and confer on the possible responses to current daily living situations. In ***supportive cooperative groups,*** during both completion of a task and ongoing discussion, members can share more personal feelings and are expected to more fully meet the emotional needs of others. Sometimes, the activity becomes secondary to the interactive aspects of the session. The leader facilitates this interaction and steps back a bit to allow members to take more active responsibility. An example might be the formation of a postsurgical cancer survivors' group in which members make bracelets to raise funds for other survivors. With the leader's guidance, they share feelings to provide support to each other.

In ***mature groups,*** members take on a variety of roles. In a mutually supportive manner, they are involved with both the task and the interpersonal challenges faced in any gathering of committed members. The occupational therapy practitioner might serve as a consultant, inside or outside the session. Sometimes there is no official leader, and a form of natural leadership emerges within the group. Examples are a book club for high-functioning adults with a history of depression or a student government group in a university program.

Using this developmental model can prove helpful when groups do not go as planned. For example, with the calendar activity mentioned earlier, suppose that the group is having a bad day and is not working together to complete the task. The occupational therapy practitioner could modify the activity and give each member their own set of supplies to work on individual sections of the calendar, and under supervision, the final product is pasted together. Essentially, the group is adjusted down one level to a parallel group. Levels can also be raised when groups make progress. Discussion of these adjustments, if appropriate, can help members understand challenges, cement new skills, mark accomplishments, or relieve stress within the group.

Group Development

Group development refers to how groups, over an extended time period, grow and change. These changes have been studied by many who have looked at both the way in which tasks are mastered and the evolution of member and leader interactions. Many occupational therapy authors, such as Posthuma (2002, p. 28) have included this material in texts to help illustrate that groups are not static. They begin, mature, may fall into crisis, and eventually end.

Social scientists have organized group development into a set of ***group stages.*** Often cited in occupational therapy texts are Tuckman (1965), who described the stages of group development as forming, storming, norming, and performing (adding a final stage, adjourning, in Tuckman & Jensen, 1977), and Lacoursier (1980), who labeled the stages as orientation, dissatisfaction, resolution, production, and termination. Both designate an initial stage with many unknowns as the group begins to take form. This is followed by the second stage, which includes some turmoil (e.g., questioning the usefulness of the group or the role of the leader). The next stage or stages involve the resolution of prior conflicts and productive accomplishment of goals (for occupational therapy groups, these stages move toward a focus on the tasks and occupations first mentioned in the group protocol). The last stage addresses ending the group, and members look back at the group's evolution and what has or has not been gained.

For practitioners to make these concepts most useful, it is important to look at group development in a flexible manner.

Some groups may not go through all stages, or the stages may occur in a different order. The important thing is to acknowledge that groups grow and change and to recognize that this can help the leader mark the development of positive, productive relationships and functional gains both for the group as a whole and for the members individually.

Tracking Progress

Assessing the group's progress and the attainment of goals, both individual and group, is an important step in providing evidence-based treatment. The practitioner may use formal and informal assessments to track progress and determine the effectiveness of the group and program. Depending on the setting, progress notes are also helpful. One example of documentation commonly seen in different settings, in electronic or written format, is provided in Exhibit 8.3.

Further explanations of outcomes for groups and communities who receive educational intervention may include improved social interaction, increased self-awareness through peer support, a larger social network, or improved employee health and productivity. For example, education interventions for groups of employees on safety and workplace wellness have been shown to decrease work injuries and increase workplace productivity and satisfaction.

Outcomes for populations are dependent on the results of the needs assessments and the gaps noted. The outcomes for the targeted population can be focused on occupational performance, engagement, and participation, and they may address health promotion, occupational justice and self-advocacy, health literacy, community integration, community living, and access to services. As a result of advocacy interventions, examples of outcomes at the population level would include the construction of accessible transportation and improved accessibility throughout nature trails at parks and facilities.

Innovative Group Approaches

Following are examples of some innovative developments in group treatments. Many include traditional aspects of group work seen over the years, but they take advantage of new approaches, new technology, or simply new ways of thinking.

Social Profile: Evaluation and Treatment

The ***Social Profile*** (Donohue, 2013) is an assessment that looks at social participation in activity groups. It can be applied to groups of many kinds, such as those in clinics, schools, clubs, sports, and the community. Using concepts from the work of Parten (1932) and Mosey (1996), group social and interactional skills are measured on the five levels described previously

EXHIBIT 8.3. Progress Note: "Can You Dig It?" Session 7

Service Provided: Members met for a 50-minute session to plant herbs and water and prune the plants in the garden. Safety precautions were reviewed. The three-step tasks were outlined in sequential order in large print on colored paper. Members were encouraged to discuss how they would share tasks (e.g., distribution of materials, choice of task, workspace), working in pairs. Discussion followed.

Results: Through discussion, members were able to form pairs and distribute tasks.

All members made at least one verbal contribution, with Mary taking a greater verbal role as leader. All members selected appropriate adapted tools, gloves, and new watering cans. Residents manipulated and calibrated tools to independently complete garden tasks, using the visuals provided in a previous session. Three-step directions were followed by all pairs except for John and Adam, who needed the leader's review and clarification. Residents were able to independently complete the motor requirements of planting, watering, and pruning through the use of adaptive equipment. Members were visibly engaged and appeared happy during the group, as demonstrated by smiles, laughter, and friendly discussion. Residents approached other residents and staff to share their experiences with gardening and show them the garden plants and adaptive tools they had been using (i.e., mini-watering cans). All agreed that the watering cans were ideal and easy to use. During the discussion, members were able to recall the activity steps and what was accomplished. One resident stated that this was "the best group" and was very happy to be a part of this group. Other members nodded in agreement. They spoke of gardening as part of their future plans.

Assessment: Residents accomplished short-term goals by collaborating with each other and completing gardening tasks. The discussion segments of this group have shown progress in social interaction within the group. Today, residents made connections between the components of gardening and how these relate to themselves, their needs, their relationships, and their personal growth. The discussion revealed cognitive strength, as they followed directions and completed tasks. Residents were able to independently complete the motor requirements of planting, watering, and pruning using adaptive equipment.

Plan: This group will continue, with one more activity session and a wrap-up session the following week. Residents expressed a desire to learn about thinning, pruning, and fertilizing plants, so this will be incorporated into next week's activity. Next week, we will follow up on how the watering schedule is to be implemented. The long-term goal of this group will be discussed and reviewed (i.e., emphasis on the use of tools to complete gardening tasks while interacting with fellow group members). Accomplishments will be noted. Starting in 2 weeks, a new group will be formed, in which new members will maintain the garden and current members will take on a leadership role.

(parallel, associative, basic cooperative, supportive cooperative, and mature). There are child and adult versions. Cole and Donohue (2011) offer many interventions to develop social participation in various age groups, including children, adolescents, adults, and older adults. With children, there are group-based social–emotional training, conflict resolution, antibullying, anger management, self-regulation (with a family group), and social competence programs, as well as many others (Donohue, 2011a). It should be noted that if the group leader is an occupational therapy practitioner, the leader will, in many cases, simply not conduct a discussion group. Instead, the leader will introduce an activity—daily living, work, educational, or leisure—and help the group look at social participation as part of the activity.

Let's Get Organized: Evaluation and Treatment

The Assessment of Time Management Skills (White et al., 2013) evaluates time management within the scope of daily routines and reports a self-evaluation of effective cognitive strategy use. This 10-minute, 30-item questionnaire can easily be administered to an individual or to individuals in a group. Let's Get Organized (Holmefur et al., 2019; White, 2007) is a 10-week manualized program, with two 1-hour sessions per week. Participants use calendars to record their daily activities. Habits, routines, and roles and all parts of performance patterns are explored. Although this program has been used with adults dealing with mental health and substance abuse disorders, it can also be used with those who have other cognitive challenges. (Research and details about this program can be found at https://www.suzannewhiteotr.com/lets-get-organized.)

Ocean Therapy Program

The short documentary film "Resurface" describes a group for returning veterans with posttraumatic stress disorder (PTSD; Izenberg & Padula, 2007). In the related TED talk and journal article (Rogers et al., 2014), occupational therapist Carly Rogers describes the Ocean Therapy program and its occupational therapy perspective. Program participants receive surfing lessons, a lunch discussion group, and focused group processing. The program aims to increase self-efficacy through an activity creating "flow" (the all-encompassing feeling of involvement in an activity; Csikszentmihalyi, 2002). In the film, participants are interviewed. They describe the therapeutic aspects of the program and how it helped them work through many issues related to PTSD.

The Alert Program

Williams and Shellenberger (1992) developed this program to help children learn to regulate their emotions by identifying their "engine" as running too low, too high, or just right. Self-regulation activities are commonly used in individual sessions, in small groups, or even in entire classrooms.

Zones of Regulation™

The Zones of Regulation is a framework designed by Kuypers (2011), an occupational therapist, to help children gain skills in self-regulation. This 18-lesson curriculum was developed to provide very clear instructions that guide students through a sequence of lessons that encourages them to learn about their needs, their regulatory system, and how to adjust. It provides tools and strategies to assist children and adults in social, emotional, and sensory development to stay in the just-right and ready-to-learn zone. A full curriculum addresses self-regulation; children and adults learn vocabulary, use emotional terms, and develop skills in reading and better understanding facial expressions. They gain a different perspective on how others see and react to their behavior, and they develop insight into emotional triggers to their behavior through calming and alerting strategies and problem-solving skills (https://www.zonesofregulation.co/). The Zones of Regulation curriculum can be combined with other tools, such as yoga, mindfulness, and the Response to Intervention Program developed by Gloria Lucker (2011).

Functional Occupational Therapy Groups

Stromsdorfer (2020) provided suggested groups for adults in physical rehabilitation, such as discharge planning, home safety, simple meal prep, orthopedics education, adaptive equipment education, falls prevention, life skills, energy conservation, stress management, health promotion, and holiday-themed craft groups. Stromsdorfer also provides information about Medicare guidelines and best-practice principles to help in forming the most effective groups.

Telehealth: Circle of Friends

Zubatsky et al. (2020) described a group, Circle of Friends, that addresses the needs of older adults at risk for isolation; loneliness; and related physical, social, and cognitive decline. The group addresses circumstances related to the coronavirus disease 2019 pandemic. The group meets online for 12 sessions during a 3-month period. Activities include exercise, creative arts, and writing. The group is conducted over Zoom, with additional support provided by phone and additional Zoom sessions for individual participants and their caregivers. Although the authors belong to other disciplines, occupational therapy practitioners can use this innovative model, and expand upon it, offering additional daily living, cognitive, or creative pursuits (see Figure 8.4).

Essential Group Concepts to Consider

Mental Health, Psychosocial, and Holistic Aspects of Groups

When considering the process of creating a new group, it cannot be stressed enough that, although groups may address very important concrete and practical task skills, the practitioner must always consider social participation (i.e., psychosocial and interpersonal) aspects of the activity to have the greatest impact. Personal factors, such as attitudes and beliefs that contribute to intrapersonal issues (psychological aspects within

FIGURE 8.4. A virtual family group was developed by fieldwork students to support physical and emotional well-being during COVID-19. This group used age-appropriate play and pre-writing activities to provide family-centered care to a child and her family.

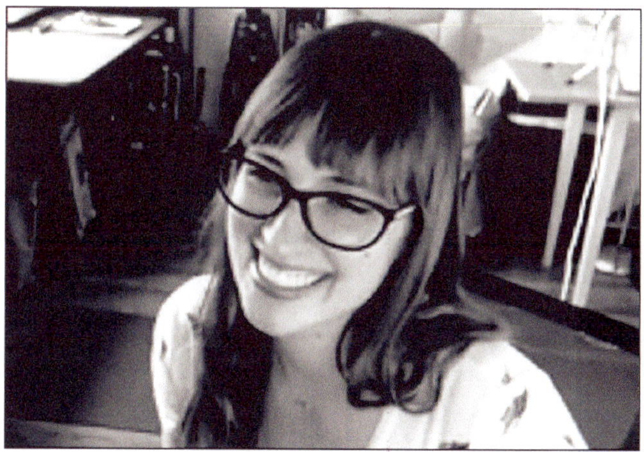

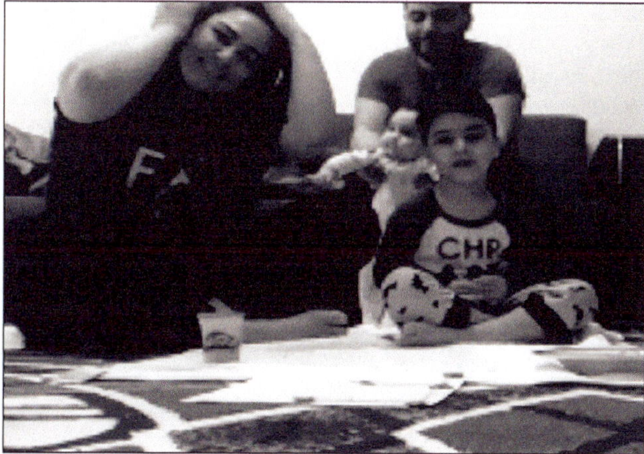

Source. H. MacAlpine. Used with permission.

the self) mentioned in the *OTPF-4*, need to be factored in when looking at the whole person. Mental health issues may take center stage or be addressed when they interfere with a member's or the group's ability to function. In any group, practitioners must acknowledge occupational therapy's insistence on treating the whole person, as opposed to focusing on a single skill or a part of an individual.

Generalization of Group Work

Equally important is the need to make sure that learning generalizes to the environment in which group members will find themselves after treatment. Group, as opposed to individual, treatment is already ahead of the game, because group work involves a greater number of individuals who can help provide insight into multiple contexts.

Evidence-Based Practice

Occupational therapy practitioners must always strive to demonstrate that what they do is effective. It is critical for practitioners to stay up to date and translate current writings and evidence into practice. One way to do this is to read and develop research studies. Other methods, such as pre- and post-evaluation, can also be helpful in ensuring effectiveness. Finally, asking clients for feedback on what they have learned or accomplished will help to document positive outcomes.

Summary

Interventions with groups, communities, and populations provide unlimited opportunities to help people achieve their goals. Occupational therapy practitioners' holistic training and deep understanding of human occupation can be among the most effective agents of meaningful change for the group members with whom they work.

References

Accreditation Council for Occupational Therapy Education. (2018). 2018 Accreditation Council for Occupational Therapy Education (ACOTE®) standards and interpretive guide (effective July 31, 2020). *American Journal of Occupational Therapy, 72*(Suppl. 2), 7212410005. https://doi.org/10.5014/ajot.2018.72S217

American Occupational Therapy Association. (2015). *Occupational therapy and universal design for learning.* https://www.aota.org/~/media/Corporate/Files/AboutOT/Professionals/WhatIsOT/CY/Fact-Sheets/UDL%20fact%20sheet.pdf

American Occupational Therapy Association. (2017). Vision 2025. *American Journal of Occupational Therapy, 70,* 7103420010. https://doi.org/10.5014/ajot.2017.713002

American Occupational Therapy Association. (2020a). Occupational therapy in the promotion of health and well-being. *American Journal of Occupational Therapy, 74,* 7403420010. https://doi.org/10.5014/ajot.2020.743003

American Occupational Therapy Association. (2020b). Occupational therapy practice framework: Domain and process (4th ed.). *American Journal of Occupational Therapy, 74*(Suppl. 2), 7412410010. https://doi.org/10.5014/ajot.2020.74S2001

American Occupational Therapy Association. (2021a). *AOTA strategic framework.* https://www.aota.org/-/media/Corporate/Files/AboutAOTA/BOD/2021%20AOTA%20Strategic%20Framework.pdf

American Occupational Therapy Association. (2021b). The Association—Improve your documentation and quality of care with AOTA's updated Occupational Profile Template. *American Journal of Occupational Therapy, 75,* 7502420010. https://doi.org/10.5014/ajot.2021.752001

Bandura, A. (1977). *Social learning theory.* Upper Saddle River, NJ: Prentice Hall.

Bandura, A. (2004). Health promotion by social cognitive means. *Health Education and Behavior, 31*(2), 143–164.

Benne, K. D., & Sheats, P. (1948). Functional roles of group members. *Journal of Social Sciences, 4,* 41–49.

Bitel, M. C. (1999). Mixing up the goulash: Essential ingredients in the "art" of social group work. *Social Work With Groups, 22,* 77–99.

Centers for Disease Control and Prevention. (2021, February 26). *Learn the signs. Act early.* https://www.cdc.gov/ncbddd/actearly/index.html

Cole, M. (2012). *Group dynamics in occupational therapy: The theoretical basis and practice application of group intervention* (4th ed.). SLACK.

Cole, M. B., & Donohue, M. V. (2011). *Social participation in occupational context in schools, clinics, and communities*. SLACK.

Crosby, R., & Noar, S. M. (2011). What is a planning model? An introduction to PRECEDE-PROCEED. *Journal of Public Health Dentistry, 71*(Suppl. 1), S7–15. https://doi.org/10.1111/j.1752-7325.2011.00235.x

Csikszentmihalyi, M. (2002). *Flow: The classic work on how to achieve happiness*. Ebury Press.

Donohue, M. V. (2011a). Interventions for children to develop social participation roles, skills, and networks. In M. B. Cole & M. V. Donohue (Eds.), *Social participation in occupational contexts: In schools, clinics, and community* (pp. 201–227). Slack.

Donohue, M. V. (2011b). Social development in infancy and childhood. In M. B. Cole & M. V. Donohue (Eds.), *Social participation in occupational contexts: In schools, clinics, and community* (pp. 99–110). Slack.

Donohue, M. V. (2013). *Social Profile: Assessment of social participation in children, adolescents, and adults*. AOTA Press.

Fazio, L. (2017). *Developing occupation-centered programs with the community* (3rd ed.). Slack.

Fertman, C. I., & Allensworth, D. D. (Eds.). (2017). *Health promotions programs from theory to practice* (2nd ed.). Jossey-Bass.

Fidler, G. S. (1969). The task-oriented group as a context for treatment. *American Journal of Occupational Therapy, 23*, 43–48.

Gately, C., & Borcherding, S. (2017). *Documentation manual for occupational therapy: Writing SOAP notes* (4th ed., pp. 57–131). Slack.

Grajo, L., & Boisselle, A. (2019). *Adaptation through occupation: Multidimensional perspectives*. SLACK.

Grim, M., & Hortz, B. (2017). Theory in health promotion programs. In C. I. Fertman & D. D. Allensworth (Eds.), *Health promotion programs from theory to practice* (2nd ed., pp. 53–81). Jossey-Bass.

Higgins, S., Schwartzberg, S. L., Bedell, G., & Duncombe, L. (2015). Current practice and perceptions of group work in occupational therapy. *American Journal of Occupational Therapy, 69*(Suppl. 1), 6911510223. https://doi.org/10.5014/ajot.2015.69S1-PO7096

Hocking, C. (2011). Occupation to health and well-being. In E. B. Crepeau, B. A. B. Schell, & E. S. Cohn (Eds.), *Willard & Spackman's occupational therapy* (11th ed., pp. 53–67). Lippincott Williams & Wilkins.

Holmefur, M., Roshanay, A., Lidström-Holmqvist, K., Arvidsson, P., White, S., & Janeslätt, G. (2019). Pilot study of Let's Get Organized: A group intervention for improving time management. *American Journal of Occupational Therapy, 73*, 7305205020. https://doi.org/10.5014/ajot.2019.032631

Howe, M. C., & Schwartzberg, S. L. (2001). *A functional approach to group work in occupational therapy* (3rd ed.). Lippincott.

Hulse-Killacky, D., Kraus, K. L., & Schumacher, R. A. (1999). Visual conceptualizations of meetings: A group work design. *Journal for Specialists in Group Work, 24*, 113–124. https://doi.org/10.1080/01933929908411423

Izenberg, J., & Padula, W. (Directors). (2007). Resurface [Documentary]. Only Humans Film.

Johnson, D. W., & Johnson, F. P. (2013). *Joining together: Group theory and group skills* (12th ed.). Pearson Education.

Kielhofner, G., Forsyth, K., Kramer, J. M., Melton, J., & Doson, E. (2003). Model of human occupation. In E. B. Crepeau, B. A. B. Schell, & E. S. Cohn (Eds.), *Willard & Spackman's occupational therapy* (11th ed., pp. 446–461). Lippincott Williams & Wilkins.

Kuypers, L. M. (2011). *The zones of regulation*. Think Social Publishing.

Lacoursier, R. B. (1980). *The life cycle of groups: Group developmental stage theory*. Human Sciences Press.

Lucker, G. (2011). *Occupational therapists and RTI: Practical ideas and strategies for working successfully with students*. Bureau of Education & Research.

Mosey, A. C. (1996). *Psychosocial components of occupational therapy*. Raven Press.

Parten, M. (1932). Social participation among preschool children. *Journal of Abnormal and Social Psychology, 28*, 136–147. https://doi.org/10.1037/h0074524

Posthuma, B. H. (2002). *Small groups in counselling and therapy* (4th ed.). Allyn & Bacon.

Price, J. H., Dake, J. A., & Ward, B. (2017). Assessing the needs of program participants. In C. I. Fertman & D. D. Allensworth (Eds.), *Health promotion programs from theory to practice* (2nd ed., pp. 85–111). Jossey-Bass.

Reik, T. (1948). *Listening with the third ear: The inner experience of a psychoanalyst*. Grove Press.

Rogers, C. M., Mallinson, T., & Peppers, D. (2014). High-intensity sports for posttraumatic stress disorder and depression: Feasibility study of ocean therapy with veterans of Operation Enduring Freedom and Operation Iraqi Freedom. *American Journal of Occupational Therapy, 68*, 395–404. https://doi.org/10.5014/ajot.2014.011221

Scaffa, M. E., Reitz, S. M., & Merryman, M. B. (2014). Theoretical frameworks for community-based practice. In M. E. Scaffa & S. M. Reitz (Eds.), *Occupational therapy in community-based practice settings* (2nd ed.). F. A. Davis.

Schwartzberg, S. L., Howe, M. C., & Barnes, M. A. (2008). *Groups: Applying the functional group model*. F. A. Davis.

Sheu, J. J., Chen, W. W., & Chen, H. S. (2017). Making decisions to create and support a program. In C. I. Fertman & D. D. Allensworth (Eds.), *Health promotion programs from theory to practice* (2nd ed., pp. 114–140). Jossey-Bass.

Soga, M., Gaston, K. J., & Yamaura, Y. (2017). Gardening is beneficial for health: A meta-analysis. *Preventive Medicine Reports, 5*, 92–99. https://doi.org/10.1016/j.pmedr.2016.11.007

Stromsdorfer, S. (2020). *10 occupational therapy group treatment ideas*. https://www.myotspot.com/ot-group-treatment-ideas/

Tomlinson, J., & White, S. (2014). Group process, occupation, and activity. In J. Hinojosa & M. Blount (Eds.), *The texture of life: Occupations and related activities* (4th ed., pp. 211–234). AOTA Press.

Touchinsky, S. (2019). Building capacity. In K. Jacobs & G. L. McCormack (Eds.), *The occupational therapy manager* (6th ed., pp. 133–140). AOTA Press.

Tuckman, B. W. (1965). Developmental sequence in small groups. *Psychological Bulletin, 63*(6), 384–399. https://https://doi.org/10.1037/h0022100

Tuckman, B. W., & Jensen, M. (1977). Stages of small group development. *Group and Organizational Studies, 2*, 419–427.

U.S. Department of Health and Human Services. (2020). *Health-related quality of life and well-being*. https://www.healthypeople.gov/2020/topics-objectives/topic/health-related-quality-of-life-well-being

White, S. M. (2007). Let's get organized: An intervention for persons with co-occurring disorders. *Psychiatric Services, 58*, 713. https://ps.psychiatryonline.org/doi/pdf/10.1176/ps.2007.58.5.713

White, S. M., Riley, A. W., & Flom, P. (2013). Assessment of Time Management Skills (ATMS): A practice-based outcome questionnaire. *Occupational Therapy in Mental Health, 29*, 1–17. http://www.tandfonline.com/doi/abs/10.1080/0164212X.2013.819481

Williams, M. S., & Shellenberger, S. (1992). *An introduction to "How Does Your Engine Run?®" The Alert Program® for self-regulation*. TherapyWorks.

World Health Organization. (1986). *The 1st International Conference on Health Promotion, Ottawa, 1986*. https://www.who.int/teams/health-promotion/enhanced-wellbeing/first-global-conference

Yalom, I. D. (1970). *Theory and practice of groups psychotherapy*. Basic books

Yalom, I. D., & Leszcz, M. (2020). *Theory and practice of group psychotherapy* (6th ed.). Basic Books.

Zubatsky, M., Berg-Weger, M., & Morley, J. (2020). Using telehealth groups to combat loneliness in older adults through COVID-19. *Journal of the American Geriatric Society, 68*, 1678–1679. https://doi.org/10.1111/jgs.16553

9

Occupations and Contexts

JULIE ANN NASTASI, ScD, OTD, SCLV, CLA, FAOTA

CHAPTER HIGHLIGHTS

- Occupations
- Contexts
- Promoting engagement
- The dark side of occupation
- Further exploration of occupations and contexts through case examples

KEY TERMS AND CONCEPTS

• ADLs • attitudes • context • dark side of occupation • education • environmental factors • health management • human-made changes to the environment • IADLs • leisure • natural environment • occupation • personal factors • play • products and technology • rest and sleep • services, systems, and policies • social participation • support and relationships • work

Introduction

The occupations we engage in are influenced by the contexts (environmental and personal factors). The ***context*** is a "construct that constitutes the complete makeup of a person's life as well as the common and divergent factors that characterize groups and populations" (American Occupational Therapy Association [AOTA], 2020, p. 76). Contexts can facilitate or prevent a person from engaging in a desired occupation. This chapter reviews occupations and then the contexts (environmental and personal factors), followed by an exploration of how contexts support or block engagement and participation in occupations. The chapter concludes with eight cases that describe various aspects of how environment and context are critical to intervention in occupational therapy.

Occupations

The *Occupational Therapy Practice Framework: Domain and Process* (*OTPF*–4; 4th ed.; AOTA, 2020), identifies nine categories of ***occupation*** that are further broken down into specific occupations. The nine categories are (1) ADLs, (2) IADLs, (3) health management, (4) rest and sleep, (5) education, (6) work, (7) play, (8) leisure, and (9) social participation. These occupations may be completed in a variety of contexts.

Activities of Daily Living

ADLs typically focus on the person's taking care of their own body. Within this category are the occupations of bathing/showering, toileting and toilet hygiene, dressing, eating and swallowing, feeding, functional mobility, personal hygiene and grooming, and sexual activity (AOTA, 2020). These daily occupations, typically completed in the home environment but possibly performed elsewhere, support the person's ability to prepare for the day before heading out into the community. Completing the activities in the home provides a sense of familiarity and knowing where items belong and how to access them.

Imagine you are on vacation: You packed your belongings, and now you need to set them up at the place where you are staying. Is it as easy to find and access the items? Is your routine the same, or is it different? How easy is it to do your normal routine? Do you forget steps or tasks that you normally would have completed?

Think about an older adult with dementia. The family no longer can take care of the person. The person has cognitive decline and is in a new living setting. How easy or difficult will it be for the person to adjust to the new environment and complete basic ADLs? How much assistance will the person need? Does the person have access to the same items they previously had? Were any items taken away for safety purposes?

Instrumental Activities of Daily Living

IADLs focus on activities that occur in the home and in the community. All of the following are IADLs: the occupations of care of others, care of pets and animals, child rearing, communication management, driving and community mobility, financial management, home establishment and management, meal preparation and cleanup, religious and spiritual expression, safety and emergency maintenance, and shopping (AOTA, 2020). IADLs typically are more complex than ADLs and require multiple activities or steps to occur in completing the task.

Imagine you have moved to a new area. Where are the stores located where you normally shop? How much time will it take to go to these places? Do you know where things are located in the community and within stores? Can you simply run in and out of stores, or do you need to scan the stores to find items?

Health Management

Health management focuses on self-care with the goal to support participation in other occupations. Health management includes social and emotional health promotion and maintenance, symptom and condition management, communication with the health care system, medication management, physical activity, nutrition management, and personal care device management (AOTA, 2020). The person develops, manages, and maintains routines that support the ability to engage in other desired occupations.

Imagine you recently moved to college. Have you found new doctors' offices and pharmacies? Will your hometown doctor be able to write a prescription in a new state? Does your insurance cover doctors where you are going to school? Will you be able to continue working with the counselor you had been receiving services from? How will you know which doctors are the best for you?

Rest and Sleep

To participate and engage in occupations, it is important to have enough sleep and be well rested. The occupation of ***rest and sleep*** includes rest, sleep preparation, and sleep participation (AOTA, 2020). Through proper sleep, the person is able to support overall health.

Think about your sleep routine. Is it the same on weekdays as on weekends? Is it the same when you are away on vacation? What would happen if you went from working days to working nights? How would your sleep change? What adjustments would you need to make? Would you need curtains to darken the room so you could sleep? Would you need to wear an eye mask to block the light? What if you were diagnosed with sleep apnea and needed to wear a machine to assist your breathing at night? Would you be able to sleep? Or, what if you broke a bone and were in a cast? Would you be able to position yourself for sleep?

Education

The occupation of ***education*** focuses on activities needed to learn and participate in an educational environment. This occupation includes formal educational participation, informal personal educational needs or interest exploration beyond formal education, and informal educational participation (AOTA, 2020). Education may lead the person to obtain a degree or learn about an area of interest.

Think about places where you have studied. For you, what characteristics make a place desirable? What characteristics are undesirable? What motivated you to pursue educational opportunities? Why might you decide not to pursue educational opportunities?

Work

The occupation of ***work*** is a labor that may or may not provide financial benefits. Work includes employment interests and pursuits, employment-seeking and acquisition, job performance and maintenance, retirement preparation and adjustment, volunteer exploration, and volunteer participation (AOTA, 2020). A person may work at one job for a lifetime or many jobs over time. Work does not have to be paid, and the person may participate in volunteer activities that benefit a group or organization.

What factors might affect the decision to take one job over another job? What qualities do you look for in employment? What qualities would make you uninterested in a job? Do work hours play a role? Do the number or specific days of the week influence your decision? Does the commuting distance or the type of commute play a role?

Play

The occupation of ***play*** is a complex and intrinsically motivating activity typically completed by children. Play includes play exploration and play participation (AOTA, 2020). Societal factors commonly influence play and the type of activities children decide to engage in.

Why might a child choose a specific type of play? Is individual or group play preferred? How does access to toys or supplies affect the activities selected? If you only had toys for older children and you had a toddler visiting, what would you do? What items in your home might you be able to use to play with the toddler? Could you use blankets and pillows to make a fort? What other items in the home could you use creatively to make toys?

Leisure

The occupation of ***leisure*** is an intrinsically motivating activity completed in free time. Leisure consists of leisure exploration and leisure participation (AOTA, 2020). Leisure typically provides some type of enjoyment or happiness as the person completes the desired occupation.

What do you like to do in your free time? Do you always choose the same things? If you choose different things, why? How do you feel when you complete certain leisure activities? Would knitting be a leisure activity for you? Would you prefer playing card games or a board game with friends over an activity by yourself?

Social Participation

The occupation of ***social participation*** involves social interactions with others. Social participation includes community participation, family participation, friendships, intimate partner relationships, and peer group participation (AOTA, 2020). Social participation supports social interdependence.

What activities do you participate in? Are the same people or different people involved in the activities? Do you like belonging to different social groups, or do you prefer socializing with a specific group of people? How do other family members and friends influence your social participation? How do other occupations influence social participation?

Contexts

The *OTPF–4* defines *contexts* as environmental and personal factors specific to the person, group, and population that influence engagement and participation in occupations (AOTA, 2020). This section discusses the broad categories and components for each.

Environmental Factors

Environmental factors include the broad categories of the natural environment and human-made changes to the environment; products and technology; support and relationships; attitudes; and services, systems, and policies (AOTA, 2020). Environmental factors include physical, social, and attitudinal aspects of where the person lives and conducts life occupations.

The category ***natural environment*** and ***human-made changes to the environment*** includes the physical geography, population, flora and fauna, climate, natural events, human-caused events, light, and time-related changes (AOTA, 2020). *Physical geography* describes physical aspects of the environment—for example, a three-story walk-up apartment in which the person would need to climb three flights of steps to access the apartment. The *population* describes groups of people in the same environment with the same pattern of environmental adaptation—for example, people with visual impairment accessing a center for the blind. All of the people attending classes at the center would have some form of visual impairment and, to participate at the center, would need to adapt to the vision loss. The component of *flora and fauna* provides information on plants and animals found in the environment. The *climate* describes the weather for the environment, and *natural events* are disruptions caused to the environment by flooding, blizzards, and other weather events. *Human-caused events* describe disturbances caused by humans from air pollution, deforestation, and chemical spills. *Light and time-related changes* describe the amount of light available in an environment and the natural and predictable changes that occur daily, weekly, monthly, seasonally, and yearly. All of these components included in the natural and human-made environment help provide key information on how the environment may facilitate or hinder engagement and participation. It is important to evaluate and address these components when working with the person, group, or population.

The category ***products and technology*** includes food, drugs, items of personal consumption, general products, and the technology used in daily living, transportation equipment, communication, education, employment, cultural and recreational and sporting activities, religion and spirituality, human-made environments for public and private use, economic assets, and virtual environments (AOTA, 2020). These components should be evaluated to determine how they support or hinder engagement and participation for the person, group, or population. They should be assessed individually as well as collectively to determine how they support or hinder engagement and participation.

The category ***support and relationships*** includes immediate and extended family, friends, peers, colleagues, neighbors, community members, people in positions of authority and subordinate positions, personal care providers, and domesticated animals (AOTA, 2020). People or animals provide support and assistance in different settings. By knowing and understanding the support system for the person, group, or population, plans can be made to facilitate engagement and participation in occupations. For example, a person with posttraumatic stress disorder may not feel safe going out into the community without a service dog. Incorporating the service dog into planned activities and occupations in the community will allow the person to complete the desired activities and occupations. Or, for a person with visual impairment who is no longer able to drive, reaching out to a neighbor who drives to and attends the senior center provides the person with the opportunity to continue to attend and participate in activities there. Maximizing the supports for the person enables engagement and participation.

The category ***attitudes*** includes the mindsets of individuals, society, and social norms held by people other than your client. The attitudes may positively or negatively affect the person—for example, a religious community joining together to pray for the health of a community member, or an employer who will not allow an employee to take time off from work on a religious holiday. The first example shows how people come together to support the person. The second example shows how the employer does not respect or honor the person's religious holiday.

The category ***services, systems, and policies*** refers to the services, systems, and policies designed to meet the needs of persons, groups, and populations (AOTA 2020). *Services* include government agencies like Social Security, Medicare, and Medicaid. *Systems* include utility companies, transportation systems, and political systems. *Policies* include rules and regulations for local, regional, and national government.

Personal Factors

Personal factors are features of a person that are part of the person's background. Personal factors include age; sexual orientation; gender identity; race and ethnicity; cultural identity and cultural attitudes; social background, social status, and socioeconomic status; upbringing and life experiences; habits and past and current behavioral patterns; individual psychological assets (e.g., temperament; character traits; coping styles; the handling of responsibilities, stress, crises, psychological demands); education; profession and professional identity; lifestyle; and other health conditions and fitness considerations (AOTA, 2020).

Personal factors may support or inhibit the person from being able to participate in an occupation—for example, a 13-year-old is not eligible to obtain a learner's permit or a driver's license, but in most states, a 16-year-old is. As another example, until recently, laws in many states prohibited same-sex marriages. This created a barrier to accessing the same rights that heterosexual couples were able to obtain through marriage. It is important to understand how personal factors affect the person and the person's ability to engage and participate in activities.

Socioeconomic status and upbringing also affect the person. A child with medical needs may not have the same type of access to standard medical interventions as others do. For example, if the child lives in a city with multiple providers, the family has a choice about who to see and what services to access. A child living in a rural area, though, may need to travel long distances to access the same medical interventions. The cost of travel and issues of time may prevent the family from taking the child to certain providers or restrict the services available. As occupational therapy practitioners, we need to understand personal factors to better serve our clients.

Promoting Engagement in Occupations and Contexts

Having discussed different occupations and contexts, this section discusses and provides examples of how occupations and contexts affect the person. In the field of occupational therapy and occupational science, engagement in occupation is viewed positively. Occupational therapy practitioners evaluate the person, the occupation, and the context to facilitate health, well-being, and participation in occupations (AOTA, 2015). Practitioners analyze the occupations and contexts to generate ways to incorporate strengths and reduce barriers through modifying and adapting the environment.

Understanding the occupations the person desires to complete and the contexts where the occupations need to be completed allows occupational therapy practitioners to design specific interventions to promote engagement in these occupations. The ultimate goal is to allow the client to successfully engage in and complete desired occupations. The following case studies further explore how occupations and context influence engagement in occupations for persons with and without disabilities.

Ernesto

Ernesto is a 40-year-old man who is married and has two children. He graduated from a university with a law degree. He has worked for the same law firm since passing his bar exam and has earned the position of partner in the firm. Ernesto enjoys spending his free time with his wife and children at their home in a Los Angeles suburb.

During recent forest fires, Ernesto's home was destroyed, and he sustained first- and second-degree burns to his upper body when trying to rescue the family's dog. Ernesto's family escaped without injury, but the family lost their home and dog in the fire. Ernesto received excellent care at a medical facility after sustaining the burns and is on the road to recovery. His wife contacted the insurance company, and arrangements were made for temporary housing until the family can have their home rebuilt. Ernesto's wife rented a furnished apartment for the family to live in for the time being.

When Ernesto was discharged from the hospital, he had no difficulties with ambulating but had problems using his upper extremities, which were affected by the burns. Ernesto was sent to an outpatient occupational therapy clinic to address the occupations that he was no longer able to complete or had difficulty completing. Ernesto's occupational therapist sat down with him during the initial evaluation to identify his goals for therapy, evaluate his strengths and barriers, and discuss occupations and the contexts in which Ernesto was having a difficult time completing his occupations.

He reported that his first goal was to be able to return to work. He was concerned because he was the primary source of income for his family, and he had a heavy caseload of clients who worked exclusively with him. Decreased range of motion, strength, and dexterity, and increased pain in his hands and upper extremities, made it difficult for him to type, dial the phone, and go through papers and files. The occupational therapist asked Ernesto to describe his work environment, the supports available, and the attitudes of his coworkers. Ernesto said that, as a partner in the firm, he had his own office, a paralegal, and an assistant. His colleagues were supportive of him and said they would make whatever accommodations were needed for him to return to work. Ernesto was concerned about the setup of his office and how he would be able to complete the physical requirements of work. Ernesto's occupational therapist made arrangements to go and visit his workplace with him.

At the workplace, the occupational therapist discovered that Ernesto primarily worked with a laptop. The therapist recommended a docking station for the laptop to ergonomically position Ernesto at the computer. An adaptive keyboard was used to position the keys in a place where Ernesto was able to sit with his arms supported while typing. The occupational therapist also had the workplace install voice-activated software to the computer to allow Ernesto to dictate his memos and notes with clients so he did not have to type all of the time. The therapist worked with Ernesto, his paralegal, and the assistant to organize files in cabinets in a way that Ernesto would be able to easily access them. The assistant would scan files and email them to Ernesto in an electronic format so he would not have to flip through the paper pages. For court cases, the paralegal and assistant would carry necessary items to and from court. For his phone, the assistant showed Ernesto how to page the assistant, and the assistant could dial and transfer the calls to him so he would not have to dial the numbers. With proper accommodations and support, Ernesto was able to return to work.

While working, Ernesto continued occupational therapy before or after work. His team of occupational therapy practitioners worked with him to build his range of motion, strength, and endurance as well as decrease his pain while addressing secondary goals that Ernesto had established for completing desired occupations with his wife and children. His team made temporary adaptations to his apartment and helped him design aspects for his new home, which would enable Ernesto to engage in his desired occupations. The new home would have doorknobs and faucets with levers to make it easier for Ernesto to access rooms and turn water on and off. A voice-activated system would be installed to turn appliances and lights on and off. Ernesto's home office would be fitted with a docking station and would be ergonomically set up like his work office so he would have the ability to work from home.

In addition, Ernesto's therapy team of occupational therapy practitioners and physical therapists felt he would benefit from aqua therapy as well as be able to enjoy time with his family in a pool, so they recommended the installation of an in-ground pool with walk down steps at their new home. Built-up grips would be put on the pool equipment so Ernesto could skim the top of the pool. A pool vacuum would enable cleaning the bottom of the pool. Through adaptations to the environment, Ernesto was able to regain participation in occupations he had enjoyed before his injury.

EXERCISE 9.1. Exploring How Context Affects Intervention

Ernesto's success in life provided him with means that others might not be afforded.

- How might occupational therapy be different for a person who has limited health care coverage or financial means?
- For a person working at a job requiring physical labor, how might therapy look different?
- Would the person be able to return to a job requiring physical demands?
- What type of housing would the person need to move into?
- Would the person be able to afford to replace everything in the fire?
- How would the person's occupational therapy sessions be different?
- What would be the same?
- What goals would become priorities?

Jill

Jill is a 16-year-old girl who survived a severe car accident in which two of her friends were killed. Jill was sitting in the back seat, and her two friends were in the front seat of the car when it hit a utility pole. Jill lives with her mother in a first-floor apartment in a four-story building, which has an elevator. Jill uses the elevator to access the laundry facilities in the basement, and because the apartment is on the first floor, she does not need to use stairs or the elevator frequently. She is a junior in high school and is in honor classes.

As a result of the car accident, Jill broke both legs and currently is non–weight bearing. Jill's medical team feels that, because of her age, it would be best to discharge her to her home. The occupational therapy practitioners working with Jill do a home visit to determine what needs to be changed for her to be able to return home. Because Jill is non–weight bearing, she will need to use a wheelchair to get from place to place. The practitioners measure the doorways in her apartment building and in her apartment to determine whether she will be able to move through the entrances. The main entrance is not a problem in terms of width, but it does not have an accessibility button to open the doors. The entrance to the apartment is wide enough to enter. The doorways in the apartment do not have enough clearance with the doors on but do have enough room if the doors are temporarily removed. The apartment has a tub–shower with sliding doors.

The occupational therapy practitioners recommend removing both the doors within the apartment and the tub–shower sliding doors temporarily; installing a curtain rod and curtain; and placing a tub bench in the shower. They also recommend switching the showerhead for an adjustable showerhead that Jill will be able to use to wash her body in the tub. They recommend having a commode to go over the toilet to assist Jill in transferring on and off the toilet. The team talks with Jill's mom, who talks to the landlord to make the temporary changes. The landlord says he can remove the doors within the apartment the next week as well as the glass doors in the shower and install a curtain rod, curtain, and detachable shower head.

During therapy at the hospital, the occupational therapists work with Jill on wheelchair mobility and transfers for the toilet and shower. They discuss with Jill what her high school environment is like. Jill needs to travel to multiple levels in the school building, which has elevators. The therapists talk to the school principal and guidance counselor to arrange temporary accommodations to allow Jill to participate at school. An aide will be assigned to Jill to help her get to her classes and to access the bathrooms, her locker, and supplies that she will need. Tables will be put in the classrooms so she can position her wheelchair there to complete schoolwork. An adaptive school bus will be sent to her apartment to pick her up and drop her off from school. In addition, Jill's occupational therapy practitioners help Jill learn to dress herself without weight bearing and teach her how to prepare snacks and meals when her mother has not yet arrived home from work.

On discharge from the hospital, the hospital makes arrangements for Jill to receive home therapy for a week before returning to school. Once at school, Jill will receive outpatient visits as needed to address any other accommodations she requires. By addressing the occupations in the contexts in which they occur, accommodations were made to support Jill's engagement in desired occupations.

Jill's mom will be responsible for the costs associated with purchasing a curtain rod, curtain, and detachable showerhead. Jill's occupational therapist will contact her insurance company to see if it will provide coverage to rent a wheelchair and issue her a commode. Jill's mom will need to purchase a shower seat and may need to cover the rental of the wheelchair and commode if the insurance will not cover them and there are no loan closets from which she can borrow them. Accommodations for school should be provided through the school district.

EXERCISE 9.2. Providing Accommodations for Jill

Jill's mother has taken responsibility for providing many of the accommodations that Jill needs.

- Consider what would happen if Jill's mother could not afford these accommodations and they are not covered by insurance. What could the occupational therapy practitioners do in this case?
- What accommodations will be needed for Jill in the school setting?
- Although the school is expected to provide the accommodations, what would happen if accommodations are too costly or not available?

James and John

James and John are 70-year-old male twin brothers. James lives with his wife in a condo, and John is widowed and lives alone in a house. The brothers both love the outdoors and fish and kayak together. They are both in great shape and work out a couple times a week. On a recent outing, James and John were caught by surprise when the weather took a turn for the worse. They made it into the cabin as the storm moved toward them. There was no basement, so they grabbed a mattress to cover themselves in the bathtub for safety. A tornado hit and completely destroyed the cabin. The brothers were crushed by the roofing and walls of the cabin. A rescue team found the brothers and was able to free them from the debris. They were taken to the local hospital to be treated for their injuries.

James and John both sustained concussions, broken ribs, a broken arm (humerus), and a broken leg (fibula). Both were evaluated by an occupational therapist at the hospital, and the occupational therapist and an occupational therapy assistant worked together with the brothers. Although the twins had similar injuries, their plan of care was different based on the contexts. See Table 9.1 for the personal factors for each brother and Table 9.2 for the environmental factors for each brother.

Although the brothers sustained the same injuries, their living environments are different. James needs to be able to travel stairs inside and outside of his home, whereas John does not. James has his wife available to help him, and John lives alone and does not have someone to regularly be with him. Both brothers are healthy and in good shape. James takes a multivitamin a day and does not require prescription drugs. John takes multiple medications to control his HIV.

Both brothers want to return to their homes from the hospital. James's wife rented a hospital bed to put in their living room until James is able to travel the flight of stairs up to their bedroom. His home has a three-quarter bath on the main floor that he is able to use. John does not have to worry about mobility on steps but needs to focus on independence in his ADLs and IADLs because he lives alone. James's wife is available to assist James with ADLs and IADLs until he gains independence in the tasks.

Bringing a hospital bed into James's home allows him to be discharged home from the hospital with home care services. John is discharged from the hospital to an acute rehab facility, where he receives 3 hours of therapy a day. After a week in rehab, John is able to be discharged home.

Both brothers are temporarily unable to drive because their right legs were broken in the accident. James relies on his wife to grocery shop and has telehealth sessions with his doctors until he is able to get out and into the car with his wife. John hires a car service to drive him places and has items delivered to his home through online shopping.

Although the brothers sustained the same injuries, the treatment plan was different based on the contexts. Personal and environmental factors influenced their discharge plans from the hospital. Both had the financial resources to support the decisions made about their care. Understanding the contexts allows occupational therapy practitioners to collaborate with their clients to best meet their individual needs.

Shawn

Shawn is a 50-year-old man who struggles with anxiety and depression. After years of counseling, his doctor has recommended that Shawn be seen for an evaluation by an occupational therapist. The doctor stated that Shawn has plateaued

TABLE 9.1. PERSONAL FACTORS FOR JAMES AND JOHN

PERSONAL FACTOR	JAMES	JOHN
Age	• 70 years old	• 70 years old
Sexual orientation	• Attracted to women	• Attracted to men
Gender identity	• Male	• Male
Race and ethnicity	• Caucasian, non-Hispanic	• Caucasian, non-Hispanic
Cultural identity and cultural attitudes	• White • Italian American	• White • Italian American
Social background, social status, and socioeconomic status	• Urban, middle-class neighborhood • Retired schoolteacher	• Suburban, upscale neighborhood • Retired vice president from a Fortune 500 company
Upbringing and life experience	• Raised by two parents • Twin sibling	• Raised by two parents • Twin sibling
Habits and past and current behavioral patterns	• Daily meals with spouse • Minimalist	• Goes out with friends to eat and socialize • Loves the arts and collects art pieces for his home
Individual psychological assets	• Calm and easygoing • Enjoys quiet times with wife • Enjoys experiences rather than things, enjoys living a minimalist lifestyle	• Outgoing and bubbly • Likes to hang out with friends • Always on the lookout for a new piece of art
Education	• Master's degree in education	• Master's degree in business administration
Profession and professional identity	• Retired schoolteacher	• Retired vice president of Fortune 500 company
Lifestyle	• Member of the homeowners' association board for condo • Quiet nights with spouse • Leisure activities • Travel	• High-end dining and socialization • Casual dating • Road trips
Other health conditions and fitness	• Regular workouts at gym	• Regular workouts at gym • HIV well controlled with medication

EXERCISE 9.3. Considering How Context Affects Intervention

Both brothers were in excellent health.

- How might occupational therapy be different if one or both brothers were not in excellent health?
- If the brothers were obese, how might occupational therapy and discharge planning be different?
- Would James's wife be able to care for him at home if he were non–weight bearing and obese?
- What type of equipment (e.g., shower seat, tub benches) would need to be ordered?
- If the brothers could not tolerate 3 hours of therapy per day and could not go home, where would you recommend they be discharged to?
- If the bothers did not have financial means, what would be different, and what would be the same?

with the counselor and that his medications have been helping, but he would benefit from occupational therapy services.

Shawn schedules an occupational therapy evaluation, not knowing what to expect. The occupational therapist sits down with Shawn and begins collecting information for his occupational profile. Shawn tells the therapist that he was a salesman. He had worked many jobs over the past 20 years and has held most jobs for 1 or 2 years. He had been married, but the marriage fell apart over time. He dated but was unsuccessful in maintaining any long-term relationships. He had friends in the past but no one whom he would call a close friend at this time. Shawn reports that when he is not working, he likes to go to sporting events, watch television, and engage on social media. He rents an apartment and leases his car.

The occupational therapist asks Shawn to describe his work environment. Shawn says he has worked in a variety of

TABLE 9.2. ENVIRONMENTAL FACTORS FOR JAMES AND JOHN

ENVIRONMENTAL FACTOR	JAMES	JOHN
Natural environment and human-made changes to the environment	• Lives in a two-story condo with steps inside and outside of the home • No outdoor responsibilities • Good lighting throughout the home	• Lives in a single-story ranch with no steps to enter • Hires people to care for 1 acre of property • Spot-illuminated lighting throughout home for art pieces
Products and technology	• Minimal items in home; lives a minimalist lifestyle	• High-end technology and voice-activated controls throughout the home
Support and relationships	• Spouse • In-laws • Twin brother • Friends	• Friends • Twin brother
Attitudes	• Overall support from family and friends	• Faces discrimination from some neighbors because of sexual orientation • Support from family and friends
Services, systems, and policies	• Social Security	• Social Security

settings. He did sales over the telephone, and he also worked the floors in retail shops. He likes interacting with his customers. He reports his biggest challenge is understanding what his bosses want from him. He knows he has to sell things and make quotas for his sales, but his bosses do not seem to be clear in their expectations of him. Multiple employers have put him on performance improvement plans. He does not think that his employers fairly assess his abilities. Customers like him and never complain about him.

The occupational therapist asks Shawn if he thinks his anxiety and depression play a role in his challenges at work. Shawn says things are fine until his employers tell him he is not meeting expectations. He does not understand why they will not spell out what they want from him. He says he gets anxious not knowing what he is supposed to be doing, and he second-guesses everything he is supposed to do. He then asks his bosses and reports that they ignore him or blow him off. He does not understand why this happens to him all of the time.

The occupational therapist asks Shawn about the supports in his life. He says his parents used to be his supports, but both have passed away. He does not have any siblings or children. In many respects, he is alone in the world. He has had friends in the past, but none live in the area. He and his ex-wife remained friends after the divorce, but she moved on with her new husband.

The occupational therapist tells Shawn they think he would benefit from a functional capacity evaluation and, specifically, a cognitive functional capacity evaluation. The functional capacity evaluation will determine his capacity to complete and participate in work activities for employment (Dorsey et al., 2019). Completing a cognitive functional capacity evaluation also will provide insight into his cognitive capacities related to his job demands.

After completing the cognitive functional capacity evaluation, Shawn's occupational therapist and an occupational therapy assistant work together with Shawn to develop strategies to assist him in meeting the demands of his current job. The occupational therapy practitioners go over his job description and requirements. They role-play different scenarios with Shawn for him to communicate better with his employers. They provide Shawn with a checklist to review while at work to ensure he addresses all components of his job. He had been successful with sales in the past; his challenges were his relationship and understanding of what employers expected of him. Role-playing scenarios prepare Shawn in how to respond to feedback from his employer as well as how to report the outcomes of his sales and records needed by his employer.

Occupational therapy played a unique role in allowing Shawn to succeed at his job. Completing a cognitive functional capacity evaluation that looked at his occupation and the context was the key to addressing Shawn's challenges at work. Understanding Shawn's personal and environmental factors

EXERCISE 9.4. Considering Other Aspects of Shawn's Environment and Context

While Shawn's work situation has improved, consider other aspects of his life:

- Identify other areas of Shawn's life where occupational therapy practitioners might intervene to help Shawn.
- Do you think there should be other priorities in Shawn's life to help with his occupational performance?
- What types of evaluations might the occupational therapist use to explore these areas?
- What kinds of interventions might the practitioners use to treat these areas?

was necessary for him to be successful. Shawn used his checklist and skills learned in role play to improve his communication and interactions with his employer. Ultimately, he found greater job satisfaction.

Jane

Jane is a 38-year-old married woman who has lived with her husband for the past 15 years. Jane teaches kindergarten at the local elementary school and is well liked by her colleagues, the parents, and her students. Jane started her job right out of college and went back for her master's degree at night while teaching full time. Jane has no children; she always wanted to have children, but she has had fertility problems and her physician does not think that she will be able to have biological children.

Jane and her husband rent a home outside of the city. The cost of living is high, and they have not been able to save money to purchase a home. Jane's family includes a sister and her mother. Her father passed away when she was young. From outside appearances, friends and family think Jane has a good life. She excels in the classroom and is active in her community.

Jane recently found out her husband is having an affair. He has decided to leave her because his girlfriend is pregnant, and he wants to be with her and the new baby. Her husband literally walked away, leaving Jane with no money or help. She is completely devastated. She went from feeling happy and safe to feeling alone and uncertain. She feels betrayed and does not know how she is going to make it with the financial demands of the home she rents and not having a second income to help pay the bills.

Jane reaches out to her principal and friends at her school. One of her friends is the school occupational therapist, Jennifer. Jennifer invites Jane out to lunch and listens as Jane shares her fears and worries. Jennifer holds Jane's hand, assuring her that things are going to work out. Jennifer offers to help her friend as she transitions from married to single life. Jane and Jennifer create a list of all of Jane's current expenses at her home. As they look at the list, they work together to see what expenses are necessary and what can be eliminated or decreased. Jane's rent is the one expense that is too challenging for her. The rent takes almost all of her monthly paycheck. Jane and Jennifer talk about the possibilities for places for Jane to rent or move to. They reach out to friends to find out whether more affordable places are available to her. One of their friends finds Jane an apartment that costs only a third of her monthly income. Jane is uncertain but knows she needs to move to a place that will allow her to have money to pay for other expenses.

The principal at Jane's school rallies her coworkers and their friends to help Jane move her furniture and personal items to the new apartment. The new apartment has a lot less space. Jane decides what items to keep, what items to sell, and what items to donate. Jane is able to sell enough items to cover the security deposit for her new apartment.

Jane and Jennifer look at Jane's other expenses. Jennifer helps Jane prioritize what things are important to her and what things are not. Identifying the meaningful activities helps Jane decide what she needs to do next. Jane tells Jennifer that she likes working out. Changing her gym membership from a couple's membership to a single membership helps decrease the cost and allows Jane to be able to have a place to exercise after work. Jane tells Jennifer that working out always makes her feel better, plus it helps Jane to stay fit and provides her with the opportunity to interact with others.

When looking at utilities and cable, Jane decides to change to a prepaid cell phone plan, which decreases her monthly phone expenses. She also decides she no longer needs a landline. Jane knows she needs money to pay the electric, water, and sewer bills. And after teaching in a hybrid format during the SARS-CoV-2 virus (COVID-19) pandemic, she also knows that she needs Internet access. Jane rarely watches television, so she decides that she does not need cable. A subscription to an online streaming platform will give her enough options for shows to watch.

Throughout the divorce, stress causes Jane to lose a lot of weight. Jennifer and other friends prepare meals for Jane to have when she does not feel motivated to cook. Her friends know finances are hard, so they invite Jane over for dinner and socialization at their homes. They want Jane to know that she is loved, is cared for, and is not alone.

Slowly, Jane begins to rebuild her life. The process is slow, but the help of friends and family provides her with the support she needs to be able to move on. Jane finds pleasure in teaching her kindergarten students, working out, and hanging out with her friends at their homes. Jane was fortunate that her friend Jennifer was an occupational therapist who was able to use her knowledge as a therapist to help her. Jennifer essentially completed an occupational profile, identified strengths and weaknesses, and provided interventions that assisted Jane in accomplishing her desire goals.

EXERCISE 9.5. Exploring Personal Factors

Thinking about your life, if you found yourself in a similar situation to Jane, what would you do?

- Who are your supports?
- What are the attitudes of the people around you?
- What services would you need?
- How would your personal factors affect you?
- What strategies would you use to allow the contexts to better enable engagement in occupations?

The Dark Side of Occupation

Up to this point, the focus of this chapter has been on how occupations and contexts support health and participation for people. In recent years, occupational therapists and occupational scientists have shed light on the "dark side of occupation" (Twinley, 2021). The ***dark side of occupation*** looks at occupations that may be harmful or maladaptive, or may decrease overall health. Excessive drinking, illegal drug use, rape, violence, murder, human sex trafficking, and other occupations and activities along these lines exist but typically are not or were not addressed in occupational therapy. By shedding light and attention on these harmful occupations, it is hoped that occupational therapy practitioners will delve into these areas and discuss topics that may be uncomfortable topics to address, thus working with their clients to promote health, well-being, and a better quality of life.

In terms of occupations, we, as occupational therapy practitioners, need to look at all occupations that people participate in. If an occupation is going to hinder health and recovery, we need to be aware of it. We need to discuss with our clients the reasons for choosing to participate in unhealthy occupations or if they are being forced into them. If our clients are being forced into them, we need to work with other professions and law enforcement to seek shelter and safety for our clients. Might our clients be choosing unhealthy occupations because they do not know of other opportunities? Maybe addiction has led them to choices they would not otherwise have made, but they have made them as a result of feeding an addiction? These are all areas that we may need to explore with our clients.

As we think about personal factors, consider how a person's social background and upbringing affects them. If a person was raised in an environment in which they only know prostitution or sex trafficking, would they know that this is not a norm for others? Think about children who have been kidnapped at a young age and are abused by their kidnappers. Will they remember life before the kidnapping? How and what mechanisms do they use to allow themselves to survive the horrific conditions and abuses that they have endured?

Think of victims of trauma. Consider how trauma affects their ability to participate in life (Lynch et al., 2021). These are all things that occupational therapy practitioners might be thinking about and addressing with their clients. Think about the occupational therapy evaluations and assessments that you have learned about or will learn about. Do any of them address the dark side of occupation? Have your professors, fieldwork supervisors, or practitioners in the field addressed these types of occupations with you or with their clients? We live in a world where abuse takes place, and there are occupations that are not healthy and safe. What is our role in this? How do we address this and work with our clients to address occupations and contexts that will better support their health and overall well-being while supporting their autonomy? The following case studies further explore the dark side of occupation and how occupational therapy practitioners can make a difference in their clients' lives.

Jasmine

Jasmine is a 14-year-old girl who has been living on the street since she ran away from home when she was 12. Her mother's boyfriend sexually assaulted her from the ages of 8 to 12 years. Jasmine's mom did not believe her when she told her what had happened. By age 12, Jasmine had endured enough and joined a local street gang. She felt she would do better on her own rather than live under her mother's roof. Jasmine took money in exchange for sex, so that she could get food. She also learned how to be a pickpocket and steal from stores.

As a member of the local street gang, Jasmine feels a sense of connection and belonging. She and her gang have managed to avoid problems with law enforcement until recently. During a recent crackdown, Jasmine and other members of her gang are arrested for prostitution and illegal drug activities, and Jasmine is appointed a public law defender. Because this is her first offense, the attorney seeks foster care, treatment, and community service for Jasmine. She is placed in foster care, and her foster parents take her to the community center to focus on getting her the help that she needs. Jasmine is also ordered to complete 10 hours of service a week at the community center.

At the community center, Jasmine meets Shannon, an occupational therapist. Jasmine connects with Shannon and opens up to Shannon about her life. Shannon learns that Jasmine left home because of sexual abuse. Jasmine, a survivor, chose to participate in activities that allowed her to meet her basic needs. Jasmine values being independent and wants to take care of herself. Shannon learns that Jasmine feels a strong sense of identity and belonging as a member of the street gang.

Shannon and Jasmine develop a good therapeutic relationship over time. Shannon involves Jasmine in group activities that she runs at the center. Shannon trains Jasmine to be an assistant in the groups. Jasmine is able to complete her community service hours in the groups while building skills and relationships with the young children coming to the center. Shannon focuses on involving Jasmine in activities in which she can build her identity and feel like she belongs and is doing something good. Jasmine's foster parents report seeing a big difference in Jasmine as she becomes more active at the community center. Jasmine shows more interest in school and talks to Shannon about plans for her future. Jasmine thinks she would like to work at a community center and become involved with children's lives. Shannon provides guidance to Jasmine and helps her to believe in herself. Jasmine begins to realize her worth and that people value her just for being the person she is at the center.

Shannon is the first person Jasmine encounters who really listens to her story and understands what she wants in life. Shannon provides Jasmine with the trauma-sensitive support and understanding that she needs. Shannon meets Jasmine where she is and helps Jasmine to see how she can build her identity and sense of belonging without being a member of a street gang. Having foster parents who provide a safe home allows Jasmine to focus on school and the community center instead of trying to figure out how to feed herself and where to stay.

Understanding the dark side of occupation, and how to approach clients about unhealthy occupations is a unique opportunity for the profession of occupational therapy. Occupational therapy practitioners understand occupations and contexts. Delving into unhealthy occupations creates a holistic picture of our clients and allows us to better understand their motivations and life circumstances.

EXERCISE 9.6. The Dark Side of Occupations

In your fieldwork and clinical experiences, have occupational therapy practitioners addressed the dark side of occupations?

- Do you think these occupations should be addressed in occupational therapy practice?
- How do you think they should be addressed?
- If you felt personal biases about such occupations, how would you deal with them?

R.J.

R.J. is a 24-four-year-old man and a former professional football player. After years of playing defense, he lives in chronic pain. R.J. started out using prescription painkillers for injuries that he sustained while playing football. Over time, the pain medications were no longer working, and his doctors would no longer prescribe additional medications. So, R.J. turned to illegal street drugs to help ease his pain.

R.J. lived with his girlfriend, but she moved out after he overdosed on multiple occasions. She decided it was too much for her. During a recent overdose, R.J. fell and hit his head, resulting in a traumatic brain injury (TBI). This is not the first brain injury for R.J. because he has a history of concussions from playing football. He was sent to an acute rehabilitation facility to address deficits from the TBI and his chronic pain.

R.J.'s rehabilitation team includes a psychiatrist, pain management specialist, occupational therapist, physical therapist, nurse, and social worker. At a meeting with his occupational therapist for his initial evaluation, the therapist asks R.J. to share a little bit about himself. He tells them that he was a former football player and talks about the lifestyle he led while playing football. The therapist asks him about his pain and how the prescription drugs and illegal drugs became a part of his life. R.J. tells the therapist that it started innocently. The physicians would give him pain medications so he could get back out on the playing field. Over time, the medications no longer worked, and the physicians would not prescribe more for him. His salary from football gave R.J. the finances to obtain illegal drugs for his pain. He knew he was taking more than he should, but it took increasing amounts to make the pain manageable. R.J. knows he lost his girlfriend because of the drugs and realizes he will lose his life if he does not get it under control.

R.J.'s occupational therapist helps him to identify goals that he wants to accomplish in acute rehabilitation and in life after rehabilitation. Because playing football is no longer an option, R.J. needs to determine, going forward, what his purpose is in life. From the time he was a boy, he has lived and breathed football. He needs to identify what else he wants to do.

The psychiatrist and pain management specialist work with R.J. to help him with his pain. R.J. joins a support group to be with others who are also battling addiction. Physical therapists and occupational therapy practitioners work with R.J. to help him overcome deficits resulting from the TBI. He decides he wants to get involved with coaching college football. He knows he needs to clean up his drug use if he wants to obtain and sustain employment at a college. Coaching at a college will provide him with the opportunity to be involved in a sport that he loves, and he knows he can make a difference in players' lives. He wants to share his story so he will be able to help others avoid following in his footsteps.

The path to coaching is not going to be easy, but R.J. knows he needs to overcome his addiction to be able to move forward. His occupational therapist works with him on strategies to use when he feels the urge to use drugs. R.J. identifies some activities he can do to distract himself. He also identifies people to serve as supports to whom he can reach out to stop himself from the habits he has developed. R.J. joins a 12-step program. He knows that his addiction is a daily battle, and he needs to address it each day to ensure he does not fall back to old ways. With his therapist, R.J. identifies the triggers and the people who enable him to use drugs. He knows he needs to end those relationships if he wants to succeed.

After finishing acute rehabilitation, R.J. joins an outpatient support group and completes a functional capacity evaluation with an occupational therapist to guide his transition to coaching football. R.J. knows if he can stay drug free, he may be able to move forward with a purposeful and meaningful life. His occupational therapist is not afraid to confront his drug use and what motivates him to use drugs. The therapist is able to treat R.J holistically because they know the whole picture of his life. Together, R.J. and his therapist create a plan for him to search for football coaching positions, create application materials, and submit applications to colleges and universities. R.J. hears from two colleges and interviews with both. He is offered a position at one of the colleges and eagerly accepts it. He knows this new position is his chance to move forward with his career and life.

R.J. received occupational therapy in several settings. Working with his rehabilitation team and occupational therapist, R.J. set goals for his future. He ultimately was able to transition to a college coaching position that motivated him to stay clean.

EXERCISE 9.7. Dealing With Difficult Topics

- Would you have been able to confront R.J. about his drug use?
- What strategies would you have used while working with him?
- How comfortable would you be addressing illegal activities?
- How can you better prepare yourself to address the dark side of occupation?
- How can you work on your own biases?

Sari

Sari is a 14-year-old girl who was kidnapped and forced into human sex trafficking at age 6 years. She lived in inhumane conditions with dozens of other girls who were forced into sex trafficking. After receiving a tip from a crime line, federal investigators started an investigation into the ring that kidnapped and forced Sari into sex trafficking. After months of investigating and planning, federal investigators swarmed the location where the girls were being held and rescued them from the sex trafficking ring. Through the database for missing children, investigators reunited Sari with her family. Although her family was made aware of what happened to her, they were not prepared to see how it affected her.

Sari's pediatrician and a team of mental health practitioners consult with each other to determine how best to care for Sari. She is withdrawn and does not speak, and she jumps at sounds and people. She is malnourished and did not receive any form of education while kidnapped. Her doctors plan for her to receive psychiatric counseling, and occupational therapy, physical therapy, speech therapy, art therapy, music therapy, and animal-assisted therapy. Her family will coordinate the services available to her where she lives. Sari's school district plans to provide her with one-on-one tutoring at home until she is ready to go to school. Because Sari was sexually violated by men, the doctors decide all her health care providers and teachers should be women. Sari remembers her family from before being kidnapped. The doctors say her family should be present with her to provide comfort and support until she is comfortable working with the health care team one-to-one.

Sari's occupational therapist meets with Sari and her family for her initial evaluation. Sari does not speak during the evaluation. The family provides her therapist with her occupational profile before the kidnapping and since her return. The family also makes the therapist aware, ahead of time, of the ordeal Sari has lived through. Taking the information learned before the meeting along with the information learned during the evaluation, Sari's therapist plans goals with Sari and her family. Goals include increasing Sari's social participation with family and friends, increasing Sari's independence in ADLs and IADLs, and Sari selecting and engaging in play and leisure activities.

During occupational therapy sessions, Sari learns how to complete ADLs and IADLs in which she is not independent. Occupational therapy addresses communication management, meal preparation, safety and emergency maintenance,

EXHIBIT 9.1. Occupations and Contexts for Jana

Jana is 28-year-old woman and single mom of 3-year-old twin girls. She works in automotive sales and lives with friends because she cannot afford rent and day care costs. Jana just purchased a used car to be able to drive her daughters to day care and other places they need to go. Finances are really tight for Jana, and she has no family in the area to help her. She wants to be able to provide her daughters with a good life but also wants to be able to spend time with them.

Answer the following questions to further understand how environmental and personal factors affect Jana's ability to participate in occupations with her children.

QUESTION	YOUR ANSWER
As a mom to twin 3-year-olds, how does the natural environment and human-made changes to the environment affect Jana's ability to participate in occupations with her children?	
What products and technology would be beneficial to Jana and her children to help engage in occupations?	
What supports and relationships are available to Jana to help her with her occupations?	
How do people's attitudes affect Jana's ability to participate in occupations with her children?	
What services, systems, and policies might be available to help Jana?	
How does Jana's age affect the situation?	
How does Jana's social background, social status, socioeconomic status, and upbringing and life experiences shape her life and occupations?	
What habits and behavioral patterns might be helpful to support Jana's ability to engage in occupations with her children?	
What assets will help Jana navigate life as a single mom to twins?	

shopping, and social and emotional health promotion. Her occupational therapist engages Sari in playing board games that build basic learning skills (e.g., taking turns, understanding directions, counting, remembering information). Over time, Sari warms up to her therapist as they build trust in each other. Sari enjoys playing the games and quickly builds basic learning skills. She starts to open up to the therapist about the trauma in her life. The therapist listens and guides future sessions based on what she hears Sari saying.

Providing Sari with a safe space and allowing her to understand that she can openly talk to her occupational therapist encourages her to open up. Her therapist uses therapeutic use of self and her understanding of trauma-informed care in her sessions with Sari. Sari feels safe with her occupational therapist; she tells the therapist about the challenges she faces when having to meet people she does not know, specifically men. Her therapist encourages Sari to join some clubs and activities for girls her age. Hesitant, Sari agrees, and she and her family look into clubs and activities just for girls her age.

Sari joins a gardening club in her town. She enjoys digging in the dirt and planting flowers, and she likes it so much that she asks her parents if she can build a garden at their house. Her parents agree, and her occupational therapist suggests adding relaxation features to the garden. Sari thinks it is a great idea, and she plans her garden with the therapist. Her therapist encourages her to invite some girls from the gardening club to join her at her house as she works on her garden. Sari invites one of the girls she likes at the gardening club. Together, the two plan and begin to plant the garden. Sari chooses a variety of brightly colored flowers for her garden. She and her friend create a colorful pattern for the flowers they are planting. After a week of planning, creating, and planting, the garden comes together. Some of the friends from the garden club come over to see the beautiful creation Sari and her friend put together. Sari's health care team chips in to purchase a bench for the

EXHIBIT 9.2. Occupations and Contexts for Laurie

Laurie is 30-year-old woman and wife and mom to two children, both boys. She works in student engagement at a college. Laurie and her husband and kids live in a large colonial house. He has a high-paying job, and their sons are in day care. Laurie has no financial worries. She has multiple sclerosis (MS) and needs to carefully schedule her day to avoid exacerbating the MS. Laurie wants to work but also wants to be able to spend time with her children.

Answer the following questions to further understand how environmental and personal factors affect Laurie's ability to participate in occupations with her children.

QUESTION	YOUR ANSWER
As a mom with MS, how does the natural environment and human-made changes to the environment affect Laurie's ability to participate in occupations with her children?	
What products and technology would be beneficial to Laurie and her children to help engage in occupations?	
What supports and relationships are available to Laurie to help her with her occupations?	
How do people's attitudes affect Laurie's ability to participate in occupations with her children?	
What services, systems, and policies may be available to help Laurie?	
How does Laurie's age affect her diagnosis and her ability to work and take care of her children?	
How does Laurie's social background, social status, socioeconomic status, and upbringing and life experiences shape her life and occupations?	
What habits and behavioral patterns might be helpful to support Laurie's ability to engage in occupations with her children?	
What assets will help Laurie navigate life as a mother with MS?	
How will Laurie's MS affect her life as an employee and mother to two small children?	

garden. Sari selects a place for the bench in the yard that gives her a perfect view of the garden. The garden provides Sari with a place to relax, listen to music, draw the beauty around her, and have friends over to help her care for the garden. Through the many therapies received, Sari begins to feel comfortable around other girls her age. Her occupational therapist plans to gradually integrate Sari into activities with boys her age to help prepare her for starting school.

EXERCISE 9.8. Working With a Client Who Has Experienced Severe Trauma

Consider Sari's situation.

- What other type of activities do you think Sari would benefit from?
- What recommendations would you make for her family?
- What recommendations would you make for school?
- Because of the sensitive nature of her abuse and age, what would be appropriate to talk about with her?
- What would a therapy session with Sari look like?
- What goals would you want her to accomplish?
- How would you determine when occupational therapy services are no longer needed?
- Which contexts might be easier for Sari, and which ones might be more difficult? Why might they be more difficult?

Further Exploration of Occupations and Contexts

Occupations and their contexts may support or hinder participation. As occupational therapy practitioners, we must fully understand our clients' desired occupations and the contexts in which they exist. See Exhibits 9.1 and 9.2 to further explore the relationship between occupations and contexts. It is important to fully understand personal factors as well as environmental factors. Although an environment may appear to support an occupation, personal factors may create problems for the person. Compare and contrast the lives of Jana and Laurie in the two exhibits. Think about the similarities and differences and how those affect their lives.

Summary

Occupations and contexts need to be viewed as interdependent. Contexts includes environmental factors as well as personal factors. Environmental factors that support one person will not necessarily support another person. Understanding each person's unique personal factors is essential to providing good occupational therapy services. Always think about occupations, environmental factors, and personal factors as you move forward in the profession. Understanding the interplay will allow you to be more successful as you work with your individual clients.

References

American Occupational Therapy Association. (2015). Occupational therapy's perspective on the use of environments and contexts to facilitate health, well-being, and participation in occupations. *American Journal of Occupational Therapy, 64*(6 Suppl.), S57–S69. https://doi.org/10.5014/ajot.2015.696S05

American Occupational Therapy Association. (2020). Occupational therapy practice framework: Domain and process (4th ed.). *American Journal of Occupational Therapy, 74*(Suppl. 2), 7412410010. https://doi.org/10.5014/ajot.2020.74S2001

Dorsey, J., Ehrenfried, H., Finch, D., & Jaegers, L. A. (2019). Work. In B. A. Boyt Schell, & G. Gillen (Eds.), *Willard and Spackman's occupational therapy* (13th ed.; pp. 779–804). Wolters Kluwer.

Lynch, A., Ashcraft, R., & Tekell, L. (Eds.). (2021). *Trauma, occupation, and participation: Foundations and population considerations in occupational therapy*. AOTA Press.

Twinley, R. (Ed.). (2021). *Illuminating the dark side of occupation: International perspectives from occupational science therapy and occupational science*. Routledge.

10

Occupations Across the Lifespan

PAULA KRAMER, PhD, OTR, FAOTA

CHAPTER HIGHLIGHTS

- Ecological developmental perspective
- Life course perspective

KEY TERMS AND CONCEPTS

• adolescence • disengagement theory • ecological developmental perspective • infancy • leisure activities • life course • life course perspective • linear developmental perspective • occupational imbalance • occupations in children • older adulthood • parenting • role playing • sandwich generation • school-age children • self-identity • toddlerhood • young adulthood • work

Introduction

Occupations develop and change over the course of people's lives. The occupations that people choose are related to their development and determined by their age, culture, background, and experiences. Some believe that development is stage specific, innate, and without outside influence (Gesell & Armatruda, 1954; Knobloch & Pasamanick, 1975; Kohlberg, 1969). Others believe that environment has a major effect on development (Bronfenbrenner, 1979, 1989; Bronfenbrenner & Evans, 2000). Still others subscribe to the life course perspective (Elder & Shanahan, 2006).

There are many ways to explore the development of occupations over the lifespan, but in this chapter I focus on two different perspectives on occupational development: (1) the traditional ecological developmental perspective and (2) the more recent view, the life course perspective. This chapter is not meant to be a full exploration of all aspects of development or a comprehensive discussion of all occupations that people may engage in over the course of their lives. It is designed to be an overview of how occupations may change over the life span and the factors that may influence those occupations that people choose to pursue.

From a personal perspective, my beliefs about occupations are that

- the personal meaning one attaches to an occupation is the most important factor, and yet that personal meaning is very much dependent on the context of the occupation and may change over one's lifetime, and
- occupations can be determined by many factors, such as innate abilities and disabilities, culture, education, socioeconomic status, and exposure to experiences.

These beliefs are reflected in this chapter.

Ecological Developmental Perspective

The ***ecological developmental perspective*** builds on the traditional linear developmental perspective. The ***linear developmental perspective*** includes theories proposed by Gesell and Armatruda (1954; Knobloch & Pasamanick, 1975) and

Kohlberg (1969), which set forth that skills are stage specific and that components must be learned or acquired before a skill can be achieved (Howe et al., 2020). Others believe that environmental experiences affect children's development and their skills and that, as in the linear approach, nurture and experiences also have an impact on development. Many occupational therapy practitioners are more comfortable with the ecological theory approach (Howe et al., 2020). Here I discuss this perspective as it relates to occupations.

At birth, infants are purely reflexive beings. They respond to sensory stimuli in the environment and their personal feeling state, such as comfort or hunger. During ***infancy,*** infants begin to form patterns of behavior based on their interactions with people in the environment. They engage with those around them and begin to recognize their parents and caretakers very early. They begin to motorically respond to people who are familiar to them by increasing the movement of their arms and legs (Kramer & Hinojosa, 1995). These initial motor reactions form the basis for patterns of behavior and patterns of movement.

Later, infants begin to respond to objects. These responses later become activities, such as continually reaching for and then swatting an object on a mobile hanging over their crib. As time progresses, the infant's repertoire of behaviors expands and forms many different patterns. These patterns depend on the individual child and what the child is exposed to. Some children enjoy items that make sounds, such as rattles, and others gravitate toward things that move (Kramer & Hinojosa, 1995).

Humphry (2002) defined ***occupations in children*** as "culturally valued, coherent patterns of actions that emerge through transactions between the child and environment and as activities the child either wants to do or is expected to perform" (p. 172). As the child's social world changes, their activities change, and their experiences increase. Some children may have pets in their home, which promote a different kind of interaction than with familiar humans. People from different cultures will expose their children to different objects and activities. Similarly, those from different socioeconomic groups may value and provide different kinds of experiences and activities for their children.

Infants' development focuses on growth, feeding, and increasing abilities. This development is often measured in length, weight, and the ability to achieve developmental milestones (Schering, 2022). Feeding is critical to growth and development, and although feeding of infants may not have the same occupational meaning as eating does to adults, it may be viewed as the infant's first occupation. When hungry, infants make their needs known through crying, and when satiated with milk, they relax and often fall asleep. Similarly, reacting to and playing with objects are meaningful occupations to infants. Although they cannot yet articulate their meaning, their involvement in and responses to repetitive play with a toy, rattle, or familiar object indicate that these occupations are both pleasurable to and have meaning for the infant. Primary occupations of infancy have been described as play,

FIGURE 10.1. This little boy is getting great joy out of playing with a mobile.

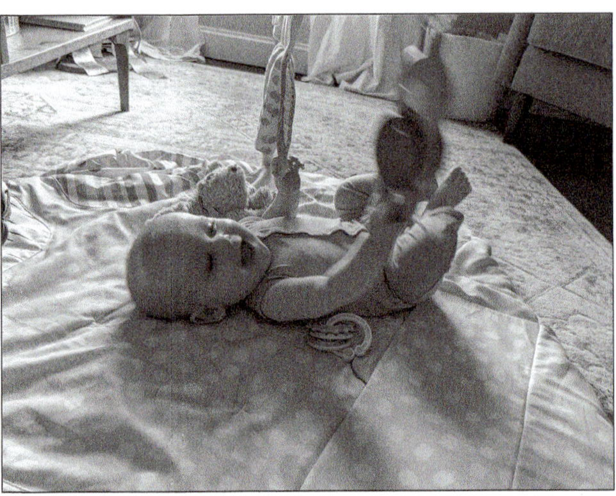

Source. J. Alfred. Used with permission.

social interaction, getting attention to have needs met, and feeding (Vergara, 2002). In her seminal work *Play as Exploratory Learning,* Reilly (1974) wrote about the importance of play to the child's development. Parham and Fazio (2008) noted that play is the most common occupation of children.

Increased motoric abilities are also critical to the development of infants and toddlers (Schering, 2022) and appear to be very meaningful to them. As a child repeatedly tries to hold their head up, reach for an object, and roll from supine to prone, this drive to change positions and become more active is inherent to their development and their ability to negotiate their environment. As they continually try to move more, children appear excited and happy with their new abilities, which may indicate that these increased motor competencies are meaningful to them (Figure 10.1). Could these motor skills be meaningful occupations? Maybe not from a cognitive standpoint but certainly from the observational perspective of adults around them. Infants and toddlers are totally engrossed in their increased motor abilities and, given the opportunity, are actively engaged in exploring their environments.

Infancy and Toddlerhood

Early childhood is a period of major change and exploration. Infants are learning basic life skills. Movement and sensory experiences are critical areas of development at this time of life. Social skills are beginning as infants come to interact with new people around them. In most cases, infants meet and experience other children. Play skills are critical as they explore items that make sounds or move when touched. Although development is somewhat innate, the way in which children develop depends on the type of experiences provided to them. Opportunities to interact with others and experience different environments promote development, especially as caregivers and others ensure the infant's needs are met.

From an occupational perspective, participation contributes to health (Hocking, 2019), so these opportunities are important to a child's development. Occupation can also be viewed as "a social determinant of health" (Pereira, 2017, p. 429), and occupational engagement is a critical component of health, well-being, and belonging (Wilcock & Hocking, 2015).

Eating, moving, sleeping, and playing are critical occupations in the first year of life (Figure 10.2). They are biological needs and also promote skill development. Eating and playing are certainly co-occupations with caregivers, and movement can be supported by caregivers.

During ***toddlerhood,*** a child's world expands with many new experiences, increased mobility, and a wider variety of play opportunities. They are creeping and beginning to walk, trying to climb, experimenting with other sensory experiences, eating solid food, and experiencing increased socialization. Culture can influence the food children eat and the clothes they are learning to take off and put on. Socioeconomic status can also influence the type of experiences the child has, such as access to safe play areas, nature, or fresh foods. Some children may be exposed to day care and have more structured socialization experiences, and other children may have family or caregivers in the home. Some children may have extended family around them. The types of experiences provided will be determined by the people caring for the child, as well as the family's ability to provide different opportunities. Some families may, for example, seek structured swimming experiences and gym classes for toddlers, whereas other families may focus on playground experiences or in-house activities. Toddlers now enjoy different foods and are beginning to self-feed. No matter what experiences are provided, the child's occupations in this period of life center around play, movement, feeding, and sensory experiences.

EXERCISE 10.1. Occupations in Infancy

Observe a child age 12 months or younger for 30 minutes.

- Describe what you see in terms of movement.
- Describe what you see in terms of play skills.
- Describe any eating or feeding that you observed.
- Do you see skills emerging? What are they?
- What can you describe in terms of occupations?

FIGURE 10.2. A first experience eating yogurt.

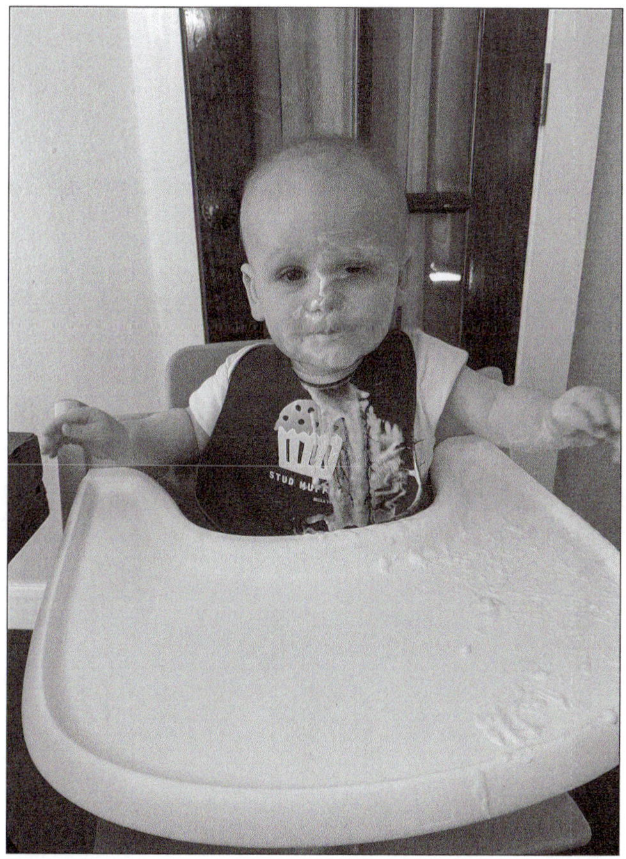

Source. J. Alfred. Used with permission.

Preschool

During the preschool years, the child is continuing to expand their repertoire of play and learning new skills. Many children are attending preschool classes, which are teaching them social skills as well as providing beginning educational experiences. Many different preschool approaches are available for children, which promote different childhood occupations (Table 10.1).

Preschoolers are also learning self-care occupations. At this age and stage (ages 2–4 years), children are usually fully toilet trained and beginning to undress and dress themselves. They still require assistance with clothes fastenings and supervision when bathing, but they are usually able to wash their hands independently (Mulligan, 2012).

While children are becoming independent in feeding, they are also identifying their food preferences, which may be related to their cultural experiences, including cultural or religious customs related to diet, and the types of food they are served (Schultz-Krohn & Wagle, 2021). They are drinking from a cup, biting, and chewing different foods, and they are able to eat more complex foods. At this stage, they often begin to exercise their independence by choosing the foods they will eat and rejecting other things served to them.

Another new occupation at this stage is that children start to become helpers. In preschool and at home, they are frequently asked to help clean up, wipe the table, and engage in helping types of activities with family and caretakers. They begin to see themselves as capable and able to contribute, which builds self-efficacy, self-esteem, and skills.

The predominant occupations seen at this stage are play, social skills, sleep and rest, and beginning self-care skills, both ADLs and IADLs. Moreover, children are beginning to assert their independence through food choices, choosing specific play activities, and doing things for themselves.

TABLE 10.1. **COMPARISON OF SELECTED EARLY CHILDHOOD EDUCATION AND EARLY CHILDHOOD SPECIAL EDUCATION APPROACHES**

APPROACH	KEY COMPONENTS	ROLE OF ADULTS/TEACHERS	ENVIRONMENT/CONTEXT
Behavior approach	• Is often used when providing special instruction for children with delays/disabilities (e.g., autism spectrum disorder) • Is based on behaviorism • Includes brief periods of one-on-one instruction	• Cue a behavior, prompt the appropriate response, and provide reinforcement • Address isolated skills with frequent and detailed progress monitoring	• Initially, "learning to learn" behaviors addressed at small tables/cubbies to reduce distractions • Skills generalized to facilitate peer play, and inclusive early childhood education settings supported
Comprehensive commercially available curricula (creative curriculum)	• Includes theme- or project-based investigations • Addresses the following areas of development: social–emotional, physical, cognition, and language • Includes scope and sequence, daily activity guides, and ongoing assessments	• Lead small and large group activities centered around interest areas	• 10+ classroom interest areas, often referred to as "centers" (e.g., blocks, dramatic play, toys and games, art, library, discovery, music and movement, sand and water, cooking, computers, outdoors)
Embedded learning opportunities (naturalistic instruction)	• Provides specialized instruction during everyday learning opportunities • Uses typically occurring activities and authentic materials across any curricular approach • Uses an activity matrix to plan what, when, and how to teach a specific learning objective throughout naturally occurring daily routines	• Plan for and implement individualized instructional sequences within routines • Teach through short interactions embedded within routine activities instead of pulling a child out or aside to address skills • Use own priorities to drive goals and activities (i.e., family or caregiver role in early intervention)	• Natural environments, including homes, preschools, and child-care contexts
HighScope curriculum	• Involves children learning by interacting with people, materials, and the environment • Focuses on executive function via "plan-do-review" methods • Uses consistent routines	• Facilitate "key experiences" with time for active exploration and learning • Document learning through child observation records	• Well-defined areas, and easily accessible materials labeled at child's level • Purposefully set-up classroom areas to explore and build social relationships
Montessori approach	• Is based on children learning best by doing, through their senses • Groups together children of multiple ages • Offers long periods of individual work time (often 2–3 hours at a time) • Focuses on independence, autonomy, and choice	• Systematically demonstrate use of learning materials (i.e., task) • Instruct didactically • Ensure that setting is prepared and aesthetically pleasing	• Specifically designed, often "errorless" learning materials • Mats or rugs to designate space for children to work

(Continued)

TABLE 10.1. **COMPARISON OF SELECTED EARLY CHILDHOOD EDUCATION AND EARLY CHILDHOOD SPECIAL EDUCATION APPROACHES *(Cont.)***

APPROACH	KEY COMPONENTS	ROLE OF ADULTS/TEACHERS	ENVIRONMENT/CONTEXT
Reggio Emilia Approach	• Focuses on social learning, collaboration, community, and democracy • Considers children with disabilities to have "special rights"	• Serve as "guides" • Emphasize documentation through portfolio data collection • Use long-term meaningful projects to teach across domains as opposed to using short weekly themes	• Aesthetically pleasing with a focus on open-ended child art and easily accessible materials • Environment considered the "third teacher" in the classroom • Use of "provocations" (experiences set up to encourage a child's interests or ideas such as photo, picture, book) and "loose parts" (natural and manufactured materials that can be used in a variety of ways, including moved, combined, and taken apart) to facilitate open-ended play

Source. From "Influences From Early Childhood Professional Organizations and Technical Assistance Centers," by S. P. Maud & S. Parks. In G. Frolek Clark & S. Parks (Eds.), 2021, *Best Practices for Occupational Therapy in Early Childhood*, p. 19. Copyright © 2021 by the American Occupational Therapy Association. Used with permission.

EXERCISE 10.2. Preschool Occupations

Observe preschoolers on a playground or at a day care or education center for about 15 minutes. What do occupations do you see? Is there anything other than play? Describe your observations.

School-Age Children

School-age children, ages 6–10 years, continue to develop cognitively, socially, and emotional as they grow older. Milestones in these areas, shown in Table 10.2, allow school-age children to engage in increasingly different types of occupations, providing more depth to their experiences. The focus in this stage of life is learning, which includes formal school learning, increased social skills, and increased independence in ADLs and IADLs. The majority of time is spent in formal education in school, online, or through home schooling. Children have to adjust to less play time in their lives; daily routines and tasks become more structured and demanding. During this period, children often engage in team sports, dance classes, music lessons, scouting, and community and religious activities that enhance both their physical and their social skills. Through their various activities, children learn about sportsmanship, working successfully with others, setting goals, improving through practice, and learning how to cooperate and develop healthy friendships (Figure 10.3). These social skills will be important later in life as they become members of a community. However, these activities can be costly and time consuming, so not all children have such opportunities. Again, development of these critical social skills is dependent on children's environment; culture; and, to some degree, the interests of their parents.

School-age children are beginning to explore ***self-identity*** (i.e., an understanding of who they are as individuals) and personal likes and dislikes. They often engage in ***role playing,*** which can involve games, and also trying out different actions and reactions with friends and family to figure out what is comfortable for them (Figure 10.4). This can be part of the self-identity process. Again, culture, family structure, and familial experiences influence what the child is exposed to at this stage of life. Peer groups become more important, and children begin to become more aware of their familial situation in comparison with those of other families (Segal, 2014). Although a parent may be more interested in soccer or cricket, a child may gravitate to baseball or football, and the neighborhood may support some sports and not others. These are areas that school-age children learn to negotiate. They learn that they will not always get their own way, figure out successful ways of getting what they want, and decide what is really important to them and where they can be more flexible.

Learning, in its broadest sense and as part of the work of the school-age child, is the major occupation at this stage of life. Other critical occupations at this stage are playing, learning to care for oneself, and becoming a member of a community (Chapparo & Lowe, 2012).

EXERCISE 10.3. School-Age Children

Interview a school-aged child (ages 6–11 years).

- What do they like to do?
- Why are these activities important to them?
- Do they like to do them alone or with others? If with others, with whom?
- How do they feel about school? Friends?
- If you choose to ask other questions, make them open ended so that you will learn more about the child, rather than getting a yes-or-no answer.

Share your experience with your classmates.

TABLE 10.2. **COGNITIVE, SOCIAL, AND EMOTIONAL MILESTONES OF CHILDREN AGES 6–11 YEARS**

AGE LEVEL	COGNITIVE DEVELOPMENT	SOCIAL AND EMOTIONAL DEVELOPMENT
6–7 years	• Participates in simple group activities or board games • Starts to see that words have more than one meaning • Remains focused on an activity in school for 15 minutes or more • Can recognize the perspective of others • Shows more independence at reading and writing	• Believes rules can be changed • Shows more independence from family • Understands the difference between reality and pretend • Is better able to tell what they feel and what they think • Develops improved self-control skills and emotional stability • Wants to please friends and be liked by peer group • Shows more independence from family
8–9 years	• Is able to focus on an activity in school for an hour or more • Uses progressively more complex strategies to solve problems • Understands more about their place in the world • Is able to follow an increased number of directions and commands	• Adheres strictly to rules and fairness • Is able to describe the cause and consequence of their emotions • Treats peers with respect when playing games • Is able to deal with their emotions better, especially in public situations • Is starting to become more balanced in coping with frustration and disappointment • Changes emotions quickly
10–11 years	• Is able to focus on an activity in school for an hour or more • Uses progressively more complex strategies to solve problems • Is able to follow an increased number of directions and commands • Understands more about their place in the world	• Adheres strictly to rules and fairness • Is able to describe the cause and consequence of their emotions • Treats peers with respect when playing games • Is able to deal with their emotions better, especially in public situations • Is starting to become more balanced in coping with frustration and disappointment • Changes emotions quickly

Source. From "Children and Mental Health," by P. Rabey & S. Kletti. In K. M. Matuska (Ed.), *Ways of Living: Intervention Strategies to Enable Participation, 5th Edition*, 2020, p. 122. Copyright © 2020 by the American Occupational Therapy Association. Used with permission.

Teen Years: Adolescence

From an occupational perspective, ***adolescence*** (ages 12–18 years) is about defining oneself and beginning to separate from one's parents. Social relationship priorities shift from family members to friends and others. Rapid changes in the brain and body occur at this time (youth.gov, 2022). Table 10.3 shows the cognitive, social, and emotional milestones that occur during adolescence and allow adolescents to engage in different types of occupations. Valued occupations vary widely depending on context, social environment, cultural background, socioeconomic status, and even geographic location. Some teens are more content to follow parental norms, and others are actively trying to define themselves as separate individuals. Adolescent leisure activities often take place outside the adult-controlled institutions of family, school, and work and provide opportunities for adolescents to structure their own time (American Occupational Therapy Association [AOTA], 2022; Fine et al., 1990). Teens will often experiment with different hairdos, hair colors, tattoos, piercings, and styles of dress that differ from their parents' norms as a way of identifying with friends or separating themselves from the norms of their families.

Sports, music, and dance are very important to some teens, and education continues to be a critical occupation for most. Others may be involved in caring for family members and doing part-time work outside of the household. This is a period of life in which teens are exploring a range of new occupations, which include increased self-care, interest in finances, moving independently through their communities, driving, and often food preparation (Rodger et al., 2015). Use of technology, video gaming, and use of social media increase at this stage. It has been reported that social media can negatively affect teens' self-esteem, especially girls, as they often compare themselves to unrealistic ideals (Abi-Jaoude et al., 2020). Occupations begin to become more individualized at this stage of life, with teens choosing what is meaningful and fulfilling to them personally.

Because teens go through puberty at this stage in their lives, they have an increased awareness of their developing bodies. Hormonal changes also affect their emotions and behavior. Adolescents begin to understand their own sexuality, develop their preferences, and possibly engage in intimate relationships or sexual activity. In later adolescence (ages 16–18 years), they often become more comfortable in relationships with others (Segal, 2014), including both emotional and physical relationships. Some teens may experiment with behaviors, including sexual activities and drug use. Some of these

FIGURE 10.3. These boys grew up in Guam, so water play and developing survival skills in the water are important for them.

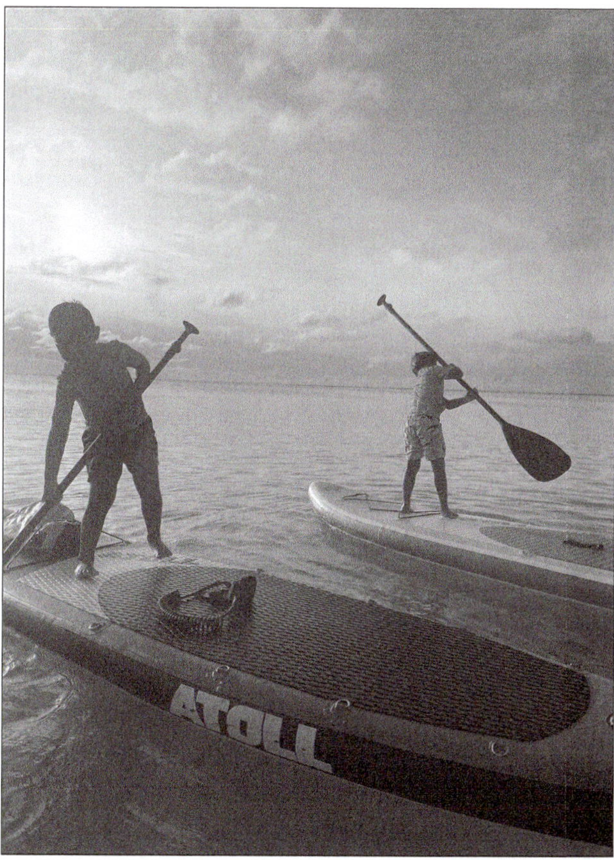

Source. J. L. Hoff. Used with permission.

FIGURE 10.4. Boys engaging in role playing.

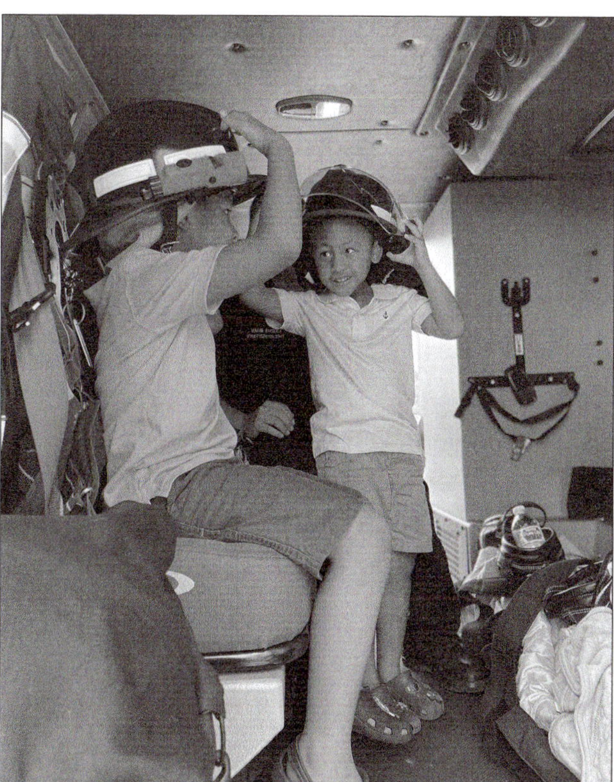

Source. J. L. Hoff. Used with permission.

occupations may be perceived as "negative occupations," or the dark side of occupations, although these types of occupations are not restricted to adolescence (Twinley, 2021). Occupational therapy practitioners believe that "active engagement in occupation promotes, facilitates, supports, and maintains health and participation" (AOTA, 2020, p. 5).

Belonging is critical at this stage of life, and many adolescents struggle to find their place amid personal change in a culture filled with norms and pressures that can be difficult to navigate. At times, it is quite acceptable to dress like everyone else, and at other times, a teen will strive to be different and stand out. Cultural rules and social dynamics seem to be fluid and sometimes difficult to grasp. Again, the sociocultural environment and socioeconomic status may affect the types of occupations in which teens engage.

EXERCISE 10.4. Exploring Occupations in the Teen Years

Think back to your own teen years.

- What occupations were important to you?
- What occupations did you try to avoid?
- In hindsight, were there occupations that were important to you that you might now consider "the dark side of occupations"? What made them so?
- Were there occupations that were generally acceptable among your social group but your parents or caregivers might not have approved of?
- Describe the experience of belonging (or not belonging) to a group

Choose a partner in your class and discuss your answers to these questions.

Adulthood

At this stage of life (ages 18–65 years), occupations are less stage specific and become more like the traditional definition of *occupation* as contributing to health, well-being, doing, and belonging (Wilcock 2006; Wilcock & Hocking, 2015). Adult occupations often focus on work and family but can be influenced by socioeconomic status, cultural background, and the region in which people live.

Major concerns in ***young adulthood*** (ages 18–30 years) center on education and training, with a focus on future work. Some social scientists (e.g., Hill & Redding, 2021; Sawyer et al., 2018) have stated that adolescence has been somewhat extended into this phase of life, because graduate and professional education has delayed many young adults' entry into the workforce. They are making decisions about their future and the life roles they want to explore. They are also exploring and establishing social and intimate relationships (Matuska

TABLE 10.3. **COGNITIVE, SOCIAL, AND EMOTIONAL MILESTONES FOR ADOLESCENTS AGES 12–17 YEARS**

AGE LEVEL	COGNITIVE DEVELOPMENT	SOCIAL AND EMOTIONAL DEVELOPMENT
12–13 years	• Starts to think hypothetically • Uses imagination to form thought • Independently reads and writes outside of school • Uses active listening in a variety of settings	• Identifies with peers • May start to psychologically distance self from parents • May overreact to parental standards • Is able to voice emotions and tries to find solutions to conflicts • Understands the consequences of their actions
14–15 years	• Thinks more hypothetically, abstractly, and logically • Demonstrates an increasing ability to reason • Investigates how living things interact with each other • Is starting to develop deeper moral reasoning	• Is embarrassed by family and parents • Is eager to be accepted by peers • May not want to talk as much, and may be argumentative • Is discovering where they belong in the world • Begins to analyze their own feelings and what caused them
16–17 years	• Begins to understand morality, philosophy, and faith • Starts developing learning and memory strategies • Understands the effects of their behavior • Starts setting realistic goals for the future	• Develops friendships based on loyalty, understanding, and trust • May participate in risky behaviors • Begins to relate to family better, and sees parents as real people • Spends a lot of time with friends • Is able to voice their emotions and find solutions to conflicts

Source. From "Children and Mental Health," by P. Rabey & S. Kletti. In K. M. Matuska (Ed.), *Ways of Living: Intervention Strategies to Enable Participation, 5th Edition,* 2020, p. 123. Copyright © 2020 by the American Occupational Therapy Association. Used with permission.

& Barrett, 2015). For some, just making a living and becoming more independent is the focus.

Work is a primary occupation in adulthood. People are beginning to establish themselves in their career and determining what they need to support themselves. Disparities can be seen between those with educational opportunities that have prepared them for a career and those who have not had that advantage. The recent SARS-CoV-2 virus (COVID-19) pandemic showed that many people adjusted and worked from home, but those with more hands-on or physical jobs were out of work for a significant period of time. Moreover, those with a higher level of education were more likely to be employed than those with a high school degree or less (Auginbaugh & Rothstein, 2022). Although some government assistance was available in the United States, it was often not enough because measures had to be taken to avoid evictions and maintain food security. The pandemic has highlighted the employment disparities that exist among those with different educational and socioeconomic backgrounds.

Although many adults focus on work to the exclusion of other activities, many others combine their work with a focus on the important occupation of parenting and caregiving. ***Parenting*** is one of the few major life occupations for which there is no formal education; parents often generally learn by doing and using whatever resources are available to them (Matuska & Barrett, 2015). Those resources may also be affected by socioeconomic status and culture. For example, some families can afford child care; others cannot. Other families may have extended family who can help with child care, and some cultures may be more supportive of these roles than others.

During adulthood, many families face the challenge of taking care of older adults as well as their children. Many families need to care for an older adult family member in their home because of the high cost of professional care, both in and outside of the home, for older adults. This has led to the term ***sandwich generation,*** which refers to those who care for their older parents while supporting and caring for their children (Merriam-Webster, n.d.). Caregiving often leads to increased stress and potentially to occupational disruption, in which people cannot manage working and caregiving at the same time, and ***occupational imbalance,*** in which people are focused on their employment and caregiving without the chance to relax or engage in leisure occupations that are important to sustaining their quality of life.

Leisure occupations are very important to life as an adult. ***Leisure activities*** are those activities in which people engage to relax and rejuvenate and are determined by personal preference, region, culture, and socioeconomic status. The activities that one chooses to engage in depend on who one is and what one likes. Some adults will choose to play baseball or more typical American sports, and others will play cricket or soccer. Some may engage in skiing and surfing; others enjoy gardening or craft activities. Still others like running, biking, or fishing. Regions and location enter into the choice of occupations, such as hunting in some rural areas or golfing in locations that stay warm through winter, and the activities one chooses can vary widely. Some leisure activities, such as golf and skiing, are costly, and others are low cost and can be done anywhere. Some people are content to just sit and watch television. Regardless of which activities one enjoys, relaxation and leisure are important parts of a healthy life.

Older Adulthood

The beginning of ***older adulthood*** has typically been thought to be at age 65 years, the traditional age at retirement. However, as life expectancies have increased over the years, the question of whether this is the proper demarcation of older adulthood has arisen (AARP, 2022). Occupations among older adults frequently depend on two things: (1) health status and (2) financial status. Those who are fortunate enough to experience good health have many more opportunities to engage in favorite occupations in older adulthood. They can continue their previous leisure activities, sometimes with mild accommodations. Again, socioeconomic status plays a large role in retirement and older adulthood. Many are fortunate enough to have been able to accumulate enough funds so that they can pursue many important occupations during their retirement years. These occupations may include active leisure occupations such sports and travel or more relaxing leisure occupations, including various types of entertainment. Other people may not be able to retire and may have to continue working to support themselves, thus limiting their leisure occupations, and others may continue to work because they enjoy it.

As people continue to age, many leisure occupations become more limited, and people tend to become more sedentary. Ludwig (1998) was one of the first occupational therapists to report that as women age, they tend to decrease their routines and reduce their number of activities. Social scientists have identified this decrease in routines and activities as ***disengagement theory*** (Perzynski, 2006). This disengagement has been observed in many older adults, although it is sometimes related to physical deterioration or cognitive decline. Many adults increase the amount of television they watch as means of leisure activity (Kuykendall et al., 2021), which also makes them more sedentary and socially isolated. The recent COVID-19 pandemic increased the isolation of many older adults (Burgoyne et al., 2022); when older adults participate less in exercise and hobbies, they experience less life satisfaction (Sherman & Lindstrom, 2022). See Chapter 13 for a more extensive discussion of leisure across the lifespan.

A Life Course Perspective

The concept of ***life course*** is defined as "a sequence of socially defined events and roles that the individual enacts over time" (Giele & Elder, 1998, p. 22). The ***life course perspective*** incorporates aspects of history, sociology, developmental psychology, economics, and demography. It became popular during the 1990s and focuses on the person's actual experiences rather the specific stages of life. Both human development (aging and developmental changes) and the experiences that a person has within their family and social group are critically important to the life course perspective. Some specific principles of this approach are the person's social history and geographic location, when the person was born and their experiences, and how the past shapes the future.

Social history and geographic location influence people's experiences as they grow up. Those who have experienced poverty have a very different perspective than those who were raised in an affluent family. Consequently, the occupations that children coming from these two different backgrounds are exposed to can be very different. Similarly, the traditions of those who grew up in a family in the northeastern part of the United States may be very different from the traditions of

EXERCISE 10.5. Comparison of Two Older Adults

Miguel retired from a life of office work. He had chronic asthma and chronic pain due to some damage to his cervical spine that affected his fine motor coordination. He also had some hearing loss and used hearing aids. When he felt good, he walked with a cane, but more often he spent time in a wheelchair. His wife continued to work. He lived in an apartment building with an elevator, so even on his bad days, he was able to go outside and socialize with his neighbors. Otherwise, he spent most of his time in the house watching television. One day, he was outside with his neighbors and had difficulty hearing what they were saying. His response to them was off topic, and they laughed at him. He became very upset and went back upstairs. From then on, he refused to go outside unless his wife took him out. He became more isolated and depressed.

LaToya retired from a career as a high school teacher. Her husband had retired but continued to teach part time at the college level. She played tennis and did needlework to pass the time. LaToya had a lot of friends and often went out to lunch with them. As she got older, she found that playing tennis was too physically taxing and gave that up, concentrating more on knitting and needlework. Then her eyesight began to fail, so she took a sculpting class. She found this very enjoyable and chose to work in stone, a very difficult medium. Her husband helped her move her artwork because she was not able to do it herself. When her husband passed away, she chose to leave her home and move into a senior community, where she explored other types of art media and was able to socialize with others.

Questions

1. Miguel and LaToya are very different and have different approaches to occupations. Compare and contrast these two people.
2. What might the role of occupational therapy be for each of them? Is occupational therapy necessary for each of them?
3. What do their occupations tell you about them?

those who grew up in the South. Those who grew up in a location with four seasons may have very different occupations and experiences than those who were raised in an area with a year-round warm climate (Figure 10.5). People who grew up in an area with a very diverse population may have a different perspective than those who did not. The life course perspective can provide a way for occupational therapy practitioners to understand how social situations affect the occupations in which people choose to engage (Crosnoe & Elder, 2002; Elder & Shanahan, 2006; Mayer, 2009).

FIGURE 10.5. Growing up on an island, many of the occupations important to these boys revolve around water.

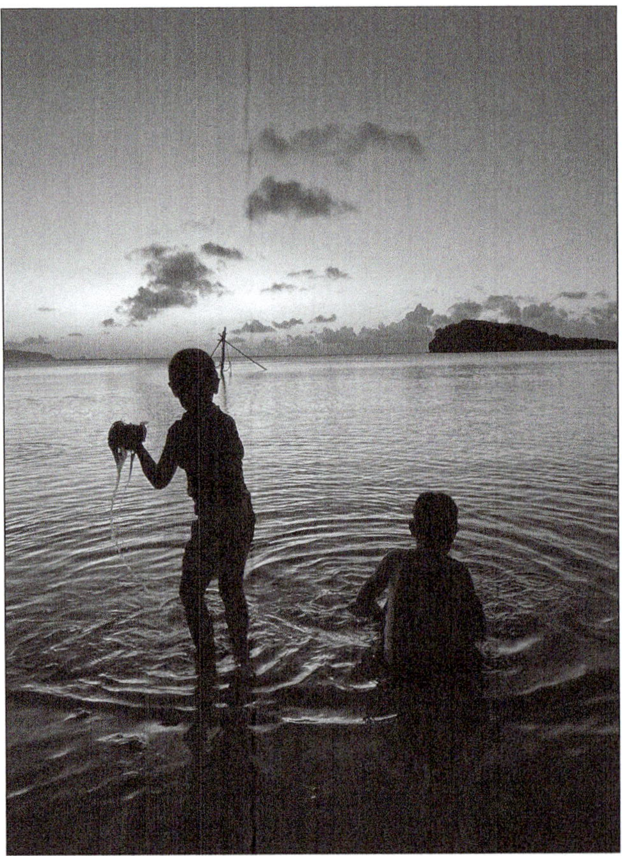

Source. J. L. Hoff. Used with permission.

The temporal context of people's lives can affect their perspective because their experiences may be very different. Those who served the country during wartime have a very different perspective on the horrors of war and service to their country than those who have not. Those who experienced the Great Depression have different ways of thinking about and spending money than those who did not. If a therapist is evaluating a teenager, they will see that the teen's way of perceiving the world is different from theirs. For example, some older adults react strongly to people with tattoos because tattoos were less prevalent 20 years ago than they are today.

People's past and upbringing shape the way they look at issues today. Every generation is different and has different values, but although people may reject some values from their upbringing, those values still influence their current and future values and occupations. For example, a person who had a great experience on a particular vacation may want to revisit that place at some time in the future, and people brought up in an environment in which art or music was valued often find themselves seeking out art or music in their lives as they grow up (see Case Example 10.1).

Humphry and Womack (2019) presented five life course principles and related them to occupation, based on the work of Elder and Shanahan (2006):

1. Past experiences transform over the lifetime, and past occupations affect future occupations;
2. Relationships have an effect on a person's occupations, because people are connected;
3. Society and historic events provide particular meaning to occupations and affect what they do;
4. People make choices about their occupations on the basis of who they are and their circumstances at the time; and
5. Past experiences, life transitions, and circumstances surrounding an event may affect how people react, and reactions will often depend on their personal life course at the time.

CASE EXAMPLE 10.1. Demonstrating How Experiences Affect Occupations and Behavior

Elsie grew up in the Midwest during World War II. Her family did not have a lot of money and rationing of food and supplies at this time made it even more difficult to meet basic needs. Despite having a comfortable life during her adulthood, she remained very frugal. She often repeated a saying that her mother taught her: "Use it up, wear it out, make it do, or do without."

Jack's father was an opera singer. Music was always played in his home, and his father encouraged everyone to sing. Jack grew up to become a physician. Although he never liked opera as a child, as an adult he enjoys all types of music, including Broadway shows, symphonic music, and opera. He considers listening to music and attending concerts to be critical occupations in his life.

The life course perspective offers a different way of understanding the lives of clients and the occupations that are important to them. It should certainly be considered when evaluating a client and gathering information for an occupational profile.

EXERCISE 10.6. Comparing Life Experiences and Occupations

Spend at least 15 minutes talking with someone whose age is at least 10 years different from your own.

- Identify their important occupations.
- Explore how their occupations have changed over time.
- Explore how their past may have (or may not have) influenced these occupations.
- Ask about their family occupations and explore how these occupations may (or may not) influence their current occupations.
- Explore the region where they grew up and where they now live, and discuss how that affects their occupations.

Summary

This chapter provided an overview of the development of occupations over the lifespan. It focused on two perspectives used by occupational therapists, the ecological developmental perspective and the life course perspective. The chapter is not meant to provide a complete review of development or of these two perspectives but rather an overview of how occupational therapy practitioners can view the development and importance of occupation to their clients through the lenses of two different approaches.

References

AARP. (2022). *Is the Social Security retirement age going up?* https://bit.ly/3BJyC2I

Abi-Jaoude, E., Naylor, K. T., & Pignatiello, A. (2020). Smartphones, social media use, and youth mental health. *Canadian Medical Association Journal, 192*(6), e136–e141. https://doi.org/10.1503/cmaj.190434

American Occupational Therapy Association. (2020). Occupational therapy practice framework: Domain and process (4th ed.). *American Journal of Occupational Therapy, 74*(Suppl. 2), 7412410010. https://doi.org/10.5014/ajot.2020.74S2001

American Occupational Therapy Association. (2022). *School mental health interventions.* https://www.aota.org/practice/clinical-topics/school-mental-health-toolkit

Auginbaugh, A., & Rothstein, D. S. (2022). *How did employment change during the COVID-19 pandemic? Evidence from a new BLS survey supplement.* U.S. Bureau of Labor Statistics. https://www.bls.gov/opub/btn/volume-11/how-did-employment-change-during-the-covid-19-pandemic.htm

Bronfenbrenner, U. (1979). *The ecology of human development: Experiments by nature and design.* Harvard University Press.

Bronfenbrenner, U. (1989). Ecological systems theory. In A. Bandura & R. Vasta (Ed.) *Annals of child development: Vol. 6. Six theories of child development: Revised formulations and current issues* (pp. 189–249. JAI Press.

Bronfenbrenner, U., & Evans, G. W. (2000). Developmental science in the 21st century: Emerging questions, theoretical models, research designs and empirical findings. *Social Development, 9,* 115–125. https://doi.org/10.1111/1467-9507.00114

Burgoyne, A., Ercanbrack, M., Wiley, S., & Kornblau, B. (2022). COVID-19's effect on social isolation and loneliness as experienced by older adults. *American Journal of Occupational Therapy, 76*(Suppl. 1), 7610505133. https://doi.org/10.5014/ajot.2022.76S1-PO133

Chapparo, C., & Lowe, S. (2012). School, participating in more than just the classroom. In S. J. Lane & A. C. Bundy (Eds.), *Kids can be kids: A childhood occupations approach* (pp. 83–101). F. A. Davis.

Crosnoe, R., & Elder, G. H. (2002). Successful adaptation in the later years: A life course approach to aging. *Social Psychology Quarterly, 65,* 309–328. https://doi.org/10.2307/3090105

Elder, G. H., & Shanahan, M. J. (2006). The life course and human development. In R. M. Lerner (Ed.), *Handbook of personal psychology* (6th ed., Vol. 1, pp. 665–715). Wiley.

Fine, G. A., Monimer, J. T., & Robens, D. F. (1990), Leisure, work, and the mass media. In S. S. Feldman & G. R. Elliott (Eds.), *At the threshold: The developing adolescent* (pp. 225–252). Harvard University Press.

Gesell, A., & Armatruda, C. S. (1954). *Developmental diagnosis* (2nd ed.). Harper.

Giele, J. Z., & Elder, G. H. (1998). *Methods of life course research: Qualitative and quantitative approaches.* Sage.

Hill, N. E., & Redding, A. (2021). *The end of adolescence: The lost art of delaying adulthood.* Harvard University Press.

Hocking, C. (2019). Contribution of occupation to health and well-being. In B. A. B. Schell & G. Gillen (Eds.), *Willard & Spackman's occupational therapy* (13th ed., pp. 113–123). Wolters Kluwer.

Howe, T. H., Kramer, P., & Hinojosa, J. (2020). Developmental perspective: Fundamentals of developmental theory. In P. Kramer, J. Hinojosa, & T. H. Howe (Eds.), *Frames of reference for pediatric occupational therapy* (4th ed, pp. 20–28). Wolters Kluwer.

Humphry, R. (2002). Young children's occupations: Explicating the dynamics of developmental processes. *American Journal of Occupational Therapy, 56,* 171–179. https://doi.org/10.5014/ajot.56.2.171

Humphry, R., & Womack, J. (2019). Transformations of occupations: A life course perspective. In B. A. B. Schell & G. Gillen (Eds.), *Willard & Spackman's occupational therapy* (13th ed., pp. 100–112). Wolters Kluwer.

Knobloch, H., & Pasamanick, B. (Eds.). (1975). *Gesell and Armatruda's developmental diagnosis: The evaluation and management of normal and abnormal neuropsychologic development in infancy and early childhood.* Harper & Row.

Kohlberg, L. (1969). Stage and sequence: The cognitive developmental approach to socialization. In D. Groslin (Ed.), *Handbook of socialization theory and research* (pp. 347–480). Rand McNally.

Kramer, P., & Hinojosa, J. (1995). Epiphany of human occupation. In C. B. Royeen (Ed.), *Human occupation* (AOTA Self-Study Series). American Occupational Therapy Association.

Kuykendall, L., Lie, X., Zhu, Z., & Hu, X. (2021). Leisure choices and employee well-being: Comparing need fulfillment and well-being during TV and other leisure activities. *Applied Psychology: Health and Well-Being, 12,* 532–558. https://doi.org/10.1111/aphw.12196

Matuska, K., & Barrett, K. (2015). Occupations of adulthood. In C. H. Christiansen, C. M. Baum, & J. D. Bass (Eds.), *Occupational therapy: Performance, participation, and well-being* (pp. 157–168). Slack.

Maud, S. P., & Parks, S. (2021). Influences from early childhood professional organizations and technical assistance centers. In G. Frolek Clark & S. Parks (Eds.), *Best practices for occupational therapy in early childhood* (pp. 13–22). AOTA Press.

Mayer, K. U. (2009). New directions in life course research. *Annual Review of Sociology, 35,* 413–433. https://doi.org/10.1146/annurev.soc.34.040507.134619

Merriam-Webster. (n.d.). Sandwich generation. *Merriam-Webster.com.* https://www.merriam-webster.com/dictionary/sandwich%20generation

Mulligan, S. (2012). Preschool, I'm learning now. In S. J. Lane & A. C. Bundy (Eds.), *Kids can be kids: A childhood occupations approach* (pp. 63–83). F. A. Davis.

Parham, L. D., & Fazio, L. S. (Eds.). (2008). *Play in occupational therapy for children* (2nd ed.). Mosby Elsevier.

Pereira, R. B. (2017). Towards inclusive occupational therapy: Introducing the CORE approach to inclusive and occupation-focused practice. *Australian Occupational Therapy Journal, 64,* 427–513. https://doi.org/10.1111/1440-1630.12394

Perzynski, A. T. (2006). Disengagement theory. In L. S. Noelker, K. Rockwood, & R. L. Sprott (Eds.), *The encyclopedia of aging: A comprehensive resource in gerontology and geriatrics* (4th ed., pp. 321–322). Springer.

Rabey, P., & Kletti, S. (2020). Children and mental health. In K. M. Matuska (Ed.), *Ways of living: Intervention strategies to enable participation* (5th ed., pp. 107–130). AOTA Press.

Reilly, M. (1974). *Play as exploratory learning: Studies of curiosity behavior.* Sage.

Rodger, S., Ziviani, J., & Lim, S. M. (2015). Occupations of childhood and adolescence. In C. Christiansen, C. M. Baum & J. D. Bass (Eds.), *Occupational therapy: Participation, performance and well-being* (4th ed., pp. 129–156). Slack.

Sawyer, S. M., Azzopardi, P. S., Wickremarathne, D., & Patton, G. C. (2018). The age of adolescence. *Lancet Child & Adolescent Health, 2*(3), 223–228. https://doi.org/10.1016/S2352-4642(18)30022-1

Schering, S. (2022, February 7). CDC, AAP update developmental milestones for surveillance program. *AAP News.* https://publications.aap.org/aapnews/news/19554/CDC-AAP-update-developmental-milestones-for?autologincheck=redirected

Schultz-Krohn, W., & Wagle, A. (2021). Best practices in supporting mealtimes and nutritional needs (adaptive skills). In G. Frolek Clark & S. Parks (Eds.), *Best practices for occupational therapy in early childhood* (pp. 243–256). AOTA Press.

Segal, R. (2014). Dimensions of occupation across the lifespan. In J. Hinojosa & M. L. Blount (Eds.), *The texture of life: Occupations and other activities* (4th ed.). AOTA Press.

Sherman, D. S., & Lindstrom, D. (2022). Activity participation and life satisfaction of older adults during the COVID-19 pandemic. *American Journal of Occupational Therapy, 76*(Suppl. 1), 7610510170. https://doi.org/10.5014/ajot.2022.76S1-PO170

Twinley, R. (2021). *Illuminating the dark side of occupations: International perspectives from occupational therapy and occupational science.* Routledge.

Vergara, E. R. (2002). Enhancing occupational performance in infants in the NICU. *OT Practice, 7*(12), 8–13.

Wilcock, A. A. (2006). *An occupational perspective of health* (2nd ed.). Slack.

Wilcock, A. A., & Hocking, C. (2015). *An occupational perspective of health* (3rd ed.). Slack.

Youth.gov. (2022). *Adolescent development.* https://youth.gov/youth-topics/adolescent-health/adolescent-development

11

Independence in Occupations

ANITA PERR, PhD, OT/L, FAOTA

CHAPTER HIGHLIGHTS

- Interdependence, independence, and ableism
- Activities and participation
- Context
- Practitioner approaches to facilitate independence and interdependence
- The natural environment

KEY TERMS AND CONCEPTS

• ableism • amelioration • compensation • context • environmental factors • immersive technologies • independence • interdependence • natural environment • participation • personal factors • restoration • simulation

"Independent living is not doing things by yourself. It is being in control of how things are done." —Judy Heumann, #DisabledWomensHistory

This chapter focuses on independence, beginning with defining what independence is and what associated terms mean. It aims to discuss independence from the point of view of both the occupational therapy practitioner and their clients. It also examines context in relation to simulation; simulation in occupational therapy; and intervention approaches, including amelioration and compensation. The chapter wraps up with a discussion of home-based therapy and a second view at independence.

Amelioration is the process of ***restoration,*** or making someone better to improve function (Merriam-Webster, n.d.-a). Occupational therapy practitioners use various techniques to facilitate amelioration, including strengthening as well as motor interventions and activities to improve cognitive processes. ***Compensation*** measures are used to fill the gap between the person's performance skills and the skills needed to accomplish a task or participate in an occupation. Compensation includes use of adaptive equipment or assistive technology, environmental modification, and alteration of the task. Compensation measures may be used at the same time as amelioration. For instance, a person may use a long-handled spoon to feed themselves until they gain the strength and motor control to be able to use a conventional spoon. When the person is no longer making progress toward amelioration, compensation measures continue to be used to improve participation.

Interdependence, Independence, and Ableism

Interdependence

Interdependence is the state of being dependent on one another or having a mutual dependence (Merriam-Webster, n.d.-c). Interdependence acknowledges that people cannot do everything—period. Even those activities that people consider independent rely on collaboration with others. Interdependence seems like a more realistic goal—for instance, people with disabilities who live a functioning, interdependent lifestyle get help for what they need, such as ADLs. They also realize their value and help others using their own expertise and skills.

This interdependence requires self-empowerment and allows for satisfaction and pride. Many clients will need to learn how to direct others in their care. The necessary skills are a balance of clarity, forcefulness, and empathy. It may take a while for a person with a disability to develop an optimal relationship with their caregiver and see results in self-empowerment and autonomy (Bourke, 2021). Occupational therapy intervention, then, should challenge the client both in their independent occupational performance and their confidence in and skill to direct assistance, when needed. Successful management is success: Not everything has to get an A+, and that's okay (J. Lee, personal communication, March 28, 2022).

Independence

People define the term "independence" differently from other people and differently at various times in their lives. ***Independence*** usually infers self-reliance and autonomy, and it is often stated in terms of the absence of dependence. Among other things, independence is used to describe a person's nonreliance on others for care or livelihood, on guidance in conduct, or on political or societal pressure (Merriam-Webster, n.d.-b).

Independence is often measured by occupational therapy practitioners on a scale from "dependent" to "independent" using an assessment like the Functional Independence Measure (FIM; Uniform Data System for Medical Rehabilitation [UDS], 1997). Originally published in the 1980s, the FIM defines the characteristics of dependence and independence for each of 13 motor and cognitive items (Dodds et al., 1993). This tool measures burden of care and does not take into account whether the person is able to direct their care, whether the activity is important to the person, the quality of the person's actions, or the importance of independence to the person. In addition, the FIM prevents people who use adaptive equipment or assistive technology or who use extra time to complete the task or activity from attaining the highest score of 7. Occupational therapy's roots in the medical model partly explain the tendency of practitioners to have rigid definitions of independence in some practice areas, such as physical rehabilitation.

Ableism

Another factor that might explain occupational therapy practitioners' view of independence is ***ableism,*** which Campbell (2001) defined as

> a network of beliefs, processes and practices that produce a particular kind of self and body (the corporeal standard) that is projected as the perfect, species-typical and therefore essential and fully human. Disability then is cast as a diminished state of being human. (p. 44)

In their evolving definition, Lewis (2022), defined *ableism* as

> a system of assigning value to people's bodies and minds based on societally constructed ideas of normalcy, productivity, desirability, intelligence, excellence, and fitness. These constructed ideas are deeply rooted in eugenics, anti-Blackness, misogyny, colonialism, imperialism, and capitalism. This systemic oppression leads to people and society determining people's value based on their culture, age, language, appearance, religions, birth or living place, "health/wellness," and/or their ability to satisfactorily re/produce, "excel" and "behave." You do not have to be disabled to experience ableism. (para. 3)

Ableism, like other forms of oppression, should be explored by occupational therapy practitioners so that it does not influence our work with clients and other members of society. We need to identify our own biases to ensure they are minimized in our client assessments, interventions, and relationships. When considering client performance, it is important to consider client perspectives, experiences, and opinions.

EXERCISE 11.1. Bias

Take a few minutes to think about your own biases—in general and in relation to disability. Answer the following questions in relation to a new client assigned to you whom you have not yet met:

- What judgments do you make when you see a new client's name? Do you know anyone else with that name? Have you read about anyone with that name? How does that influence you?
- What judgments do you make when you find out where a client lives?
- What judgments do you make regarding their age, diagnosis, comorbidities, and so forth?

People make judgments; sometimes they are right, and sometimes they are wrong. By making yourself aware of your own biases, you may be able to develop strategies so as not to let these judgments overpower your therapeutic relationship. Think about why you have your own biases and what you want to do about them.

Think of a time when you prejudged a person and (1) your expectations were met and (2) your expectations were disproved. What were the differences in these instances? Sometimes there are no identifiable differences in the reasoning for your judgments. This reinforces the need to control your judgments and not let them cloud your therapeutic relationships. Take a few more minutes to think about strategies you can use to either lower your tendency to prejudge or to improve your ability to notice when you do this and then to consciously prevent yourself from using those judgments.

Now, let's take it to the next step. What expectations do you have when you learn of a new client's age, gender, diagnosis, and comorbidities? Thinking about our expectations can help us to prepare for patient treatment. Your expectations may reflect your ableist thinking. This can happen in all practice areas when working with people with any type of disability. It is important, however, to make sure that ableism and other prejudgments do not overpower your assessments or interventions. What strategies can you put into place to accomplish this when working with children in a classroom? When working in a community-based summer camp for children with autism and related diagnoses? When working in a residential treatment program for teenagers and young adults with anorexia? When working on a locked psychiatric unit? Or in a hospital-based acute rehabilitation setting?

Again, it is important to be aware of your own judgments and biases so that you can manage them. You may find that certain functional abilities, such as the ability to communicate, bring out your biased impressions regarding a client's interest, intelligence, and capacity for improved participation. If you find there are certain things that are more likely to affect you, think about why that is and be aware of it so you do not mistreat people in your practice.

Activities and Participation

Just as we occupational therapy practitioners aspire to be nondiscriminatory in our interactions with clients, we should also aspire to be broad in our expectations for what is usual or typical performance or practice. I often use the activity in Exercise 11.2 to demonstrate how to broaden my expectations. As you can see, there are many *right* ways to perform tasks.

When you work with clients, broaden your perspective and ask questions to learn the reasons behind their strategies. Go with their preferences whenever you can. That being said, as occupational therapy practitioners, we are deeply concerned with safety, so if your client suggests a method you feel is unsafe, work with them to find acceptable, alternative strategies, even when compromise is necessary. You may also suggest other strategies that are more efficient, more thorough, or otherwise more desirable. As your relationship deepens, clients may be more apt to consider your suggestions (Enemark Larsen et al., 2018).

The previous discussion about interdependence, independence, and ableism reflects goals that refer to participation in activities of choice in environments of choice. Your therapeutic relationships are likely to help as you focus on each client's individual needs. Considering ableism and other prejudgments may help you to develop strong relationships that lead to positive outcomes.

The United Nations Convention on the Rights of Persons with Disabilities is based, in part, on the principle of full and effective participation and inclusion in society (United Nations, 2006). Participation is central to the functioning described in the *International Classification of Functioning, Disability and Health* (*ICF*; World Health Organization [WHO], 2001). The *ICF* model of functioning and disability describes the interactions among the person, activities, and contexts. The *ICF* acknowledges that biological and societal influences cannot be addressed separately; rather, both must be addressed when discussing participation. The fourth edition of the *Occupational Therapy Practice Framework: Domain and Process* (4th ed.; American Occupational Therapy Association [AOTA], 2020) uses WHO's definition of ***participation***: involvement in a situation. Occupational therapy and this chapter both are based in the belief that people should be able to participate fully and effectively in their society.

EXERCISE 11.2. Broadening Expectations

Take a few minutes to write down the steps you take when you put on your shoes and socks. After doing that, consider the following, each of which demonstrates that there is usually more than one right way of performing a task.

One way: I put on my socks and then my shoes.
Rationale:

- I don't know. I just do it.
- If there is an emergency, I don't want to get caught with one bare foot.

Another way: I put on the sock and shoe for one foot first and then the sock and shoe for the other foot.
Rationale:

- I don't know. I just do it.
- It seems more efficient. Less leg movement is needed.

A third way: I put on my socks and then put on slippers (or just wear socks) until I leave the house.
Rationale:

- I don't know. I just do it.
- I don't like walking in shoes in my home because
  - they get the floors dirty,
  - they are noisy, or
  - they are too hot.

In my culture, we don't wear outside shoes in the home. The shoes stay at the door.

A fourth alternative: I put on my socks and shoes while I'm standing.
Rationale:

- I don't know. I just do it.
- I do this as a meditation. I work on yoga poses to improve my balance. I focus my eyes on a spot on the wall, and I pay attention to my breath as I stand on one leg while putting the sock and shoe on the other.
- There is no chair near my door.

A fifth alternative: I put on my socks and shoes while I'm sitting.
Rationale:

- I don't know. I just do it.
- I would fall if I did this in standing.
- I sit on the floor because there is no room for a chair near my door.

Context

Occupational therapy practitioners assume a critical role in the process of integrating a client into their natural contexts.

Context comprises both environmental factors and personal factors. ***Environmental factors*** comprise the physical, social, and attitudinal surroundings. ***Personal factors*** are "the particular background of a person's life and living" (AOTA, 2020, p. 81) and comprise the unique features of the person other than their state of health. Personal factors include features like age, social background, and education (AOTA, 2020). In this chapter, the ultimate goal is participation at a desired level in the natural environment, the usual place where the activity or occupation occurs—perhaps the client's home or any other place the client visits.

Using the therapeutic value of simulated activities and a variety of contexts, the occupational therapy practitioner works in collaboration with the client, caregivers, significant others, and other professionals to match the client's engagement in an activity with particular therapeutic goals. Throughout occupational therapy practice, simulation is used when the natural environment, real tools, and actual contextual factors are unavailable or inappropriate as a result of the client's tolerance and functional abilities. ***Simulation*** is the copied representation of functioning by other means (Merriam-Webster, n.d.-d).

Practitioner Approaches to Facilitate Independence and Interdependence

To help clients to participate in desired occupations in natural environments, occupational therapy practitioners use a variety of evidence-based approaches that are based on numerous theories. This section describes a number of practitioner approaches used in rehabilitation: amelioration, compensation, immersive technologies and robotics, and online intervention or telerehabilitation.

Practitioner Approach: Amelioration

Occupational therapy practitioners need to be flexible in their response to the client's abilities and needs. The practitioner sets goals and expectations in conjunction with the client based on a wealth of information, including the practitioner's previous experiences and knowledge and the client's current level of functioning, context, and expectations. The practitioner adjusts the interventions and revises the goals in response to the client's progress.

Occupational therapy is often a combination of amelioration (restoration) and compensation. At the point when occupational therapy is initiated, practitioners often use contrived activities in a clinical environment; interventions may not resemble real life at this point. For instance, instead of working on an occupation like self-feeding, the practitioner may develop an activity in which the client grasps objects of various shapes and sizes, placing and releasing these objects on various planes, and performing certain movement patterns while sitting or lying in bed. These activities, although contrived, may promote joint range of motion and muscle flexibility in the upper extremities, which will allow the person to hold utensils and feed themselves later on. Sometimes clients and families misunderstand the use of contrived activities; they may not realize the relationship to real life, and they may become frustrated. Practitioners need to explain how each activity prepares the client for the real-life activities. As the client progresses, the intervention is designed to more closely reflect real-life occupations.

Clients may be working individually or in groups, and the environment may not reflect any aspects of the natural context. Conversely, interventions may simulate real-life environments. For instance, clients may be wearing hospital gowns and participating in intervention individually in their own hospital or facility room. Later, clients may wear street clothes and leave their rooms for occupational therapy in central settings like clinics or activity rooms.

When they are able, clients may participate in interventions in spaces designed to replicate home or community settings. For instance, occupational therapy practitioners may start working on meal preparation and self-feeding at bedside. Initially, the practitioner may need to set up the food, including opening sealed packets of condiments. Later, the client may join a cooking group in which tasks are assigned, and the client takes responsibility for a portion of the tasks, such as setting a table with dishes and silverware rather than paper and plastic, and using condiments in more homelike packages like salt and pepper shakers rather than small, paper packets. The meal prep may take place in a kitchen area with a refrigerator, stove, and sink, and the meal may be shared in a dining space that looks and feels more contextual than eating in bed or at the bedside using a hospital table.

Practitioner Approach: Compensation

In general, two broad categories of compensation in occupational therapy intervention are (1) alternative strategies and (2) adaptive equipment or assistive technology.

Let's continue talking about the client who has difficulty self-feeding. Previously we talked about developing interventions to improve arm and hand use. Let's say that the client also has difficulty maintaining the posture and trunk control to use their arms for activities. Ameliorative interventions might include the use of activities that require the client to move from their base of support progressively. Initially, perhaps a second occupational therapy practitioner provides external support and relaxes that support as the client's sensory and motor function improves.

In addition to working to regain sensory and motor function outside of mealtime, the client may use alternative strategies during self-feeding. For instance, perhaps the client will use bimanual strategies for tasks that they previously performed single-handedly, like wiping their mouth. Or perhaps they will rest their elbows on the table to provide support so that they can bring their hand to their mouth.

This same client might also use adaptive equipment until they are able to attain and maintain an optimal posture for self-feeding. Perhaps seating supports are added to a dining chair so that the client does not have to use their arms to maintain a balanced, seated position or rely on an occupational therapy practitioner to provide that external support. These seating supports provide external trunk support so the client can use their hands and arms for the feeding activity. The same client may also find that the addition of utensils with built-up handles makes it possible for them to hold their utensils during self-feeding.

Ameliorative and compensatory strategies are often used simultaneously. As the person's function improves, the use of alternative strategies or adaptive equipment or assistive technology can be reduced. Satisfactory performance—in this case, feeding oneself—would still reflect the client's expectations and preferences to be able to perform the actual feeding activity on their own.

With the ubiquitous nature of mobile technologies and the ever-present applications, many people use applications (apps) to assist with their everyday function. For instance, a person may use a phone- or computer-based calendar, a warning or notification app, apps to measure heart rate, apps for maintaining their to-do lists, and texting rather than face-to-face or telephone communication. Often, everyday apps can also work for people with physical, cognitive, or social limitations. Many apps and operating systems have controls to personalize most aspects of the technology's function. These settings may be found in the general preferences areas or in accessibility features.

The successful use of these technologies also relies on the developers and creators to provide the information needed for accessibility features to work. For instance, notifications can be set as visual prompts, auditory prompts, or haptic prompts. Depending on the person's preference or need, the notification can be personalized for people with hearing impairments or blindness/low vision. Captions are available for people with hearing impairments or for using an app in a noisy environment. Audio description apps provide descriptions of what is seen in video and are useful to people who are blind or have low vision; they also are useful to people who may miss parts of the visual display because of limited attention or processing difficulties. Many people with limited attention or processing skills benefit from both enhanced visual and auditory input. Grigorenko et al. (2020) suggested that many factors should be considered when working with children with specific processing disorders. Based in part on work by Mathes et al. (2005) and Fuchs et al. (2014), comprehensive interventions, such as those that address both visual and auditory input, adjustable intensity, and intervention in the academic environment, are more effective than isolated skills training (Grigorenko et al., 2020).

When selecting apps for clients, it is important to identify the client's specific needs. Sometimes everyday technologies are sufficient, but sometimes specialty apps with more advanced or individualized programming are needed. For instance, some people with learning disabilities find that a word processing program with spell check or grammar check is all they need. Other people may benefit from a program that also has word prediction, sentence rephrasing, or text-to-speech functions.

Practitioner Approach: Immersive Technologies and Robotics

Immersive technologies are sometimes used to improve the simulation of real-life situations or to improve the person's cognitive, sensory, or motor function. For instance, virtual reality may more closely resemble a natural setting than a clinic, allowing the client to work on performance skills. Use of immersive technologies is still relatively new in occupational therapy. Studies have demonstrated the feasibility of virtual-reality and robotic-based technologies in poststroke, upper-limb rehabilitation. Use of these technologies has been found to be feasible and potentially efficacious (Norouzi-Gheidari et al., 2020).

In addition, numerous teams of researchers have developed hand-based robotics for hand rehabilitation of stroke survivors (Jiralerspong et al., 2018; Yap et al., 2017). Based on their earlier work, Heung et al. (2019) improved the design of their Soft-Elastic Composite Actuator, a 3D printed—rather than elastomer molded—soft robotic hand with pneumatic components to control finger movement in stroke survivors. Two stroke survivors tested the 3D printed, soft robotic hand three times weekly for a total of 20 sessions, with each session lasting 45 minutes plus a 5-minute break. The participants initially practiced opening and closing their hand. Later sessions included grasping, moving, and releasing objects. Improvement of hand function was noted when the robotic hand was removed. Using an iterative design process, these researchers were able to develop a method of making the robotic hand in various sizes. They reported that they plan to use their iterative learning process to control the actuation of the robotic hand, which can then alter the range of motion and tip force to improve function during ADLs (Heung et al., 2019).

Virtual-reality–based interventions may also be effective in cognitive rehabilitation. In their 2019 study, De Luca et al. compared traditional cognitive rehabilitation with virtual-reality cognitive retraining. They found that although participants in both treatment approach groups demonstrated significant improvement, the participants in the virtual-reality cognitive retraining group demonstrated a significant improvement in cognitive flexibility, ability to shift tasks, and selective attention (De Luca et al., 2019).

This research by DeLuca et al. (2019) used BTS Bioengineering technology called Nirvana, a "medical device based on virtual reality designed to support motor and cognitive rehabilitation" (BTS Bioengineering, n.d.). The researchers suggested that the multisensory approach of virtual reality may be more effective because it provides global stimulation as well as dual cognitive and motor tasks. In addition, virtual reality may increase motivation and speed of information processing (De Luca et al., 2019).

Practitioner Approach: Telerehabilitation

With the exception of services provided in acute care hospitals, the global impact of the SARS-CoV-2 virus (COVID-19) pandemic brought nearly all occupational therapy intervention to online platforms. Since 2020, much has been written about telehealth in occupational therapy. Guney Yilmaz and Onal (2021) investigated telerehabilitation in providing sensory processing and functional independence interventions in children. Using the Sensory Profile (Dunn, 1999) and the Functional Independence Measure for Children (Ottenbacher et al., 1996; UDS, 2004), they were able to demonstrate improvements in the children's function and visual, vestibular, tactile, and multisensorial processes. In this study, materials were sent to families via email before the intervention. Phone calls were used to ensure that the families could apply the sensory activities correctly. Occupational therapy practitioners guided sessions that were carried out by the family member with the child. This method of telerehabilitation allows the practitioner to observe the relationship between the parent and child and to provide meaningful, real-time feedback (Guney Yilmaz & Onal, 2021).

Torpil and Kaya (2022) compared telerehabilitation with in-person rehabilitation of 48 people ages 65 to 75 years who underwent total knee replacement surgery. Participants were divided into two groups: (1) face-to-face intervention in a treatment center and (2) telerehabilitation. Participants in each group identified the same areas of greatest concern: going up or down stairs, toileting, bathing, moving from one room to another, sitting in and rising from a chair, meeting family and friends, and engaging in social activities. Although the authors reported that the socialization problems could have been caused by pain, changes in sleep patterns, and limited mobility, they also reported that the problems could have been caused by measures taken to prevent the spread of COVID-19. Family or other caregivers participated in the telerehabilitation sessions to ensure safety. Limitations in telerehabilitation included Internet connection problems and difficulty of the participants in adapting to the telerehabilitation environment. Participants in the face-to-face group reported fear of getting sick and difficulties with transportation. Those in both groups made significant gains in quality of life and perceived occupational performance and satisfaction. No differences in progress were noted between the two groups (Torpil & Kaya, 2022).

The Natural Environment

Let's explore context in relationship to participation, satisfaction, independence, and interdependence. Occupational therapy in the natural environment is optimal. The term ***natural environment*** relates to the real environment in which the client lives. Up to this point, simulated environments played proxy for natural environments and included working in a hospital room, a clinic space, or even a simulated community or home environment. Occupational therapy intervention addresses occupations, personal factors, and context. Working in a contrived environment may actually negatively affect clients by presenting unrealistic situations. For instance, a client may think or say something like, "Oh, this room isn't anything like my room at home. I'll be able to do it at home." This is often not the case. Conversely, a clinical environment in which everything is accessibly designed and all of the fixtures work as they should may cause the client to be concerned that they won't be able to function at home because of the difficulties in the spaces themselves.

We all face any combination of quirks in our own natural environments. The following list includes just a few common quirks that are not accounted for in simulated, clinical settings:

- A shower faucet that has to be set in a precise location; otherwise, the water will freeze or burn you.
- A door lock that requires you to wiggle the key in just the right way for the door to unlock.
- A creaky flight of steps that requires you to stay far to the right for the first few steps, then skip a step. and then continue to ascend the flight. If you do not follow these patterns, the creaking is likely to wake the baby.
- A broken door buzzer that causes delivery people to call you so that you can toss your key out of the window—wrapped in a sock, of course.
- A garden that needs to be tended daily, ensuring that the fencing prevents animals from eating the yield.

These quirks are difficult to simulate in a clinical environment. It is unrealistic that clients will even be aware of many of the quirks in their own natural environments for occupational therapy practitioners to even consider simulating. When intervention takes place in the natural environment, the focus of intervention becomes occupations and personal factors. It is often necessary and effective to make contextual changes or environmental modifications to further the person's abilities.

Simulation is effective in working toward participation, but it may be more effective to turn this around and aim to provide more intervention in natural environments. An example of where this has already taken place is in school-based occupational therapy. In many locations, push-in services have replaced many of the services involving pulling the child from their classroom. It makes sense to work with students on school-based issues in the classroom. Changes can be made to the classroom context to facilitate participation, and the child can learn effective ways to enhance participation.

Home-based intervention also allows the client to maintain nearby friendships and activities as they are able, thus decreasing loneliness and disempowerment (J. Lee, personal communication, March 28, 2022). The natural environment or home is also the place where the client's meaningful belongings are located. Perhaps they will perform their hand coordination and endurance exercises by shelling peas for dinner, or by picking up a knitting project put aside years ago, or by going out to the yard and starting a garden.

CASE EXAMPLE 11.1. Shameka Andrews

FIGURE 11.1. Shameka Andrews.

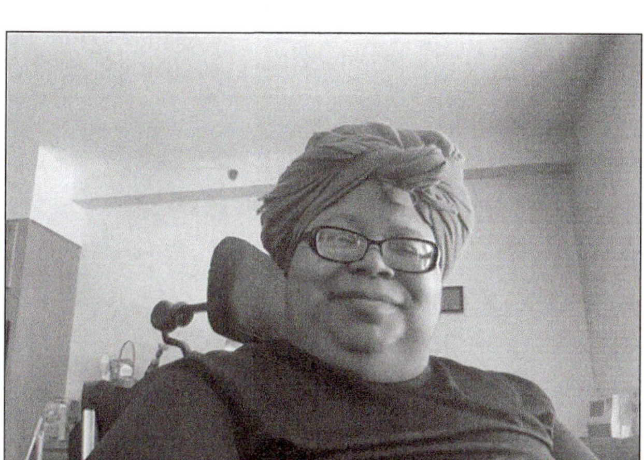

Note. S. Andrews. Used with permission.

Shameka works as an advocate in New York State (see Figure 11.1). She is the founder of Disability Empowered Consulting and is the community outreach coordinator of the Self-Advocacy Association of New York State, Inc. She advocates for women's rights; housing rights; and human rights, including disability issues. She is also the New York State coordinator of the Ms. Wheelchair NY program and has written a children's book, *Butterfly on Wheels*.

In the Zoom discussion she and I had in March 2022, Shameka shared her insights on independence, community living, and changes resulting from the pandemic. She talked about her own personal experiences and about disability issues in a more expansive way as a result of her advocacy work.

Shameka said that her own view of independence has developed over the years. She used to think that independence meant doing everything without assistance. She attributed this to a health care and social system in the United States that values independence as measured by doing things by yourself and alone.

Now, though, she believes that people should be able to choose what they do by and for themselves and what they do with assistance. She describes it as knowing that none of us can do everything by ourselves and that the same should hold true for people with disabilities: "You are on this earth, and you are going to need help someday, and that's okay." The important part is knowing when and how to ask for help. Shameka told the story of how she had to be, literally, hit on the head to realize this. Shameka was reaching for something on a high shelf using a broom to extend her reach. The item hit her on the head as it fell from the shelf. It was then that she says she realized it was okay to ask for help.

We talked about how the pandemic changed her shopping habits and how she thinks about that in terms of disability. Like many people, Shameka completed most of her shopping online while staying at home to protect herself and others from COVID-19 transmission. She likes to do her own shopping, however, and has returned to completing many shopping errands on her own. Even when shopping in stores, she often asks for assistance, such as when items are out of her reach. In addition to shopping in stores, Shameka also often shops online. Tied into shopping, she also talked about using public transportation again. The public transport system provides Shameka with the ability to move about in her community independently. For her, independence is not one way or the other; rather, it is a continuum through which she moves under her own control. In speaking with other people with disabilities, Shameka finds that people have found their own balance—from completing errands on their own, using delivery services, or via assistance from others.

(Continued)

CASE EXAMPLE 11.1. Shameka Andrews (*Cont.*)

It seems like her lifelong self-advocacy and advocacy on behalf of others has resulted in a powerful woman who is independent, interdependent, and able to accept assistance when needed and desired. When working with clients, occupational therapy practitioners can facilitate this kind of empowerment during their treatment sessions through collaboration with and respect for client needs and desires. Shameka suggests that practitioners ask questions, listen more, talk less, and build their alignment with their clients.

As of March 2022, Shameka has continued to work from her home office. She is active in social media, is passionate about the lives of people with disabilities, and is a strong advocate for people with disabilities.

Follow Shameka on social media:

- Instagram: instagram.com/disabilityempowered
- Facebook: https://www.facebook.com/ShamekaLAndrews
- LinkedIn: https://www.linkedin.com/in/shameka-andrews-4a010430/
- Self-Advocacy Association of New York State: https://sanys.org/
- Ms. Wheelchair America: https://www.mswheelchairamerica.org/

Right now, most home-based occupational therapy intervention is provided because the person cannot leave to participate in outpatient therapy, because of their own abilities, because of transportation difficulties, or because of inaccessibility in the home. Szanton et al. (2016) demonstrated the effectiveness of home-based care and contended that it may improve older adults' ability to age in place. Imagine how much more effective it would be to work with a very tall client with arthritis and back pain in that person's own kitchen. Instead of suggesting moving things around in the kitchen, the occupational therapy practitioner could actually guide and assist with the reorganization. This might also lead to the practitioner noticing the foot mats in front of the stove top and countertop that might be tripping hazards for this client.

Summary: Independence Reconsidered

This chapter reflects a concerted effort to consider people with disabilities as knowledgeable about their conditions, needs, preferences, and goals. Occupational therapy practitioners can support their clients by developing close relationships and being open to individual definitions of independence, while considering interdependence and avoiding ableism.

When that respect and professional, therapeutic relationship is present, the team of occupational therapy practitioner and client can focus on occupations, personal factors, and contexts to meet the clients' goals. Case Example 11.1 gives a client's perspective on independence.

References

American Occupational Therapy Association. (2020). Occupational therapy practice framework: Domain and process (4th ed.). *American Journal of Occupational Therapy, 74*(Suppl. 2), 7412410010. https//doi.org/10.5014/ajot.2020.74S2001

Bourke, J. A. (2021). The lived experience of interdependence: Support worker relationships and implications for wider rehabilitation. *Brain Impairment,* 1–7. https://doi.org/10.1017/BrImp.2021.24

BTS Bioengineering. (n.d.). *Nirvana.* https://www.btsbioengineering.com/project/nirvana/

Campbell, F. A. K. (2001). Disability's date with ontology and the ableist body of law. *Griffith Law Review, 10*(1), 42–62.

De Luca, R., Maggio, M. G., Maresca, G., Latella, D., Cannavo, A., Sciarrone, F., . . . Calabro, R. S. (2019). Improving cognitive function after traumatic brain injury: A clinical trial on the potential use of the semi-immersive virtual reality. *Behavioural Neurology, 2019,* Article 9268179. https://doi.org/10.1155/2019/9268179

Dodds, T. A., Martin, D. P., Stolov, W. C., & Deyo, R. A. (1993). A validation of the functional independence measurement and its performance among rehabilitation patients. *Archives of Physical Medicine and Rehabilitation, 74*(5), 532–536. https://doi.org/10.1016/0003-9993(93)90119-U

Dunn, W. (1999). *The sensory profile.* Pearson.

Enemark Larsen, A., Rasmussen, B., & Christensen, J. R. (2018). Enhancing a client-centred practice with the Canadian Occupational Performance Measure. *Occupational Therapy International, 2018,* Article 5956301. https://doi.org/10.1155/2018/5956301

Fuchs, L. S., Powell, S. R., Cirino, P. T., Schumacher, R. F., Marrin, S., Hamlett, . . . Changas, P. C. (2014). Does calculation or word-problem instruction provide a stronger route to prealgebraic knowledge? *Journal of Educational Psychology, 106*(4), 990–1006, https://doi.org/10.1037/a0036793

Grigorenko, E. L., Compton, D. L., Fuchs, L. S., Wagner, R. K., Willcutt, E. G., & Fletcher, J. M. (2020). Understanding, educating, and supporting children with specific learning disabilities: 50 years of science and practice. *American Psychologist, 75*(1), 37–51. https://doi.org/10.1037/amp0000452

Guney Yilmaz, G., & Onal, G. (2021). The effectiveness of telerehabilitation-based occupational therapy interventions on sensory processing and functional independence in the COVID-19 pandemic: A case series. *International Journal of Disabilities Sports and Health Sciences, 4*(2), 160–165. https://doi.org/10.33438/ijdshs.1008690

Heung, K. H. L., Tang, Z. Q., Ho, L., Tung, M., Li, Z., & Tong, R. K. Y. (2019). Design of a 3D printed soft robotic hand for stroke rehabilitation and daily activities assistance. *2019 IEEE 16th International*

Conference on Rehabilitation Robotics (ICORR), 65–70. https://doi.org/10.1109/ICORR.2019.8779449

Jiralerspong, T., Heung, K. H. L., Tong, R. K. Y., & Li, Z. (2018). A novel soft robotic glove for daily life assistance. *2018 7th IEEE International Conference on Biomedical Robotics and Biomechatronics (Biorob)*, 671–676. https://doi.org/10.1109/BIOROB.2018.8488060

Lewis, T. A. (2022, January 1). Working definition of ableism—January 2022 update. *Talila A Lewis*. https://www.talilalewis.com/blog

Mathes, P. G., Denton, C. A., Fletcher, J. M., Anthony, J. L., Francis, D. J., & Schatschneider, C. (2005). The effects of theoretically different instruction and student characteristics on the skills of struggling readers. *Reading Research Quarterly, 40*(2), 148–182. https://doi.org/10.1598/RRQ.40.2.2

Merriam-Webster. (n.d.-a). Ameliorate. In *Merriam-Webster.com dictionary*. https://www.merriam-webster.com/dictionary/ameliorate

Merriam-Webster. (n.d.-b). Independent. In *Merriam-Webster.com dictionary*. https://www.merriam-webster.com/dictionary/independent

Merriam-Webster. (n.d.-c). Interdependence. In *Merriam-Webster.com dictionary*. https://www.merriam-webster.com/dictionary/interdependence

Merriam-Webster. (n.d.-d). Simulation. In *Merriam-Webster.com dictionary*. https://www.merriam-webster.com/dictionary/simulation

Norouzi-Gheidari, N., Hernandez, A., Archambault, P. S., Higgins, J., Poissant, L., & Kairy, D. (2020). Feasibility, safety and efficacy of a virtual reality exergame system to supplement upper extremity rehabilitation post-stroke: A pilot randomized clinical trial and proof of principle. *International Journal of Environmental Research and Public Health, 17*(1), Article 113. https://doi.org/10.3390/ijerph17010113

Ottenbacher, K. J., Taylor, E. T., Msall, M. E., Braun, S., Lane, S. J., Granger, C. V., . . . Duffy, L. C. (1996). The stability and equivalence reliability of the Functional Independence Measure for Children (WeeFIM)®. *Developmental Medicine & Child Neurology, 38*(10), 907–916. https://doi.org/10.1111/j.1469-8749.1996.tb15047.x

Szanton, S. L., Leff, B., Wolff, J. L., Roberts, L., & Gitlin, L. N. (2016). Home-based cared program reduces disability and promotes aging in place. *Health Affairs, 35*(9), 1558–1563. https://doi.org/10.1377/hlthaff.2016.0140

Torpil, B., & Kaya, O. (2022). Effectiveness of client-centered intervention delivered with face-to-face and telerehabilitation method after total knee arthroplasty: A pilot randomized control trial. *British Journal of Occupational Therapy, 85*(6), 392–399. https://doi.org/10.1177/03080226211070477

Uniform Data System for Medical Rehabilitation. (1997). *FIM clinical guide, version 5.01.* State University of New York at Buffalo.

Uniform Data System for Medical Rehabilitation. (2004). *WeeFIM II®*. State University of New York at Buffalo.

United Nations. (2006). *Convention on the Rights of Persons with Disabilities.* https://treaties.un.org/Pages/ViewDetails.aspx?src=TREATY&mtdsg_no=IV-15&chapter=4&clang=_en

World Health Organization. (2001). *International classification of functioning, disability and health.* Author.

Yap, H. K., Khin, P. M., Koh, T. H., Sun, Y., Liang, X., Lim, J. H., & Yeow, C.-H. (2017). A fully fabric-based bidirectional soft robotic glove for assistance and rehabilitation of hand impaired patients. *IEEE Robotics and Automation Letters, 2*(3), 1383–1390. https://doi.org/10.1109/LRA.2017.2669366

12

Self-Care Occupations

TSU-HSIN HOWE, PhD, OTR, FAOTA,
AND ANITA PERR, PhD, OT/L, FAOTA

CHAPTER HIGHLIGHTS

- What are self-care occupations?
- Contextual factors
- Self-care evaluation
- Self-care intervention
- Group versus individual treatment

KEY TERMS AND CONCEPTS

• acquisitional frames of reference • activity • activity limitation • adaptation/compensation approach • attitudinal settings • BADLs • behavior theory • body functions • body structures • compensatory frame of reference • context • disability • dynamic theory • environmental factors • functioning • habit training approach • IADLs • impairment • learning theories • occupations • participation • participation restriction • personal factors • physical settings • self-care occupations • self-determination theory • social settings

Introduction

This chapter defines and describes self-care occupations and their categories, including basic activities of daily living (BADLs) and instrumental activities of daily living (IADLs), as well as their relationship to occupations. It also explains how BADLs and IADLs are evaluated in the context of occupations.

Because self-care occupations make up a large part of everyone's life, the occupational therapy practitioner's focus on a person's ability to engage in self-care occupations is vitally important. Self-care occupations are fundamental to human existence and affect people's ability to function. By addressing self-care with clients, practitioners shape the daily lives of those they serve. In this chapter, the terms used to organize the discussion of self-care are adopted from the *Occupational Therapy Practice Framework: Domain and Process* (4th ed.; *OTPF-4;* American Occupational Therapy Association [AOTA], 2020) and the *International Classification of Functioning, Disability and Health* (*ICF;* World Health Organization [WHO], 2001).

First, the importance of self-care on the individual level is discussed, and then the factors that influence the efficacy of self-care are examined. Elements that influence participation in self-care include client factors (i.e., values, beliefs, body function and structure), contexts (i.e., environmental and personal factors), performance patterns, and performance skills.

The chapter provides a framework for occupational therapy practitioners to organize a self-care evaluation and design appropriate interventions for a person who has difficulty with self-care. It emphasizes the importance of addressing a person's self-care occupations when evaluating and designing interventions related to BADLs and IADLs.

Case examples (for Aisha and Jon) throughout the chapter demonstrate factors that need to be considered during self-care evaluations and interventions. The case examples also explain how a person's values, priorities, and preferences are taken into consideration during these processes. Aisha and Jon lead very different lives and have distinctive patterns of daily living, interests, values, and needs. Their occupational profiles describe various aspects of self-care that practitioners can address.

What Are Self-Care Occupations?

In this chapter, ***self-care occupations*** are defined as everyday life activities that people do to take care of themselves. BADLs and IADLs are discussed in the context of occupation. ***BADLs*** are activities oriented toward taking care of one's own body and are completed on a routine basis (e.g., bathing, dressing, eating, grooming, toileting; see Exhibit 12.1). ***IADLs*** are activities to support daily life in the home and community (AOTA, 2020). Examples of IADLs are care of others, community mobility, financial management, meal preparation, safety and emergency maintenance, and shopping (Exhibit 12.2).

Occupations are "the everyday activities that people do as individuals, in families, and with communities to occupy time and bring meaning and purpose to life" (AOTA, 2020, p. 30). Moreover, in the *OTPF–4, occupation* denotes personalized and meaningful engagement in daily life events by a specific client. Thus, occupations are unique to everyone, providing personal satisfaction and fulfillment as a result of engaging in them (AOTA, 2020). Therefore, this chapter includes personal values, preferences, and priorities in the examination of a client's abilities to perform BADLs and IADLs.

EXHIBIT 12.1. Basic Activities of Daily Living

- Bathing and showering
- Toileting and toilet hygiene
- Dressing
- Eating and swallowing
- Feeding
- Functional mobility
- Personal hygiene and grooming
- Sexual activity

Source. American Occupational Therapy Association (2020, p. 30).

EXHIBIT 12.2. Instrumental Activities of Daily Living

- Care of others (including selecting and supervising caregivers)
- Care of pets and animals
- Child rearing
- Communication management
- Driving and community mobility
- Financial management
- Home establishment and management
- Meal preparation and cleanup
- Religious and spiritual expression
- Safety and emergency maintenance
- Shopping

Source. American Occupational Therapy Association (2020, pp. 30–31).

Self-care occupations are fundamental to human existence and affect people's ability to function. Providing interventions to improve a person's self-care occupations has always been an important part of occupational therapy practice. By addressing self-care occupations with clients, occupational therapy practitioners contribute to improving clients' quality of life. The terms and emphasis of these interventions, however, have shifted over time as populations and the needs of society have changed and various occupational therapy interventions have gone into and out of vogue.

Early in the profession's history, intervention focused on the mechanics of daily activities. That is, practitioners focused on the acquisition of specific skills. Theoretical rationales and explanations were not used at that time, and interventions were developed and carried out through trial and error. For example, practitioners developed various strategies to establish daily routine skills, as evidenced by Eleanor Clarke Slagle's ***habit training approach,*** which introduces routines to help individuals learn skills to be productive and maintain a balanced daily schedule. During World Wars I and II, interventions became more oriented toward adaptation because of the influence of the medical model and the increasing number of wounded veterans returning home. In the 1980s, the compensatory frame of reference embraced the use of environmental adaptation, adaptive equipment, and alternative strategies to promote a person's level of independence. Today, the profession has a renewed emphasis on the importance of ADLs and has added new meanings to the term.

To explain this further, the importance and scope of ADLs are identified in both the *OTPF–4* (AOTA, 2020) and the *ICF* (WHO, 2001). During the evaluation and intervention process, occupational therapy practitioners consider not only a client's activity performance but also the surrounding context and its impact on self-care occupations. In other words, occupational therapy practitioners include the client's experience and physical and social contexts when they perform evaluations of and develop interventions for self-care occupations.

A person's specific routines vary by age, culture, ethnicity, gender, and many other factors. Occupational therapy practitioners should address these differences, or preferences, when planning and implementing interventions. Case Example 12.1, Part 1, and Case Example 12.2, Part 1, describe the self-care activities that are important to two occupational therapy clients, Aisha and Jon.

As the field of occupational therapy further explores the definitions of *occupation, activity,* and *task,* it makes sense to think about ADLs in terms of these definitions. At the most basic level, the category of self-care can be considered the occupation. If occupation can be thought of as a collection of activities, then the various components of self-care can be considered activities. In this paradigm, examples of activities are

CASE EXAMPLE 12.1. Part 1. Aisha: Important Self-Care Activities

Aisha is a 45-year-old woman who underwent surgery to repair a brain aneurysm. During the surgery, the aneurysm ruptured, resulting in a hemorrhagic stroke. Aisha's right upper extremity is paralyzed with a flaccid tone. Aisha is right-hand dominant. Although the right lower extremity has some areas of abnormal tone and weakness, she can ambulate for about 10 feet on level surfaces without using an ambulation aid, such as a cane. She also has slight memory impairment and limited memory and problem-solving skills.

Upon meeting Aisha, her occupational therapist is struck by her precise dressing and grooming. Aisha reports that it is important that she look well put together. Before her stroke, she wore her hair in long braids, which she braided herself. She jogged 1 to 3 miles at least 3 times a week. She showered each morning before leaving for work. An important occupation was cooking, during which she attended to nutritional advice and enjoyed the challenges of preparing dinner for others.

CASE EXAMPLE 12.2. Part 1. Jon: Important Self-Care Activities

Jon is a 16-year-old Asian American boy who broke his right arm while skateboarding. He has compound fractures of the humerus (midshaft) and of the ulna and radius. An external fixator is in place at the humerus. Internal fixators, plates, and screws are in place in the forearm. Jon is right-hand dominant.

Jon is a social teenager who spends a great deal of time getting ready to go out with friends. He wants to look and dress the part, just like his friends and their role models, who are mainly hip-hop artists. Jon reports that since breaking his arm, he has great difficulty putting gel in his hair and getting it to look the way he wants. Before the injury, Jon showered at school after his gym class 3 times weekly. During his evaluation, Jon revealed that he is uncomfortable dressing and undressing after gym class (both before and since his accident). He worked out about 4 times a week before the accident, primarily lifting weights and working to improve his physique. Regardless of his effort, he still perceives himself as scrawny. He does not want his classmates to see that he is skinny. He thinks he looks like a little kid and does not understand why he is not bulking up like most of the other teens he is friendly with.

Jon has no interest in cooking or preparing meals. His mother prepares meals at home for the whole family. Jon buys lunch in his school cafeteria and says he really does not care about nutrition. He eats pizza for lunch on a nearly daily basis.

combing hair, brushing teeth, toileting, eating, and expressing sexuality.

The way each person puts the activities of self-care together becomes the occupation and is grounded in personal meanings. Continuing the paradigm, if brushing teeth is the activity, then opening the toothpaste cap, putting toothpaste on the toothbrush, brushing the teeth, and rinsing the mouth are the tasks.

Contextual Factors

Everything takes place within a ***context,*** which is the setting in which an event occurs. Changing the context changes the ways the activity is performed. Context includes environmental factors and personal factors. ***Environmental factors*** are aspects of the physical, social, and attitudinal surroundings in which people live and conduct their lives. Examples of environmental factors include animate and inanimate elements of the natural or physical environment, products and technology, physical or emotional support, attitude, service, and policy (AOTA, 2020). ***Personal factors*** are the particular background of a person's life and living. They consist of the unique features of the person that are not part of a health condition or health state (WHO, 2001). These factors may include age, sexual orientation, gender identity, race and ethnicity, social background, upbringing and life experiences, past and current behavioral patterns, individual psychological assets, education, and profession and professional identity (AOTA, 2020). Personal factors are reported to have the potential to determine functioning and disability outcomes (e.g., participation in work or communication; Geyh et al., 2011).

Contextual factors need to be identified during the ADL evaluation and included during the intervention. Note that for people with disabilities, the impact of contextual factors may be magnified compared with their impact on people without disabilities. Occupational therapy practitioners need to keep in mind that for people to truly achieve full participation, meaning, and purpose, they must not only function but also engage comfortably in their own distinct combination of contexts (AOTA, 2020).

Contextual factors can be facilitators that help people perform an activity, and they can also be barriers that limit or prevent performance. For example, for a person with limited hand grip, long, lever-style door handles can facilitate performance because the person can open the door just by pushing down the handle. The design of the door handles facilitates easier access to the room. Some contextual factors, however, are barriers that restrict or prevent performance. Imagine the same person living in an apartment with knob-shaped door handles. Here, the person is unable to open the doors and needs help, making the design of the door a barrier to performance. These examples show that contextual factors affect people's ability to participate. By understanding each client's contextual factors, occupational therapy practitioners are better able to prioritize treatment and determine what is important for each client.

Environmental Factors

Environmental factors include physical, social, and attitudinal settings. ***Physical settings*** include the natural or human-made products or systems of products, equipment, and technology in a person's immediate environment. ***Social settings*** include support and relationships that a person has in their own environment. These supports may be physical or emotional in nature. A person may seek support, nurturing, protection, and assistance from others or pets. A person may establish relationships with other people at home, work, or school or during play (Schneidert et al., 2003). ***Attitudinal settings*** are the observable consequences of customs, practices, ideologies, values, norms, and religious beliefs. After reading Case Example 12.1, Part 2, and Case Example 12.2, Part 2, readers can list these factors as noted by each client's occupational therapist.

During intervention, occupational therapy practitioners use environmental facilitators to improve participation in self-care occupations and address environmental barriers to alleviate or lessen their effect. For example, the height of the cabinet shelves could be an environmental barrier for a man in a wheelchair because he cannot reach his kitchen items. A seat-elevating feature for his wheelchair would allow him to easily reach his kitchen items (see Figure 12.1).

Personal Factors

Personal factors are the particular background of a person's life and living and consist of the features of the person that are not part of a health condition or health state. They include age,

CASE EXAMPLE 12.1. Part 2. Physical, Social, and Attitudinal Settings for Aisha

Physical

Aisha lives in a studio apartment in an urban East Coast city. The apartment is on the second floor, up a flight of 18 steps. The building has no elevator. Aisha sleeps on a waterbed that is against the wall at the head and left side. She has a small closet where she keeps the current season's clothing and outerwear. She also has a small dresser for undergarments. Aisha's bathroom is very small (5 ft × 8 ft). The only storage space she has in the bathroom is a small medicine cabinet over the sink. She has a clawfoot tub with a shower extension attached to the tub spout.

Social

Aisha is engaged and planning to be married about 6 months after her surgery. She has no immediate or extended family nearby except for her fiancé, Tony. Aisha has four or five close friends with whom she spoke or spent time about 5 times a week before her stroke. Since then, they have visited her regularly in the hospital, and it is expected that they will remain supportive and be available to help Aisha. Aisha is very pleasant, and somewhat quiet. She has many acquaintances at work, her gym, and church. Aisha does not have pets. Before the aneurysm, Aisha had never had any medical problems. She goes for a physical checkup annually.

Attitudinal

Aisha values her social and economic independence. Although she is in love with Tony, they both plan to continue to spend time with their own friends and pursue their own interests in addition to building new friendships and developing new pursuits together. Aisha belongs to a church in her neighborhood. She attends services regularly and participates in other church activities. She met Tony during a fund raising activity sponsored by the church. Aisha enjoys yoga and meditation and is learning about Eastern religions. She celebrates her African heritage, celebrates Kwanzaa, and plans to jump the broom at her wedding.

CASE EXAMPLE 12.2. Part 2. Physical, Social, and Attitudinal Settings for Jon

Physical

Jon lives in the suburbs, about 2 hours from the city in which Aisha lives. He lives in a two-story, four-bedroom house in which all the bedrooms are on the second floor. Jon shares a bedroom with his 14-year-old brother. He sleeps on the bottom bunk of a set of bunk beds. Jon keeps his clothes folded in dresser drawers or hung on hooks or hangers in a closet, but he reports that his room is usually messy, and he usually puts the clothes he wears on the floor or on a chair. The bathroom Jon most frequently uses for his morning routine is shared with his three siblings and has a stall shower. As previously stated, Jon usually showers at school and says it is because if he showers at home, his siblings might not have enough hot water.

Social

Jon lives with his parents and three brothers. His extended family lives in nearby states and in Taiwan. The family in the area gets together regularly. He has cousins with whom he is very friendly. Jon has a group of about 15 close friends from school. None of these boys live near Jon because the catchment area for the school is large. Jon has one neighborhood friend, a boy who lives next door and who is about 2 years younger than Jon. His school friends do not know about his neighborhood friend because Jon is afraid his friends will tease him for being friends with a younger boy.

Attitudinal

Jon's family believes in Buddhism, but they only go to temple on special occasions. His family is generally conservative in their political views. Jon views his family as too traditional and boring. He says that they are sometimes worried about him because he is the "wild" one in the family. Jon and his friends tend to use curse words when they are with each other, but Jon does not curse when he thinks his family members might hear him. Jon's family places a high value on education and believes that effort, rather than innate ability, is the key to success. They expect him to go to college after graduating from high school.

EXERCISE 12.1. Think About Environmental Factors

In the profiles for Aisha and Jon, what are the physical, social, and attitudinal facilitators of and barriers to participation in daily activities? Think about your own life. What are the environmental facilitators and barriers? How do you use the facilitators? How do you deal with the barriers?

gender, social status, life experiences, and so on. It is easy to see that the daily activities of a 3-year-old differ from those of a teenager, which differ from those of an adult, which further differ from those of an older adult.

Young children may be focusing on learning to dress themselves. Their parents may let them wear clothing with an elastic waist or shoes with hook-and-loop closures to minimize hand manipulation and encourage early independence. Most teens have mastered grooming and dressing and focus on conforming to their peer group. Teens may also be more focused on other activities, such as learning to drive or shopping. Gender-specific and sexual activities are also important activities and occupations for teenagers. Sexual activity, an often-ignored daily life activity, is extremely important for people during the developmental stages of adolescence, young adulthood, and adulthood. Once in the adult stage, the focus of daily activities may shift further toward IADLs, such as care for others and budgeting. The nature and performance of IADLs change with aging (Ishizaki et al., 2000; Tabira et al., 2020). Older adults may carry out their IADLs differently because of changes in their physical or cognitive status or their environment. For example, depending on the nature of their residence, they may have to drive to a mall for grocery shopping if they live in a suburban home. After their children move out, they may choose to move to an urban dwelling where stores are within walking distance or offer delivery services. Case Example 12.1, Part 3, and Case Example 12.2, Part 3, discuss personal factors for each client.

In the *ICF*, ***functioning*** "is an umbrella term encompassing all body functions and structure, activities and participation. Similarly, ***disability*** serves as an umbrella term for impairments, activity limitations or participation restrictions" (WHO, 2001, p. 3, bold and italics added). ***Body functions*** include physiological and psychological actions of body systems, whereas ***body structures*** describe anatomical parts of the body such as organs, limbs, and their components. ***Impairment*** is a problem in body functions or structures. ***Activity*** and ***participation*** describe a person's performance at the

FIGURE 12.1. **A seat-elevating wheelchair allows this man to reach items in his kitchen cabinet.**

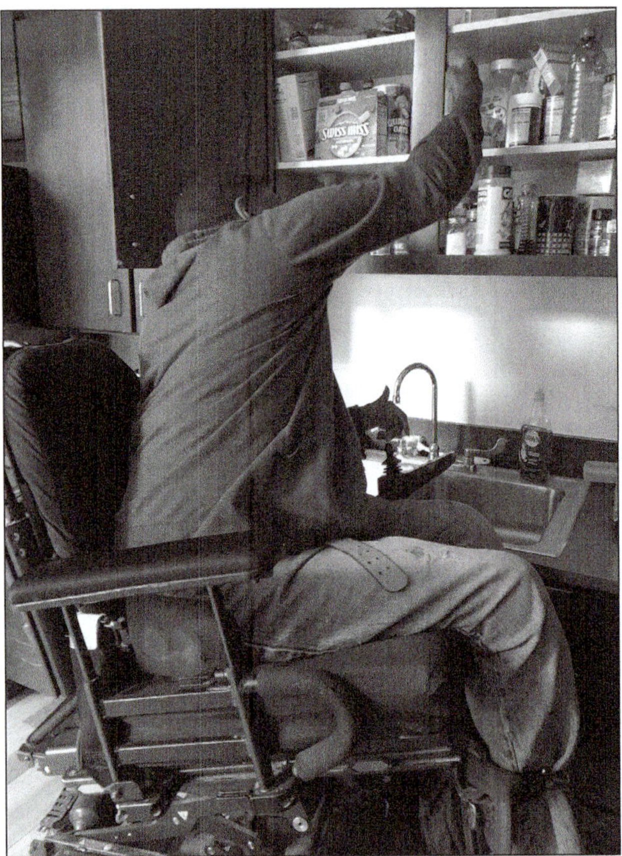

Source. A. Perr. Used with permission.

person or societal level. ***Activity limitation*** is a difficulty at the person level. ***Participation restriction*** refers to societal-level impediment. Case Example 12.1, Part 4, and Case Example 12.2, Part 4, describe body structure and function factors for Aisha and Jon.

According to the *ICF,* functioning and disability are the outcomes of the interaction between health conditions and contextual factors (environmental and personal). When a person's interactions result in their functioning at a less-than-optimal level, the person is experiencing a disability or is disabled (Schneidert et al., 2003).

The term *disability* applies in cases in which a person has problems at different or combined levels. A person can have a problem only at the body level (an impairment) but no activity limitation or participation restrictions; have problems at all three levels of functioning, that is, body (impairments), person (activity limitation), and society (participation restrictions); or have an impairment and activity limitation but no participation restriction; and so forth.

For example, a fourth-finger amputation on the nondominant hand (impairment) may not have any influence on a person's participation at the personal level (no activity limitation) or societal level (no participation restrictions). However, a person who has a double below-knee amputation (impairment) can perform all dressing, bathing, and grooming independently (no activity limitation) but may have difficulty navigating in their community (participation restrictions).

Self-Care Evaluation

Occupational therapists must complete a thorough evaluation to develop an appropriate intervention plan. A comprehensive evaluation identifies areas of limited participation. Moreover, it identifies how the impairments limit participation. Therapists usually complete an evaluation in the following sequence. They begin the evaluation with an assessment of the client's potential capacity, functional status, and actual abilities. In this part of the evaluation, therapists assess a client's physical, psychological, sensory, perceptual, and cognitive functions. After therapists have a general understanding of the client's baseline, they conduct a thorough assessment of the client's performance of BADLs. If appropriate, they also assess

CASE EXAMPLE 12.1. Part 3. Personal Factors for Aisha

At age 45 years, **Aisha** cannot believe that she is middle aged, does not like to think about it, and does not want to think about getting older. She is African-American and grew up in a small southern town. She has lived on her own since high school. She earned an undergraduate degree and a Master of Business Administration degree from a prestigious New England university. Her fiancé, Tony, is Brazilian and not yet a U.S. citizen. The couple has been together for 3 years.

Aisha says that before her stroke, their love life was healthy, and they had sex regularly. She says that she liked to experiment a little more than Tony does. Since the stroke, Tony is still caring and compassionate, and they have talked about resuming sexual intimacy. Aisha currently works for a small business that imports gift items from Africa. She loves to travel and has many responsibilities at work that require her to travel to West Africa. She is somewhat concerned about how she will be able to travel once she returns to work.

CASE EXAMPLE 12.2. Part 3. Personal Factors for Jon

Jon is a high school student, and his grade point average is 2.42. He and his male friends often skip school. He has lived his entire life in the same house. He has slept over at friends' houses but not for more than a night. Jon does not have a girlfriend and is extremely hesitant to talk about close personal relationships. Jon says that he is not sexually active. He denies the use of drugs and alcohol.

CASE EXAMPLE 12.1. Part 4. Body Structure and Function Factors for Aisha

Body structure

Aisha had a left parietal lobe infarct during a planned surgery to clip an aneurysm. She presents with decreased trunk control and extremely low tone in the right arm. She has decreased movement in her right leg, but in comparison with her right arm, the tone change is less significant.

Body function

Since the stroke, Aisha has become quieter and now perceives herself as shy. She does not know how people will react to her new medical condition and is concerned about whether she will be able to follow conversations and understand their nuances. She is somewhat downhearted about her condition and her impending wedding. Her motivation fluctuates from day to day. She tends to be sleepy most of the time and cannot tell whether it is a side effect of her medication, a side effect of the stroke, or her feelings of low energy. She says she just feels "crummy." She has mild memory deficits and has some trouble carrying out complex activities that require planning, organizing, problem solving, and decision making. Her sensory functions are intact. Aisha has a mild gait and balance impairment and mild to moderate impairment in endurance.

CASE EXAMPLE 12.2. Part 4. Part 4. Body Structure and Function Factors for Jon

Body structure

Jon experienced multiple fractures in his right arm and has an external fixator in place for 5 to 7 weeks. He also uses a sling and a bolster to support his arm when standing. Jon's arm should also be raised and supported when he is seated, but he says that he is not usually able to do this. Open wounds exist at the pin sites where the external fixator protrudes from his arm.

Body function

Jon's mental and sensory functions are intact and age appropriate.

specific IADLs applicable to the client. The evaluation process should be contextual and client specific, focusing on the daily living skills identified by the client. That is, therapists should listen to the client and to what the client needs to do, wants to do, or expects to do (Law, 1993).

Occupational therapists gather information about self-care occupations through self-report, proxy report, direct observation of behavior in settings in which clients live, and performance-based measures that use tasks in clinical settings. Each of these methods has strengths and weaknesses. A consensus in the literature stresses the need to apply both self-report and observation methods because both assess different but complementary aspects of ADL ability (Decker et al., 2017; Nielsen & Wæhrens, 2014).

Occupational therapists obtain the most reliable information when the client performs an activity in their usual or natural environment. Therapists who work in home-based practice have the advantage of using the client's own environment and materials during evaluations and when developing interventions. However, because most evaluations and interventions occur in a clinic or hospital setting, an alternative is to have the client perform the activity in a closely simulated environment using their real tools, such as their own clothing or toothbrush. Care should be taken to bring as much of the real-life environment into the evaluation and intervention context as possible, including considering the client's values and beliefs and their roles and responsibilities.

A person's performance of self-care occupations is a major predictor of their dependence, morbidity, mortality (Millán-Calenti et al., 2010), and quality of life (Andersen et al., 2004). Estimating the number and characteristics of self-care occupations performed by an occupational therapy client is important because an increasing number of third-party payers rely on these measures to determine whether a person qualifies for service coverage. Depending on the purpose of the evaluation, therapists should choose a standardized assessment with adequate psychometric properties and supplement it with a nonstandardized assessment of salient characteristics of client's activity performance either observed by the therapists or obtained through client or caregiver descriptions (James & Pitonyak, 2019). Regardless of the nature of the assessment, it should include information about BADLs, IADLs, and mobility (see Exhibits 12.1 and 12.2), and the tasks selected for assessment should be consistent with clients' needs and priorities.

Semantic and numeric rating methods can be used to describe self-care performance. For example, terms such as *independent, moderate assistance,* and *dependent* are used to rate the amount of assistance a client needs during self-care. The *ICF* uses qualifiers such as *no problem, mild problem, moderate problem, severe problem,* and *complete problem* to rank the level of difficulty that a person encounters when performing self-care (WHO, 2001). A numeric scale, such as one ranging from 1 to 7, is also used in some circumstances to delineate levels of independence. The occupational therapist can use any type of rating scale as long as the measures are identified and each level is clearly defined. The measures should also make sense for the clients being evaluated and for the environment in which they are evaluated.

At times, occupational therapists may rely on reports from the client, the client's family, and others involved in the client's care. Using these methods of self-report or proxy report, therapists gain more understanding of clients' perceived physical competence and learn the coping strategies used in daily activities. These methods, used in conjunction with other evaluation methods, provide a more comprehensive view of the client.

EXERCISE 12.2. Evaluation

Before moving on to intervention, think about Aisha and Jon and perform an imaginary evaluation with them. What areas of self-care are going to be limited? What are the causes of the limitations? Are they body structures? Body functions? Environmental factors? Personal factors?

Self-Care Intervention

Occupational therapy practitioners provide intervention to improve a client's ability to participate in activities; in this case, self-care. Areas of disability should be addressed during goal setting before implementing interventions. Interventions are developed to remedy impairments in body structures and body functions, to maximize the facilitation of contextual factors, and to eliminate or lessen barriers. The ultimate goal of intervention is to enhance clients' participation in self-care occupations. The evaluation will help to identify the problem areas. Once an occupational therapist completes the evaluation, the next step is to identify priorities, because it may be impossible to address everything simultaneously. Setting priorities helps the therapist and client focus on the most critical areas to target first.

Client preferences should strongly influence the priorities for intervention, but safety is more important than client preference. Although safety is often the client's highest priority, the client may sometimes put themselves at risk because they are unable to recognize or they underestimate their own physical or cognitive deficits. The prevalence of falls among community-dwelling older adults, for instance, may be caused in part by an inability to recognize environmental hazards (Gell et al., 2020). A client with a spinal cord injury may express a strong desire to learn to propel their wheelchair and identify it as the first goal they want to work on. The occupational therapy practitioner, however, recognizes that because of the impairments to body structures, the client cannot reach and use the emergency call bell in the hospital room. Being able to use the call system to alert a nurse that help is needed is the first safety priority for all patients. Thus, it should be the first ADL task addressed with all hospitalized patients. The practitioner and the client should have candid, honest discussions when collaborating on identifying and prioritizing goals.

After completing Exercise 12.3, recall whether you identified toileting as a priority. What are the limitations that

EXERCISE 12.3. Priorities of Self-Care for Aisha and Jon

What are the self-care priorities for Aisha and Jon? Are there safety concerns? First, list as many problems as you can, considering Aisha's and Jon's conditions. Then put the list in order of priority. Examine your list and think about why you set the priorities as you did and what rationales support your decision. To do this, use your imagination to fill out the occupational profiles for these individuals. For this exercise, it is fine to fill in the blanks regarding Aisha's and Jon's values, priorities, and interests as you develop your rationales for setting priorities. When working with clients, you should ensure that rationales reflect the client's priorities and input.

CASE EXAMPLE 12.1. Part 4. Part 5. Aisha's Priorities

Aisha is having a difficult time dealing with the changes she is experiencing. The stress of her upcoming wedding and the possibility that she may still have residual disabilities at that time sometimes overwhelm her. Through conversation, Aisha and the occupational therapist decide that her depression must be addressed immediately, and intervention strategies specific to depression must be incorporated into every activity they work on.

Other priorities Aisha identifies are learning to hold objects in both hands when walking (she wants to be able to carry her bouquet as she walks down the aisle without losing her balance) and being able to dress, bathe, and groom herself so she does not have to rely on others for help. Improving her ability to complete self-care activities independently is especially important to her because she knows how particular she is, and she thinks others will be bothered by her idiosyncrasies.

Moreover, Aisha prefers not to change the type of clothing she likes to wear. Therefore, instead of wearing sweatpants with an elastic waist, she learns to use a button aid and zipper pull to fasten her pants after toileting. She is also thinking about what her priorities are for her job and realizes that working on these tasks will be useful in her job as well.

CASE EXAMPLE 12.2. Part 5. Jon's Priorities

Jon identifies being able to put gel in his hair as his priority. However, the therapist knows that one ADL task that must be addressed is cleaning the pin sites on Jon's arm. If these sites are not kept clean, infections can develop, which would slow recovery and perhaps lead to further disability. The therapist is not sure whether Jon is mature enough to realize the threat of infection, so one of the first things the therapist does is to discuss this potential problem with Jon and his parents, emphasizing the importance of wound care in healing. Jon agrees to make wound care a top priority, which includes washing and drying his right arm, caring for the sling and bolster, and addressing issues of positioning in sitting and standing.

The occupational therapist then discusses toileting with Jon. Jon is embarrassed and admits he does not use the bathroom at school because it is too difficult for him. However, after discussing it with the therapist, Jon agrees that working on toileting is a higher priority than hair care.

Jon's therapist asks about the pants he likes to wear, and Jon decides to put away his button-fly jeans until his arm heals. He chooses to wear sweatpants or loose-fit zipper-fly jeans rather than use an alternative technique such as a button aid or other adaptive device to help with buttoning. Jon is so happy with his decision that he initiates switching to boxer shorts because briefs are too difficult for him to manage with one hand. If the therapist had not addressed toileting, Jon might not have developed compensatory strategies for this activity.

affect both Aisha's and Jon's ability to use a bathroom independently? Read Case Example 12.1, Part 5, and Case Example 12.2, Part 5, and compare your list from the exercise with the priorities in the case examples.

In the case examples, note how communication between the client and the occupational therapist can lead to mutually agreed-upon goals and priorities. For example, applying hair gel remains a priority for Jon, but both Jon and the therapist agree that they should address wound care and toileting first. In these situations, it is also important for the occupational therapy practitioner to emphasize the connection between improvement in one area and improvement in other areas. For instance, the therapist explains to Jon that working on wound care and toileting would lead to Jon's ability to apply hair gel more easily because both tasks involve improving Jon's coordination using his nondominant hand.

Occupational therapy practitioners may use several theory-based approaches to help clients choose priorities and make decisions about how to implement intervention. ***Acquisitional frames of reference,*** those frames of reference that are based on a teaching–learning approach, are the favored approach of many occupational therapy practitioners. The theoretical base for these approaches is often not only drawn from teaching and learning theories but also considers performance in the context of ***self-determination theory.*** These acquisitional frames of reference share the theoretical postulates that learning and performance can be enabled by the provision of appropriate learning support, and demonstration, practice, repetition, and positive reinforcement are essential elements of increasing the client's competence in and mastery of tasks (Deci & Ryan, 1985, 2008).

In this situation, the occupational therapy practitioner begins by using an acquisitional frame of reference that combines principles of learning and self-determination (Greber et al., 2013). It involves promoting a person's self-initiation in identifying their learning needs, formulating learning goals, choosing and implementing appropriate learning strategies, and evaluating learning outcomes. This approach was used when the therapist and Jon were deciding between using a button aid or wearing sweatpants. The therapist did not tell Jon that buttons would be too difficult; instead, she suggested that many other clients have found that wearing sweatpants is more manageable and comfortable. This approach allowed Jon to make the final decision and increased his sense of competence and control.

The ***adaptation/compensation approach*** to improve occupational performance (Gillen, 2019) involves the practitioner providing the client with various adaptive devices or compensatory strategies to complete a task. For example, Aisha was given the opportunity to decide which button aid and zipper pull she felt comfortable using. Once she made the decision, the therapist used an acquisitional frame of reference to teach her how to use the devices.

Activities are rarely addressed individually. Most activities occur in combinations. For instance, although one focus for Aisha and Jon was toileting, dressing also had to be addressed. This example illustrates a common occurrence in occupational therapy practice settings: Single treatment sessions frequently address multiple problem areas and multiple goals.

Where to Start Intervention

The client's goals guide the intervention. These goals should be established through a collaborative process between the client and occupational therapy practitioner that is based on a synthesis of the evaluation and client's preference. Practitoners first select intervention approaches that have a sound theoretical rationale for their use with the client, the limitation, the environment, and all the other factors influencing participation. Included in this rationale is the understanding of how a person develops self-care competencies. On the basis of the theoretical postulates, practitioners are able to articulate the reason for the clients' self-care problems in terms of their activity limitations and participation restrictions. The intervention process is illustrated in Figure 12.2.

FIGURE 12.2. Theoretically based intervention.

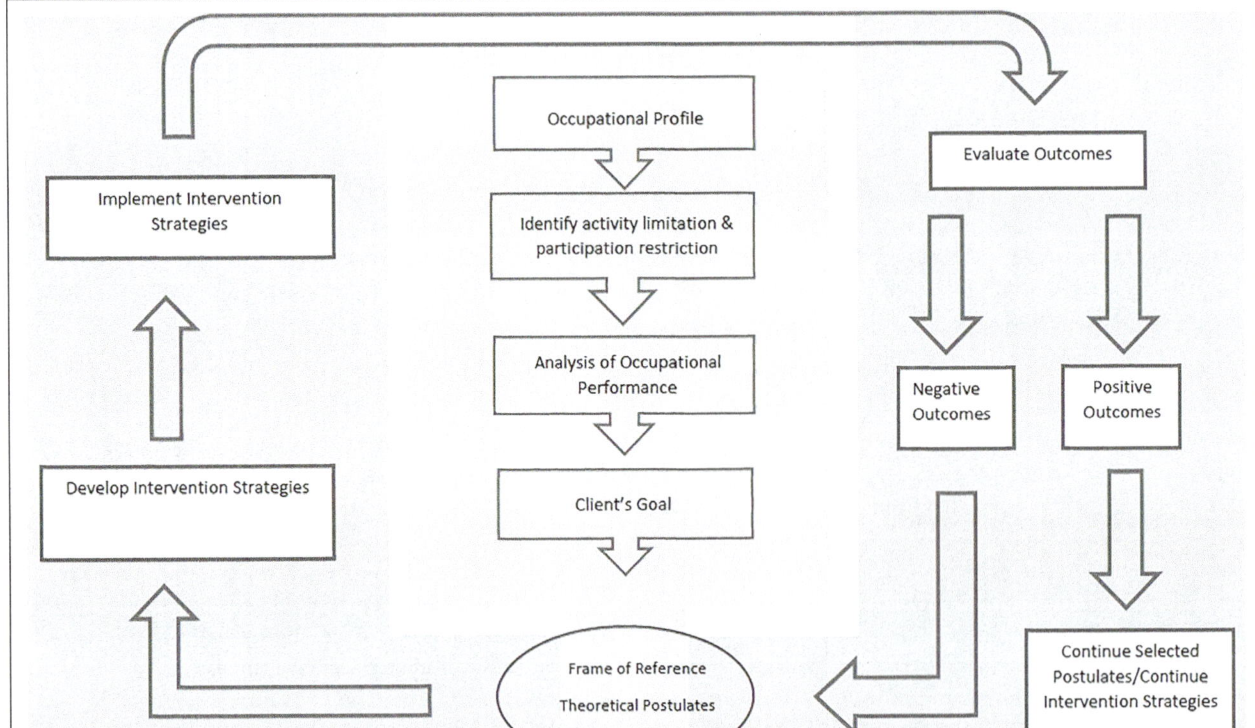

Note. The shaded blocks indicate different phases of the occupational therapy process: evaluation (left), intervention (middle), and outcome (right).
Source. T.-H. Howe. Used with permission.

Next, the occupational therapy practitioner identifies a specific dynamic theory to facilitate change. A ***dynamic theory*** explains how change will occur. Practitioners will be able to apply treatment principles derived from this dynamic theory and choose the optimal activities to promote changes in problem behaviors and progress clients toward their goals.

Learning theories are the most common dynamic theories used to address the facilitation of ADL competencies. These theories explain how the occupational therapy practitioner should provide instruction to bring about positive outcomes or shape specific behaviors. For example, the practitioner might use a ***behavior theory,*** which refers to procedures that change the consequences of behavior (Spiegler, 2016), to guide the shaping of skills for a person who has limited cognitive abilities.

With self-care, the occupational therapy practitioner bases the intervention on some combination of improving function and compensating for a permanent disability. Compensation involves two approaches: (1) changing the strategy used to complete the activity and (2) using adaptive equipment or technology. In Figure 12.3, the client uses tenodesis for hand position and a custom utensil holder to position the utensil. Because of the paralysis that occurred as a result of a spinal cord injury, he is unable to hold his utensil in the usual way. In this example, the client places the utensil in the holder using his mouth and hands. The fork tines are in his mouth while he places the handle in the holder and positions it where he needs it. The purpose of this intervention approach is not to change a client's physical abilities but to provide an appropriate tool so the client can perform an occupation.

Addressing Body Structure and Body Function During Intervention

The occupational therapy practitioner uses information on body structure to determine diagnosis. Anatomical structures, including the presence and extent of impairment, set the foundation for occupational therapy intervention. It is more straightforward to see that a person with a missing body part may have difficulty performing self-care occupations or will need to perform self-care occupations using an alternative technique. The same is true for impairment of any body structure.

During the evaluation, the extent of impairment is identified, and the expected recovery is determined. Goals

FIGURE 12.3. With the appropriate tool (compensation), the client is able to feed himself.

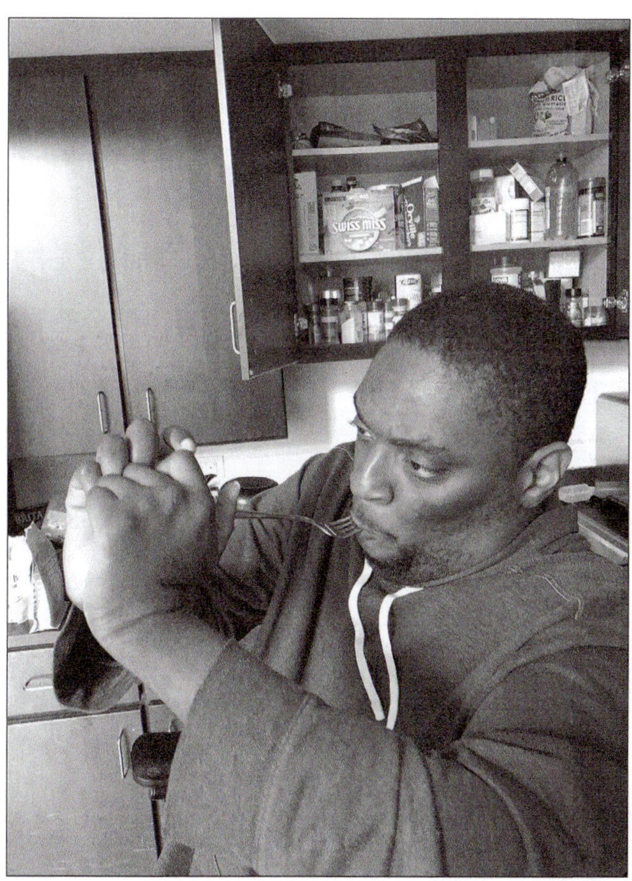

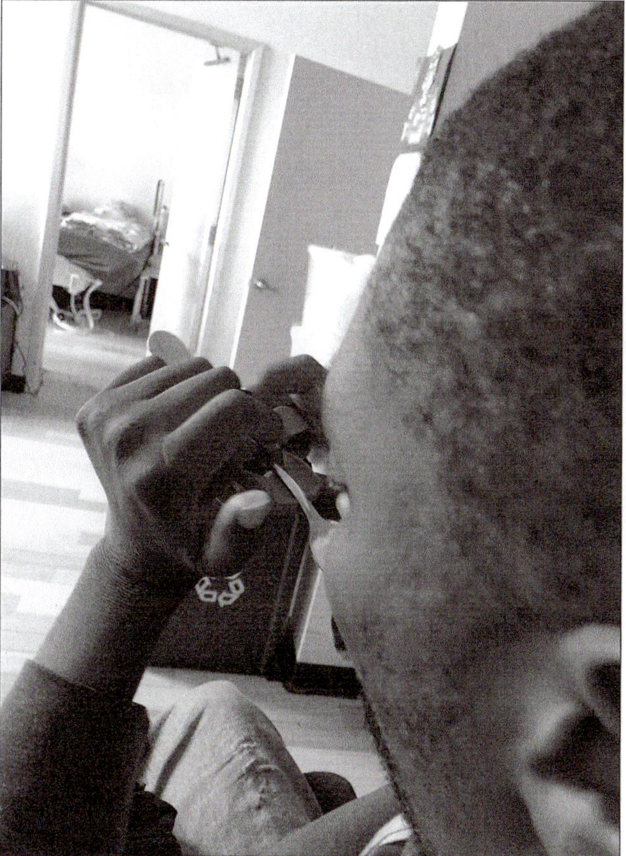

Source. A. Perr. Used with permission.

EXERCISE 12.4. Theoretical Rationale for Intervention

Identify a theoretical rationale that you might use to guide your interventions for Jon and Aisha. Create an intervention strategy based on a theoretical rationale that would be appropriate for Jon and Aisha and specific to their self-care goals.

are set according to the client's anticipated recovery and expected ability to compensate for any residual impairment while considering the client's preference. Related to body structures are body functions. How is the person able to function within the confines of the extent of impairment in any of the body structures? The occupational therapy practitioner focuses their intervention at this level by extracting

CASE EXAMPLE 12.1. Part 6. Aisha's Interventions

Aisha had a hemorrhagic stroke during surgery. At the time of her intervention, she presented with a flaccid right arm. There was some neurological involvement in her right lower extremity and her trunk, but she could stand and walk. Although some cognitive deficits were noted, Aisha's overall program was designed to allow medical recovery of body structures to occur, which meant that occupational therapy intervention would include activities and occupations to improve Aisha's ability to use her right arm.

Aisha's diagnosis is complicated. There is no way to know how much of the blood in her brain will be reabsorbed or how much residual damage there will be. How much the neurological system will recover is not known. Brain function may improve as the blood is reabsorbed and the swelling resolves, or the associated areas of the brain may take over for the damaged areas. Because of these variables, the occupational therapist will have difficulty predicting how much recovery will occur in Aisha's flaccid right arm and in her cognitive functioning, so intervention must be flexible to address her changing needs.

The theoretical rationale supporting this occupational therapy intervention was derived from dynamic system theory and central nervous system plasticity (Maier et al., 2019). In addition, the occupational therapist simultaneously uses another frame of reference to encourage Aisha to learn alternative techniques. To guide Aisha to use her left arm, the therapist uses postulates from the ***compensatory frame of reference,*** which describes using alternative actions to complete tasks and to participate in activities. For instance, Aisha is guided to use her left arm as the dominant arm during activity and to position her right arm to act as a stabilizer. Another example is when the therapist demonstrates to Aisha how to stabilize her toothbrush while applying toothpaste with her left hand. The therapist then gives Aisha time to practice. One-handed techniques are also taught on the chance that Aisha might not recover full function in her right arm. This frame of reference is based on learning theories that highlight the importance of demonstration, practice, and repetition to learn new skills.

Aisha is depressed. A goal of occupational therapy intervention is to address her depression with treatment strategies that are integrated with her other goals. To address Aisha's psychosocial functioning, the occupational therapist uses a frame of reference based on Bandura's (1977) social learning theory. The therapist applies the theoretical postulates from Bandura's theory along with other frames of reference (i.e., acquisitional or compensatory), depending on the goal Aisha is working on. According to Bandura's social learning theory (1977), modeling behaviors and activities that are viewed as helpful to change her mood are an important strategy for learning and improving self-efficacy, so the therapist helps Aisha to express positive attitudes, which then initiate and model the constructive behaviors.

CASE EXAMPLE 12.2. Part 6. Jon's Interventions

Jon has a mostly temporary disability. It is likely that his bones will heal. He should recover fully, although a chance exists that he will have limited mobility in his forearm, affecting his ability to supinate and pronate. Jon is also at risk for developing infection at the wound sites. Therefore, the occupational therapy program for Jon focuses on the level of body functions by learning alternative techniques to promote self-care independence while his body structures mend.

CASE EXAMPLE 12.1. Part 7. Aisha's Summary

Aisha is now on an inpatient rehabilitation unit in an acute-care hospital and is likely to stay there for about 3 weeks before she goes home. Her personal self-care issues are being addressed here. This environment is not like her home because Aisha lives in a small apartment, so it does not address her care of her home or how to adjust to things in a small apartment.

CASE EXAMPLE 12.2. Part 7. Jon's Summary

Jon is treated in an outpatient occupational therapy setting. This environment is not like his home because Jon lives in a large single-family house. His personal self-care is being addressed in the outpatient setting.

theoretical rationales from acquisitional frames of reference to guide the intervention. Consistent with the theoretical postulates, the occupational therapy practitioner encourages a client to learn specific skills required for optimal performance in the client's environment. The practitioner uses activities to improve body function while maintaining body structures under the best conditions. Case Example 12.1, Part 6, and Case Example 12.2, Part 6, describe clients' interventions.

Guided by the compensation approach to improve occupational performance, both Aisha and Jon will use alternative techniques to complete their self-care occupations. Part of the intervention for both clients may include training in upper-extremity range-of-motion exercises. To have the potential for the highest level of independence, both Jon and Aisha need to maintain the structural integrity of their arms so that when they are able to, they can use them as fully as possible.

As stated earlier, during evaluation occupational therapy practitioners must gather information about the contextual factors affecting a client's participation in self-care by considering how the physical environment could influence participation. For example, the person pictured in Figure 12.4 has motor impairment secondary to a spinal cord injury. The man uses the overhead method by

1. laying the jacket on his lap with the collar near his body and placing his hands and arms in the sleeves (Figure 12.4a),
2. swinging the arms and jacket up and over his head (Figure 12.4b),
3. wriggling the jacket down his back (Figure 12.4c),
4. leaning to pull the jacket down fully at the back (Figure 12.4d), and
5. wearing the jacket.

The treatment environment influences how the occupational therapy practitioner formulates treatment activities, as shown in Case Example 12.1, Part 7, and Case Example 12.2, Part 7. A discussion of treatment that occurs in simulated and real settings is provided in Chapter 11, "Independence in Occupation." Practitioners must consider the meaningfulness of activities to clients and how to simulate natural environments in the inpatient or outpatient setting when developing the most optimal interventions for their clients. Many other factors must be considered when developing interventions, including personal factors, such as the client's age and gender, which influence the focus of the treatment, the types of activities or occupations the practitioner brings into treatment, and the client's priorities.

It would be important, for example, to know that a client is vegetarian so that cooking activities used in therapy include ingredients the client will eat. It is just as important to know whether the person has dietary restrictions related to religion or personal taste and preferences. By tying personal factors to body functions and structures, a practitioner can, for example, see that a client wears dentures or has dysphagia and would prefer soft foods that are easier to manage.

Group Versus Individual Treatment

Occupational therapy intervention can be delivered in both individual and group settings. Occupational therapy practitioners work individually with clients when one-to-one attention and assistance are required. After the client has mastered a certain level of independence in their newly acquired skill, they can be treated in a group setting with others who have similar goals. Groups also emphasize the social nature of people, fostering physical and emotional supports among clients. Self-care activities can be addressed effectively in groups. A common example is self-feeding groups, which exist in many settings. A group of clients with dysphagia may eat together, with a speech–language pathologist, an occupational therapy practitioner, or a nursing assistant available for cuing and assistance. Similarly, routine participation in a grooming group may be effective in helping a client with mental illness resume

FIGURE 12.4. **A four-step method used by a man with a spinal cord impairment to put on his jacket.**

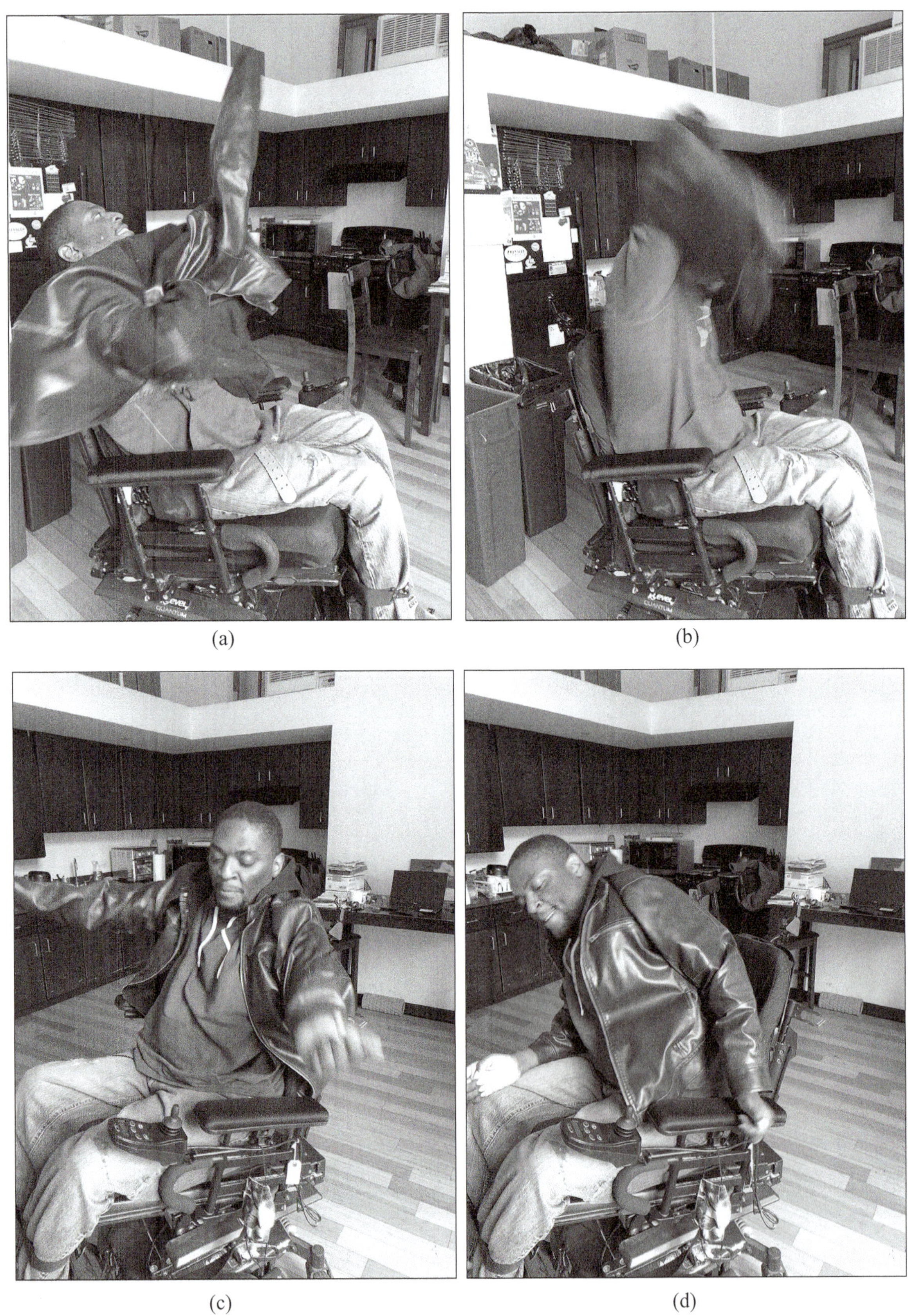

Source. A. Perr. Used with permission.

grooming activities. This routine group daily life activity uses Slagle's concept of rebuilding routines and allows each participant to develop and refine interpersonal communication skills and appropriate social behaviors (Schwartz, 2003).

Summary

Self-care intervention is central to successful occupational therapy. The occupational therapy practitioner can address clients' activity limitations and participation restrictions by focusing on ADLs. Intervention involves identifying the factors that influence the client's ability to participate in self-care, making the most of the factors that facilitate participation and lessening or eliminating the effect of barriers. The end result should be the highest level of independence or the highest degree of participation in self-care that the practitioner and clients are set to achieve.

References

American Occupational Therapy Association. (2020). Occupational therapy practice framework: Domain and process (4th ed.). *American Journal of Occupational Therapy, 74,* 7412410010. https://doi.org/10.5014/ajot.2020.74S2001

Andersen, C. K., Wittrup-Jensen, K. U., Lolk, A., Andersen, K., & Kragh-Sørensen, P. (2004). Ability to perform activities of daily living is the main factor affecting quality of life in patients with dementia. *Health and Quality of Life Outcomes, 2*(1), 52. https://doi.org/10.1186/1477-7525-2-52

Bandura, A. (1977). *Social learning theory.* Prentice-Hall.

Deci, E. L., & Ryan, R. M. (1985). *Intrinsic motivation and self-determination in human behavior.* Plenum.

Deci, E. L., & Ryan, R. M. (2008). Facilitating optimal motivation and psychological well-being across life's domains. *Canadian Psychology, 49,* 14–23. https://doi.org/10.1037/0708-5591.49.1.14

Decker, L., Träger, C., Miskowiak, K., Ejlersen, W. E., & Vinberg, M. (2017). Ability to perform activities of daily living among patients with bipolar disorder in remission. *Edorium Journal of Disability and Rehabilitation, 3,* 69–79. https://doi.org/10.5348/D05-2017-33-OA-9

Gell, N. M., Brown, H., Karlsson, L., Peters, D. M., & Mroz, T. M. (2020). Bathroom modifications, clutter, and tripping hazards: Prevalence and changes after incident falls in community-dwelling older adults. *Journal of Aging and Health, 32,* 1636–1644. https://doi.org/10.1177/0898264320949773

Geyh, S., Peter, C., Müller, R., Bickenbach, J. E., Kostanjsek, N., Üstün, B. T., . . . Cieza, A. (2011). The Personal Factors of the International Classification of Functioning, Disability and Health in the literature—A systematic review and content analysis. *Disability and Rehabilitation, 33,* 1089–1102. https://doi.org/10.3109/09638288.2010.523104

Gillen, G. (2019). Occupational therapy intervention for individuals. In B. A. B Schell & G. Gillen (Eds.), *Willard and Spackman's occupational therapy* (13th ed., pp. 413–435). Wolters Kluwer.

Greber, C., Hinojosa, J., & Ziviani, J. (2013). Achieving success: Facilitating skill acquisition and enabling participation. In J. Ziviani, A. Poulsen, & M. Cuskelly (Eds.), *The art and science of motivation: A therapist's guide to working with children* (pp. 123–158). Jessica Kingsley.

Ishizaki, T., Kobayashi, Y., & Kai, I. (2000). Functional transitions in instrumental activities of daily living among older Japanese. *Journal of Epidemiology, 10,* 249–254. https://doi.org/10.2188/jea.10.249

James, A. B., & Pitonyak, J. S. (2019). Activities of daily living and instrumental activities of daily living. In B. A. B. Schell & G. Gillen (Eds.), *Willard and Spackman's occupational therapy* (13th ed., pp. 714-752). Wolters Kluwer.

Law, M. (1993). Evaluating activities of daily living: Directions for the future. *American Journal of Occupational Therapy, 47,* 233–237. https://doi.org/10.5014/ajot.47.3.233

Maier, M., Ballester, B. R., & Verschure, P. F. (2019). Principles of neurorehabilitation after stroke based on motor learning and brain plasticity mechanisms. *Frontiers in Systems Neuroscience, 13,* 74. https://doi.org/10.3389/fnsys.2019.00074

Millán-Calenti, J. C., Tubío, J., Pita-Fernández, S., González-Abraldes, I., Lorenzo, T., Fernández-Arruty, T., & Maseda, A. (2010). Prevalence of functional disability in activities of daily living (ADL), instrumental activities of daily living (IADL) and associated factors, as predictors of morbidity and mortality. *Archives of Gerontology and Geriatrics, 50,* 306–310. https:/doi.org/10.1016/j.archger.2009.04.017

Nielsen, K., & Wæhrens, E. (2014). Occupational therapy evaluation: Use of self-report and/or observation? *Scandinavian Journal of Occupational Therapy, 22,* 13–23. https://doi.org/10.3109/11038128.2014.961547

Schneidert, M., Hurst, R., Miller, J., & Üstün, B. (2003). The role of environment in the International Classification of Functioning, Disability and Health (ICF). *Disability and Rehabilitation, 25,* 588–595. https://doi.org/10.1080/0963828031000137090

Schwartz, K. B. (2003). History of occupation. In P. Kramer & J. Hinojosa (Eds.), *Perspectives in human occupation: Participation in life* (pp. 18–31). Lippincott Williams & Wilkins.

Spiegler, M. D. (2016). *Contemporary behavior therapy* (6th ed.). Cengage.

Tabira, T., Hotta, M., Murata, M., Yoshiura, K., Han, G., Ishikawa, T., . . . Ikeda, Y. (2020). Age-related changes in instrumental and basic activities of daily living impairment in older adults with very mild Alzheimer's disease. *Dementia and Geriatric Cognitive Disorders Extra, 10*(1), 27–37. https://doi.org/10.1159/000506281

World Health Organization. (2001). *International classification of functioning, disability and health.*

13

Leisure Occupations

WENDY E. WALSH, PHD, OTR/L, FAOTA

CHAPTER HIGHLIGHTS

- Expertise of occupational therapy practitioners in leisure development
- Leisure through a cultural lens
- Leisure's role in human development
- Leisure needs
- Disability and leisure
- Leisure occupations
- Leisure across the lifespan
- Factors affecting leisure participation
- Occupational therapy assessment of leisure engagement
- Barriers to participation in leisure occupations for individuals, groups, and populations
- Leisure interventions for health promotion and prevention of secondary health issues

KEY TERMS AND CONCEPTS

• cognitive status • culture • environmental press • equipment • eudaimonic well-being • extrinsic motivation • extroverts • flow • gerotranscendence • intrinsic motivation • introverts • invigorating activities • leisure • leisure pursuits • modeling • nonobligatory tasking • occupational balance • occupational imbalance • opportunities • personality • physical status • play activities • relaxing • resources • self-development • stereotype • temperament • vocations • Zoom fatigue

"If you are losing your leisure, look out! It may be you are losing your soul."

—Virginia Woolf

"A life of leisure and a life of laziness are two different things."

—Benjamin Franklin

"All work and no play makes Jack a dull boy."

—American proverb

Introduction

As established across history and many times within this very text, humans are occupational beings. How we engage and what we engage in are main focus points in the field of occupational therapy. Activity choices are sometimes required of us, such as in work or vocational settings. Work occupations and work tasks have requirements demanded on the individual, such as start and stop times, deadlines, and mandated work partners. Self-care tasks (e.g., grooming, meals, hygiene) and sleep are also obligated activities. One cannot just decide not to sleep! Thus, these activities must be completed on a regular basis to exist and survive in society.

Activities that are nonobligatory are generally self-selected, internally driven, and individually chosen. These ***leisure pursuits,*** much like work, self-care, and sleep, also have the capacity to vastly influence our lives. Occupational therapists can measure engagement in these pursuits as data points through life satisfaction evaluations and can use engagement to assess an individual's overall health. The general trend supported by research and evidence-based practice is that the more satisfied one is with their life, the better their health outcomes. This concept was articulated in the American Occupational Therapy Association's (AOTA's) 1962 Eleanor Clarke Slagle lecture by Mary Reilly, titled "Occupational Therapy Can Be One of the Great Ideas of 20th Century Medicine," in the following quotation: "Man, through the use of his hands, as they are energized by mind and will, can influence the state of his own health" (Reilly, 1962, p. 2). When Mary Reilly made this statement, she was referring to all activities in which an individual engages. In this chapter, I focus specifically on ***leisure*** as a general group of tasks undertaken in an avocational frame and also referred to as leisure, leisure pursuits, leisure tasks, and leisure occupations. This chapter focuses on the nuances of these engagements and how the types of activity choices affect persons, groups, and populations.

Expertise of Occupational Therapy Practitioners in Leisure Development

Occupational therapy practitioners are uniquely qualified to incorporate leisure into therapeutic interventions. Engagement in leisure pursuits is clearly outlined in the fourth edition of the *Occupational Therapy Practice Framework: Domain and Process* (*OTPF–4*; AOTA, 2020) as a main occupational category. Engagement in leisure pursuits, whether alone or with others, is a way to structure the attainment of independence for clients. This can be done as a singular goal for independence in a specific leisure pursuit or be interdependent with other categories of occupational pursuits identified in the *OTPF–4*. For example, to travel away from home, you would need to manage work tasks to free up your time (work), pack needed items ahead of time (ADLs), and get sufficient rest before beginning the travel experience (sleep). Complex interweaving between areas of occupation supports the need for the practitioner's expertise to address disruption or the need for increased independence in the occupational area of leisure or leisure development across the lifespan.

Importantly, the occupational therapy practitioner's knowledge is not just for singular client intervention but can be shared with groups of people, communities, and agencies to promote the skills and abilities of their constituents. These could be individuals with disabilities, people who are marginalized, or individuals who are of various socioeconomic strata. Using their expertise, the practitioner can evaluate and assess a person, group, or population to then use evidence-based interventions to address areas of concern. Designing leisure occupations that bring independence and function to the client in a pleasurable way may require remediation, adaptation, or compensation.

Leisure Through a Cultural Lens

Culture and cultural interpretation of activities inevitably shapes how an individual or group views ***nonobligatory tasking*** or occupations that are internally driven and individually chosen. Interpretation of leisure through a cultural lens can be different for similar activities. For example, urban dwellers may describe movie watching as catching the newest film at the crowded Cineplex, whereas the rural dweller may look forward to a night at the local drive-in theater that is playing the most recent films. Both activities are nonobligatory, but the environment in which they exist is influenced by the geographic culture of the individuals.

Similarly, mealtimes are an area that can seem obligatory or nonobligatory depending on one's cultural interpretation. Cooking for someone or a family can carry different cultural contexts versus cooking for one's self solely for nutritional satisfaction. Many other leisure pursuits are influenced by the beliefs of persons, groups, or populations. Consider the things you do for leisure and how they would change if you had a differing cultural belief.

Leisure's Role in Human Development

When people are engaged in nonobligatory activities, laypersons sometimes interpret these actions as nonessential, a "waste of time," or as "goofing off." To the trained professional, these activities are essential to humans because they provide vital balance to the individual for growth (physical, social, emotional, spiritual) and overall development.

For the first few months of life, there is little distinction between obligatory and nonobligatory activities. This is a wondrous state of integration of systems as they exist for the first time outside the womb. As an infant's sensory and motor systems mature, visual–motor integration begins, and sensory input is better regulated and interpreted by the central and peripheral nervous systems. Occupational therapists and other health professionals measure maturity of the infant in the following areas: social and emotional health, language and communication, cognitive functioning, and motor and physical development. These "milestones" help providers monitor the health and development of the infant (Centers for Disease Control and Prevention, n.d.).

As the infant matures, there is a typical and expected increase in capacity for them to engage in more demanding and complex activities. For example, a 2-month-old infant is just beginning to pay attention to faces and people and has smoother motoric abilities of arms and legs. A 9-month-old infant, though, has the ability to point at things, plays peekaboo, crawls, and may even begin walking. This comparison shows how maturation and integrations of body systems allow a developing human to begin to engage in the world around them.

Later in childhood begins a differentiation of obligatory and nonobligatory tasking as overall development continues. Children learn to tie their shoes and zip up coats (obligatory) but spend time dressing dolls or opening and closing containers to access molding dough or other craft supplies (nonobligatory). Task refinement occurs, and individual decision making about what they "have to" do versus "want to" do becomes clearer as a child ages. Once formalized educational activities start, usually around the kindergarten level (typically ages 5 to 6 years), children's cognitive functions have evolved to incorporate personality and desires that support self-selected choice of activities to engage in.

Choosing activities is an integral part of leisure engagement. By definition, leisure is generally free from obligation: Someone can decide if they want to do a specific activity—or not—merely for the pleasure of doing the activity. Psychologist Mihaly Csikszentmihalyi (2008) described the pursuit of happiness as full engagement in the positive aspects of life, referring to this feeling as "flow." ***Flow*** happens when one's mind is fully invested in the activity at hand. As recipients of therapeutic interventions, clients can often view therapy as "work"; however, a skilled occupational therapy practitioner can tap into the elements of flow and craft intervention services to maximize therapy effect. When interventions are "fun," that is, they bring happiness to a client, occupational therapy can positively influence health outcomes.

Free from obligations, leisure pursuits often allow the person to experience the flow concept, thereby highlighting the importance of nonobligatory engagements. When self-directed, nonobligatory tasks or activities are undertaken, time feels altered. Did you ever look at the clock and say, "Gee, have I been doing this activity for that long?" or "It's already 2 hours later!"? Flow frees the mind to wholly commit to the activity at hand and alters one's perception of time.

Leisure Needs

Tracing back to the age of Aristotle, such pursuits as health, money, or power were expected to bring a state of satisfaction akin to good work being inherently satisfying. Pursuing happiness for happiness' sake was a separate and elevated concept and was seen as a choice. However, philosophers recognized that free time was inherently more difficult to enjoy because it took much more energy to craft meaning in a way that brought about joy or the flow referenced earlier (Csikszentmihalyi, 2008).

So, what does one need to pursue nonobligatory tasks? First, and most importantly, is the opportunity to engage in these types of tasks. Referencing the proverb at the start of this chapter, if someone is solely focused on work or vocational activities, elementary tasks like ADLs, or dedicated activities required of them that do not consist of paid work or self-management, they do not have any time left in the day to engage in activities of choice. By opening up opportunity to self-direct activity choice or simply be allowed the choice to limit engagement in any tasking at all gives an individual the space to direct their own time. It is in this space that the pursuit of happiness, flow, and the influence of the health state that Mary Reilly (1962) spoke of can occur.

One does not engage in any activity without thought to the resources and equipment the activity would require. If you are employed and wanted to go away on vacation, you need the proper amount of time off accrued with your employer. These time resources need to be requested and approved for you to take time away from your job and still collect a paycheck for this time off work. Resources are critical in releasing an individual from work obligations to allow them to pursue leisure activity choices. Infringement on time resources, such as when one works more than the standard 40-hour work week or more than the typical 5 days per week can lead to dire consequences. When individuals work multiple jobs to pay their bills and meet their financial commitments, there is a direct and negative effect on social relations, life roles, and health status. Heavy workloads with many hours and high achievement expectations, in addition to other job stressors, can lead to "burnout," a term American psychologist Herbert Freudenberger coined in the late 1970s (Freudenberger & Richelson, 1980). Without proper resources, leisure pursuits become less of a priority. The concept of burnout supports that time off to pursue leisure is not a "luxury" but rather a necessity for balance-of-life occupations. Prioritizing leisure engagement can lead to a healthier lifestyle.

Travel is an example that often requires an equipment need for successful leisure engagement (see Figure 13.1). You would not choose to go on vacation to a colder climate without taking proper clothing to protect you from the elements. You would also need to get your clothes and other packed items to the location of choice, so there is a need for a substantial suitcase or other container to transport your goods. Clothes and suitcases are essential pieces of equipment necessary for you to engage in your chosen leisure pursuit of traveling to a specific cold destination. Without either of these pieces, the leisure occupation of travel would be substantially more difficult and certainly become less enjoyable because you would not have warm clothes or a way to get them there.

Opportunities, resources, and equipment are all tied to money. An individual's economic situation greatly influences what types of leisure pursuits are available to them. A minimum wage earner might not even consider travel or a weekend skiing because of the financial investment required to participate in these leisure activities. Although many leisure choices

FIGURE 13.1. Winter sports are traditional leisure activities.

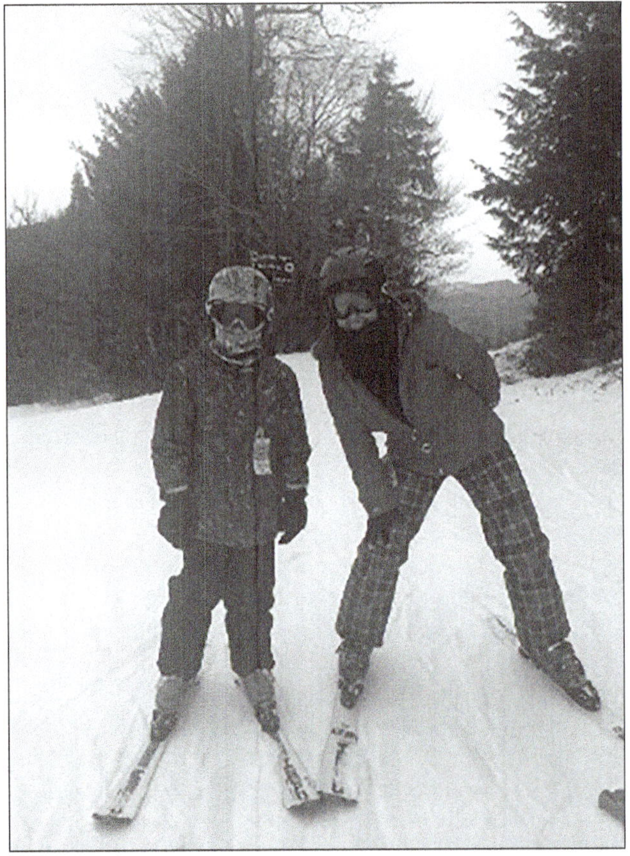

Source. J. Fadgen. Used with permission.

are available, occupational therapy practitioners should consider what is financially feasible for their clients to access and participate in when generating a plan of care that includes leisure pursuits.

Disability and Leisure

Whether a disability is acquired at a particular point in life or involves a developmental delay of the maturing individual, disability status affects pursuit, engagement, and satisfaction of leisure occupations. The degree of the effect is often part of an occupational therapy plan of care or reason a client (or client's family) seeks the services of an occupational therapy practitioner. Research supports that those living with a disability often experience decreased levels of leisure engagement and high levels of social isolation (Abbott & McConkey, 2006). Understanding the disability and the nature of its effects is a key part of therapy intervention as well as the incorporation of more nonobligatory activity choices for individuals with disabilities and leads to improved life satisfaction (Law, 2002).

Choosing nonobligatory activities is an integral part of leisure engagement for everyone. Research supports that people who identify as disabled have lower expectations for leisure and an overall lower amount of engagement in leisure; they tend to engage in solitary activities and rely less on social groups for enjoyment. When leisure engagement is down, individuals are more inactive and isolated, putting them at greater risk for mental health and physical dysfunction (Alma et al., 2011; Law, 2002).

However, social inclusion activities like membership in community-based clubs are highly valued by the population of people with disabilities, yet they rarely seek out membership without significant family or other social supports in place first (Pitt et al., 2020). The International Classification of Functioning, Disability and Health and the American Association on Intellectual and Developmental Disabilities include in their models social participation as a primary factor of good overall health (Schalock et al., 2010; World Health Organization, 2001). Lack of social inclusion is detrimental not only to leisure participation but to overall functioning and health status.

Leisure needs of opportunities, resources, and equipment also play a large role in leisure engagement for people with disabilities. For individuals to engage in leisure, there must be available chances to do so. These are ***opportunities.*** There must also be supports for that individual to engage. These are ***resources.*** Proper tools to complement the engagement in leisure must also be present. This is ***equipment.*** For those with physical disabilities, the occupational therapy practitioner may focus on opportunities to access types of gear to engage in age-related leisure pursuits. In 2018, Microsoft launched the Xbox Adaptive Controller, which enables people of all ages to adapt the inputs on the control panel for Xbox gaming (Xbox, 2018, 2021). Body differences had prohibited potential gamers from engaging in this popular leisure activity, so technology modification of equipment increased accessibility to all games in the Microsoft system. Inclusivity in gaming builds capacity for the individual in confidence, self-determination, self-identity, social belonging, and quality of life (Abbott & McConkey, 2006; Schreuer et al., 2014).

Individuals with developmental and intellectual disabilities take longer to pick up novel activities and even longer to develop fluency with new tasking. Often because of these learning differences, they are delayed in skills related to social participation and experience social isolation (Alma et al., 2011). Being accepted by a peer group is important to those with disabilities; inclusive conversations and being made to "feel safe" are means to use resources (peers) and create opportunities for expanding leisure interests (Abbott & McConkey, 2006, p. 280). With increased practice and time, mastery of everyday technologies like cell phones and iPads can help those with developmental and intellectual disabilities achieve leisure goals that are both client centered and individually meaningful (Ullenhag et al., 2020). Mastery of activity is a concept that applies to most leisure pursuits, not just those involving technology.

Acquired disability can lead to similar barriers in leisure engagement and occupational disruption. Because the disability may be new, physical, emotional, and cognitive aspects of

CASE EXAMPLE 13.1. Rosemary: Leisure After Stroke

Rosemary, age 47 years, has been married to Tony for 26 years and is the matriarch of a large Italian family with extended family members (aunts, uncles, and cousins) who live in the local vicinity. She does not work outside the home, and her main occupations outside of self-care are caring for the family and managing the home. She spends most of her days cleaning, preparing meals, and handling the family's appointments. She has always had an interest in French baking, but with five teenager-to-early-adult children who live with her and her spouse, she had not pursued this leisure activity. During a home care visit months after a stroke that left her with moderate paralysis, she identified with the occupational therapist that she would like to engage in this leisure pursuit.

activity engagement, participation and satisfaction, along with the opportunities, resources, and equipment of leisure needs, are considerations occupational therapy practitioners should incorporate as they plan interventions (see Case Example 13.1).

Regardless of how an individual has come to have participation differences, feelings of social belonging and inclusion are significant. Badia et al. (2013) reported that subjective preferences for activity choice and perceived constraints to that activity choice were the best indicators of life satisfaction for persons with a disability, as opposed to merely participation in lots of leisure activities. To address these findings, society must delve deeper into the unique opportunities and resources that are offered for greater disability inclusion in local communities. Angell et al. (2020) added that for the population of people with disabilities, community engagement is an ongoing process that requires long-term supports for success and integration.

EXERCISE 13.1. Rosemary's Opportunities, Resources, and Equipment

Explore these questions:

- What are some considerations Rosemary should think about relative to the opportunities, resources, and equipment needed to engage in this new leisure pursuit?
- What considerations would be relevant given her cultural background and family structure?
- In your community, what types of supports exist for a person with Rosemary's type of disability?

Leisure Occupations

This section discusses three types of leisure activities: those that are (1) relaxing, (2) invigorating, and (3) providing self-development. Both obligatory and nonobligatory activities serve meaningful purposes in the social, emotional, and physical development of humans across the lifespan. Seeking pleasure or enjoyment can come in a variety of ways, and the satisfaction one receives through leisure engagement is up to the individual to determine.

To that end, what one person sees as obligatory, another may define as a nonobligatory leisure pursuit. An example is clothes shopping at a large retail mall. Some people view the activity of driving to the location, finding the correct store, trying on items, and the entire experience as a notch just above loathsome. Then there are the folks who plan trips to new shopping locations, inhale on entry to the mall, and say, "Ahh, this is heaven!" The occupation of shopping occurs in the same location, but it is a very different personal experience for each individual. The takeaway here is the type of activity experience occurring and how the individual views it; one considers it leisure, the other considers shopping a necessary ADL or obligatory task.

Relaxing

Much like the specific hormones in the human body that are primarily responsible for the metabolism, growth, and reproduction of tissue and tissue healing, ***relaxing*** involves engaging in activities that are perceived as bringing a calming sensation to the individual. Relaxing can bring healing through regulation of demands on the body.

The sympathetic and parasympathetic nervous systems are responsible for maintenance of our body's systems for homeostasis (Chung et al., 2019; Jänig, 2006). Individuals who experience stress and do not counter the stressors with equally relaxing or calming activities risk a prolonged imbalance in the homeostatic condition and the formation of a diseased state. Prolonged stress, that is, *press,* is highly detrimental to the physical body.

Health professionals and laypersons alike confirm the benefits calming activities have on the physical body. A relaxing activity triggers the parasympathetic nervous system, which can lower heart rate, increase lung volume, and elongate musculature, thereby placing the individual in a calm state. Research by Kuykendall et al. (2021) indicated that television watching is a leisure pursuit that brings pleasure but is more of a relaxing activity; it fosters detachment from stressors versus fulfills needs of skill mastery or association with others. The authors went on to say that improvements to well-being are stronger with self-determining activities, whereas watching television is "less conducive to fulfilling a number of psychological needs and to promoting general well-being" (Kuykendall et al., 2021, p. 554). Does this mean that watching television should be avoided in favor of other types of leisure pursuits? No. As mentioned before, the perceived benefit, or pleasure factor, of leisure engagement is an individual decision. Thus, the individual's choice of activities can be in any type combination they feel benefits them the most. Notably, health care professionals, supported by Kuykendall et al.'s work, agree that varied types of leisure activities are best for overall well-being.

Invigorating Activities

Invigorating activities bring energy to the individual; they excite, raise body system activity (circulation, heart rate), and elevate endocrine production of "feel good" hormones like endorphins (Rogers, 2012). These activities may be through physical, cognitive, or emotional invigoration. Each can bring a sense of pleasure without regard to the utility of the activity to those other than one's self. Examples of invigorating activities are running, dancing, playing an instrument, or riding amusement park rides.

One point of clarification is that responses evoked from invigorating activities are different from those generated by stressors. A stress response can also raise body system activity, specifically with increased neurotransmitter production, elevation of blood glucose levels, and more cortisol production in preparation for a fight-or-flight response aimed at species survival (Rogers, 2012). Instead, invigorating activities stem from the concept of ***eudaimonic well-being***; that is, living a life of contentment, virtue, and belonging that brings pleasure to the individual (Joshanloo, 2018; Pöllänen & Weissmann-Hanski, 2020). Leisure pursuits that are eudaimonic can balance other areas of life occupations that may not always be as pleasurable, such as mundane ADLs or instrumental ADLs, general health management, rest and sleep, typical education and work, or obligatory social participation (AOTA, 2020).

Joshanloo (2018) reported the top three predictors of eudaimonic well-being are (1) positive affect, (2) standard of living satisfaction, and (3) level of education, and all have very little to do with financial prosperity. Occupational therapy practitioners should keep these predictors in mind when constructing plans of care that include leisure exploration or novel leisure pursuits.

Self-Development

The ***self-development,*** or personal skill or character building, category of leisure pursuits is an interesting one because task pieces of a larger activity may not all be "pleasurable," but the totality of the activity is. Self-development relates to any activity that helps one learn a new skill or enhance a previously developed sklll. Take, for example, the popular paint-and-sip craze (Figure 13.2). For about 2 hours, you receive all the supplies and direct instruction on how to use paints to make a portrait or picture of a tabletop canvas. The palm trees and finer details are hard to master, and your performance may not be what you want; inevitably, for novice painters, the degree of accuracy is low. This can be incredibly frustrating. One may challenge, "Is this leisure then?"

FIGURE 13.2. A paint-and-sip student.

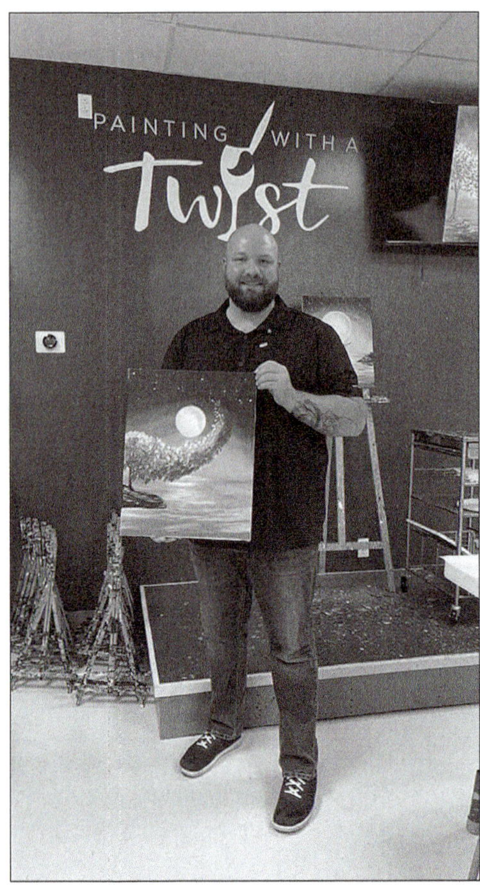

Source. D. Wykes. Used with permission.

The activity must be considered in the larger context of a night out versus painting palm trees. Friends (old and new) have gathered, laughs are exchanged, and the participants get to take home their work to show others. The level of satisfaction is not only in the task of painting but in the experience of the night as a whole. Frequently, participants report that they would attend another paint-and-sip. Having this experience may prompt someone to pursue formal painting classes or advance their skills as an artist through other classes or experiences.

EXERCISE 13.2. Types of Leisure

Think of relaxing, invigorating, and self-development leisure pursuits you enjoy:

- Why do you enjoy them?
- What opportunities, resources, and equipment do you need to successfully engage in them?

Leisure Across the Lifespan

Over the course of a lifetime, an individual's obligatory responsibilities shift mainly because of developmental maturity, role transition, or a change to one's overall capacity. Leisure pursuits and their ranked importance change over time as well.

Consider the high adrenaline activity of motorcycle riding. As a very young person, mastery of the activity may seem too scary to even attempt. As a mature and physically fully developed adult, mastery comes easier with practice, making this leisure choice an exhilarating sensory experience. In addition, mastery of this form of vehicle may also be utilitarian if used as one's primary mode of transportation. Older adults frequently recognize the danger that aging brings. Their reaction times are slower, and the bike has progressively become too heavy to manage safely. Detachment from this leisure pursuit often occurs in later life when the "need for speed" or high adrenaline activities pose more risk than reward.

Early Life: Infant, Child

Much of the focus in early life is on physiological development. For the first 6 months, body systems are maturing and integrating. As humans develop, they begin to explore their surroundings. Exploring and interacting with their environment are ways of learning and the main ways children develop motor, cognitive, and social skills (Besio, 2022; Parham & Fazio, 2008). A child's main occupation is play. ***Play activities*** are ones that do not have a structured teaching purpose; they are meant to be experiential, discovery based, and for general enjoyment. Children engage in play because it is fun. For example, giving infants a "busy box" with various items allows them to inspect, trial, and use a toy as they see fit. In first or early exposure to that item, it does not matter if it used correctly. Parents can instruct infants and children on the purpose of an item later, and through practice, the youngster can master the toy at hand. Often with mundane tasks like dressing or hygiene, parents and caregivers will make it fun to complete such basic ADLs. Consider toilet training. Any big-box baby store will have countless items to make toileting and toilet hygiene "fun," such as toilet water colorant, interesting seats, "sinkable" targets, and colorful underwear. In reality, the routine task of toileting just needs to be mastered and can take time. Learning through play is a method for capacity building and improving a child's independence in daily life skills (see Figure 13.3).

The degree of playfulness of a child is derived from their motivation for a leisure task. Motivation can either be driven internally or drawn out with an external locus of control. A child's internal drive to engage with objects and persons in the surroundings is called ***intrinsic motivation.*** Here, a child manages the degree and depth to which they participate in an activity. When intrinsic motivation is high, it displays as focused, outgoing, or excited behavior. Caregivers and parents can supply ***extrinsic motivation*** to a child by coaching or directing parameters of the leisure task. A good example of extrinsic motivation can be illustrated in the swimming pool (Figure 13.4). The adult coaches a youngster to jump in from the side deck. They hold their hands out, assure the child that it is safe, and can demonstrate how cool the water is and what a fun sensation jumping and swimming can be. This positive external pressure is applied to raise the child's intrinsic motivation level to take a new risk, thereby experiencing new skills and abilities. The parent or caregiver support and guidance in this example provides the child with the confidence that they can be successful while having fun.

FIGURE 13.3. A young child plays with a mirror.

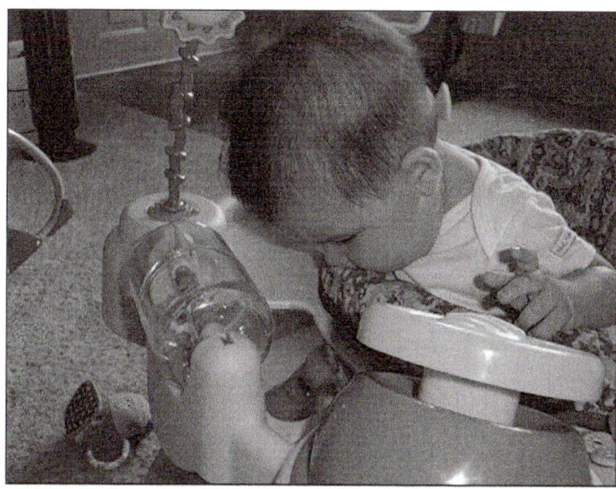

Source. W. Walsh. Used with permission.

FIGURE 13.4. Motivation to engage in swim leisure is both internally and externally driven.

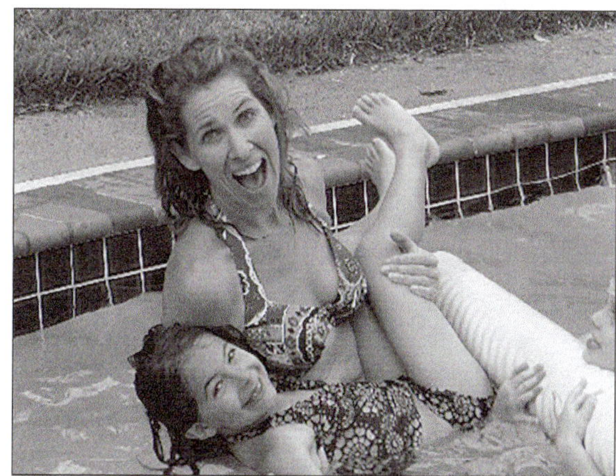

Source. W. Walsh. Used with permission.

Middle Life: Adolescents, Early Adult

As children grow and mature into adolescents, play becomes leisure as the depth and breadth of exposure to different occupations has deepened. They begin to engage in work roles; formal education becomes their primary work with paid, part-time jobs often in the later teen years. Adolescents and young adults exercise more individual choice when it comes to leisure pursuits and seek out preferences like organized sports, after-school activities, or social clubs.

Sport, activity, and social clubs serve two main purposes for adolescents and teens. First, they provide experiences with navigating interpersonal relationships. The development of a network of friends (close and distant) helps young people adjust to new roles and responsibilities; explore or experience leadership; and navigate social dynamics, especially the ups and downs of teen relationships. Second, dealing with peer pressure, experiencing conflict, and beginning to pursue romantic interests lay the foundation for adult relationships.

Leisure pursuits are the context in which much of the interpersonal experiences occur. Going to movie theaters, group "dates," and high school pep rallies or Friday night football games bring young people together such that they are exposed to social pressures. Conversely, having leisure choices like after-school open art or book clubs can be a refuge from overbearing social pressures. Exposure to the different types of leisure (relaxing, invigorating, self-development) contributes to teen or young adult life satisfaction (Law, 2002). Regulation of self through leisure is also an important part of middle life. Disproportionate engagement in leisure (too much or too little) shifts the stressors so that dysregulation of systems occurs; this is a barrier to leisure engagement. An overabundance of negative types of leisure pursuits (e.g., drinking alcohol, using drugs, excessive "hanging out," smoking, racing cars, using too much social media) sets up young individuals for difficulties with school and community administration or law enforcement. Adults who role model work–leisure balance and a variety of leisure occupations help adolescents and young adults develop confidence, positive self-identity, belonging, and self-direction (Abbott & McConkey, 2006; Schreuer et al., 2014).

Later Life: Middle Adult, Older Adult

A hallmark of adult relationships is increased individual independence that generally occurs toward the end of early adulthood. One may move out of the parental dwelling or purchase a home or car; or a single person may partner up, indicating a transition to middle adulthood. A shift is seen in their life focus, which is now on work (for financial stability) and family (partner, spouse, children). In this life phase, availability of leisure pursuits may increase, but participation in choice activities may decline. Available time for leisure is relegated to weekends and with decreasing frequency as more "adult" or individual responsibilities emerge.

Role shifts also affect leisure engagement. Single people often have the means and availability to engage in leisure that holds more risk (e.g., skydiving), has more grandiose components (month-long travel), or requires larger budgets. People who are partnered, and especially those with children, have different priorities for leisure. These may be family focused, fostering interpersonal relations between the older and the next generations, or smaller endeavors, saving on both time and overall cost.

Becoming parents changes the dynamic between partners. Although both parents may be responsible for child care and home upkeep, one usually emerges as the main caregiver, even if both work outside the home. Leisure time for the main caregiver is less than for their partner and markedly less than before they had children.

As time progresses and responsibilities of family and work become more stable, exploration of leisure pursuits sees a resurgence. Interest may become more actioned by the individual and can have dividends that benefit others as well. For example, an interest in history and politics may have someone run for an open position on the local school board, or a pastime of thrift shopping could turn into an online resale store venture that creates additional income.

Older adults transition out of work and into the retirement phase. To a greater extent, intrinsically motivated leisure pursuits begin to occupy their days. These individuals now have the time and supports to expand leisure as work obligations have decreased. Adults ages 70 years or older dedicate more time in hours to leisure tasking like reading, games, and computer use than those ages 60 to 69 years. And, as is supported by much evidence, elders who engage in various and plentiful leisure pursuits have better mental health and hold a longer life expectancy (Bureau of Labor Statistics, 2015; Kuykendall et al., 2015, 2021; Rivera-Torres et al., 2021).

A phenomenon occurs in later life when leisure and other activities decline. Social theorists attribute this to a disengagement from social constructs (i.e., relationships, attitudes, meanings), whereas other theorists describe feeling connected to those close to the individual while letting go of materialistic and control areas in their lives. This phenomenon is termed ***gerotranscendence***; that is, a social withdrawal (Perzynski, 2006). Physical deterioration or cognitive decline undoubtedly contribute to disengagement and social isolation. Regardless of the reasons, the removal of activities, including leisure pursuits, can be problematic for our clients. Long periods of being sedentary (e.g., television watching) or limited cognitive stimulation (e.g., one type of activity only, napping) is not good for overall health and well-being. These are the areas occupational therapy practitioners should consider targeting interventions.

EXERCISE 13.3. Elder Leisure

Think of elder family members or friends who are older than age 65 years:

- What types of leisure activities do they engage in?
- Ask them whether their leisure pursuits have changed over time. What are your thoughts on their answers?
- If they were under your care as an occupational therapy practitioner, where would you focus intervention for increasing leisure engagement? Think carefully, and consider the client as a whole being, inclusive of all roles, values, and beliefs they hold.

Factors Affecting Leisure Participation

Several factors are responsible for leisure participation across the lifespan, including personal traits, family and cultural traits, and technology. As stated earlier, leisure engagement and the variety (and complexity) of activities is not static as a person grows and ages. Infants and children need exposure to leisure for development of body systems. For them, leisure is about discovery of skills and abilities.

Adolescents and early adults use leisure to explore their personality, wants, desires, and dislikes. They find meaning in purpose and may view some obligatory activities, such as employment, as more of a leisure pursuit until they gain more responsibilities within the pursuit and in their life contexts (Figure 13.5).

Adults use leisure to connect with others, engaging a sense of familial and societal belonging. They also use leisure to disconnect from societal responsibilities at times. Balance of these two types of engagement is important for overall mental well-being.

Elder adults begin to pull back from societal interactions and activity engagement in leisure as they age and enter a phase of gerotranscendence. It is safe to say that no matter where in life a person is, their contexts affect the degree of leisure participation.

FIGURE 13.5. **A teen sees power washing a patio as "fun." Adult homeowners typically consider this to be work.**

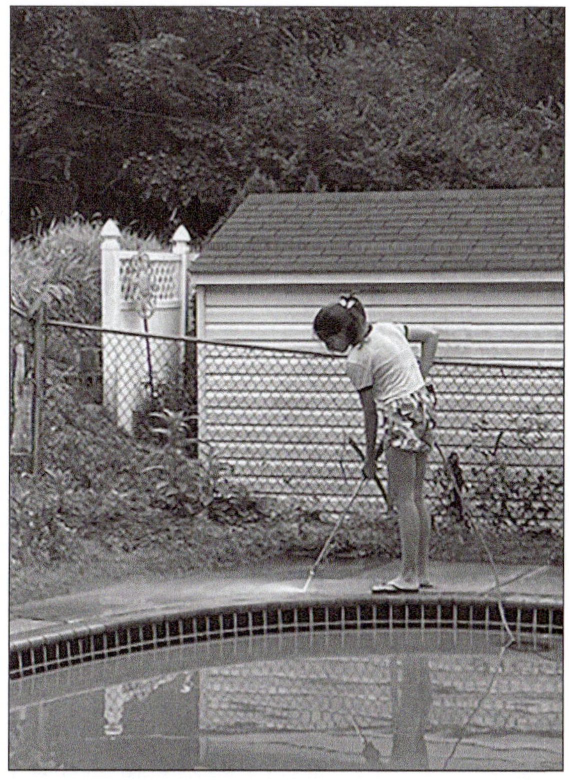

Source. W. Walsh. Used with permission.

Personal Traits

Temperament and personality are factors that drive engagement in all occupational pursuits, especially leisure activities. Activity choice and level of commitment to a leisure activity have a lot to do with the incorporation of these two factors. ***Temperament*** is best defined as the style of engagement and how one reacts to the environmental context of an activity. People can be high threshold or low threshold for activity engagement. Often, activation of our sensory systems is involved with choices driven by one's temperament. When an individual is a sensory seeker, activity choices mimic excitement and high-energy tasks. Conversely, low-threshold and low-sensory individuals typically seek out more sedentary activities with lesser demand on one's sensory system. Individuals who fall in between these two extremes are comfortable in high- and low-energy activities but may choose either.

Personality of an individual refers to introvert or extrovert qualities that can guide leisure choice. For example, ***extroverts*** gravitate toward group activities and social situations in which leisure pursuits have many individuals contributing to the energy of overall task. ***Introverts***, on the other hand, often present as shy and prefer solitary or partnered leisure to bring them enjoyment. If extroverted individuals engage in low-threshold activities for too long, they can become bored, whereas introverted individuals might leave a leisure activity early, finding it overwhelming with too many people present to continue to engage in that leisure task.

The ***physical status*** of an individual is a personal factor that also drives engagement in leisure pursuits. Fitness, stamina, flexibility, strength, coordination, and balance either allow or disallow the development of skills and overall abilities for some tasks within a leisure pursuit. Strenuous activities require high demand on the body and the components of physicality. Level of physical status can dictate the degree to which one can engage in a leisure pursuit of choice. That is not to say that a low-physicality person cannot participate in a physically challenging pursuit, but they must consider safety and skill levels as they explore the leisure task demands and resultant leisure choice satisfaction.

Likewise, ***cognitive status*** (i.e., the individual's ability to think, analyze, and reason) plays a major role in the participation of leisure pursuits. Occupational therapy practitioners must evaluate the cognitive demand of a chosen leisure activity with the cognitive capacity of the person who wants to engage in that activity. Individuals with high cognitive capacity might naturally gravitate toward choosing high cognitive–demand activities like chess or problem-solving tasks, such as furniture assembly, electrical circuitry, or spatial design. After an injury with cognitive disability or a condition like neurodegenerative disease, when an occupational therapy practitioner engages their client in new or reattempted leisure pursuit, clients can sometimes report that the activity is "boring." A clinician must consider if the cognitive demand for a beloved leisure pursuit is now just too high for the client to derive enjoyment and satisfaction from it like they did before. Finding the correct challenge level for the temperament, personality, physicality, and cognitive demand a leisure activity places on the individual helps to facilitate the flow and derivation of pleasure and satisfaction Csikszentmihalyi (2008) described.

EXERCISE 13.4. Challenges to Leisure Engagement

Think back to a time you attempted to do a leisure activity that was "too difficult":

- Can you consider why you thought this way?
- Were the barriers physical? Cognitive? Related somehow to exposure, practice, or a mastery of the task?
- How did this experience prepare you for other similar experiences in your lifetime?
- How can occupational therapy practitioners incorporate the challenges of leisure occupations into client-centered interventions?

Family and Cultural Traits

Family and cultural traits are important persuasive factors when considering leisure engagement. ***Modeling*** is the experience of observing others and trying out the activities and is how young people discover leisure pursuits and make decisions about whether they want to participate; families are powerful models for exploring types and kinds of leisure activities. Family size may play a role in leisure choice. If an individual is raised in a larger family that values participatory activities, inclusion, and productive outcomes from their efforts, members tend to gravitate toward leisure that has similar characteristics of community engagement and industriousness. For smaller families, activities focused on creating quality family time with one-on-one leisure pursuits may be preferred (see Figure 13.6).

Culture, which is a combination of shared values, practices, and beliefs of a particular group, can also play a role in the leisure choices and pursuits of different gender categories or ages. For example, in the Jewish religion, strict Orthodox followers frequently practice gender segregation at social gatherings, with swimming, and at parks and recreation facilities. These are accepted practices within this culture and align with their views of modesty and purity. Other cultures like the Romany gypsies of Europe maintain different perspectives on the roles of men and women. Marriage between men and women happens much younger—usually around age 16 years—than in other Western countries. Women are expected to keep the home immaculately clean and raise the children, leaving little time for anything else. The men are the sole financial support of the family, often working long hours at manual jobs. Formal education is not a priority in this nomadic culture and typically stops before the high school grades.

The role of family and culture in the pursuit and engagement of leisure is an important concept for occupational therapy practitioners to understand. Incorporating the client's beliefs, values, and roles is critical for well-rounded and appropriate client-centered provision of care.

FIGURE 13.6. A mom and daughter share a family tradition of coffee treats when shopping.

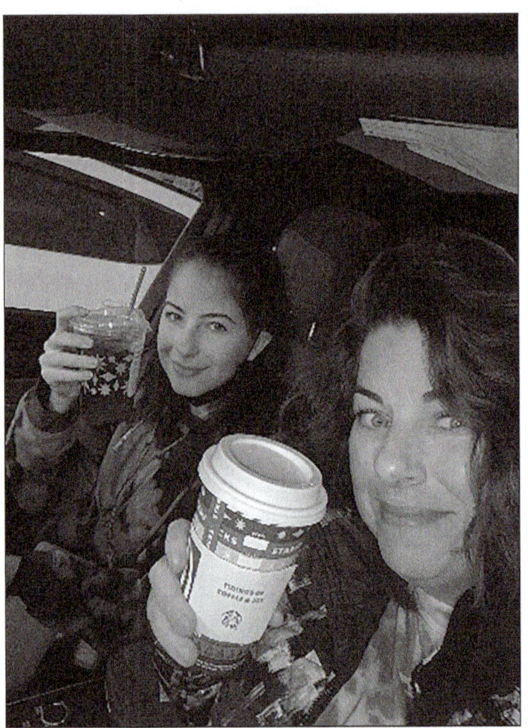

Source. W. Walsh. Used with permission.

Technology and Leisure

Depending on the age of the client, technology likely plays some role in their leisure engagement. Social interrelationships and the maintenance of a social network have been made infinitely easier with recent technology developments. Smartphones and tablets with Internet capability allow individuals to remain connected to family and loved ones virtually 24/7. A recent study by von Humboldt et al. (2020) reported that 71% of Mexican elders (ages 67 to 72 years) used some form of smart technology like social applications or video calling. The ease and accessibility of smart-designed homes and smart technologies make in-home leisure easier to coordinate or engage. For example, robot floor sweeping, touch-free faucets, smart speakers, motion beds, auto-lift recliners, and app-controlled lights, doors, and media systems are now available and within the budgets of many.

Using social media for leisure engagement is a phenomenon that has seen tremendous growth since around 2010. People, especially adolescents and teens, use social media for thought exchange, entertainment, and the acquisition of information by following individual or group accounts. The platforms of Facebook and Instagram have morphed over recent years so users can interface more easily with "stories" and direct messaging. New social media platforms have emerged as well. Snapchat allows users to exchange pictures that disappear after viewing, and TikTok permits video replies and response "duet" videos between users. Use of these platforms can hold much enjoyment and discovery. They also help with feelings of interconnectedness when users create online relationships with family and friends far away or grow their social network of likeminded individuals.

However, not all use of social media comes with positive experiences. As adolescent demand for access to technologies like tablets, smart watches, and smartphones becomes more socially acceptable (and financially accessible), parents *must* be vigilant. Earlier and earlier exposure to mature content or cyberbullying can occur behind the protective anonymity of online profiles. Someone who claims to be a 10-year-old schoolmate could easily be a predatory adult with nefarious intentions. Alternatively, when young people are presented with situations they are not mature enough to handle, behaviors and responses could set a maladaptive baseline for relationship expectations in real life. It is safe to say that with access to leisure technology for younger children, caution and supervision should be a priority.

There are additional downfalls to having technology at our fingertips. There is a point at which connectedness with friends and social networks for leisure interferes with open access availability for obligatory activities. This was evident during the SARS-CoV-2 virus (COVID-19) pandemic in 2020, when the world essentially went virtual. This phenomenon in relation to leisure engagement during a pandemic is described in more detail later in the section "Environmental Press as a Barrier (Population)."

Occupational Therapy Assessment of Leisure Engagement

Assessment of leisure engagement should be considered at the beginning of occupational therapy services with the initial evaluation of a client. The initial evaluation should be comprehensive, covering all areas of occupational engagement, and should be client centered. Leisure engagement or lack of leisure engagement may not be the highest-ranking issue or problem the client is currently encountering, but consideration of the person as a whole is fundamental and can be traced to the philosophical base of the occupational therapy profession, which puts occupation as an integral part of a person's health and (occupational) participation (Meyer, 1922).

At the initial evaluation, some clients may not believe that leisure assessment is fundamental to their recovery. Communication by occupational therapists about the holistic value of occupational therapy services is an important component of the therapeutic relationship between practitioners and clients. Therapeutic use of self (Taylor, 2020) and open and honest communications not only help clients see occupational therapy's value in their recovery but allow trust to develop between client and practitioner, which strengthens the breadth and depth of living with and after disability.

A well-known and easily administered client-centered performance overview is the Canadian Occupational Performance Measure (COPM; Law et al., 2019). The COPM is composed of a semistructured interview format investigating three areas of occupation: (1) self-care, (2) productivity, and (3) leisure. Clients rate activities identified on a 10-point-scale, ranging from 1 (poor performance and low satisfaction) to 10 (very good performance and high satisfaction) for their perception of satisfaction with their performance in each activity. This reliable and valid standardized assessment can help occupational therapists begin a conversation that addresses the most acute areas of occupational disruption as well as assesses meaningful areas to the client. Boredom and loneliness are often concepts that are brought up when disability affects engagement in leisure pursuits. The therapist should investigate further during their assessment of the client.

Many assessments of leisure occupations are available today, so how does an occupational therapist choose which one to administer? Context-specific deficit areas and age of the client help to guide that choice. In addition to the COPM, the following are a few of the broad leisure assessments in adults that can be used for evaluative purposes:

- Activity Card Sort (Baum & Edwards, 2008) uses 89 photographs of instrumental ADLs, social activities, and leisure activities that subjects (ages 60 years and older) sort according to their levels of participation. Changes in levels of activity are investigated as clients discuss their occupational history with the evaluator. There are three versions of the instrument: (1) Institutional, (2) Recovering, and (3) Community Living.
- Life Balance Inventory (LBI; Matsuka, 2009) attempts to measure desired time spent doing chosen activities and actual time spent doing those activities (electronic administration and scoring preferred). Clients answer "yes" or "no" for activities and then input the perceived satisfaction for time associated with doing the activity. Results are scored immediately via the web-based interface and have good reliability and construct validity.
- The QuiLL (Quality in Later Life; Evans et al., 2005) is a short (10- to 15-minute) self-report questionnaire in which the client rates their quality-of-life perceptions in 10 domains: (1) Life, (2) Family, (3) Finances, (4) Health, (5) Living Arrangements, (6) Neighborhood, (7) Occupy Time, (8) Safety, (9) Self, and (10) Social. This questionnaire has good reliability and validity and excellent interrater reliability.
- The Volitional Questionnaire (de las Heras et al., 2007) is a tool that uses a 14-item rating scale, scoring *passive, hesitant, involved,* or *spontaneous* for each item. Minimum score is 14 and a maximum score is 56. The therapist evaluates an individual's motivation and how the environment affects their participation in meaningful occupations. It is used for people ages 8 years and older and has online and paper scoring.
- The World Health Organization developed a self-reporting measure of quality of life across international cultural contexts (WHOQOL). This tools has existed for many years, is

translated into 75+ languages, and has good reliability and validity across cultures. The translated versions of WHOQOL-BREF and WHOQOL-100 are commonly used in the United States (WHOQOL Group, 1998).

Cognitive, motor, or sensory issues can affect leisure engagement, too. The following assessments specifically focus on one of more of these areas:

- Barth Time Construction (Barth, 1998) is a visual tool useful for adolescents through adults to categorize their allotted time spent per week using four colored categories: (1) Sleep, (2) ADLs, (3) Work, and (4) Leisure. This tool can be administered individually or with multiple persons at one time. The percentage of daily time per category is calculated. This is an older assessment but is useful for visual representation of life activity participation, specifically leisure.
- The Behavior Rating Inventory of Executive Functioning–Adult Version™ (Isquith et al., 2006) is a standardized rating scale that looks at 75 items with nine scales, two summary scales, and a global functioning scale. These scales inform self-regulation abilities with everyday functioning (including leisure). It includes client report forms and informant; that is, caregiver, report forms.
- The Sensory Profile™ 2 (Dunn, 2014) and the Adolescent/Adult Sensory Profile (Brown & Dunn, 2002) are assessments that measure processing of sensory information in daily life. The Sensory Profile 2 is appropriate for ages birth through 14 years, with an Infant version ages (birth through 6 months); Toddler version (ages 7 to 35 months); and Child, Short, and School Companion version (ages 3 to 14 years). The Adolescent/Adult Sensory Profile is appropriate for ages 11 to 65 years. Both evaluations are standardized and have strong reliability and validity measures. Scores are determined for the four quadrants of the Sensory Processing Framework: (1) Seeking/Seeker, (2) Avoiding/Avoider, (3) Sensitivity/Sensor, and (4) Registration/Bystander. Results indicate if sensory processing is interfering with functional performance of the individual.

Children spend much of their time in play. For them, play is synonymous with leisure. There are many play assessments, and some of them are targeted for specific age groups or certain aspects of play:

- Children's Assessment of Participation and Enjoyment & Preferences for Activities of Children (CAPE/PAC; King et al., 2004) is a two-part assessment for children's (ages 6 to 21 years) participation and enjoyment of certain leisure pursuits. It looks at diversity, intensity, and location (CAPE) and their preference for identified activities (PAC). Typically developing children have been reported to have adequate to excellent test–retest reliability (the *n* was small).
- Pediatric Volitional Questionnaire (Basu et al., 2008) is similar to the Volitional Questionnaire, but this tool assesses children (ages 2 to 12 years) on 14 behavioral items on a 4-point scale (Spontaneous, Involved, Hesitant, Passive) in three stages of volitional development (exploration, competency, achievement) to support leisure pursuits.
- Children's Leisure Assessment Scale (Rosenblum et al., 2010; Schreuer et al., 2014) assesses school-age children on six dimensions of nonobligatory activities: (1) Variety (which), (2) Frequency (how often), (3) Sociability (with whom), (4) Preference (how much [activity] is liked), (5) Time Consumption (invested time), and (6) Desired Activities (desired, but not currently undertaken). The tool was found to be reliable and valid. When children with and without disabilities were compared, effect of disability status limited participation and variety of leisure occupations the most, followed next by gender, with girls at most risk for limiting variety.
- The Preschool Activity Card Sort (Berg & LaVesser, 2006) measures parent report on the participation of children (ages 3 to 6 years) from photographic cards depicting typical play activities in seven domains: (1) Self-Care, (2) Community Mobility, (3) High Demand Leisure, (4) Low Demand Leisure, (5) Social Interaction, (6) Domestic Activities, and (7) Education. Results help to understand the occupational profile of a child through the parental report. The child's level of independence in participation or their length of time in participation is not the focus of this assessment. Test-retest and interrater reliability are excellent.

If you are uncertain which assessment might be appropriate for your client, consult references that annotate and index many assessments available for practitioner use (e.g., Asher, 2014). Or visit online database websites that are dedicated to housing information about assessments of a specific nature for various populations. These resources are highly informative and helpful for both students learning about assessment and seasoned occupational therapy practitioners who are looking for specific help in identifying an appropriate assessment of their client.

Barriers to Participation in Leisure Occupations for Individuals, Groups, and Populations

As discussed earlier in the chapter, leisure needs of opportunities, resources, and equipment each play an integral role in occupational engagement and leisure pursuit. Having a balance of the three is optimal for exploring leisure interests. An imbalance creates an environment in which barriers to exploration and participation in leisure activities exist.

This section explores three areas that are significant barriers to an individual's, group's, or population's ability to more fully engage in leisure pursuit: (1) stereotypes, (2) vocational influence, and (3) environmental press.

Stereotypes as a Barrier (Individual)

What if you really wanted to engage in a particular leisure occupation but were hesitant because you have a belief that "people like you don't do [that specific leisure occupation]"?

CASE EXAMPLE 13.2. Franco: Automobile Technician

You are working in a subacute inpatient hospital setting, and a new client, **Franco,** is put on your service after his open heart surgery 2 weeks ago. His anticipated length of stay is 4 to 6 weeks because of some preexisting conditions and a need to return home independently. Franco is 6 feet, 3 inches; 240 pounds; has an extremely muscular physique; and is tattooed from his wrists to his neck, with complete coverage of his chest, stomach, and back. Many tattoos are related to his motorcycle club. He works as a mechanic in a busy automobile dealership.

After a few weeks, it becomes clear that his healing has not been optimal and he will need to be non–weight bearing in his bilateral upper extremities for another few months. Although he will be headed home soon, he will not return to work for a little more time. In addition, he is unable to manage the weight of his Harley Davidson motorcycle, which is necessary to drive it. He asks his occupational therapy practitioner for suggestions to occupy his time at home now that he is extremely limited in his prior leisure choices.

Would you do it anyway, or would you abandon the idea? Would you try out for that team, play, or spot regardless of what others think? This is a good example of how a social ***stereotype***; that is, social perception, can influence what or when people or groups engage in various leisure pursuits. Stereotyping can occur across the lifespan and is a major factor that can prohibit engagement in an identified leisure occupation. Younger children might view a schoolmate as "weird" because of their learning disability and exclude them from recess activities. Older adults in an independent living community may choose to avoid the hallway of a particularly politically vocal resident because they always ask to join in whatever the planned activity is. It is the stereotype by the friends' group that prevents the school child and elder resident from participating in certain leisure occupations (see Case Example 13.2).

EXERCISE 13.5. Franco's Leisure

Read Case Example 13.2 and answer the following questions about Franco:

- What activities can you think of that would be enjoyable to him and still adhere to his precautions?
- Did you consider art-based activities? Why or why not?
- How would you begin the conversation about new leisure pursuit exploration?
- Do you think stereotyping would be a concern for Franco?

Consider the leisure activity of knitting. When thinking of a person who knits, an image of an older woman in a rocking chair with her cat by her side may come to mind. Elders are perceived to have more available time for leisure, and knitting is a quiet, solitary activity that does not require much other than working hands and some knowledge of stiches. Countless articles describe the health and societal benefits of knitting, and knitting is often reported to be a relaxing form of leisure. It takes little in terms of materials (equipment) and can be done almost anywhere (opportunities) for very little cost—usually just the yarn supply and knitting needles (resources). Pöllänen and Weissmann-Hanski (2020) reported that in modern society, the need to create things for living no longer exists; however, the desire to create things by hand remains strong, with a resurgence every few years. An investment in textile crafting has the power to raise overall contentment and quality of life for the individual through eudaimonic well-being, or the "doing, belonging, becoming, and being are expressed in crafting" (Pöllänen & Weissmann-Hanski, 2020, p. 350; see Case Example 13.3).

Additionally, knitting has become popular with men in prison. What makes knitting for the population of incarcerated men in prisons or detention centers unique? Accounting for equipment, opportunities, and resources, a main reason is that male individuals who are incarcerated or detained generally do not have any experience with knitting. Their exposure to the leisure pursuit of knitting (or other textile crafting) may be limited because of societal beliefs about male roles, gender norms, and forced-choice leisure across the lifespan.

However, by products from knitting while incarcerated are plentiful. Knitting relaxes the individual and brings a calmness to the prison atmosphere, even outside the knitting group. Communication between participants is improved, and knitting has even been linked to reduced recidivism rates (Wiltenburg, 2012). In the 1943 "A Theory of Human Motivation," Abraham Maslow spoke of the highest level of human development as *self-actualization,* or the realization of one's potential, stating, "What a man *can* be, he *must* be" (cited in Green, n.d., para. 34 of "II. The Basic Needs"). Through knitting, the prison inmates can see their potential, something that may not have ever been revealed to them through other lifetime activities.

Another benefit for this group is in societal giveback. The actual product created is representative of the person who made it, and how the product is used carries meaning, too. Often, group knitting projects like those found in prisons have a purpose that raises the meaning of the completed activity. Programs like Knitting Behind Bars allows inmates to give of themselves in their work product. Completed blankets may go

CASE EXAMPLE 13.3. Tom: Athlete and Knitter

Tom Daley, 27, a British diver and gold medalist, was frequently spotted in the stands at the Olympic pool knitting in his downtime during the 2020 Summer Olympics Games in Tokyo (hosted in 2021 as a result of the COVID-19 pandemic; Daley, 2021a). The @madewithlovebytomdaley Olympic Cardigan Reveal! (Daley 2021b) on Instagram gained 755,000 likes across the globe and is an example of how one man's individual passion for leisure knitting can inspire an image of one who knits to include many types of people. As an athlete and advocate of the LGBTQ+ community, Daley is breaking down the stereotype of one who knits.

to a local neonatal intensive care unit, or small sweaters can be donated to agencies like Children of the Night, a federal program to assist victims of child prostitution. Giving back equates to reparation for their crimes.

Vocational Influence as a Barrier (Group)

Vocations are personal desires toward a specific type of career or employment field. As humans, we often define ourselves by the kinds of vocations we are drawn to. Vocations help to meet the humanistic need for interpersonal relationships, and employment in chosen fields is often personally fulfilling and provides a satisfaction beyond just financial rewards. Diversity in vocational pursuits leads to a larger functioning of society and accomplishment of tasks for the whole versus the individual. ***Occupational balance*** (also called *work–life balance*) occurs when there is a positive relationship between one's work and other areas of one's life that lead to a positive outcome. Conversely, ***occupational imbalance*** occurs when there is a lack of balance between work and other areas of one's life that leads to unhappiness and potentially unhealthy outcomes. Careers or employment that sustains a good work–life balance is related to good health outcomes; conversely, lack of good employment is detrimental to health outcomes (Isaacs, 2016; Schalock et al., 2010). Heavy vocational demands (capabilities), rigid agency requirements (flexibility), and gender inequality can contribute to an imbalance of work and life tasks and can lead to life dissatisfaction (Hobson, 2014). These are barriers to the "life" part of work–life balance and prohibit full engagement in leisure pursuits.

Work–life imbalance can occur across the lifespan. The influence of agency presses the worker role. For example, in school-age children, educational work is prioritized. Often, they have only weekends or evenings to engage in chosen leisure, and that is after they have completed their homework and other obligated tasks. An example of poor work–life balance in the overscheduled teen is evident in their struggle to meet societal expectations for extracurricular activities, volunteering, and part-time employment if they want to gain acceptance into a prestigious college. Where is leisure for pleasure? Unfortunately, this is a common phenomenon in today's competitive society.

For most adults, paid employment takes the lion's share of time so they can meet financial obligations or provide for themselves and others. When someone is not working, they theoretically can engage in leisure, but there still must be consideration for opportunities, resources, and equipment. In modern society, there is a mass market for leisure advertisement. Television, radio, and Internet bombard us, touting the "perfect" vacation or need for escape. These often come with hefty price tags, making them desirable but unreachable for many, especially those in lower socioeconomic strata. These folks are the ones who may work two jobs or longer hours to afford such leisure (resources and equipment), and it is the working that proves the biggest barrier to specific leisure pursuits (opportunities). Again, socioeconomic status and stratum are big influencers to leisure choice and engagement.

As clients transition throughout the lifespan, occupational therapy has a unique role to address dysfunction in leisure

CASE EXAMPLE 13.4. David: Retired CEO

David retired from his top-tiered chief executive officer role at a Fortune 100 company 3 years ago. Two years before retiring, he and his wife of 35 years divorced at her request. After retiring, David gained 75 pounds; he reports low mood and has some medical issues (obesity and high blood pressure, possible depression). His primary physician referred him to a mental health counselor to address mood-related concerns. His doctor also prescribed outpatient occupational therapy to address his maladaptive role shift and lack of occupational engagement after retiring.

attainment. How can this be more fully understood by society at large? What steps would the profession need to take to assure reimbursement for occupational therapy services that address leisure engagement?

EXERCISE 13.6. David's Occupational Imbalance

Referring to Case Example 13.4, answer the following questions about David:

- Why do you think David is experiencing such occupational imbalance?
- What do you think are David's most critical areas of occupational disruption?
- What types of occupational therapy assessments might be appropriate for this case?
- What is your rationale for choosing these assessments?
- How will these assessments inform goals and a plan of care?

Environmental Press as a Barrier (Population)

Leisure activity choice is personal; reliant on opportunities, resources, and equipment; and highly dependent on environmental context. In March 2020, the United States entered a global shutdown because of spread of COVID-19. In a weekend, the population of most major cities were subject to stay-at-home orders that limited any activity outside of one's dwelling. As the virus spread, ***environmental press*** (i.e., the external pressures that the environment places on the individual) of the now pandemic-level situation caused people to drastically alter how they went about most daily activities; leisure pursuits were no exception. "Occupational disruption" was a term aptly applied to our everyday lives reimagined through the lens of a public health crisis. Occupational therapy practitioners emerged as essential personnel to help persons and, by association, the entire population dealing with COVID-19 restrictions deal with the new "normal" occupations of living and leisure (Whitney & Walsh, 2020). Dealing with occupational disruption changed us as a population and engendered new environmental contexts for education, work, home, and leisure.

In 2020, individuals were forced to function in vastly different ways than before the pandemic for school, work, daily life, and leisure. Schools shifted to virtual platforms, and bedrooms became classrooms. Telecommuting was not an option for many industries before 2020, but many of them were able to harness Internet-based platforms like Zoom® or Microsoft Teams® to continue workplace productivity. Unfortunately, not all industries could go virtual. There was increased demand for sanitizing and home-based products, and there were supply chain issues, proving that pandemic heroes are also truck drivers and grocery workers. COVID-19 brought about serious occupational disruption for nearly everyone.

Later in 2020, businesses and marketplace industries had to pivot to remain viable, even with a governmental subsidy. Work and vocational activities either ramped up, attempting to manage virus exposure, operating costs, and employees, or took a serious decline as we headed into a period of marked unemployment with layoffs necessary for some businesses. This dramatic environmental press caused significant changes to how people were employed and subsequently met their financial obligations like rent, mortgage, food bills, utilities, and leisure money. Changes in the work environment also affected home life and the leisure environment. In some cases, leisure time was increased but without the opportunity to engage in typical leisure activities. For others, leisure time was diminished because working from home did not provide the typical "workday" boundaries.

As a society, we became innovative. Curbside pickup was a concept yet to be applied (or even considered) for many restaurants and dining establishments before the pandemic. Outdoor dining was instituted even in subfreezing temperatures, with "dining bubbles" made from heavy plastic sheeting and portable heaters. Many who worked during the pandemic conditions had job expectations changed or were forced to leave their job because they were unable to manage the new demands. Work in pandemic times was dramatically different. Leisure activities also changed as the pandemic limited opportunities to socialize with others and typical activities, like going to the movies, were not available.

There were some benefits to the altered work expectations. With the unfortunate loss of employment and a need to remain at home during lockdown, society saw a surge in leisure type activities: crafting groups online, stoop barbecues with neighbors, bread making and other types of baking, and eventual outdoor dining. When obligatory work was removed, many found their time occupied by things they "discovered" they like to do or "hadn't had the time" to engage in before. Occupational disruption created space for leisure exploration or engagement to a much larger degree than before the pandemic. Greater opportunities for leisure were only limited by the resources and equipment available to supply the pursuit of leisure activity choices, returning to the consideration of economic status and stratum of the individual or family during this time.

Conversely, some individuals had obligatory work activities that ramped way up during lockdown. These folks lost commuting time but gained many more hours of daily work and more responsibilities expected of them to keep their industry afloat. They experienced, and are still experiencing, great workplace stress. With longer hours and more responsibilities, they experienced a blurring of work–home distinction, when work was now in their home and existed almost 24/7. Long hours plus less physical activity equals an opportunity for the decline of overall health. Increased weight during 2020 was a real thing for many people and was named "the COVID 10 [or 20 or 25]" in reference to the amount of extra pounds gained. Less active, overworked people had to be careful to balance their obligatory and nonobligatory activities and increase physical activities lest they allow a dangerous opportunity for decline of overall health outcomes over time.

Leisure deprivation occurred during the pandemic and continues to affect leisure choice from prepandemic times.

CASE EXAMPLE 13.5. Dr. Patel: College Professor

Dr. Patel is an associate professor at a midsized urban university. She teaches in a graduate health science professional program. On Thursday, March 12, 2020, in Week 8 of the spring semester, Dr. Patel got word that her university was going virtual the following Monday. She had exactly 3 days to prep her classes for the rest of the semester and familiarize herself with this new virtual meeting technology called Zoom. All of her hands-on laboratory work needed to shift to virtual engagement, and it would be impossible to assess clinical skills through video.

She spent many hours in the next few months crafting meaningful experiences for her students. She reported that although she no longer had a commute, she found herself seated in front of her screen for 8 to 10 hours a day (and some time on the weekend days, too) preparing her classes and having virtual meetings with her colleagues and administration. In addition, student requests for one-on-one meetings skyrocketed because they needed connection with their instructor. Dr. Patel's scholarship writing halted, she began to decline "virtual happy hours" with peers and friends, and she no longer was leisure reading.

Personal leisure time is critical for maintaining a balance of obligatory and nonobligatory activities. Consider that, for many people, "old" leisure choices (prepandemic) may have been computer based, such as social media scrolling, Internet gaming, or virtual shopping. For quite a few months after March 2020, everyday activities and tasks were done online: Groceries and other household items were bought online, Internet banking was done to pay the bills, doctor appointments were via telehealth, and the like. The paradox is that when planning leisure, that was done online, too.

Many did not want to watch television or movies or participate on social media platforms because they had already been at a screen for 8-plus hours for obligatory work (Lovink, 2020). ***Zoom fatigue*** was a term that had been defined but was not a mainstay in the American vernacular until after March 2020. It refers to the feeling of exhaustion that one gets after many virtual meetings. Social groups that could not meet in person attempted to meet virtually, which posed tremendous problems for younger children who, developmentally, do not have long attention spans. Virtual education did not keep pace well because of technology access and implementation difficulties, home distractions, and boredom; so many hours in front of a computer were visually and cognitively taxing; and it was developmentally inappropriate for many age groups. Additionally, virtual education was not necessarily appropriate for all age groups. Girl Scout troop leaders reported that keeping 20 Girl Scouts ages 6 to 8 years old engaged in an evening virtual badge activity in later spring that year was nearly impossible (C. Besseler, personal communication, May 4, 2020). At the time of publication, Zoom fatigue is still a problem for some, while others prefer the flexibility of working from home. Even as we have emerged from some aspects of the pandemic, some children are struggling to catch up with skills that were affected during virtual education and a lack of opportunities to develop socialization skills (see Case Example 13.5).

EXERCISE 13.7. Work–Life Balance

Consider these questions:

- What is the effect of Zoom fatigue on workplace and personal relationships?
- What are some assessments that could be helpful for improving work–life balance?
- What are two interventions for leisure deprivation that would be appropriate for Dr. Patel in Case Example 13.5?
- How could prolonged work affect Dr. Patel's health outcomes?

Leisure Interventions for Health Promotion and Prevention of Secondary Health Issues

Throughout this chapter, the focus has been on discovering the role that leisure occupations hold in our lives. By understanding typical development and when impairment or disability enters the picture, the occupational therapy practitioner can efficiently and holistically plan treatment and interventions using a client-centered approach. Intervention becomes a means to independence, and by addressing opportunities, resources, and equipment needs (or adaptations), the practitioner can more fully engage clients in meaningful occupations to influence the state of their own health, as Mary Reilly (1962) spoke of at the beginning of this chapter.

Developing and maintaining social relationships, a sense of inclusion, and perceived social achievements (friends, success, advancement) are critical to experience throughout the lifespan for a high quality of life. Leisure deprivation not only suppresses physical wellness but also suppresses emotional and social well-being. Children and adolescents may avoid certain leisure activities or limit themselves because of a fear of failure. The occupational therapy practitioner should focus on interventions that offer opportunities to build skills and on low-risk challenges to build confidence and allow for self-perceived successes. Doing so will translate into the client's improved sense of well-being and feelings that they are a functioning member of society. Adults may experience an imbalance in their time or ability to be available for leisure pursuits from a variety of sources, such as work, family pressures, financial hardships, or disability status. All can impair emotional well-being through lack of engagement, deprivation, and isolation as a result of these conditions.

An example of leisure intervention can be seen in this example: With the role shift to "new mother," a person may not have the same resources to continue to engage in running, a leisure activity of choice. They may not have a babysitter at their disposal, or they may not fit in the same running sneakers because pregnancy has caused their foot to spread, making their shoes too tight. Without the available safety for their child, such as a sitter, or the proper equipment, like well-fitting sneakers, the leisure occupation of running loses its meaningfulness. The occupational therapy practitioner can offer interventions like a new time configuration for the activity, adapting the stroller so baby can accompany the running mother, or a discussion about running in different footwear. Without alternatives, the new mom may keep her focus on daily housekeeping (an increased obligatory activity), limiting leisure and pleasurable activities. Over time and without intervention, the mother can become lethargic, fatigued, and irritable, which undoubtedly will negatively affect her relationship with baby, family, and social circles.

By participating in meaningful leisure, individuals can self-actualize and increase their overall quality-of-life satisfaction. Elders who use leisure pursuits in the transition from work to retirement have improved "worth, purpose, or perception of usefulness and status" (Heaven et al., 2013, p. 274). Skillfully exploring leisure occupations can have unanticipated health benefits, too, such as improved cognition, stress relief, improved mental health status, and optimal aging, and they can bring enjoyment to the participant (Heaven et al., 2013; Mihaila et al., 2020; Thomson et al., 2003).

Any given day has only 24 hours. How an individual chooses to or is required to fill those hours defines their state of homeostasis. When a balance of obligatory and nonobligatory activities or life needs is spread over those hours, a state of satisfaction is generally reported by the individual. By using assessments like the Barth Time Construction (Barth, 1998), or the Life Balance Inventory (Matuska, 2009), a person can see where and when obligatory activities or requirements may dominate. An imbalance that leaves little leisure creates a high-stress state. Humans cannot operate indefinitely in a high-stress state without our bodies breaking down and opening the door to various diseases and sick conditions. Overwork reduces the body's immunity. Lack of sleep or poor-quality sleep results in chronic fatigue. Sleep is when our bodies heal, and if we are robbed of the precious time of rest, systems remain inflamed, are slow to recover, or cannot function at optimum performance. We gain weight, become sedentary, and age more quickly. Over time, the imbalance of obligatory and nonobligatory time brings on secondary health issues like diabetes, cardiovascular disease, and vision changes. One can certainly see how the American proverb "all work and no play make Jack a dull boy" (cited at the chapter's inception) has real meaning, even today.

An active, stress-free lifestyle is one that supports and promotes health. Stults-Kolehmainen and Sinha (2013) performed a systematic search of scholarly evidence and consistently found that with increased stressors, physical activity declined significantly. Prevention of secondary health issues resulting from stress and lack of activity is critical for reducing health care dollars spent in one's lifetime.

The occupational therapy practitioner has expertise in evaluation, assessment, intervention, and implementation of plans of care that address leisure exploration and attainment. Leisure interventions can rebalance time configurations; improve skills, abilities, and capacity; or adapt supplies and craft new tools to achieve leisure participation goals.

EXERCISE 13.8. Recalling Client Leisure Pursuits

Think about past clients you have encountered during your schooling or in your occupational therapy practice:

- How was leisure brought into the evaluation conversation and then through the intervention phase of treatment (if appropriate)?
- Can you recall how engagement in leisure was supported?
- Were there barriers to fully participate in leisure pursuits?
- Are you more comfortable with examples of leisure across the lifespan after reading this chapter?
- If leisure was not addressed, how might you have handled the situation differently?

Summary

This chapter summarizes leisure pursuits and the engagement of nonobligatory activity choices across the lifespan and effects of leisure on life satisfaction and health outcomes. Although often thought of secondarily, the importance of leisure choice and engagement in an individual's life should not be underestimated. Stressors can impair one's development of self, belonging, and self-actualization, which are derived from leisure pursuits.

Leisure must be attended to. Where, how, and when we engage in leisure is very personal. It requires opportunities, resources, and equipment for maximal engagement. An imbalance in leisure needs leads to a lack of exploration and low participation. Consideration of socioeconomic status and stratum is essential for parity in leisure engagement, limiting a divide resulting from financial means. For these reasons, community supports and investments are crucial, especially for successful inclusion of persons with disabilities into leisure and social settings.

Our clients are whole beings, rich with needs for recovery or development that absolutely includes leisure exploration and engagement. It is important for occupational therapy practitioners to articulate their expertise in areas of leisure assessment and intervention. Development of leisure-incorporated intervention leads to improved health outcomes and must be reimbursed by all payers of occupational therapy services. In addition, it is imperative for the client-centered, evidence-based profession of occupational therapy that every practitioner advocate the need for leisure to be addressed more strongly in daily interventions and more broadly in larger health promotion policy developments (Heaven et al., 2013).

References

Abbott, S., & McConkey, R. (2006). The barriers to social inclusion as perceived by people with intellectual disabilities. *Journal of Intellectual Disability, 10*(3), 275–287. https://doi.org/10.1177/1744629506067618

Alma, M. A., van der Mei, S. F., Melis-Dankers, M. J. M., van Tilburg, T. G., Groothoff, J. W., & Suurmeijer, T. P. (2011). Participation of the elderly after vision loss. *Disability and Rehabilitation, 33*(1), 63–72. https://doi.org/10.3109/09638288.2010.488711

American Occupational Therapy Association. (2020). Occupational therapy practice framework: Domain and process (4th ed.). *American Journal of Occupational Therapy, 74*(Suppl. 2), Article 7412410010. https://doi.org/10.5014/ajot.2020.74S2001

Angell, A. M., Goodman, L., Walker, H. R., McDonald, K. E., Kraus, L. E., Elms, E. H. J., . . . Hammel, J. (2020). "Starting to live a life": Understanding full participation for people with disabilities after institutionalization. *American Journal of Occupational Therapy, 74*(4), Article 7404205030. https://doi.org/10.5014/ajot.2020.038489

Asher, I. E. (Ed.). (2014). *Asher's occupational therapy assessment tools: An annotated index* (4th ed). AOTA Press.

Badia, M., Orgaz, M. B., Verdugo, M. Á., Ullán, A. M., & Martínez, M. (2013). Relationships between leisure participation and quality of life of people with developmental disabilities. *Journal of Applied Research in Intellectual Disabilities, 26*(6), 533–545. https://doi.org/10.1111/jar.12052

Barth, T. (1998). The Barth Time Construction. In B. Hemphill (Ed.) *Mental health assessment in occupation therapy: An integrative approach to the evaluative process* (pp. 117–129). Slack.

Basu, S., Kafkes, A., Schatz, R., Kiraly, A., & Kielhofner, G. (2008). *Pediatric Volitional Questionnaire Version 2.1*. University of Illinois at Chicago.

Baum, C., & Edwards, D. (2008). *Activity Card Sort* (2nd ed.). AOTA Press.

Berg, C., & LaVesser, P. (2006). The Preschool Activity Card Sort. *OTJR: Occupation, Participation and Health, 26*(4), 143–151. https://doi.org/10.1177/153944920602600404

Besio, S. (2022). The need for play for the sake of play. In S. Besio, D. Bulgarelli, & V. Stancheva-Popkostadinova (Eds.), *Play development in children with disabilities* (pp. 9–52). De Gruyter Open Poland. https://doi.org/10.1515/9783110522143

Brown, C., & Dunn, W. (2002). *Adolescent/Adult Sensory Profile*. NCS Pearson.

Bureau of Labor Statistics. (2015, June 29). *Time spent in leisure activities in 2019, by gender, age, and educational attainment*. TED: The Economics Daily. https://www.bls.gov/opub/ted/2015/time-spent-in-leisure-activities-in-2014-by-gender-age-and-educational-attainment.htm?view_full

Centers for Disease Control and Prevention. (n.d.). *Milestone checklist*. https://www.cdc.gov/ncbddd/actearly/pdf/checklists/Checklists-with-Tips_Reader_508.pdf

Chung, Y. M., Lou, S. L., Tsai, P. Z., & Wang, M. C. (2019). The efficacy of respiratory regulation on parasympathetic nervous system appraised by heart rate variability. *Journal of Medical and Biological Engineering, 39*(6), 960–966. https://doi.org/10.1007/s40846-019-00472-z

Csikszentmihalyi, M. (2008). *Flow: The psychology of optimal experience*. Harper Perennial Modern Classics.

Daley, T. [@madewithlovebytomdaley]. (2021a, August 7). *Knitting my way to Olympic medal number 4! I can't believe it! Thanks for all your support and I am* [Photographs]. Instagram. https://www.instagram.com/p/CSRMHfLDAbr/

Daley, T. [@madewithlovebytomdaley]. (2021b, August 4). *Olympic cardigan reveal!* JPGB (fire emoji, ball of yarn emoji). [Video]. Instagram. https://www.instagram.com/p/CSLEbbuAh4e/

de las Heras, C. G., Geist, R., Kielhofner, G., & Li, L. (2007). *The Volitional Questionnaire (version 4.1)*. The University of Illinois at Chicago.

Dunn, W. (2014). *Sensory Profile™ 2*. NCS Pearson.

Evans, S., Gately, C., Huxley, P., Smith, A., & Banerjee, S. (2005). Assessment of quality of life in later life: Development and validation of the QuiLL. *Quality of Life Research, 14,* 1291–1300. https://doi.org/10.1007/s11136-004-5532-y

Freudenberger, H., & Richelson, G. (1980). *Burn-out: The high cost of high achievement. What it is and how to survive it*. Bantam Books.

Green, C. D. (n.d.). *A theory of human motivation [by] A. H. Maslow (1943)*, originally published in *Psychological Review, 50*[4], 370–396. Classics in the History of Psychology. http://psychclassics.yorku.ca/Maslow/motivation.htm

Heaven, B., Brown, L. J. E., White, M., Errington, L., Mathers, J. C., & Moffatt, S. (2013). Supporting well-being in retirement through meaningful social roles: Systematic review of interventional studies. *The Milbank Quarterly, 91*(2), 222–287. https://doi.org/10.1111/milq.12013

Hobson, B. (2014). *Worklife balance: The agency & capabilities gap*. Oxford University Press.

Isaacs, D. (2016). Work–life balance [Editorial]. *Journal of Paediatrics and Child Health, 52*(1), 5–6, https://doi.org/10.1111/jpc.13110

Isquith, P. K., Roth, R. M., Gioia, G. A., & PAR Staff. (2006). *The Behavior Rating Inventory of Executive Functioning—Adult Version™ (BRIEF-A™) interpretive report*. Psychological Assessment Services.

Jänig, W. (2006). *The integrative action of the autonomic nervous system: Neurobiology of homeostasis*. Cambridge University Press.

Joshanloo, M. (2018). Optimal human functioning around the world: A new index of eudaimonic well-being in 166 nations. *British Journal of Psychology, 109*(4), 637–655, https://doi:10.1111/bjop.12316

King, G. A., King, S., Rosenbaum, P., Kertoy, M., Law, M., & Hurley, P. (2004). *CAPE/PAC manual: Children's Assessment of Participation and Enjoyment & Preferences for Activities of Children*. PsychCorp.

Kuykendall, L., Lie, X., Zhu, Z., & Hu, X. (2021). Leisure choices and employee well-being: Comparing need fulfillment and well-being during TV and other leisure activities. *Applied Psychology: Health and Well-Being, 12*(2), 532–558. https://doi.org/10.1111/aphw.12196

Kuykendall, L., Tay, L., & Ng, V. (2015). Leisure engagement and subjective well-being: A meta-analysis. *Psychological Bulletin, 14*(2), 364–403. https://doi.org/10.1037/a0038508

Law, M. (2002). Participation in the occupations of everyday life. *American Journal of Occupational Therapy, 56*(6), 640–649. https://doi.org/10.5014.ajot.56.6.640

Law, M., Baptiste, S., Carswell, A., McColl, M., Polatajko, H., & Pollock, N. (2019). *Canadian Occupational Performance Measure* (5th ed., rev.). COPM, Inc.

Lovink, G. (2020, November 2). The anatomy of Zoom fatigue. *Eurozine*. https://www.eurozine.com/the-anatomy-of-zoom-fatigue/

Matuska, K. (2009). *Life Balance Inventory*. http://minerva.stkate.edu/LBI.nsf

Meyer, A. (1922). The philosophy of occupation therapy. *Archives of Occupational Therapy, 1*(1), 1–10.

Mihaila, I., Handen, B., Christian, B. T., & Hartley, S. L. (2020). Leisure activity in middle-aged adults with Down syndrome: Initiators, social partners, settings and barriers. *Journal of Applied Research in Intellectual Disabilities, 33*(5), 865–875. https://doi:10.111/jar.12706

Parham, D., & Fazio, L. (2008). *Play in occupational therapy for children* (2nd ed.). Mosby/Elsevier.

Perzynski, A. T. (2006). Disengagement theory. In L. S. Noelker, K. Rockwood, & R. L. Sprott (Eds.), *The encyclopedia of aging: A comprehensive resource in gerontology and geriatrics* (4th ed., pp. 321–322). Springer Publishing.

Pitt, H., Thomas, S. L., Watson, J., Shuttleworth, R., Murfitt, K., & Balandin, S. (2020). Weighing up the risks and benefits of community gambling venues as recreational spaces for people with lifelong disability. *BMC Public Health, 20,* Article 916. https://doi.org/10.1186/s12889-020-08654-0

Pöllänen, S. H., & Weissmann-Hanski, M. (2020). Hand-made well-being: Textile crafts as a source of eudaimonic well-being. *Journal of Leisure Research*, 51(3), 348–365. https://doi.org/10.1080/00222216.2019.1688738

Reilly, M. (1962). Occupational therapy can be one of the great ideas of 20th century medicine. The 1961 Eleanor Clarke Slagle Lecture. *American Journal of Occupational Therapy, 16*(1), 1–9.

Rivera-Torres, S., Mpofu, E., Keller, M. J., & Ingman, S. (2021). Older adult's mental health through leisure activities during COVID-19: A scoping review. *Gerontology and Geriatric Medicine, 7*. https://doi.org/10.1177/23337214211036776

Rogers, K. (Ed.). (2012). *The endocrine system*. Britannica Educational Publishing.

Rosenblum, S., Sachs, D., & Schreuer, N. (2010). Reliability and validity of the Children's Leisure Assessment Scale. *American Journal of Occupational Therapy, 64*(4), 633–641. https://doi.org/10.5014/ajot.2010.08173

Schalock, R. L., Borthwick-Duffy, S. A., Bradley, V. J., Buntinx, W. H. E., Coulter, D. L., Craig, E. M., . . . Yeager, M. H. (2010). *Intellectual disability: Diagnosis, classification and systems of support* (11th ed.). American Association on Intellectual and Developmental Disabilities.

Schreuer, N., Sachs, D., & Rosenblum, S. (2014). Participation in leisure activities: Differences between children with and without physical disabilities. *Research in Developmental Disabilities, 35*(1), 223–233. https://doi.org/10.1016/j.ridd.2013.10.001

Stults-Kolehmainen, M. A., & Sinha, R. (2013). The effects of stress on physical activity and exercise. *Sports Medicine, 44,* 81–121. https://doi.org/10.1007/s40279-013-0090-5

Taylor, R. (2020). *The intentional relationship: Occupational therapy and the use of self* (2nd ed.). F. A. Davis.

Thomson, H., Kearns, A., & Petticrew, M. (2003). Assessing the health impact of local amenities: A qualitative study of contrasting experience of local swimming pool and leisure provision in two areas of Glasgow. *Journal of Epidemiology & Community Health, 57,* 663–667. https://doi.org/10.1136/jech.57.9.663

Ullenhag, A., Granlund, M., Almqvist, L., & Krumline-Sundholm, L. (2020). A strength-based intervention to increase participation in leisure activities in children with neuropsychiatric disabilities: A pilot study. *Occupational Therapy International, 2020,* Article 1358707. https://doi.org/10.1155/2020/1358707

von Humboldt, S., Mendoza-Ruvalcaba, N. M., Arias-Merino, E. D., Costa, A., Cabras, E., Low, G., & Leal, I. (2020). Smart technology and the meaning in life of older adults during the Covid-19 public health emergency period: A cross-cultural qualitative study. *International Review of Psychiatry, 32*(7–8), 713–722. https://doi.org/10.1080/09540261.2020.1810643

Whitney, R. V., & Walsh, W. E. (2020, May). Occupational therapy's role in times of disaster: Addressing periods of occupational disruption. *OT Practice, 25*(5), Article CEA0520.

WHOQOL Group. (1998). The World Health Organization Quality of Life assessment (WHOQOL): Development and general psychometric properties. *Social Science & Medicine, 46*(12), 1569–1585. https://doi.org/10.1016/S0277-9536(98)00009-4

World Health Organization. (2001). *International classification of functioning, disability and health*.

Xbox [@xbox]. (2018, September 5). *Introducing a more inclusive way to play. The #Xbox Adaptive #Controller is available now.* [Photograph]. Instagram. https://www.instagram.com/p/BnXICZNAGik/

Xbox. (2021). *Gaming for everyone*. Microsoft Xbox. https://www.xbox.com/en-US/community/player-spotlight/spencer

14

Work Occupations

JEFF SNODGRASS, PhD, MPH, OTR, FAOTA,
AND JYOTHI GUPTA, PhD, OTR/L, FAOTA

CHAPTER HIGHLIGHTS

- History and trends in work, workers, and the workplace
- Policy, regulations, and programming in the workplace
- Development of worker role and identity
- Role of occupational therapy in the workplace

KEY TERMS AND CONCEPTS

• Americans with Disabilities Act of 1990 • contingent workforce • Employee Retirement Income Security Act of 1974 • engaged worker • Equal Employment Opportunity Commission • ergonomics • Fair Labor Standards Act of 1938 • Family and Medical Leave Act of 1993 • functional capacity evaluation • hybrid work • injury prevention • Job Accommodation Network • job analysis • knowledge workers • Occupational Information Network • Occupational Safety and Health Administration • remote work • sheltered workshop • supported employment • telecommuting • Ticket to Work Program • transition services • transitional employment services • work • work conditioning • work hardening • work-related stress • workers' compensation

Introduction

An updated chapter on ***work*** occupations, defined as employment with financial remuneration, cannot ignore the deep disruptions to the very nature of work and workplaces wrought by the SARS-CoV-2 virus (COVID-19) pandemic (Bennett, 2021; Kaushik & Guleria, 2020). Its impact was felt across the globe as a collective existential crisis that led many people to examine their values, beliefs, and life priorities and question the meaning and purpose of work (Schwab, 2021). Work, its related routines, and sometimes its roles were disrupted. One certainty is that the role of work in the context of everyday living has altered deeply, and many occupations will not return to their prepandemic conditions.

Most people spend a considerable part of their lives, nearly 90,000 hours, at work. It is not surprising that in a society that places a high premium on productivity, Americans appear to live to work (Okulicz-Kozaryn, 2010) and, living in a "no-vacation nation" (Maye, 2019), take minimal time off from work. Americans' attitudes toward work appear to have shifted postpandemic as workers question the importance of work in their lives; its relation to health, relationships, and work–life balance; and how, with whom, and where they spend their time. In the past year, 1 in 5 workers in the United States has changed careers (Schwab, 2021). For the first time in recent memory, workers are critically evaluating the importance and role of work in their lives relative to other occupations.

The obvious benefits of work are that it is a source of income to provide for people's needs, shapes their identity, uses their capabilities in a variety of ways, and challenges and promotes growth, to mention a few. The dynamic new economy requires workers who are engaged in and passionate about their work.

However, 87.7% of American workers do not have a passion for their work (Hagel et al., 2014). Moreover, only 36% of workers are engaged at work; this means that 64% of workers are disengaged, which costs the United States nearly $350 billion in losses per year as a result of lost productivity (Pendell, 2022). An ***engaged worker*** is one who is enthusiastic and highly involved in their work and workplace. In the early 2020s, the percentage of engaged workers reached an all-time high of 38%, and the level of engagement remained near this level (36%) until the early half of 2021 (Pendell, 2022). This level of engagement is remarkable, given that the pandemic meant that workers had to contend with major life disruptions. The pandemic experience did, however, make explicit, in particular to highly educated and professional American workers, the depth of their unhappiness with the structure of workplaces (Lipman, 2021; Schwab, 2021).

Workers experience a great deal of work-related stress, which leads to billions of dollars lost, a lack of productivity, and increased injuries and health care costs (Michie, 2002; National Institute for Occupational Safety and Health [NIOSH], 2017). ***Work-related stress*** is the harmful physical and emotional responses that can happen when there is a conflict between job demands on the employee and the amount of control an employee has over meeting these demands. In general, the combination of high demands in a job and a low amount of control over the situation can lead to stress (Teasdale, 2006). Occupational therapy can influence the well-being of workers and workplaces, and work and industry is one of occupational therapy's areas of practice (American Occupational Therapy Association [AOTA], 2021). During the pandemic, nearly 50% of workers with advanced degrees worked remotely, whereas 90% of those with high school diplomas had to report to a workplace (Lipman, 2021). Stress, anxiety, and decline in mental health have been reported among workers in both groups as a result of stressors such as social isolation, fear of exposure to the virus, job insecurity, suspension of work, and an uncertain future (Giorgi et al., 2020). Occupational therapy should take the lead on behavioral health in the workplace.

In this chapter, we consider a broad overview of work as a central occupation, important work policies and programs, and the various roles that occupational therapy fills in this area of practice.

History and Trends in Work, Workers, and the Workplace

Work has a high value in most societies. It is seen as integral to people's lives, contributing to their identity and self-efficacy (Gupta & Sabata, 2012; Harpaz & Fu, 2002). Article 23 of the United Nations' (1948) Universal Declaration of Human Rights states that work is a basic human right; it confers dignity on the individual and is a means to self-sufficiency, self-efficacy, and being a productive member of society, and it contributes to the overall economy. Kantartzis and Molineux (2011) attributed the centrality of work, and the unquestioned belief in its inherent positive influence on one's identity and health, to the Protestant work ethic of many Western societies. Occupational therapy also subscribes to this view of work, although productivity is viewed as a continuum across the life span, ranging from conventional paid employment to volunteerism (AOTA, 2020). In fact, the profession's historical roots in moral treatment make clear its intent "to replace brutality with kindness and idleness with occupation" (Gordon, 2009, p. 203). In other words, the profession values productive occupation of time for its positive influences on the health and well-being of individuals and society.

The nature and world of work have changed considerably since occupational therapy's beginnings. The late 19th century saw the rise of mechanization and the beginning of mass production of goods in the United States. This era changed not only the way work was done but also the meaning of work to the worker. Before this, skilled craftspeople, often working from their homes, had the satisfaction of and pride in creating a product from start to finish. In the manufacturing assembly line, work was broken down into smaller tasks, with each worker contributing in a small way to the larger whole. This breakdown of production to its component tasks meant that work became monotonous, repetitive in nature, and faster paced, and the worker was removed from the final outcome of production (Meyer, 2004).

Modern work also compartmentalized people's daily routines and habits in spatial and temporal terms, ushering in the notions of schedules, planners, and deadlines (Larson & Zemke, 2003). Workplaces demanded increased efficiency and productivity from workers, sometimes at the cost of worker health and safety. By the late 20th century, manufacturing accounted for about 30% of gross domestic product, and that percentage has steadily declined as more manufacturing has been outsourced (Glandrea & Sprague, 2017). Alongside these trends, workplace safety issues and worker activism propelled legislation aimed at equity and nondiscrimination in the workplace. The Equal Employment Opportunity Commission (EEOC) and the field of occupational safety and health came into existence as a result (Occupational Safety and Health Administration [OSHA], 2020).

More recently, two major forces that have transformed the economy and employment are globalization and technology. After the shift of manufacturing to overseas, anxiety over outsourcing of jobs to nations with cheaper labor costs was uppermost in the minds of workers in advanced industrialized countries. The nostalgia over the glory days of manufacturing was coupled with concern for an unemployed workforce that does not have the skills to meet the demands of jobs in the new digital economy. Blue-collar factory jobs placed a lot of physical demands on workers but did not require a college education or sophisticated training. These jobs are being replaced in large part by "pink-collar" service sector jobs, performed by a largely female workforce, with limited to no benefits, less job security, and lower wages. Technology has changed the way goods are manufactured, and in the 1970s spawned the Information Age that continues to the present. The management of information and information systems is an industry that demands white-collar workers, whom Drucker (1999) termed ***knowledge workers.*** Information is being efficiently packaged with minimal use of materials; thus, workers are manipulating information more than materials. These jobs differ from manufacturing because the demands on the worker are no longer physical but largely cognitive and psychosocial in nature. This is the future of work in advanced economies (Esmaeilian et al., 2016; Hausmann, 2013).

Technology and global connectedness have altered work and workplaces such that anything that can be digitized can be outsourced, and a workday does not need to end, because work can go on around the globe 24 hours a day. This requires workers to be competent in teamwork across multiple cultures; process information at a fast pace; and demonstrate convergent, divergent, and creative thinking (Reinhardt et al., 2011). Other ways in which workplaces have changed is increased ***telecommuting*** and a ***contingent workforce*** (independent contractors, freelancers). Both instances isolate the worker, spatially and temporally. In the next section, we discuss the impact of technology and the digital economy on the nature of work, the worker, and the workplace, using examples from the measures adopted to deal with the pandemic.

The World Health Organization (WHO; 2020a) declared the COVID-19 outbreak a public health emergency on January 30, 2020; on March 11, 2020, COVID-19's status was changed to a global pandemic (WHO, 2020b). The pandemic instantaneously accelerated workplace trends that had been predicted to occur in the future. In *The Future of Work: Robots, AI, and Automation,* West (2018) discussed how technology would alter work, the economy, and the way people live; this was realized during the pandemic. Three business trends that COVID-19 fast-tracked and that are most likely to persist post-pandemic are (1) remote work and virtual interactions, (2) e-commerce and digital transactions, and (3) automation and use of artificial intelligence (Lund et al., 2021). The disruptions caused by technology that were predicted before the pandemic were underestimated, and more than 100 million workers may be required to change occupations by 2030 (Lund et al., 2021). The most vulnerable workers are those who are less educated and lowest paid; they will bear the brunt of this fallout because they will not have the necessary job skills, which will require higher levels of education and different skill sets.

The pandemic has highlighted the physical dimensions of work by altering the physical environment and changing the physical proximity of work, including the virtual environment, as the factor most likely to influence future work trends. Before the pandemic, the impact of technology and globalization pertained to certain business sectors, mostly manufacturing, information technology (IT), and technology, and the backroom operations of business could be outsourced to cheaper labor. During the pandemic, all business sectors and industry had to contend with safety measures such as lockdowns, business shutdowns, limited travel and transportation, hygiene regulations, social distancing, school and university closings, and so forth. These measures necessitated an immediate shift to remote work. A retrospective analysis showed that nearly 70% of computer-based office work can be done remotely with no loss of productivity (Lund et al., 2021). Obviously, some aspects of work that require physical proximity or for which better outcomes occur with in-person interactions will revert to prepandemic conditions. Medical, education, and health and beauty occupations are some examples. During the pandemic, telemedicine was a means to access routine health care and rehabilitation services that would normally occur in a physician's office or an outpatient clinic. Because of changes that occurred during the pandemic, all occupations will be analyzed to understand the degree to which technological innovations such as remote work, automation, artificial intelligence, and robotics can perform tasks and replace workers; perhaps this will soon become the new normal (Lund et al., 2021; West, 2018).

The paradox of remote work is that it usually results in an increase in productivity and improved work–life balance and overall quality of life. Many employees are not motivated to revert to previous working conditions and prefer a ***hybrid work*** arrangement in which one works part-time from home and part-time in the office, that limits the need to go in to work daily. The benefits of ***remote work,*** in which one works off-site, include reduced transportation costs; fewer commuting hours; improved work–life balance, productivity, autonomy, and flexibility; more family time to participate in family roles; and control over time. Employers also benefit from cost savings, with reduced real estate costs, ability to access talent without geographical limitations, and, in relation to increased control in managing the work, reduced employee turnover and more satisfied workers. It must be noted that these trends will negatively affect urban real estate, transportation, and all services associated with a large number of workers going to a different location to work.

The success of remote work coupled with no negative impact on productivity and a positive impact on worker well-being has already led to policy changes. In Iceland, 86% of the workforce has now moved to a 4-day work week; some reported benefits are improved home life, reduced stress, participation in home management, ability to run errands and exercise, and higher quality weekends because errands can be spread over weekdays (Haraldsson & Kellum, 2021). Many IT businesses have also adopted a 4-day work week; Microsoft Japan has actually reported increased productivity (Chappell, 2019). This appears to be a win–win situation for both employers and employees and will, in the long run, improve the health and well-being of society by creating the conditions for occupationally balanced lifestyles.

Obviously, remote work does not suit every worker. Some negative aspects of telework that have been reported are isolation, decreased interactions and communications with managers, and reduced relationships with peers at work

(Diab-Bahman & Al-Enzi, 2020). However, good communication, time off through disconnecting, and other work best practices can benefit both worker and employer (Perlow, 2012). Remote work allows for greater autonomy, which comes with the expectation that work will be done independently with limited supervision, structure, and support. Remote work also requires that workers be disciplined and mindful of the ways to maintain boundaries between work and home life. Employers will have to revise their human resources operations and management strategies to support a large number of teleworking employees and novel job demands unique to remote work with minimal social interactions.

This change in the nature of work and the manner in which work gets done is important for occupational therapy practitioners to heed: Interventions aimed primarily at physical job demands are less relevant today because cognitive and psychosocial demands exacerbate stress at workplaces (Gupta, 2008). Industrial rehabilitation will become less needed as manufacturing and factory work is automated or performed by robots. Work stressors will be caused by social isolation from the workplace, limited supervision, lack of structure, and scheduling of work hours and meetings, among others. Work-related stress is strongly associated with workplace injury, musculoskeletal disorders, and chronic pain (Clauw & Williams, 2002). Such workplace injuries are a great opportunity for occupational therapy practitioners to work with employers to develop programs and policies that help workers develop habits and routines that are sustainable to minimize the impact of stressors through policy, appropriate supervision, and interpersonal dynamics.

Like many industrialized nations, the United States has an aging workforce. With advances in medicine and improved living conditions, people are living longer and aging well. Older workers who are healthy and active want to work past the traditional retirement age. Others have to delay retirement for a variety of reasons and are thus dealing with age-related changes in workplaces that are transforming at an alarming rate. The nature of work is ever changing, and workers are expected to adapt quickly and be nimble and flexible on the job. Occupational therapy has a lot to offer older workers and employers, so the interactions of occupational therapy practitioners and workers can be mutually beneficial (Gupta & Sabata, 2012).

Policy, Regulations, and Programming in the Workplace

Policies, regulations, and programming in the workplace are essential for occupational therapy practitioners to understand. Important legislation and programming have been enacted, implemented, and modified over the years to protect employers and employees, to ensure that hiring practices are fair, and to promote safe working conditions. It is incumbent on occupational therapy practitioners to be aware of and understand the workplace regulatory and policy environment in which they provide services to effectively serve their clients. In this section, we present a historical review of work-related policies and legislation and consider the most contemporary and relevant workplace policies, regulations, and programs that have had the most influence and impact on the practice of occupational therapy.

A variety of work-related legislation has been enacted in the past 110-plus years before, during, and after the Industrial Revolution in the United States (Library of Congress, 2021). See Table 14.1 for an overview of pertinent legislation that has influenced and continues to influence the practice of occupational therapy (AOTA, 2017).

Americans with Disabilities Act of 1990

The ***Americans with Disabilities Act of 1990*** (2000; ADA; P. L. 101-336) was signed into law on July 26, 1990. The enactment of the ADA was the result of many years, in fact decades, of advocacy by the disability and civil rights communities. The ADA was modeled after the Civil Rights Act of 1964 (P. L. 88-352), which prohibits discrimination on the basis of race, color, religion, sex, or national origin (Aiken et al., 2013). The ADA is still considered "the most comprehensive legislation for people with disabilities ever passed in the United States" (Karger & Rose, 2010, p. 74). Its broad and inclusive scope was intended to socially integrate people with disabilities; it prohibit discrimination in employment on the basis of disability and require accessibility of state and federal government programs and services, specifically in public accommodations, transportation, and telecommunications. Yet implementing the ADA, in its true intention, has been a challenge. One reason for this has been a critique of the definition of *disability* and its interpretation, with arguments ranging from the definition being too restrictive to the definition being too broad. Nonetheless, the ADA defines a *person with a disability* as someone with a recorded physical or mental impairment that substantially limits their participation in one or more life activities, such as work (ADA.gov, n.d.).

Employers are prohibited from discriminating against workers with disabilities who qualify for employment as long as they can meet the essential job functions with or without reasonable accommodations in the workplace (Sprong et al., 2019). Other challenges have been the vagueness of language, such as *substantially limits* and *reasonable accommodation,* and perceived hardships on the part of employers in providing accommodation. Under the ADA, employers fearful of lawsuits may choose not to hire a person with a disability, which defeats the purpose of this legislation (ADA.gov, 2015; Sprong et al., 2019). The enactment of the ADA Amendments Act of 2008 (ADAAA; Pub. L. 110-325) was in response to the narrowing of the definition of *disability* by the courts, which it explicitly rejects, and to clarify the language so that courts can consistently apply the Act according to its broad intent and purpose. Essentially, the Act's focus is discrimination related to people with disabilities rather than their disability (Job Accommodation Network, 2021).

TABLE 14.1. **KEY WORK-RELATED POLICIES**

POLICY	SUMMARY DESCRIPTION
Federal Employers' Liability Act	Protected and compensated railroad workers injured on the job
Age Discrimination in Employment Act of 1967 (P. L. 90-202)	Prohibited employment discrimination against people age 40 years or older
Rehabilitation Act of 1973 (P. L. 93-112)	Eliminated discrimination against people with disabilities in programs or activities receiving federal funding; the Act and its subsequent amendments were precursors to the Americans with Disabilities Act of 1990
Americans with Disabilities Act (ADA) of 1990 (P. L. 101-336)	Prohibited discrimination and ensured equal treatment for people with disabilities in employment, state and local government services, public accommodations, commercial facilities, and transportation
ADA Amendments Act of 2008 (P. L. 110-325)	Placed the emphasis on discrimination rather than on a person's disability. Retained the ADA definition of a *disability* as an impairment that substantially limits one or more life activities; however, it changed how the statutory terms should be interpreted. Expanded the definition of *major life activities* and clarified that an impairment that is episodic or in remission is a disability if it would substantially limit a major life activity when active
Ticket-to-Work and Work Incentives Improvement Act of 1999 (P. L. 106-170)	Provided Social Security beneficiaries with disabilities with more choices for receiving employment services and increased provider incentives to serve beneficiaries with disabilities who want to maximize their economic self-sufficiency through work opportunities; these services may include training, career counseling, vocational rehabilitation, job placement, and ongoing support services necessary to achieve a work goal
Rehabilitation Act Amendments of 1992 (P. L. 102-569)	Included numerous amendments designed to increase the choice and control of people with disabilities over rehabilitation services, both individually and systemically; emphasizes the presumption of ability that people can achieve employment and other rehabilitation goals regardless of the severity of the disability, if appropriate services and supports are made available
Education of the Deaf Act of 1986 (P. L. 99-371)	Reauthorized educational programs for deaf individuals to foster improved educational programs for deaf people throughout the United States
Omnibus Budget Reconciliation Act of 1987 (P. L. 100-203)	Gave states the option to offer prevocational educational and supported employment services to people institutionalized at any time before the waiver program

Source. Adapted from "Occupational Therapy Services in Facilitating Work Participation and Performance," by the American Occupational Therapy Association, 2017, *American Journal of Occupational Therapy, 71*(Suppl. 2), S12–S13 (https://doi.org/10.5014/ajot.2017.716S05). Copyright © 2017 by the American Occupational Therapy Association. Adapted with permission.

Equal Employment Opportunity Commission

The ***Equal Employment Opportunity Commission*** (EEOC) is the federal agency that, since 1965, has enforced antidiscrimination laws and protected workers from being discriminated against on the basis of their race, color, religion, sex (including pregnancy), national origin, age (40 years or older), disability, or genetic information (EEOC, n.d.). Title I of the ADA, for instance, is enforced in the workplace by the EEOC, which applies to employers who have 15 or more employees (ADA.gov, n.d.). When the ADAAA was enacted in 2008, the EEOC was directed to make the necessary changes to the Title I ADA regulations and interpretive guidance documents (U.S. EEOC, n.d.). Besides preventing discrimination through community outreach, education, and technical assistance, the agency also assesses allegations and complaints and, in the event of a clear case of discrimination, the EEOC may, in certain instances, litigate against employers in the interest of the public good.

Overview of Major Employment Laws

The ***Fair Labor Standards Act of 1938*** (FLSA) prescribes standards for wages and overtime pay, which affect most private and public employment. Under the FLSA, employers must pay covered employees at least the federal minimum wage and overtime pay of at least 1.5 times the regular rate of pay. It also restricts the number of hours that children younger than age 16 can work in nonagricultural operations and prohibits the employment of those younger than age 18 in certain jobs considered to be too dangerous (U.S. Department of Labor, n.d.).

The ***Employee Retirement Income Security Act of 1974*** (P. L. 93-406) regulates employers who offer pension or benefits plans to their employees. The Labor-Management Reporting and Disclosure Act of 1959 (P. L. 86-257), also known as the Landrum–Griffin Act, deals with the relationship between a union and its members. The act requires labor organizations to file annual financial reports and reports on certain labor relations practices, and it sets forth standards for the election of union officers. The ***Family and Medical Leave Act of 1993*** (Pub. L. 103-3) requires employers of 50 or more employees to provide up to 12 weeks of unpaid, job-protected leave to eligible employees for the birth or adoption of a child or for the serious illness of the employee or a spouse, child, or parent.

The reader is encouraged to consult the U.S. Department of Labor website (https://webapps.dol.gov/elaws/#) for a summary of these and other employment-related laws.

Workers' Compensation and Disability Insurance

Workers' compensation is a social insurance program. Workers' compensation varies by state and between federal and state systems. In the United States, the majority of states adopted workers' compensation laws between 1910 and 1920; Mississippi was the last state to pass a workers' compensation law, in 1948 (National Academy of Social Insurance [NASI], n.d.). The only other disability benefits programs larger than workers' compensation are the federal Social Security Disability Insurance (SSDI) program and Medicare.

Workers' compensation provides injured workers with four categories of benefits:

- *medical care for work-related injuries and illnesses:* 100% of medical costs and cash benefits for lost work time after a 3- to 7-day waiting period
- *temporary disability benefits:* paid to a worker when a work-related injury or illness temporarily prevents them from returning to their job
- *permanent partial and permanent total disability benefits:* paid to workers who have long-term disabilities as a result of work
- *vocational training:* covers the costs of services to facilitate a worker's return to gainful employment if they are unable to return to their preinjury job (Murphy et al., 2020).

Benefits for workers' compensation are paid by private insurance, by state or federal workers' compensation funds, or by self-insured employers.

According to the latest data from NASI (Murphy et al., 2020),

- The number of U.S. jobs covered by workers' compensation continues to grow, with that growth slowing slightly from 4% between 2014 and 2016 to 3% between 2016 and 2018. A different trend is seen with respect to covered wages, which grew by 8.7% between 2014 and 2016 and then by 10% in the 2 subsequent years.
- In 2018, total workers' compensation benefits paid were $62.8 billion, a decrease of 1.2% from 2014. After falling by 1.9% from 2014 to 2016, benefits increased by 0.8% from 2016 to 2018.
- In 2018, employers' costs for workers' compensation were $98.6 billion, a 5% percent increase since 2014. When adjusted for the increase in covered wages, however, employers' costs were $1.21 per $100 of covered wages, down $0.16 (12.2%) from 2014.

Occupational therapy practitioners need to stay abreast of their state workers' compensation laws for legislative changes, which occur on a regular basis. These changes can influence reimbursement in both amount and method, the type of services that will be covered, who may provide the services, and other issues that may potentially affect the coverage of occupational therapy services (Dorsey et al., 2019).

Occupational Safety and Health Administration

The federal agency responsible for overseeing safe and healthful workplaces is the ***Occupational Safety and Health Administration*** (OSHA), which operates under the U.S. Department of Labor. The Occupational Safety and Health Act of 1970 (P. L. 51-596; OSH Act) was passed into law on December 29, 1970. The stated purpose of the act is

> to assure safe and healthful working conditions for working men and women; by authorizing enforcement of the standards developed under the Act; by assisting and encouraging the States in their efforts to assure safe and healthful working conditions; by providing for research, information, education, and training in the field of occupational safety and health; and for other purposes.

OSHA has a two-pronged mission: (1) to ensure safe and healthful workplaces by setting and enforcing standards, and (2) to provide training, outreach, education, and assistance to employers and employees. Employers are required to comply with all applicable OSHA standards and must also comply with the General Duty Clause of the OSH Act, which stipulates that employers must maintain a safe workplace free any of known and serious hazards. In addition to the General Duty Clause, OSHA has four primary industry standards that cover general industry, construction, maritime, and agriculture. The

OSH Act encourages states to develop and administer their own job safety and health programs, although OSHA must approve and monitor all state plans. OSHA's jurisdiction covers private-sector employers but excludes self-employed, family farm, and government workers except in states that have approved state plans. As of 2021, there are 22 OSHA-approved state plans covering private-sector and state and local government workers, and 6 state plans covering only state and local government workers (OSHA, n.d.-d).

As part of the requirements for employers to comply with the OSH Act, employers are required to record and report work-related fatalities, injuries, and illnesses (OSHA, n.d.-b). OSHA normally conducts inspections without advance notice. Although OSHA states that it cannot inspect all 7 million workplaces it covers each year, the agency focuses its inspection efforts on the most hazardous workplaces (OSHA, n.d.-a).

According to OSHA (2020),

> Occupational injuries and illnesses cost American employers more than $97.4 billion a year in workers' compensation costs alone. Indirect costs to employers, including lost productivity, employee training and replacement costs, and time for investigations following injuries can more than double these costs. Workers and their families suffer great emotional and psychological costs, in addition to the loss of wages and the costs of caring for the injured, which further weakens the economy. (p. 5)

Some of the OSHA standards most frequently violated include lack of adequate fall protection in the construction industry, poor hazard communication in general industry, electrical wiring hazards in general industry, and improper operation of powered industrial trucks (e.g., forklifts).

Social Security Administration's Ticket to Work Program

The Social Security Administration's (SSA's) ***Ticket to Work Program*** was created in 1999 for people ages 18 through 64 with a disability who receive SSDI or Supplemental Security Income benefits. According to the SSA (n.d.), the goals of the Ticket to Work Program are to

- offer beneficiaries with disabilities expanded choices when seeking service and supports to enter, reenter, or maintain employment;
- increase the financial independence and self-sufficiency of beneficiaries with disabilities; and
- reduce and, whenever possible, eliminate reliance on disability benefits.

Eligible beneficiaries with disabilities may voluntarily participate in the program by signing up with an approved provider. An approved provider can be an employment network or a state vocational rehabilitation agency. Occupational therapy practitioners may apply to become a designated employment network to provide services to beneficiaries who are enrolled in the Ticket to Work Program.

The SSA (2020) publishes a reference source titled *The Red Book—A Guide to Work Incentives,* which provides a summary guide that provides employment supports for people with disabilities under the SSDI and Supplemental Security Income Programs. This is a good general reference source for educators, advocates, rehabilitation professionals, and counselors who serve people with disabilities.

Occupational Information Network

The ***Occupational Information Network*** (O*NET) is a primary source of U.S. occupational information. The O*NET database (https://www.onetonline.org/) contains almost 1,000 standardized and occupation-specific job descriptors of occupations. The database also contains an interactive application for searching occupations as well as a set of assessment tools for workers and students looking to find or change careers.

Occupational therapy practitioners may find the O*NET useful when performing a job analysis or working with a client on vocational exploration activities. For example, a practitioner may be performing a job analysis for a specific occupation and use the O*NET to find the occupation-specific descriptors to assist with developing a comprehensive job analysis.

EXERCISE 14.1. O*NET Job Search

Go to the O*NET website at https://www.onetonline.org/ and search for an occupation of your choice. Take a few minutes to review the summary for your selected occupation, including the job description, task requirements, knowledge, skills, education requirements, work styles, values, and so forth. You will also find information about wage and employment trends. For instance, you can search for *occupational therapy assistants* (Code 31-2011.00) and read the summary report.

Job Accommodation Network

The ***Job Accommodation Network*** (JAN; https://askjan.org/) is a resource for guidance on workplace accommodations and disability employment issues. The JAN is an especially useful tool for occupational therapy practitioners working with employers and people with disabilities. A practitioner may be consulting with an employer who is trying to provide reasonable accommodations for an employee who is returning to work after an accident that left them with a permanent limitation in upper-extremity dexterity and coordination. The JAN would be a good resource to assist both the consulting practitioner and the employer in developing appropriate accommodations for the employee. According to the JAN, it provides free consulting services for rehabilitation professionals such as occupational therapy practitioners about all aspects of job accommodations, including the accommodation process, ideas for accommodations, vendors for related products, referral to other resources, and ADA compliance assistance.

EXERCISE 14.2. Job Accommodation Network

Go to the JAN at https://askjan.org/ and navigate to the Searchable Online Accommodation Resource (SOAR) to explore various accommodation options for people with disabilities. For example, an occupational therapy practitioner may have a client with carpal tunnel syndrome who is a produce manager in a grocery store. Through the SOAR system, the practitioner can select *osteoarthritis* and choose a limitation that corresponds with that of the person needing an accommodation, such as limitations related to joint immobility, fatigue, and weakness. The SOAR provides accommodation recommendations, such as scheduling periodic rest breaks, providing adjustable workstations, antifatigue matting, and so forth.

Development of Worker Role and Identity

One of the most important choices a person has to make as they transition from adolescence to adulthood is choosing a career. Numerous underlying contextual factors influence and affect choice of career, such as gender, family or group influence, ethnicity, and socioeconomic status (Lent & Brown, 2020). To make an informed choice, one must consider a complex array of information and data and ultimately choose from among many occupational alternatives.

From an occupational science and occupational therapy perspective, people's occupational choices contribute to their identity—in other words, who they are and who they become. In his Eleanor Clarke Slagle Lecture, Christiansen (1999) posited that occupational engagement is the means by which people develop and express their identities and have identities conferred on them by others in their context. To be identified as a worker is critical in any society and more so in American society, which places high value on independence and personal responsibility. Working-age adults are expected to work so that they can take care of themselves and fulfill their family obligations and their responsibility to society as tax-paying citizens. By doing so, people fully participate and experience a sense of belonging in their society. Earnings determine one's socioeconomic status and class identity. Work is also a means to experience self-efficacy and display competence, which contribute to one's overall well-being. The negative consequences of chronic unemployment and underemployment on health have been well documented in the literature and are beyond the scope of this chapter (Bartelink et al., 2020; Voss et al., 2020).

Several career choice and development theories have been introduced over the past century, beginning with the first textbook on vocational choice by Frank Parsons in 1909. Although presenting a comprehensive and detailed examination of all career choice and development theories is beyond the scope of this chapter, a review of the most commonly cited theories is presented in Table 14.2 (Braveman & Page, 2012; Kornblau et al., 2000). It synopsizes several of the models most commonly cited and used over the past century that help to explain career development and career choice, including the process and stages of career development and exploration. Although the theories presented in Table 14.2 are not occupational therapy theories, they are important for occupational therapy practitioners to know and understand to support work-related practice.

Role of Occupational Therapy in the Workplace

History of Occupational Therapy in the Workplace

The profession of occupational therapy traces its roots to the notion of work as a central occupation in people's lives. The founders of the profession emphasized work-related practice as an integral part of the profession's scope of practice. Before the official adoption of *occupational therapy* as the profession's name, *work cure* and *ergotherapy* were entertained as possibilities. From the profession's initial founding until the present day, work has been and continues to be an important area of practice. In 1923, the first educational standards for occupational therapy were generated; they emphasized the influence of occupation (work) as therapy and the need for occupational therapy practitioners to engage in work-related practice (Jacobs & Baker, 2000). Occupational therapy took a prominent role during World War II as part of the military's reconditioning program. However, after the war, the profession's focus shifted to more reductionist techniques with less involvement in work-related programming. During the 1950s and 1960s, vocational rehabilitation services were emphasized as the result of new federal policies and the overall change in attitudes toward and treatment of people with disabilities. Federal laws introduced during the 1950s, such as the Vocational Rehabilitation Amendments of 1954 and the Medical Facilities Survey and Construction Act of 1954, facilitated renewed interest in and emphasis on work-related programming for the profession. In 1959, Lilian Wegg (1960) delivered the Eleanor Clarke Slagle lecture "Essentials of Work Evaluation." In her lecture, Wegg (1960) outlined essential skills for performing work evaluation that continue to serve as a foundation for contemporary work capacity evaluation.

By the early 1980s, AOTA (1980) had developed a position paper, "The Role of the Occupational Therapist in the Vocational Rehabilitation Process," asserting the prominence and importance of work-related practice in occupational therapy. During the 1980s, the need for industrial rehabilitation services grew considerably. This need created new and expanded opportunities for occupational therapy practitioners in industrial rehabilitation and work hardening. By 1992, AOTA had published an update to the aforementioned position paper titled "Statement: Occupational Therapy Services in Work Practice" that has since been revised several times. The current version is "Occupational Therapy Services in Facilitating Work Participation and Performance" (AOTA, 2017).

TABLE 14.2. **VOCATIONAL THEORIES OF CAREER CHOICE AND DEVELOPMENT**

THEORY	OVERVIEW AND KEY POINTS
Parsons' (1909) Choosing a Vocation	Widely regarded as the first theory that attempted to explain occupational choice. Parsons viewed occupational choice as something that happened just before an individual's entry into the labor market. He asserted that occupational choice involved three elements: understanding oneself, understanding the merits of various occupations, and understanding the relationship between these two things to make an informed choice.
Holland's (1997) Career Typology	Considers congruence of one's personality, skills, and abilities with the occupational environment and posits that congruent interactions facilitate stability and incongruent interactions create change in behaviors. Holland classified personality types into 6 categories: realistic, investigative, artistic, social, enterprising, and conventional. This theory serves as basis for many standardized vocational assessments.
Super's (1953) Theory of Vocational Development (lifespan, life space)	Identifies 6 life and career development stages: crystallization, involving tentative vocational goals (ages 14–18); specification, involving development of focused vocational goals in preparation for adulthood (ages 18–21); implementation, which includes training and obtaining gainful employment (ages 21–24); stabilization, which is validation of and engaging in one's career choice (ages 24–35); consolidation, which is advancing one's career (ages 36–54); and readiness for retirement, which is the preparation for retirement (ages 55 and older). Emphasis is placed on the relationship between self-concept and choice of work and career.
Developmental Theory: Ginzberg's developmental stages of vocational development (Howell et al., 1997)	Postulates that career development occurs over an 8- to 10-year period. Individuals search for a fit between their career preferences and opportunities in the job market. Expenditure of time and resources are important components of career choice that may serve as a deterrent to change a career.
Social Learning Theory/Krumholtz's Learning Theory of Career Choice and Counseling (Mitchell & Krumholtz, 1996)	Attempts to explain career choice by answering the question, "Why do people express various preferences for different occupations at different points in their lives?" Examines 4 factors that influence the answer to this question: (1) genetic endowment and special abilities, (2) environmental conditions and events, (3) learning experiences, and (4) task approach skills.
Lent et al.'s (1994) Social Cognitive Career Theory	Framework for career development that includes the interactions among personal attributes, external environmental factors, and behavior in career decision making. Also recognized as important factors are educational and vocational interests, career-related choices, and performance. This theory proposes 3 models that facilitate career-related interests: interest development, choice, and performance.
Life Career Development Theory (Chen, 2003)	Considered to be more holistic than other previous theories, it encompasses all domains of concern to the person and the environment. This theory has many similarities to the basic theoretical underpinnings of occupational therapy. This theory outlines how individuals can visualize and plan their careers, referred to as *career consciousness*, by examining future life roles, life settings, and life events while thinking about the effect of gender, ethnicity, religion, race, and socioeconomic status on their development.

Note. Based on information from Braveman & Page (2012) and Kornblau et al. (2000).

Process of Occupational Therapy in Work

The *Occupational Therapy Practice Framework: Domain and Process* (4th ed.; *OTPF–4;* AOTA, 2020) presents a summary of interrelated constructs that define and guide occupational therapy practice. The *OTPF–4* describes the various occupations or activities considered by occupational therapy practitioners when working with clients. These areas of occupation include activities of daily living, instrumental activities of daily living, health management, rest and sleep, education, play, leisure, social participation, and work. According to the *OTPF–4,* work includes activities needed to engage in paid employment or volunteer activities and involves the following:

- *employment interests and pursuits:* identifying and selecting work opportunities based on assets, limitations, likes, and dislikes relative to work
- *employment seeking and acquisition:* identifying and recruiting for job opportunities; completing, submitting, and reviewing appropriate application materials; preparing for interviews; participating in interviews and following up afterward; discussing job benefits; and finalizing negotiations
- *job performance and maintenance:* Identifying work skills and patterns; time management; relationships with

coworkers, managers, and customers; creation, production, and distribution of products and services; initiation, sustainment, and completion of work; and compliance with work norms and procedures

- *retirement preparation and adjustment:* determining aptitudes, developing interests and skills, selecting vocational pursuits, securing required resources, adjusting lifestyle
- *volunteer exploration:* identifying and learning about community causes, organizations, and opportunities for unpaid work consistent with personal skills, interests, location, and time available
- *volunteer participation:* performing unpaid work activities for the benefit of selected people, causes, or organizations.

The process of delivering occupational therapy services includes referral, evaluation (occupational profile and analysis of occupational performance), intervention (intervention plan, intervention implementation, intervention review), and outcomes. Occupational therapy practitioners work with clients experiencing work dysfunction or those promoting workplace health and injury prevention in various and diverse settings, including business and industrial environments, general hospitals, psychiatric and mental health facilities, outpatient clinics, community health centers, schools and universities, vocational programs, U.S. military Vocational Rehabilitation and Employment divisions now known as Veteran Readiness and Employment, and rehabilitation hospitals (AOTA, 2017). The focus of work-related evaluation and intervention is primarily on facilitating workers' functional and work capacity to meet the demands of the job (Dorsey et al., 2019; Kaskutas & Snodgrass, 2009).

Referral

The occupational therapy process typically begins with a referral from a physician. Although some states do not require a physician referral, most settings and third-party payers do. For instance, most workers' compensation insurance carriers will not reimburse for occupational therapy services without a physician referral. Ultimately, occupational therapy practitioners must adhere to their state licensure laws. Referrals are, however, often initiated not just by physicians but also by many other professionals, such as case managers; employers and their representatives, such as safety managers and occupational health nurses; workers' compensation carriers; psychologists; vocational counselors; and case managers (Dorsey et al., 2019; Kaskutas & Snodgrass, 2009).

Evaluation

After a referral, the occupational therapist conducts a work-focused evaluation. In addition to the typical assessment methods, the occupational therapist must focus on the worker's capacity to meet the unique demands of the job; for example, lifting, pushing, pulling, carrying, time management, stress management, executive functioning, positional tolerances (e.g., overhead work, crouching, bending), endurance, and safety. The occupational therapist may need to conduct a thorough job site analysis to determine the demands of the job. A unique aspect of a work-focused evaluation is that the occupational therapist must determine the client's potential for returning to work, which is accomplished through work performance testing. The therapist may have the client perform a battery of tests that simulate their work and may even observe the client performing the actual work tasks after an evaluation of underlying client factors (e.g., range of motion, strength, endurance, attention to task). Typical questions that need to be answered during the evaluation process include the following:

- Who is the client (person, including family and significant others), population (e.g., workers with musculoskeletal injuries), or organization (e.g., manufacturing plant)?
- In what occupations does the client feel successful, and what barriers are affecting the client's success in desired occupations?
- Why is the client seeking services, and what are the client's current concerns relative to engaging in the occupation of work and ability to return to work?
- What areas of occupation are successful, and is the area of work the primary area causing problems or risks?
- What work contexts and environments support or inhibit participation and engagement in desired occupations?
- Is the client capable of returning to the preinjury job or of acquiring the necessary skills to obtain gainful employment?
- What is the client's employment history?
- What are the client's priorities and desired outcomes?
- Can the client return to work after disease or disability?
- How can the workplace be modified to support the worker in returning to work or staying at work after disease or disability?
- What can be done to make hazardous work safer for a group of workers?
- What can be done to improve the mental and physical health and wellness of employees?
- What vocational opportunities exist for young adults with disabilities looking to enter the workforce? (AOTA, 2017, 2020).

Intervention

The occupational therapist collaborates with the client, and often with the referral source or sources (e.g., physician, case manager, employer's representative), to develop goals and objectives that address targeted work-related outcomes such as return to work and modification of the work (AOTA, 2017; Dorsey et al., 2019; Kaskutas & Snodgrass, 2009). The intervention plan typically focuses on the client returning to a preinjury job in either a full or limited (restricted) capacity and explores vocational options, including work skill reacquisition; for example, for a client who can no longer return to the work they once performed, or the acquisition of a work skill, such as gainful employment skills.

Intervention approaches can be conceptualized as falling into one of five categories or a combination thereof:

- create, promote
- establish, restore
- maintain
- modify
- prevent (AOTA, 2020; Dunn et al., 1998).

Table 14.3 describes intervention approaches and includes examples of occupation-based interventions.

To determine success in reaching targeted outcomes (e.g., goals and objectives), outcome assessment information is used to plan the next steps for the client and to evaluate program delivery (i.e., program evaluation; AOTA, 2017; Dorsey et al., 2019; Kaskutas & Snodgrass, 2009). Typical outcomes that are targeted as part of the occupational therapy intervention process include job acquisition, vocational skill acquisition or reacquisition, unrestricted return to work, or restricted return to work (e.g., light duty, restricted duty, alternative job duties). The occupational therapist must possess knowledge of the job duties and the work environment to understand the context of the client's work (or anticipated work) and the required demands. The mismatch between the client's capacities and the work requirements is the focus of the intervention process and the discharge decision process (AOTA, 2017; Dorsey et al., 2019; Kaskutas & Snodgrass, 2009). Discharge planning begins at initial evaluation and continues through the delivery of occupational therapy services. It is important to note that part of measuring outcomes is the need to determine the continuation or discontinuation of services or referral to other professionals and services, including vocational counseling, psychology, physical therapy, and so forth.

Practice Areas: Traditional and Nontraditional

Occupational therapy practitioners work in diverse settings in which work-related services are provided and with a wide

TABLE 14.3. INTERVENTION APPROACHES AND EXAMPLES OF OCCUPATION-BASED INTERVENTIONS

APPROACH	EXAMPLES OF OCCUPATION-BASED INTERVENTIONS
Create or promote	An intervention approach designed to provide enriched contextual and activity experiences that will enhance performance for all people: • Provide barrier-free solutions in the workplace • Deliver an injury prevention course for employees • Assist with design and set-up of computer workstations • Provide a workplace stress management program
Establish or restore	An intervention approach designed to influence client variables, such as a skill or ability that has not yet been developed, or to restore a skill or ability that has been impaired: • Provide vocational exploration activities • Instruct in time management skills • Address lifting and carrying capacity with work simulation
Maintain	An intervention approach designed to provide the supports that will allow clients to preserve current functioning and abilities: • Teach home exercise program for flexibility and strength • Instruct in proper body mechanics while lifting heavy boxes
Modify	An intervention approach that modifies the environment or activity to facilitate performance; includes compensatory techniques: • Provide ergonomic interventions to reduce amount of forceful exertion required • Sequence work tasks for employees with permanent cognitive or processing restrictions • Collaborate with employer to alter work schedule and work tasks
Prevent	An intervention approach designed to reduce or eliminate potential occupational performance problems and barriers: • Collaborate with employer to develop reasonable accommodation policies • Develop a "no lift" policy at the worksite, including hydraulic lifting equipment • Create ergonomically designed workstation for all administrative staff in an organization

Sources. American Occupational Therapy Association (2017, 2020); Kaskutas and Snodgrass (2009).

variety of populations, including people with developmental disabilities, adolescents and younger workers, older workers, and people with mental illness. In this section, we consider areas of traditional and nontraditional work programs and services.

Supported and Alternative Employment

Occupational therapy practitioners contribute expertise and provide skilled services to a variety of populations, including clients with developmental disabilities and people living with mental illness. These services are provided along a continuum of work-related assessment and intervention contexts, including supported employment at sheltered workshops, transitional employment, and supported jobs with one-on-one job coaching (AOTA, 2017; Dorsey et al., 2019).

At a ***sheltered workshop,*** the occupational therapy practitioner will evaluate the client to determine their capacity to meet the demands of work in a structured, controlled environment and provide interventions to address the identified mismatches between current capacity and required capacity for the targeted job. The sheltered workshop approach is intended to move the client from simulated or hypothetical situations to real-life work experiences and contexts (AOTA, 2017).

Transitional employment services engage the client in paid positions for businesses or industries on a part-time, limited, and temporary basis while the client continues to receive ongoing training and support from a job coach and others, which may include an occupational therapy practitioner who collaborates with not only the client but also the employer to facilitate the client's engagement in work, modify the job and environment, and teach specific job-related skills (AOTA, 2017).

Supported employment typically engages the client in competitive, gainful employment with support and guidance from occupational therapy practitioners and other team members. Supported employment involves placements in employment settings that provide fully integrated roles and responsibilities with greater job longevity and no time restrictions. In other words, these placements offer the greatest chance for the client's long-term success in gainful employment (AOTA, 2017).

Transition Services (School to Adult Life)

Transition services are provided to adolescents who require supportive services to make the transition from childhood to adulthood (AOTA, 2017; Dorsey et al., 2019). Occupational therapy practitioners play an important role in facilitating a person's transition to adulthood as related to community participation and employment (Dorsey et al., 2019). Transition services are covered as part of the Individualized Education Program, as stipulated in the Individuals with Disabilities Education Act Amendments of 1997 (P. L. 105-117; IDEA). The purpose of IDEA is

> (a) to ensure that all children with disabilities have available to them a free appropriate public education that emphasizes special education and related services designed to meet their unique needs and prepare them for further education, employment, and independent living;
>
> (b) to ensure that the rights of children with disabilities and their parents are protected;
>
> (c) to assist States, localities, educational service agencies, and Federal agencies to provide for the education of all children with disabilities;
>
> (2) to assist States in the implementation of a statewide, comprehensive, coordinated, multidisciplinary, interagency system of early intervention services for infants and toddlers with disabilities and their families;
>
> (3) to ensure that educators and parents have the necessary tools to improve educational results for children with disabilities by supporting system improvement activities; coordinated research and personnel preparation; coordinated technical assistance, dissemination, and support; and technology development and media services;
>
> (4) to assess, and ensure the effectiveness of, efforts to educate children with disabilities.

Occupational therapy's contributions to the transition process related to work include evaluating job-related interests and abilities, planning and decision making regarding job placement, assessing mismatch between job demands and students' performance, modifying jobs to accommodate students' abilities and needs, and providing job site training of support personnel, including job coaches or coworkers (Dorsey et al., 2019).

Job Analysis

Occupational therapy practitioners provide job analysis for people who want to engage in gainful employment or who are returning to the workplace after an injury or illness. A ***job analysis*** consists of three major components: the work, the workers, and the workplace. It may also include an evaluation of the organizational culture, productivity expectations, and job requirements both internal and external to the organization, including regulatory issues (Gupta & Sabata, 2012). Often referred to as a *job demands analysis* (JDA), the analysis includes interviews with the incumbent or supervisors regarding the job requirements (AOTA, 2017; Dorsey et al., 2019).

In addition to interviews, the occupational therapy practitioner may conduct an on-site JDA that includes observation of the actual job being performed; on-site interviews with supervisors and employees; direct measurements of tasks, such as lifting, pushing, pulsing, and carrying; and positional requirements (e.g., bending, stooping, reaching, standing).

A standardized classification is used to ensure consistency in terminology. The U.S. Bureau of Labor Statistics (2020) provides categories for physical demands of work, including overall level of work, strength demands, and frequency of the physical demands. For instance, a job that requires lifting,

TABLE 14.4. PHYSICAL DEMAND CATEGORIES OF WORK

PHYSICAL DEMAND LEVEL	OCCASIONAL (0%–33%), LB	FREQUENT (34%–66%), LB	CONSTANT (67%–100%), LB
Sedentary	10	Negligible	Negligible
Light	10–20	10	Negligible
Medium	20–50	10–25	≤10
Heavy	50–100	25–50	10–20
Very heavy	≥100	≥50	≥20

Note. Adapted from U.S. Bureau of Labor Statistics (2020).

pushing, pulling, or carrying up to 100 pounds on an occasional basis (up to one-third of the day) would be categorized in the heavy physical demand category. Table 14.4 provides a snapshot of the physical demand categories of work.

The JDA allows the occupational therapy practitioner to identify the essential functions or tasks of the job. The essential functions of a job are those tasks that all employees must be able to perform with or without reasonable accommodation. The ADA has set forth guidelines for determining whether a task is essential or marginal (nonessential), including

- whether the reason the position exists is to perform that function;
- the number of other employees available to perform the function or among whom the performance of the function can be distributed;
- the degree of expertise or skill required to perform the function;
- the actual work experience of present or past employees in the job;
- the time spent performing a function;
- the consequences of not requiring that an employee perform a function; and
- the terms of a collective bargaining agreement (ADA.gov, n.d.).

EXERCISE 14.3. Job Analysis

Referring to Table 14.4, estimate the level of work (i.e., sedentary, light, medium, heavy, or very heavy) for each of the following jobs on the basis of the stated requirements:

1. *Construction laborer:* Load and unload building materials up to 110 pounds, distributing them to the appropriate locations, according to project plans, 3 hours per 10-hour workday.
2. *Certified nursing assistant:* With a team member (e.g., another certified nursing assistant), transfer patients weighing up to 300 pounds requiring moderate physical assistance from bed to wheelchair and from wheelchair back to bed.
3. *Stocker:* Pack and unpack items weighing up to 25 pounds to be stocked on shelves in stockrooms 5 hours per 8-hour workday.
4. *Mail clerk:* Lift and unload containers of mail or parcels weighing up to 35 pounds onto equipment for transportation to sort stations up to 6 hours per 9-hour workday.

Ergonomics

Ergonomics builds on job analysis by taking what is learned from the JDA and identifying work conditions and job demands associated with the onset of fatigue, overexertion, injuries, and chronic musculoskeletal disorders (Grant, 2012). *Ergonomics* is the scientific discipline that deals with the worker; the tools, equipment, and machines that the worker uses; and the environment in which the worker interacts and operates (Snodgrass, 2015). The literature includes numerous definitions of *ergonomics.* A holistic definition that best captures the broad scope of ergonomics is provided by the International Ergonomics Association (IEA; n.d.):

> Ergonomics (or human factors) is the scientific discipline concerned with the understanding of interactions among humans and other elements of a system, and the profession that applies theory, principles, data, and methods to design in order to optimize human well-being and overall system performance. The terms ergonomics and human factors are often used interchangeably or as a unit. (p. 1)

The objective of the application of ergonomics is to fit the work to the worker rather than the worker to the work. Occupational therapy practitioners use an ergonomic approach with their clients to minimize, if not eliminate, hazards in the workplace. An analogy can be drawn to reducing a person's cholesterol through diet and exercise to reduce, if not eliminate, the hazard of cardiovascular disease. By using a holistic approach that involves physical, cognitive, and organizational ergonomics, occupational therapy practitioners can work with employees and employers to create a culture of wellness and health that can lead to improved productivity and increased job satisfaction among older workers while reducing operational costs and workers' compensation claims. OSHA (n.d.-c) has a $afety Pays tool, an online calculator that uses data on workplace injury and prevention costs, that allows one to select from among 40 types of injuries and illnesses to estimate the direct and indirect costs of each injury. For instance, according to the tool, a single case of work-related carpal tunnel syndrome would have a direct cost of $30,930 and an indirect cost of $34,023, for a total cost of $64,953 (OSHA, n.d.-c).

The process of ergonomics includes hazard identification and assessment, which requires the occupational therapist to engage in two overarching tasks:

1. review an employer's history of injuries and accidents and employee turnover, as well as injury records (e.g., OSHA log of work-related injury and illness [OSHA 300 log], accident reports, workers' compensation claims, dispensary logs)
2. assess job tasks, processes, tools, and equipment in each work area (Dorsey et al., 2019; Snodgrass, 2015).

Once ergonomics hazards have been assessed and identified, hazard control and prevention efforts must be undertaken to eliminate or reduce identified hazards, including changes and modifications to the process, work methods and tasks, workstations, equipment, and work organization policies. Hazard control and prevention efforts by the occupational therapy practitioner are generally focused on one or more of the following categories:

- *work practice controls:* Examples include modifications of work methods such as proper body mechanics (e.g., lifting techniques; pacing; employee conditioning, including stretching before and during shift; and job coaching). This category includes education and training of workers with approaches such as continuing education courses to enhance job performance, safety seminars, and on-the-job training.
- *engineering controls:* This category is considered the most effective hazard control and includes workstation redesign, modification of tools and equipment to better fit the worker, purchase of new equipment, use of hydraulic lifts and rolling carts, suspension of heavy hand tools, and increased tool handle size.
- *administrative controls:* This category includes organizational policies and procedures related to shift work, overtime, rest breaks, number of employees assigned to a task or job, mandatory retirement age, authority and responsibility, productivity rates, equipment maintenance, incentive pay, light duty, restricted duty, and job rotation.
- *personal protective equipment:* Although not technically an ergonomic control measure, this category includes protective equipment such as gloves; respirators; chemical aprons; hard hats; eye protection; ear plugs; steel-toed footwear; and protection against cold, vibration, and contact stress (Snodgrass, 2015).

Work Hardening and Work Conditions

Work hardening is a multidisciplinary rehabilitation program focused on maximizing a person's work capacity with the overarching goal of returning the person to work. The typical disciplines involved in a work hardening program focused on rehabilitating an injured worker include occupational therapy practitioners, physical therapists and assistants, exercise physiologists, vocational counselors, psychologists, licensed counselors, and dieticians. In 1986, AOTA published "Work Hardening Guidelines," which defined and described this area of practice, and the language from those guidelines persists today in current AOTA documents, such as "Occupational Therapy Services in Facilitating Work Participation and Performance" (AOTA, 2017).

A work hardening program should lay the foundation for a return to work and typically requires the client to be engaged in the program several hours per day, 3 to 5 days per week for 4 to 8 weeks, including pretesting and posttesting, such as a functional capacity evaluation (described the next section of this chapter). The program is focused on simulating the target job with actual equipment from the job, if possible, to create realistic work simulation activities.

Work conditioning is a more generalized approached to rehabilitation that usually consists of only one discipline (i.e., occupational or physical therapy, exercise physiology) focused on physical conditioning, including strength, endurance, cardiopulmonary fitness, range of motion and flexibility, and coordination. Work conditioning may precede work hardening (AOTA, 2017; Dorsey et al., 2019).

Regardless of the approach, the goals of work rehabilitation programs are to

- maximize level of functioning after an injury or illness to maintain the worker's desired quality of life;
- facilitate the safe and timely return of people to work after injury or illness;
- remediate or prevent future injury or illness; and
- assist people in resuming their role as a worker, which can contribute to self-confidence and a view of self as a productive member of society and can prevent deconditioning as well as the negative psychosocial consequences of unemployment (AOTA, 2017; Dorsey et al., 2019).

Functional Capacity Evaluation

The ***functional capacity evaluation*** (FCE) plays an important role in work programs and services. The FCE is recognized as comprehensive evaluation that makes use of objective and reliable processes to determine a person's capacity for work. FCEs are typically performed by occupational or physical therapists. Occupational therapists are qualified to conduct FCEs because of their extensive training in activity and task analysis and focus on function (AOTA, 2017; Dorsey et al., 2019). A study conducted a number of years ago (Soer et al., 2008) sought to achieve consensus on an operational definition of FCE; the following definition had the most agreement: An *FCE* "is an evaluation of capacity of activities that is used to make recommendations for participation in work while considering the person's body functions and structures, environmental factors, personal factors and health status" (p. 394).

Various FCE approaches and methods are used in practice; thus, an FCE can vary in scope and duration. Regardless of the approach used, an FCE may be used for a variety of purposes, including to determine work rehabilitation intervention plans and goals, establish return-to-work status, quantify limitations as part of a disability determination, and resolve a case for the purpose of determining a settlement (Haruka et al., 2013). An FCE can answer the following questions regarding a person's work performance and tolerance:

- Is the client capable of performing their preinjury job?
- What are the client's physical work tolerances?
- Can the client return to work full time? If not, at what level can the client return to work?
- What limitations will require reasonable accommodation?
- What light-duty or job restrictions are necessary?
- What are the client's baseline abilities? (Page, 2012).

The FCE process includes a thorough review of medical, social, and work history; pain assessment and musculoskeletal screening; strength and endurance testing; evaluation of work simulation and tolerance to work over the course of a day; matching job demands with actual performance; and reliability of subjective reporting and level of effort (validity) by the client (Kaskutas & Snodgrass, 2009). The occupational therapist must monitor the client's responses and reactions to testing through observation, client report, and monitoring vital signs, including heart rate and blood pressure (Page, 2012). An FCE is typically conducted in 2 to 6 hours, although the evaluation can span 2 days.

Injury Prevention Programs

A focus on ***injury prevention*** is a necessary part of what occupational therapy practitioners are concerned with in work settings. For instance, a client with a diagnosis of carpal tunnel syndrome may be receiving traditional therapy services for splinting, stretching, and work modifications, but a focus on preventing an exacerbation of the condition and future injury (secondary prevention) should always be an important component of the occupational therapy intervention plan.

Injury prevention is an approach that occupational therapy practitioners may use in a variety of work settings. The *OTPF–4* (AOTA, 2020) states that the ultimate outcome of the occupational therapy process is for the client to engage in their desired occupations. Prevention efforts should be focused on

> education or health promotion efforts designed to identify, reduce, or stop the onset and reduce the incidence of unhealthy conditions, risk factors, diseases, or injuries. Occupational therapy promotes a healthy lifestyle at the individual, group, population (societal), and government or policy level. (p. 66)

Injury prevention has three tiers:

1. *Primary prevention:* The goal is to prevent disease or injury from occurring. For example, a person uses a scissor jack cart to transport 100-pound boxes in order to prevent the possibility of a low back injury.
2. *Secondary prevention:* The goal is to minimize or slow the progression of disease or injury. For example, someone recently diagnosed with mild carpal tunnel syndrome rearranges their computer workstation to decrease awkward postures of the neck and upper extremity to minimize its progression.
3. *Tertiary prevention:* The goal is to manage existing diseases or injuries, prevent further complications, and maximize participation in life. For example, a person with chronic pain participates in a pain management program and implements strategies to minimize pain responses, such as relaxation techniques.

Injury prevention programs are often part of a comprehensive rehabilitation program that includes other interventions discussed in this section, such as work conditioning and ergonomics. A program focused on injury prevention in the workplace and delivered by occupational therapy practitioners may include programs and activities focused on improving workers' fitness and comfort on the job and workplace safety initiatives. On-site injury programs from an occupational therapy perspective typically emphasize education related to health, safety, and injury prevention; proper body mechanics; postural awareness; joint protection; ergonomic considerations; symptom awareness; and stress and pain management strategies applicable to work and productive activities (AOTA, 2017; Dorsey et al., 2019). Practitioners may serve as consultants to employers to assist in establishing, implementing, and evaluating injury prevention programs (AOTA, 2017; Dorsey et al., 2019).

Welfare to Work and Ticket to Work Programs

According to the U.S. Census Bureau (2021), the poverty rate in the United States in 2020 was 11.4%, up 1.0 percentage point compared with 2019. This is important to note because it was the first increase in poverty after five consecutive annual declines. In 2020, 37.2 million people were living in poverty—approximately 3.3 million more than in 2019. Those living in poverty are disproportionately represented by female-headed families on welfare and people with disabilities (U.S. Census, 2021).

Employment is the goal of the Welfare to Work and the Ticket to Work Programs; both offer community-based practice opportunities for occupational therapy practitioners. Employment enhances social integration and empowers people who experience stigma and discrimination and reside on the fringes of society. These people have limited work history and have experienced chronic unemployment, and many have not obtained a high school diploma. Occupational therapists can develop comprehensive community-based programs that address the continuum of seeking, finding, and keeping a job. They can help people identify their interests and skills, workplace expectations and behaviors, interpersonal skills, life–work balance, and life skills in general. These types of services are covered by Welfare to Work Programs (Wilson, 2000, as cited in Mowrey & Riels, 2014), and occupational therapists are ideally suited to empower and enable participants to engage in work. In the current economy, many social programs are fiscally strained, which places vulnerable people at further risk. Mowrey and Riels (2014) noted that occupational therapy practitioners are uniquely suited to serve these two groups and can play a variety of roles from educator to consultant and broker–advocate.

Summary

This chapter provided a broad overview of work as a central occupation, important work policies and programs, and the various roles that occupational therapy fills in this area of practice. Occupational therapy practitioners are found in diverse settings in which work-related services are provided with a wide variety of populations, including people with developmental disabilities, adolescents and younger workers, older workers, and people with mental illness. Work-related services are delivered in a variety of settings, including, but not limited to, sheltered workshops, schools, community settings, industrial environments, and outpatient and inpatient settings (AOTA, 2017). Work as a central occupation has, and always will be, essential to people's health and well-being, and it is an important area of practice for the profession of occupational therapy.

References

ADA Amendments Act of 2008, Pub. L. 110-325, 122 Stat. 3553.

ADA.gov. (2015). *Fighting discrimination in employment under the ADA*. https://www.ada.gov/employment.htm

ADA.gov. (n.d.). *Introduction to the American With Disabilities Act*. https://beta.ada.gov/topics/intro-to-ada/

Age Discrimination in Employment Act of 1967, Pub. L. 90-202, 81 Stat. 602, 29 U.S.C. 621 *et seq*.

Aiken, J. R., Salmon, E. D., & Hanges, P. J. (2013). The origins and legacy of the Civil Rights Act of 1964. *Journal of Business and Psychology, 28*, 383–399. https://doi.org/10.1007/s10869-013-9291-z

American Occupational Therapy Association. (1980). The role of occupational therapy in the vocational rehabilitation process. *American Journal of Occupational Therapy, 34*, 881–883. https://doi.org/10.5014/ajot.34.12.881

American Occupational Therapy Association. (1986). Work hardening guidelines. *American Journal of Occupational Therapy Association, 40*, 841–843. https://doi.org/10.5014/ajot.40.12.841

American Occupational Therapy Association. (1992). Statement: Occupational therapy services in work practice. *American Journal of Occupational Therapy, 46*, 1086–1088. https://doi.org/10.5014/ajot.46.12.1086

American Occupational Therapy Association. (2017). Occupational therapy services in facilitating work participation and performance. *American Journal of Occupational Therapy, 71*(Suppl. 2), 7112410040. https://doi.org/10.5014/ajot.2017.716S05

American Occupational Therapy Association. (2020). Occupational therapy practice framework: Domain and process (4th ed.). *American Journal of Occupational Therapy, 74*(Suppl. 2), 7412410010. https://doi.org/10.5014/ajot.2020.74S2001

American Occupational Therapy Association. (2021). *Special Interest Sections: Work and industry*. https://www.aota.org/community/special-interest-sections/work-and-industry

Americans With Disabilities Act of 1990, Pub. L. 101-336, 42 U.S.C. §§ 12101–12213 (2000).

Bartelink, V. H. M., Zay Ya, K., Guldbrandsson, K., & Bremberg, S. (2020). Unemployment among young people and mental health: A systematic review. *Scandinavian Journal of Public Health, 48*, 544–558. https://doi.org/10.1177/1403494819852847

Bennett, R. (2021). A year into the COVID-19 pandemic: What have we learned about workplaces and what does the future hold? *National Law Review, 12*(187), 284. https://www.natlawreview.com/article/year-covid-19-pandemic-what-have-we-learned-about-workplaces-and-what-does-future

Braveman, B., & Page, J. (Eds.). (2012). *Work: Promoting participation and productivity through occupational therapy*. F. A. Davis.

Chappell, B. (2019, Nov. 4). 4-day workweek boosted workers' productivity by 40%, Microsoft Japan says. National Public Radio. https://www.npr.org/2019/11/04/776163853/microsoft-japan-says-4-day-workweek-boosted-workers-productivity-by-40

Chen, C. P. (2003). Integrating perspectives in career development theory and practice. *The Career Development Quarterly, 51*(3), 203–216. https://doi.org/10.1002/j.2161-0045.2003.tb00602.x

Christiansen, C. (1999). Eleanor Clarke Slagle Lecture—Defining lives: Occupation as identity: An essay on competence, coherence, and the creation of meaning. *American Journal of Occupational Therapy, 53*, 547–558. https://doi.org/10.5014/ajot.53.6.547

Civil Rights Act of 1964, Pub. L. 88-352, 78 Stat. 241, 42 U.S.C. §§ 1981–2000.

Clauw, D. J., & Williams, D. A. (2002). Relationship between stress and pain in work-related upper extremity disorders: The hidden role of chronic multisymptom illnesses. *American Journal of Industrial Medicine, 41*, 370–382. https://doi.org/10.1002/ajim.10068

Diab-Bahman, R., & Al-Enzi, A. (2020). The impact of COVID-19 pandemic on conventional work settings. *International Journal of Sociology and Social Policy, 40*, 909–927. https://doi.org/10.1108/IJSSP-07-2020-0262

Dorsey, J., Ehrenfried, H., Finch, D., & Jaegers, L. (2019). Work. In B. A. B. Schell & G. Gillen (Eds.), *Willard & Spackman's occupational therapy* (13th ed., pp. 779–804). Wolters Kluwer.

Drucker, P. F. (1999). *Management challenges of the 21st century*. HarperBusiness.

Dunn, W., McClain, L. H., Brown, C., & Youngstrom, M. J. (1998). The ecology of human performance. In M. E. Neistadt & E. B. Crepeau (Eds.), *Willard & Spackman's occupational therapy* (9th ed., pp. 525–535). Lippincott Williams & Wilkins.

Education of the Deaf Act of 1986. 100 Stat. 781.

Employee Retirement Income Security Act of 1974, Pub. L. 93-406, 88 Stat. 829.

Esmaeilian, B., Behdad, S., & Wang, B. (2016). The evolution and future of manufacturing: A review. *Journal of Manufacturing Systems, 39*, 79–100. https://doi.org/10.1016/j.jmsy.2016.03.001

Fair Labor Standards Act of 1938, ch. 676, 52 Stat. 1060, 29 U.S.C. 201 *et seq*.

Family and Medical Leave Act of 1993, Pub. L. 103-3, 107 Stat. 6, U.S.C. 6381 *et seq*. 29 U.S.C. 2601 *et seq*.

Federal Employers' Liability Act, 45 U.S.C. § 51 *et seq*. (1908).

Giorgi, G., Lecca, L. I., Alessio, F., Finstad, G. L., Bondamimi, G., Lilli, L. G., . . . Mucci, N. (2020). COVID-19-related mental health effects in the workplace: A narrative review. *International Journal of Environmental Research in Public Health, 17*(21), 7857. https://doi.org/10.3390/ijerph17217857

Glandrea, M. D., & Sprague, S. (2017, February). *Estimating the U.S. labor share.* https://www.bls.gov/opub/mlr/2017/article/estimating-the-us-labor-share.htm

Gordon, D. (2009). The history of occupational therapy. In E. B. Crepeau, E. Cohn, & B. A. B. Schell (Eds.), *Willard & Spackman's occupational therapy* (11th ed., pp. 202–215). Lippincott Williams & Wilkins.

Grant, K. (2012). Job analysis. In A. Bhattacharya & J. McGlothlin (Eds.), *Occupational ergonomics: Theory and applications* (2nd ed., pp. 273–292). CRC Press.

Gupta, J. (2008). Promoting wellness at the workplace. *Work & Industry Special Interest Section Quarterly, 22*(2), 1–4.

Gupta, J., & Sabata, D. (2012). Older workers: Maintaining a worker role and returning to the workplace. In B. Braveman & J. J. Page (Eds.), *Work: Promoting participation and productivity through occupational therapy* (pp. 172–197). F. A. Davis.

Hagel, J., Brown, J. S., Ranjan, A., & Byler, D. (2014). *Passion at work: Cultivating worker passion as a cornerstone of development.* https://www2.deloitte.com/us/en/insights/topics/talent/worker-passion-employee-behavior.html

Haraldsson, G. D., & Kellum, J. (2021, June 4). *Going public: Iceland's journey to a shorter working week.* https://autonomy.work/portfolio/icelandsww/

Harpaz, I., & Fu, X. (2002). The structure and meaning of work: A relative stability amidst change. *Human Relations, 55,* 639–667. https://doi.org/10.1177/0018726702556002

Haruka, D., Page, J., & Wietlisbach, C. (2013). Work evaluation and work programs. In H. Pendleton & W. Shultz-Krohn (Eds.), *Pedretti's occupational therapy practice skills for physical dysfunction* (pp. 337–380). Elsevier.

Hausmann, R. (2013, May 1). The short history of the future of manufacturing. *Scientific American.* https://www.scientificamerican.com/article/manufacturing-short-history-of-future/

Holland, J. L. (1997). *Making vocational choices: A theory of vocational personalities and work environments* (3rd ed.) Psychological Assessment Resources.

Howell, F. M., Frese, W., & Sollie, C. R. (1977). Ginzberg's theory of occupational choice: A reanalysis of increasing realism. *Journal of Vocational Behavior, 11*(3), 332–346. https://doi.org/10.1016/0001-8791(77)90029-X

Individuals With Disabilities Education Act Amendments of 1997, Pub. L. 105-117.

Individuals With Disabilities Education Act of 1990, Pub. L. 101-476, renamed the Individuals With Disabilities Education Improvement Act, codified at 20 U.S.C. §§ 1400–1482.

International Ergonomics Association. (n.d.). *What is ergonomics?* https://iea.cc/what-is-ergonomics/

Jacobs, K., & Baker, N. (2000). The history of work-related therapy in occupational therapy. In B. Kornblau & K. Jacobs (Eds.), *Work: Principles and practice* (pp. 1–11). American Occupational Therapy Association.

Job Accommodation Network. (2021). https://askjan.org/

Kantartzis, S., & Molineux, M. (2011). The influence of Western society's construction of a healthy daily life on the conceptualisation of occupation. *Journal of Occupational Science, 18,* 62–80. https://doi.org/10.1080/14427591.2011.566917

Karger, H., & Rose, S. R. (2010). Revisiting the Americans With Disabilities Act after two decades. *Journal of Social Work in Disability and Rehabilitation, 9,* 73–86. https://doi.org/10.1080/1536710X.2010.493468

Kaskutas, V., & Snodgrass, J. (2009). *Occupational therapy practice guidelines for individuals with work-related injuries and illnesses.* AOTA Press.

Kaushik, M., & Guleria, N. (2020). The impact of pandemic COVID-19 in workplace. *European Journal of Business and Management, 12*(15), 9–18. https://www.iiste.org/Journals/index.php/EJBM/article/view/52883

Kornblau, B., Lou, J., Weeder, T., & Werner, B. (2000). Occupational therapy and theories of career choice and vocational development. In B. Kornblau & K. Jacobs (Eds.), *Work: Principles and practice* (pp. 12–23). American Occupational Therapy Association.

Labor-Management Reporting and Disclosure Act of 1959, Pub. L. 86-257, 73 Stat. 519, 29 U.S.C. 401 *et seq.*

Larson, E., & Zemke, R. (2003). Shaping the temporal patterns of our lives: The social coordination of occupation. *Journal of Occupational Science, 10*(2), 80–89. https://doi.org/10.1080/14427591.2003.9686514

Lent, R. W., & Brown, S. D. (2020). Career decision making, fast and slow: Toward an integrative model of intervention for sustainable career choice. *Journal of Vocational Behavior, 120,* 103448. https://doi.org/10.1016/j.jvb.2020.103448

Lent, R. W., Brown, S. D., & Hackett, G. (1994). Toward a unifying social cognitive theory of career and academic interest, choice, and performance. *Journal of Vocational Behavior, 45,* 79–122. https://doi.org/10.1006/jvbe.1994.1027

Library of Congress. (2021). *List of federal laws related to work and healthcare.*

Lipman, J. (2021, June 1). The pandemic revealed how much we hate our jobs. Now we have a chance to reinvent our work. *Time.* https://time.com/6051955/work-after-covid-19/

Lund, S., Madgavkar, A., Manyika, J., Smit, S., Ellingrud, K., Meaney, M., & Robinson, M. (2021, February 18). *The future of work after COVID-19* (McKinsey Global Institute Report). https://www.mckinsey.com/featured-insights/future-of-work/the-future-of-work-after-covid-19

Maye, A. (2019, May 22). *No-vacation nation, revised.* Center for Economic and Policy Research. https://cepr.net/report/no-vacation-nation-revised/

Medical Facilities Survey and Construction Act of 1954, ch. 471, 68 Stat. 461.

Meyer, S. (2004). *The degradation of work revisited: Workers and technology in the American auto industry, 1900–2000.* Automobile in American Life and Society. http://www.autolife.umd.umich.edu/Labor/L_Overview/L_Overview.htm

Michie, S. (2002). Causes and management of stress at work. *Occupation and Environmental Medicine, 59,* 67–72. https://doi.org/10.1136/oem.59.1.67

Mitchell, J. K., & Krumholtz, J. D. (1996). Krumholtz's learning theory of career choice and development. In D. Brown & L. Brooks (Eds.), *Career choice and development* (3rd ed.). Jossey-Bass.

Mowrey, E. W., & Riels, L. A. (2014). Welfare to work and ticket to work programs. In M. E. Scaffa & S. M. Reitz (Eds.), *Occupational therapy in community-based practice settings* (2nd ed., pp. 257–270). F. A. Davis.

Murphy, G. T., Patel, J., Boden, L. I., & Wolf, J. (2020). *Workers' compensation benefits, costs, and coverage: Executive summary.* National Academy of Social Insurance.

National Academy of Social Insurance. (n.d.). *Workers' compensation and disability.* http://www.nasi.org/learn/workerscomp

National Institute for Occupational Safety and Health. (2017, April 13). *Stress at work.* https://www.cdc.gov/niosh/topics/stress/

Occupational Safety and Health Act of 1970, Pub. L. 91-596, 84 Stat. 1590, 29 U.S.C. 651 *et seq.*

Occupational Safety and Health Administration. (2020). *All about OSHA.* https://www.osha.gov/sites/default/files/publications/all_about_OSHA.pdf

Occupational Safety and Health Administration. (n.d.-a). *Occupational Safety and Health Administration (OSHA) inspections* [OSHA Fact Sheet]. https://www.osha.gov/sites/default/files/factsheet-inspections.pdf

Occupational Safety and Health Administration. (n.d.-b). *OSHA injury and illness recordkeeping and reporting requirements.* https://www.osha.gov/recordkeeping

Occupational Safety and Health Administration. (n.d.-c). *OSHA $afety Pays Program.* https://www.osha.gov/safetypays/estimator

Occupational Safety and Health Administration. (n.d.-d). *State plans.* https://www.osha.gov/stateplans

Okulicz-Kozaryn, A. (2010). Europeans work to live and Americans live to work (who is happy to work more: Americans or Europeans?). *Journal of Happiness Studies, 12,* 225–243. https://doi.org/10.1007/s10902-010-9188-8

Omnibus Budget Reconciliation Act of 1987, Pub. L. 100-203, 101 Stat. 1330.

Page, J. (2012). Physical assessment of the worker. In B. Braveman & J. Page (Eds.), *Work: Promoting participation and productivity through occupational therapy* (pp. 263–282). F. A. Davis.

Parsons, F. (1909). *Choosing a vocation.* Houghton Mifflin.

Pendell, R. (2022, January 1). *7 Gallup Workplace insights: What we learned in 2021.* Gallup Workplace. https://www.gallup.com/workplace/358346/gallup-workplace-insights-learned-2021.aspx

Perlow, L. A. (2012). *Sleeping with your smartphone: How to break the 24/7 habit and change the way you work.* Harvard Business Review Press.

Rehabilitation Act Amendments of 1992, Pub. L. 102-569, 106 Stat. 4344.

Rehabilitation Act of 1973, Pub. L. 93-112, 29 U.S.C. §§ 701–796l.

Reinhardt, W., Schmidt, B., Sloep, P., & Drachsler, H. (2011). Knowledge worker roles and actions—Results of two empirical studies. *Knowledge and Process Management, 18,* 150–174. https://doi.org/10.1002/kpm.378

Schwab, K. (2021, May 4). *Reevaluating your career? You're not alone.* https://www.marketplace.org/2021/05/04/reevaluating-your-career-youre-not-alone/

Snodgrass, J. (2015). Ergonomics and the older person. In L. A. Hunt & C. Wolverson (Eds.), *Work and the older person: Increasing longevity and wellbeing* (pp. 75–88). Slack Incorporated.

Social Security Administration. (2020). The red book—A guide to work incentives (SSA Publication No. 64030). https://www.ssa.gov/redbook/index.html

Social Security Administration. (n.d.). *Welcome to the Ticket to Work Program!* https://www.ssa.gov/work/

Soer, R., van der Schans, C., Groothoof, J., Geertzen, J., & Reneman, M. (2008). Towards consensus in operational definitions in functional capacity evaluation: A Delphi survey. *Journal of Occupational Rehabilitation, 18,* 389–400. https://doi.org/10.1007/s10926-008-9155-y

Sprong, M. E., Iwanaga, K., Mikolajczyk, E., Cerrito, B., & Buono, F. D. (2019). The role of disability in the hiring process: Does knowledge of the Americans With Disabilities Act matter? *Journal of Rehabilitation, 85,* 42–49.

Super, D. E. (1953). A theory of vocational development. *American Psychologist, 8,* 185–190. https://doi.org/10.1037/h0056046

Teasdale, E. L. (2006). Workplace stress. *Psychiatry, 5*(7), 251–254. https://doi.org/10.1053/j.mppsy.2006.04.006

Ticket to Work and Work Incentives Improvement Act of 1999, Pub. L. 106-170, 113 Stat. 1860.

United Nations. (1948). *The Universal Declaration of Human Rights.* https://www.un.org/en/about-us/universal-declaration-of-human-rights

U.S. Bureau of Labor Statistics. (2020). *Strength levels.* https://www.bls.gov/ors/factsheet/strength.htm

U.S. Census Bureau. (2021, September 14). *Income, poverty and health insurance coverage in the United States: 2020.* https://www.census.gov/newsroom/press-releases/2021/income-poverty-health-insurance-coverage.html

U.S. Equal Employment Opportunity Commission. (n.d.). https://www.eeoc.gov/

Vocational Rehabilitation Amendments of 1954, ch. 655, 68 Stat. 652.

Voss, M. W., Wadsworth, L. L., Birmingham, W., Merryman, M. B., Crabtree, L., Subasic, K., & Hung, M. (2020). Health effects of late-career unemployment. *Journal of Aging and Health, 32,* 106–116. https://doi.org/10.1177/0898264318806792

Wegg, L. (1960). Eleanor Clarke Slagle Lecture—The essentials of work evaluation. *American Journal of Occupational Therapy, 14,* 65–69, 79.

West, D. M. (2018). *The future of work: Robots, AI, and automation.* Brookings Institution Press.

World Health Organization. (2020a, February 12). *COVID-19 public health emergency of international concern (PHEIC)* global research and innovation forum. https://www.who.int/publications/m/item/covid-19-public-health-emergency-of-international-concern-(pheic)-global-research-and-innovation-forum

World Health Organization. (2020b, March 11). *WHO Director-General's opening remarks at the media briefing on COVID-19.* https://www.who.int/director-general/speeches/detail/who-director-general-s-opening-remarks-at-the-media-briefing-on-covid-19---11-march-2020

15

Care of Others in the Context of Occupation

KRISTINE HAERTL, PhD, OTR/L, FAOTA, ACE

CHAPTER HIGHLIGHTS

- Applying evaluation and intervention and determining the role of the therapist
- Care and caregiving
- Caregiver burden, stress, and coping in different contexts
- Caregiving and occupation
- Evaluation
- Gender and cultural influences
- Intervention
- Models of caregiving
- Parenting
- Role of occupational therapy in caregiving

KEY TERMS AND CONCEPTS

• authoritarian style of parenting • authoritative style of parenting • Belsky's Process Model • care • care transition • caregiver • caregiver burden • Caregiver Health Model • caregiving • childrearing • culture • culture care theory • emotional care • emotional caring • family systems approach • formal caregiving • hospice care • household care • informal caregiving • informational caring • instrumental caring • medical care • Multi-Level Structural Caring Model • noninvolvement • palliative care • parenting • permissive style of parenting • personal care • Post-Caregiving Health Model • professional caring

Introduction

This chapter presents an overview of the concepts of care, care of others in the context of occupation, and implications for occupational therapy practitioners. The chapter begins with an summary of definitions of *care* and *caregiving* and the differences between the two. Gender and cultural differences within caring roles are discussed along with parenting and caregiver models, including those described in the works of Belsky (1984); Belsky, Vandell et al. (2007) and Baumrind (1967, 1971, 1996) involving parenting styles and determinants. The chapter concludes with information on the roles of occupational therapists and occupational therapy assistants in working with clients and families to assess and develop caregiving skills. The chapter also includes accompanying exercises for the reader to explore their own personal and professional experiences in caring for others as they relate to the chapter content.

Care and Caregiving

Humans are social beings who give and receive care throughout life, sharing in daily activities, while working to create meaning and satisfaction. From the arrival of a newborn to the passing of a valued elderly grandparent, we rely on one another to survive and thrive in the world. Consider a mother raising a toddler, a health practitioner looking after a dying patient, a sister babysitting for a brother with a developmental disability, and partners caring for one another. All these examples encompass acts of care and caregiving. Our earliest memories often revolve around our parents and caregivers. Memories of engaged occupations with a parent may include playing with a favorite toy, sharing a favorite meal, or learning to ride a bike. Such experiences shape our development and worldview (Figure 15.1).

For many, those in caring positions take on the most significant caregiver roles during the beginning and end of the lifespan. When relationships shift as a result of increases in caregiving needs, services from a paid caregiver, health care practitioners, or educators may be needed to facilitate improved care. Knowledge of the concepts of care and caregiving are integral to the role of occupational therapy practitioners in providing holistic services. Caregiving needs change over time; occupational therapists and occupational therapy assistants bring expertise to individuals and families through their knowledge of physical, psychological, sensory, cognitive, and contextual elements that affect caregiving (AOTA, 2020a).

The terms *care* and *caregiving* usually refer to one person taking care of another, as in a parent caring for a child or a child looking after an elderly parent. Although the literature often denotes *parenting* as the roles and functions of biological or adoptive parents with their children and *caregiving* as the care for someone older or ill (e.g., caring for an elderly parent or a loved one with a chronic disease or injury), these terms are broader and more complex than that. For example, *care* and *caregiving* can refer to looking after others or the self as well as tending plants and animals.

FIGURE 15.1. Important occupational experiences shape children's memories of caregivers.

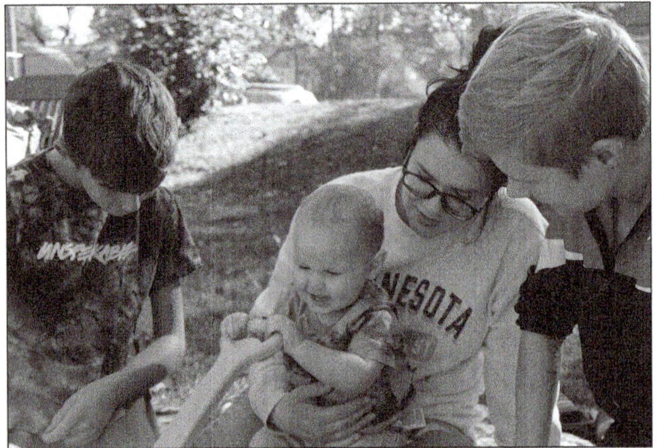

Source. K. Haertl. Used with permission.

Definitions of the term *care* often include descriptions such as "concern for" or "anxiety about" others. Merriam-Webster (n.d.) defines care to include "a disquieted state of mixed uncertainty, apprehension and responsibility" and "painstaking or watchful attention." Yet, this same definition also includes characterizations such as "regard coming from desire or esteem" and "responsibility for or attention to health, well-being and safety." Additional descriptions of *care* include words and phrases such as "concern about," "affection for," and "if you care for someone or something, you look after them and keep them in a good state or condition" (Collins Essential English Dictionary, n.d.). Thus, definitions of *care* are dependent on the context in which the term is used. In the *Occupational Therapy Practice Framework: Domain and Process* (4th ed.; *OTPF-4;* AOTA, 2020b), care of others, child care, and care of pets and animals are all occupations considered under the category of IADLs.

Leininger (1988b), a well-known nurse who was the founder of cultural care theory, differentiated between general care and professional care. She defined *care* and *caring* as "those assistive, supportive, or facilitative acts toward or for another individual or group with evident or anticipated needs to ameliorate or improve a human condition or lifeway" (p. 9). She defined ***professional caring*** as "those cognitive and culturally learned action behaviors, techniques, processes, or patterns that enable (or help) an individual, family, or community to improve or maintain a favorably healthy condition or lifeway" (p. 9). Key commonalities in the definitions of *care* and *caring* transcend the feelings associated with the terms and generally focus on the actions required for caregiving. Leininger's work in the villages of New Guinea was the foundation of her cultural care theory and emphasized that professional care should include the practitioner's knowledge of the cultural background of the client (Post University, 2020). Thus, understanding the terms *care* and *caregiving* must take into consideration the context in which they occur.

Caregiving, with the root word *care,* refers to the process of providing care for another. Generally, the concept of ***caregiver*** refers to the person who provides the primary care and support to a person (Awad & Voruganti, 2008), yet definitions vary based on culture, context, and formal versus informal caregiving. A caregiver is one who tends to the needs of another regardless of whether they are related; caregivers of all kinds, including family caregivers and those caring for close friends, contribute significantly to our health care system (Johns Hopkins Medicine, 2021). Thus, informal and paid caregiver roles may blend; all play an integral role in society throughout the lifespan. Typically, one person is the caregiver and the other person is the care receiver, yet in many situations, the role of caregiver may change. For example, a mother and father care for a child, but later in life, the roles may change as the child takes care of an aging parent. Caregiving may also occur temporarily during instances of brief illness or disability, such as when a teenager requires extra care for a broken bone sustained in a ski accident or a sibling requires extra care during a bout of the flu.

Conceptualizations of caregiving in the literature include both formal and informal caregiving. ***Formal caregiving*** is professional paid care; that is, care provided by a nurse, home health aide, or occupational practitioner. ***Informal caregiving*** is unpaid care provided by a relative or friend. However, the distinction between paid and unpaid caregiving has blurred (European Commission, 2018) because some places, such as the United States and Europe, have systems of payment for family caregivers.

Drentea (2007) defined *caregiving* as "the act of providing unpaid assistance and support to family members or acquaintances who have physical, psychological, or developmental needs" (para. 1). She identified three forms of care: instrumental, emotional, and informational. ***Instrumental caring*** includes the facilitation of tasks such as cooking or providing transportation for a loved one. ***Emotional caring*** involves providing mental support, assistance, counseling, and companionship. Finally, ***informational caring,*** a key type found in health care, may include education, adaptation of the environment, or training in compensatory techniques. Despite the differences in types of caregiving, similarities between familial, or informal, and professional caregiving often include an intense experience with few caregivers providing the care of an individual over a 24-hour period (Hayes, 2021; Lynch & Lobo, 2012). Thus, supports for both the caregiver and the individual cared for are important for maximizing the health and well-being for everyone in the caregiving relationship.

Although care and caregiving are related concepts, they are not identical. The term ***care*** is often used primarily to denote emotional feelings, affection for, and concern for the well-being of another. ***Caregiving,*** however, encompasses the actions and occupations required to meet the daily needs of another (Hayes, 2021). Caregiving may embody aspects of caring, yet a person may experience the emotion to care for another without providing the actual daily caregiving, as in the instance of an elderly relative living in a long-term-care facility. Similarly, a person may take on a formal caregiving role in a health care setting but not have the same affection for the patient as would a family member or friend. It is, however, advantageous if the caregiver maintains an unconditional positive regard and has sincere concern for the well-being of the person cared for. Caregiving takes on different forms based on the context of the caregiving situation as well as individual client factors of both the caregiver and the individual receiving care (Broese van Groenou et al., 2013).

EXERCISE 15.1. Caregiver and Care Receiver Roles

Identify the primary roles and occupational activities that you have taken on as a caregiver and care receiver in your life. Answer these questions:

- How did these roles change over the course of time?
- What specific occupations were involved in these caregiving relationships?
- What performance skills and client factors were used in these occupations?
- Consider your daily schedule and occupational demands. Do the roles of caregiver and care receiver have a prominent place, or do other occupational roles such as being a student require most of your time?
- Do you have competing responsibilities and caregiving roles that create role conflict?
- How can you work to balance your roles?
- How will your experiences as a caregiver and care receiver affect you as an occupational therapy practitioner?

Caregiving and Occupation

Who are caregivers, and what are their roles and functions? Although context greatly influences the nature of caregiving across Western cultures, there are many similarities among all caregivers. Statistics cited by the Caregiver Action Network (2021) indicate that more than 65 million Americans (29% of the U.S. population) care for in any given year. According to the same source, the caregiving value of services provided by family members is estimated at $375 billion a year, nearly twice as much as is paid for formal health care. Yet, disparities exist based on race and socioeconomic status.

According to the Centers for Disease Control and Prevention (2019), 94.3% of White caregivers had health care coverage in the United States, whereas 94.1% of Asian, 89.1% of Black, and 85.2% of Hispanic caregivers had such coverage. In addition, of those over age 65 years requiring home health care, more than 80% had a caregiver outside of a formal agency, and males in this cohort were nearly three times as likely as females to have a spouse as their primary caregiver (Jones et al., 2012). Unpaid relatives and friends will likely continue to be a significant provider of long-term-care services, thus often necessitating education from members of educational and health care teams, including occupational therapy practitioners.

Although people of all ages, genders, and sociocultural backgrounds may be called upon to take on caregiving roles, in the United States and globally, women are the predominant providers of care (Sharma et al., 2016). In Canada, the number of reported informal caregivers indicates that about one in four Canadians over the age of 15, or greater than 7.8 million people, were providing caregiving services to a family member or friend with a disability or health condition (Statistics Canada, 2018). In Europe, the familial statistics of caring are even higher. Family members provide more than 80% of care needs, with two-thirds of the caregivers being female (European Commission, 2018; Hoffman & Rodrigues, 2010). Although these statistics reflect the fact that the term *caregiving* is often used to describe providing assistance for elderly people or a person with a disability or temporary illness, caregiving also includes taking care of infants, children, and even plants and animals. In addition, such care involves both emotional challenges and personal satisfaction.

The process of caregiving is relational between those giving care and those receiving care. It can be formal (i.e., in a professional capacity) or informal (i.e., carried out by a friend or family member) and be done in the context of parenting, providing care for an individual with a disability, or caring for someone with an acute or long-term illness. The occupations surrounding caregiving vary depending on the relationship, context, and type of care. Caregiving is its own occupation, but it also requires a variety of occupational functions, including facilitating daily self-care ADL tasks and assisting with high-level IADL activities such as cooking and financial management. It can also include educational responsibilities as well as leisure engagement.

Such functions often occur as co-occupation, by which both the caregiver and receiver are sharing in the occupation in a particular time and space. Familial and systems shifts affect occupational patterns and the environment in which caregiving occurs, as in the case of a public health crisis such as the recent SARS-CoV-2 virus (COVID-19) pandemic. This pandemic caused increased social isolation, changed the nature of caregiving activities, and put a strain on both informal and formal caregivers. It also brought awareness of the importance of the health and well-being of both the caregiver and the care recipient (National Alliance for Caregiving, 2021).

In the case scenario below, the nature of caregiving is formal and multifaceted. John has lived in several foster homes and receives care for his basic physical, cognitive, emotional, and academic needs. The role of primary caregiver in a parental relationship is easy to identify, whereas in John's situation, it is far more complex because the staff members at the crisis home, his case manager, and the special education professionals all have unique roles in John's care. Moreover, during a public health crisis such as the pandemic, John's caregivers would have to shift the nature of care coordination to largely virtual. Emphasis of care is placed on supporting his daily personal, psychological, educational, and wellness needs within the home.

EXERCISE 15.2. Case Scenario: John, Caregiving Issues

John is a 7-year-old child with moderate intellectual and developmental disability (cerebral palsy, fetal alcohol syndrome, and oppositional defiant disorder). His biological mother used illicit drugs during pregnancy and abandoned him at birth, and his father's identity is unknown. John has lived in various foster care homes throughout his life. Because of recent assaultive behaviors, he was placed in a crisis home and is currently receiving services through the home, school, and county. Answer these questions:

- Who are the caregivers in this situation?
- Are they formal or informal caregivers?
- What can be done to facilitate the coordination of care in this instance?
- How might the COVID-19 pandemic have shifted the caregiving activities for John?
- As an occupational therapy practitioner, what supports do you believe would be important for John and for his caregivers to maximize occupational performance and personal satisfaction?
- How would these supports shift during the pandemic?

Caregiving may be categorized according to the relationship and the informal versus formal nature of the care provided. For example, Lackey and Gates (2001) classified caregiving for a family member with an illness into four broad categories: (1) provision of personal care, (2) provision of medical care, (3) provision of household care, and (4) spending time (emotional care) with the care receiver. ***Personal care*** includes such tasks as assistance with bathing, grooming, dressing, and feeding. ***Medical care*** includes the daily activities that assist a person in meeting health needs such as wound care or medication administration. ***Household care*** includes assistance with daily tasks such as cooking and cleaning, and ***emotional care*** provides support by spending time with, talking to, or praying with the care receiver.

Drentea's (2007) caregiving categorizations, discussed previously, differ from Lackey and Gates' (2001) by broadening their scope to include instrumental, emotional, and informational tasks. Perhaps one of the most comprehensive conceptualizations of caregiving is by Sellick (2005), who identified six domains of wellness that are crucial to both the caregiver and the care receiver. Sellick asserted the importance of maintaining wellness within the caregiver–care receiver relationship in these six domains:

1. *Physical:* physical needs, finances, nutrition, lifestyle, health and medical
2. *Emotional:* expression of feelings, control of stress, problem solving, self-efficacy
3. *Social:* relational; respect for self and others; interaction with the environment, people, peers, and community; social cause
4. *Spiritual:* purpose in life, morals and ethics, self-determination, love, hope, faith
5. *Intellectual:* lifelong learning, cognition, exploration
6. *Vocational:* skill development, work, volunteerism, personal interests.

The number of caregiving tasks and perceived difficulty may affect caregiver stress (Castellanos et al., 2019), thus con-

EXERCISE 15.3. Primary Caregiving

Consider your own life course. Who have been your primary caregivers in each of the six domains outlined by Sellick (2005)? Notice that in some situations there may be role differences (e.g., in the intellectual domain, a teacher may have played a key role but was not considered a formal caregiver). Which domains have relied more heavily on other people, and which have required self-care and self-determination? As an occupational therapy practitioner, how would you ensure that each of the domains is addressed for your clients?

sideration of each of these domains of well-being for both the caregiver and the care receiver is crucial to enhancing quality of life and the caregiver–care receiver relationship.

Gender and Cultural Influences

Gender and culture heavily influence roles and functions of caregiving and the development of related skills. From our early years, we learn about our culture and ourselves through our caregivers, with our parents often being the primary role models.

Gender

Parents are generally the socializing agents for gender roles within society (Leaper, 2002). Whereas primary childrearing responsibilities traditionally have focused on the mother, in recent years, fathers have increased their role in childrearing (Riina & Feinberg, 2012; Figure 15.2). Yet, parenthood continues as one of the most gender-typed adult roles (Roskam & Mikolajczak, 2020) because differences exist between mothering and fathering, and parents often differentiate how they treat their children based on gender; for example, through the way they dress their children or the toys they give them.

The blending of gender roles has occurred over time, as evidenced, for example, in the increase in numbers of female doctors and lawyers and of men taking on significant roles in parenting and child care or careers in nursing. In addition, the number of adoptions of children by gay and lesbian couples has increased (Geisler, 2012). Thus, familial and parenting structures have changed over time. Although the marriage rate for the general population has declined; the rate of marriages in the lesbian gay bisexual transgender queer (LGBTQ) community has increased (Family Equality Council, 2017); and in addition to adoption, in many countries in vitro fertilization (IVF) provides LGBTQ couples with options for parenting (Figure 15.3).

Despite progressive changes, Western cultures still maintain distinct differences between genders, as exemplified in the toy aisles of department stores or in television advertisements aimed at audiences of a particular gender. Parents often teach girls to care for and nurture dolls, and boys to play with trucks, cars, and action figures. Such socialization may lend itself to differing roles for caregivers. Research has suggested that fathers engage in play that is more physical with their children, whereas mothers tend to engage in more imaginary play (Lindsay & Mize, 2001). Men have also been shown to use more technological approaches (e.g., tablets, video games) in socializing their children, whereas women tend to use creative and pretend forms of play (Abrahamy et al., 2003). Gender roles further extend to the socialization of emotion, involving gender differences in emotional expression and the responsiveness to emotion based on gender (Kennedy Root & Denham, 2010), thus influencing gender expression physically, socially, and emotionally. Moreover, Lee and Hofferth (2017) conducted a data analysis of the American Time Use Survey to determine how much time single fathers and mothers spend parenting. They found that single fathers spend slightly less time than single mothers in child-care tasks and teaching; however, time spent in play was comparable in both genders. Contextual and cultural differences also influence parenting tasks between genders.

Gender differences are also noted as people age and take on responsibility for spouses, or parents, regarding tasks, responsibilities, and psychological responses to caregiving (Coutinho et al., 2006; Swinkels et al., 2019). Some of these caregiving roles are planned, such as when a couple decides to have chil-

FIGURE 15.2. Gender and culture often influence caregiving. Women continue to provide the majority of caregiving worldwide yet the role of fathers has increased in the past couple of decades.

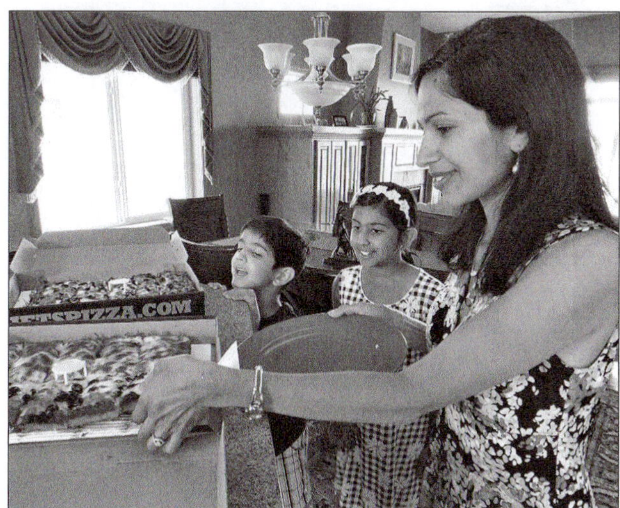

Source. K. Haertl. Used with permission.

FIGURE 15.3. The number of LGBTQ couples parenting children is increasing. Mikaela and her wife Bri care for their two children.

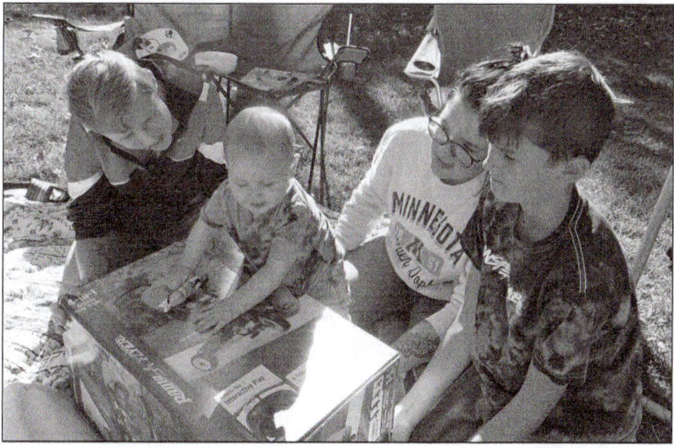

Source. K. Haertl. Used with permission.

EXERCISE 15.4. Caregivers in Life

Consider two caregivers in your childhood. What were the gender and cultural differences you experienced? Compare and contrast your experience of caregiving with that of someone from a different cultural background (e.g., ethnic, rural–urban, socioeconomic). What are the similarities and differences between your experience and theirs? Why is this important knowledge for an occupational therapy practitioner?

dren or chooses to assist in caring for a grandchild. Other caregiving roles are unplanned, such as caring for a spouse with a traumatic brain injury or an aging parent after a stroke.

Culture

Social behaviors of caring reflect expectations of relationships through the cultural milieu in which the caregiving takes place. The phenomenon of caring is universal, yet it is uniquely expressed across cultures and time. ***Culture*** includes the human beliefs, values, and activities existing within a particular setting or group. Given the multitude of cultural groupings as well as heterogeneity within in-group differences, culture is difficult to universally define (Cardemil, 2010; Jahoda, 2012), yet Mironenko and Sorokin (2018) asserted that continued interdisciplinary efforts should seek to find commonality in its definition. Although often referred to in relation to ethnic background, the term *culture* is far more comprehensive and may include socioeconomic status, geographical locale, gender, sexual orientation, ability status, age, and even a particular professional cohort (Figure 15.4).

Despite the various cultural groupings, much of the literature and research on similarities and differences in caregiving practices is based on ethnic groups. The meaning of caregiving within the familial structure is often ethnocentrically based (Napoles et al., 2010), and therefore an understanding of the interface of cultural values and caregiving is essential to providing quality services (McCleary & Blain, 2013).

FIGURE 15.4. In addition to traditional caregiving in education, ADL and IADL activities, play and leisure are integral in caregiving relationships in all cultures.

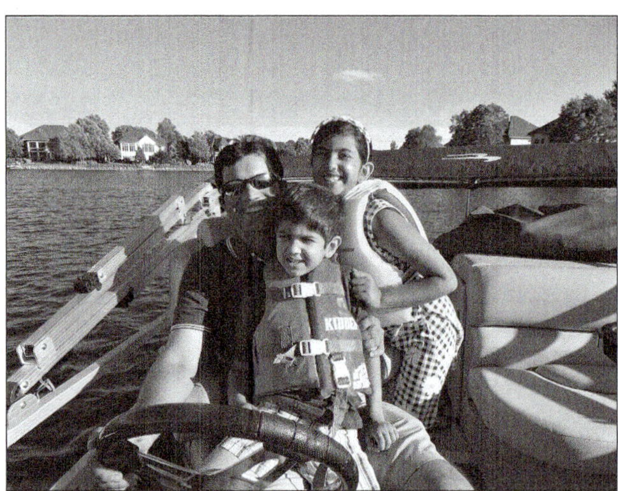

Source. K. Haertl. Used with permission.

In the United States, elderly people from ethnic minorities are more likely to be taken care of by an extended family network than are their European American counterparts because informal caregiving is more prevalent among ethnic minority groups (Rote & Moon, 2018). In addition, Latinx persons tend to spend more time in caregiving of elders than non-Latinx Whites and Blacks as a result of the higher percentage of co-residence situations (Pharr et al., 2014; Rote & Moon, 2018). Level of integration into U.S. society and socioeconomic factors may also affect the extent to which financial and personal responsibility are met in extended family caregiving (Sarkisian et al., 2007; see Figure 15.5). Despite these differences, common variables exist across cultures, including learning caregiving roles from parents and other kin during the developmental years; developing personal and cultural beliefs about the responsibility for taking care of family or extended family; and incorporating personal and familial beliefs, attitudes, and behaviors into caretaking (Ayalong, 2004).

Leininger's (1996) ***culture care theory*** emphasizes the importance of the clients' perception that the care delivered is

FIGURE 15.5. Siblings may help with family caregiving responsibilities.

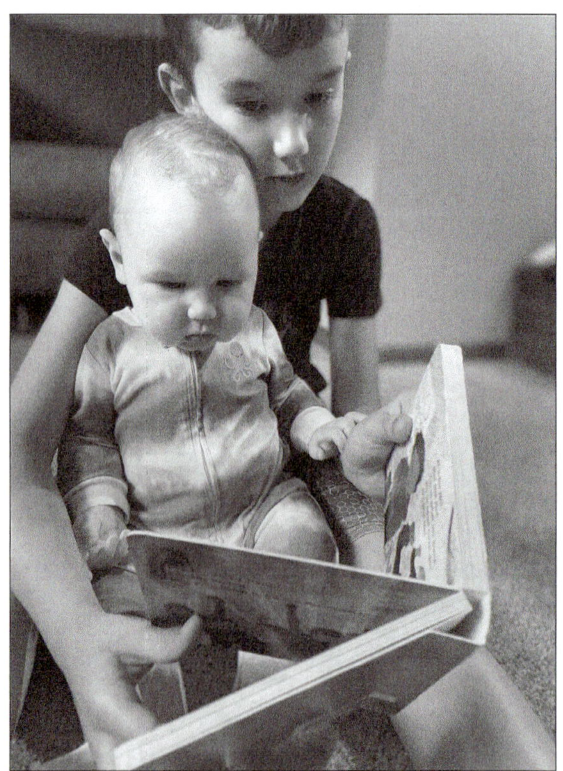

Source. K. Haertl. Used with permission.

congruent with their personal values and beliefs. This theory focuses on care that assists others' needs; care that is actively directed toward attention to culture; the actions, beliefs, and norms that guide thinking and action; and culture care diversity, which refers to types of care for different groups (Post University, 2020). According to this theory, the foundation of care in occupational therapy must be sensitive to the unique background of the client.

Models of Caregiving

Although a comprehensive presentation of caregiving models transcends the scope of this chapter, a general understanding is important for occupational therapy practitioners. Just as the *OTPF–4* addresses clients at the level of persons, groups, and populations (AOTA, 2020b), caregiving theories apply to all levels of service delivery. Caregiving models vary in their conceptual focus, from a global perspective on the systems and structures that support and govern caregiving to a more individualized emphasis on practitioner care and the relationship between caregivers and care receivers. Experts have described micro and macro factors that affect caregiving at all levels (e.g., Leininger, 1988a; Mak, 2005).

The ***Multi-Level Structural Caring Model*** as proposed by Leininger (1988a) is a hierarchical model used to conceptualize the scope, nature, and structures of caring. This model's highest level is a worldwide multicultural societal focus of caring. Leininger asserted that studies on this level generate information regarding broad views and theoretical underpinnings of care. At the mid-level, specific cultures and systems are emphasized, providing information about the systemic aspects of culture that influence care, such as legal, political, health care, and economic systems. At the lowest level are the individual or group foci, conceptualizing caring structures and functions within family or small interpersonal groups.

In contrast to large groupings, authors have also identified multilevel factors that influence caregiving on an interpersonal level. Mak (2005) identified macro factors affecting individual caregivers, including sociocultural factors such as ethnicity, age, gender, and income; interpersonal factors such as marital factors and kinship ties; structural factors such as managed care and health care systems; and clinical factors such as the caregiver and care receiver health. Micro influences on caregiving include individual experiences, day-to-day encounters, and occupational patterns within the caregiving relationship. A caregiving relationship may have strengths in certain factors, such as a close caring relationship, yet be negatively affected by lack of resources, exacerbation of illness, role strain, or limited health care coverage.

Other newer models such as the ***Post-Caregiving Health Model*** (Corey Magan et al., 2020), a model related to post-caregiving of those with dementia, and the ***Caregiver Health Model*** (Weierbach & Cao, 2016) emphasize the importance of personal appraisal, health beliefs and attitudes, coping, emotion, and the environment on the personal health of the caregiver. To provide holistic client-centered services, health practitioners must take all levels of caregiving into consideration when planning evaluation and interventions.

Parenting

Adding a child to a family is always an adjustment. Adding in the complexities of a child or parent with a disability may require the service of a health care team and occupational therapy practitioner during the adjustment process. Knowledge of parenting models is important in supporting the parent–child relationship. Parenting includes familiar ADLs and the development of performance patterns that incorporate children into familial life. The term ***parenting*** is distinguished from child rearing in that it denotes the actions taken by a parent to support and influence a child's development (Lee et al., 2014). ***Childrearing*** may encompass activities beyond the family, including those involving societal and educational systems. Although this section of the chapter focuses on classic research on parenting, it is important to note that most of this research is from developed countries and Western society (Ashdown & Faherty, 2020) and, thus, it is important to also consider the wider cultural lens.

Many parenting models emphasize an ecological theoretical framework that acknowledges multiple factors that influence parenting and child development (Farnfield, 2008). Parenting research and subsequent frameworks and models are often focused on the relationship between parent and child through attachment theory (Bowlby, 1982), styles of parenting (Baumrind, 1967, 1971, 1996), and parental processes (Belsky, 1984; Belsky, Fearon, & Bell, 2007; Belsky, Vandell et al., 2007). A comprehensive description of attachment styles and temperament may be found in the psychology literature. Given that the works of Baumrind and of Belsky and colleagues have largely stood the test of time (Taraban & Shaw, 2018), they will be the focus of this section. Consideration of these prominent models should include a bio-ecological perspective that acknowledges individual factors as well as the interactions of the parent, child, and the environment (Kiff et al., 2011; Taraban & Shaw, 2018).

Baumrind's Parenting Styles

In her seminal work, Baumrind (1967, 1971) found that parents differ in their expressions of maturity, communication, discipline, and warmth. Based on these dimensions, she identified distinct parenting styles, including permissive style, authoritative style, and authoritarian style. The ***permissive style of parenting*** governs children in an accepting, affirmative, and nonpunitive manner. In this style, parents generally make few demands of the child and maximize child input yet do not seek to model antisocial behaviors or behaviors that result in disobedience or have low tolerance for challenge. Over time, children with permissive parents may lack self-control and may struggle with the firm demands later placed on them in school.

The ***authoritative style of parenting*** emphasizes autonomy and self-will; values the child's gifts, talents, and individuality; and sets clear expectations for standards. This type of parenting often leads to well-adjusted children with the ability to regulate emotion and positive social skills. In this style of parenting, parents value the child's individuality but continue to maintain their parental authority and role in setting limits.

The ***authoritarian style of parenting*** seeks to shape the child's behaviors through discipline, firm expectations, and a set code of conduct. This type of parent is often strict and may use external forces and rules such as those derived from religion, specific philosophies, or an external set of beliefs to help guide parenting. Authoritarian styles involve more control and less flexibility than other styles and may lead to children with anxious and withdrawn demeanors and poor frustration tolerance.

A final style of parenting includes ***noninvolvement,*** which may result in low responsiveness, low involvement, and low demands. In extreme cases, children may be neglected or left without necessary care.

Over decades of research, Baumrind (1967, 1971, 1996) concluded that the authoritative parenting style, which seeks to use warmth and guidance through listening and shaping the child's behaviors, is most effective and results in happier, better adjusted children than the other parenting styles.

Although contextual cultural variations occur in parenting styles, Sorkhabi's (2005) work concluded that Baumrind's (1967, 1971) four parenting styles are applicable to both individualistic and collectivist cultures. She asserted, however, that the manifestations of parenting styles may not result in similar outcomes in collectivist cultures and that more research is needed to confirm this position.

Recent research on culturally diverse youth has suggested that parenting styles influence adolescent development and response to conflict (McKinney & Renk, 2011). However, multiple variables, including the dynamics of relationships within the family, the environment, the nature of conflict, and the presence of psychological difficulties, must be considered in determining the influence of parenting styles. A study in Iran affirmed the importance of the warm, positive authoritative parenting style versus the more hostile, strict authoritarian style in supporting children's development and emotional well-being (Kooraneh & Amirsardari, 2015). Pinquart and Rubina (2018) conducted a meta-analysis of parenting styles throughout the world. Despite some slight differences, particularly in cultures that may have slightly higher authoritarian versus authoritative styles, the authors concluded that parents around the globe could be recommended to use an authoritative parenting style. Thus, although Baumrind's work applies to diverse populations, care must be taken to apply holistic client-centered practices to working with families. Baumrind's seminal work on parenting styles continues to be upheld and used in a variety of studies to investigate the effects of parenting practices (e.g., Dehyadegary et al., 2012; Woolfsen & Grant, 2006).

Belsky's Process Model

Research has revealed a link between the quality of parenting and subsequent child development (Belsky, Vandell et al., 2007). Whereas Baumrind (1967, 1971) emphasized parenting styles, Belsky (1984) developed a process model that sought to explain the determinants or factors that influence parenting and their subsequent effects on child development. ***Belsky's Process Model*** asserts that "parents' developmental histories, marital relations, social networks, and jobs influence individual personality and general psychological well-being of parents and, thereby, parental functioning and, in turn child development" (p. 84). Belsky identified three domains or determinants influencing the parental process: (1) personal and psychological resources of the parents, (2) characteristics of the child, and (3) contextual sources of stress and support. Parental personality and psychological well-being were found to be the most powerful determinants in supporting parental function and child development.

This model assumes that parenting is influenced by forces both internal and external to the parent and child, along with the contextual factors in which the parenting takes place. Major contextual influences on stress and support include the marital relationship, social networks, and work. The model concludes that parenting is influenced by a multitude of factors, determinant factors do not equally influence the parenting process, and personality and developmental history indirectly shape the parenting process through the broader context.

Subsequent to Belsky's original research and model, Belsky, Fearon, and Bell (2007) found that although parenting is most influential in determining child development, the quality of early child care experiences external to the home also affects child development, performance, and behavior. Recent research has also used Belsky's model to explore early child care education (Swindle et al., 2017) as well as maternal emotion socialization (Bao & Kato, 2020). In addition, it appears that cultural differences influence some of the determinants of parenting. Cardosa et al. (2010) found that patterns of parental maternal stress in non-Hispanic White and non-Hispanic Black populations were consistent with Belsky's model, yet for Mexican American mothers, social support rather than spousal support helped ameliorate parental stress. Taraban and Shaw (2018) asserted that although Belsky's work has stood the test of time, additional research is needed to consider the role of culture as it interfaces with other contextual factors that influence parenting. Therefore, determinant factors of parenting should include a cultural lens, and through an understanding of the determinants of parenting and caregiving, occupational therapy practitioners can work to teach skills designed to enhance the relationship between caregiver and care receiver.

Caregiver Burden, Stress, and Coping in Different Contexts

Models of caregiving for the elderly or people with an illness or disability differ in their approach from parenting models. Many focus on the burden, stress, and coping demands of the caregiving situation. Some researchers, however, have argued that models of caregiving that focus only on these factors are inadequate given the complexity of caregiving situations (Upton & Reed, 2006).

The term ***caregiver burden*** refers to the emotional, financial, and physical strains resulting from a caregiving situation. This stress increases with additional external demands. Many contextual variables influence caregiver stress and burden, yet researchers have particularly emphasized the importance of the subjective perceptions of family members and caregivers in determining levels of caregiver burden (Murray et al., 2011). Given similar illnesses and family situations, differences occur in perceived stress. This variability is based on familial relationships, external supports, and attitudes toward the caregiving situation. Some families and individuals are more resilient regarding the stressors of caregiving roles, and others struggle to meet their typical daily obligations along with caregiving demands. As populations age and there is an increased need for familial caregivers, policy changes and education can help support familial and other informal caregivers (Harding et al., 2015).

Positive coping strategies, caregiver mastery, social support, cognitive appraisal, and education have been shown to mediate the stress caused by caregiver burden (Ergh et al., 2002; Liu & Huang, 2018; Murray et al., 2011; Pioli, 2010; Wells et al., 2005). Feeling that one has the ability to respond to stress by using effective coping strategies is important in maintaining caregiver health and decreasing burden (Kazemi et al., 2021; Tsai & Pai, 2016). Perceived self-efficacy and the ability to handle caregiver situations also influence caregiver burden (Liu & Huang, 2018).

In occupational therapy, emphasis is placed on skill building and creating a good client–environment fit to maximize occupational performance and reduce stress. Everyday occupational involvement between caregivers and care receivers has been found to create meaning and help mitigate disruption and stress in caregiving situations (Cruz & Caro, 2017; Hasselkus & Murray, 2007). For practitioners working with caregivers, emphasis is placed on providing family supports to reduce stress and maximize quality of life for both caregivers and care receivers. Therefore, a family perspective and a clear understanding of the complexities of the relationship between practitioner and family are integral to maximizing health and quality of life for clients (Klein & Liu, 2010). Note that the cognitive model of caregiving, often used with people with a psychiatric disorder, emphasizes the importance of caregivers' emotions and reactions, particularly in the presence of psychosis, and how such a disorder affects the well-being of both the caregiver and care receiver (Kuipers et al., 2018). Thus, education and support are important in working with caregivers.

Home Care

Models of caregiving consider the caregiver, the care receiver, and the context in which caregiving takes place (Figures 15.6 and 15.7). For example, care for the ill, infirmed, or elderly occurs in a multitude of environments, including institutional settings, small group homes, health care settings, and family homes. With the number of elderly people increasing globally, many nations have re-emphasized aging in place and family-based care (Bhattarai, 2013). Home-based caregiving may include specialized in-home services in addition to caregiver and family education to maximize quality of life for all and decrease caregiver and care-receiver stress.

In recent years, emphasis has been placed on encouraging research and models of care that provide support for family caregivers and emphasize the preservation of meaning and quality of life for both the caregiver and the care receiver (e.g., Kuipers et al., 2018; Sellick, 2005; Vellone et al., 2008). For example, Meidenbauer et al. (2019) found that occupational therapists providing an educational approach to caregivers delivering care in the home resulted in a significant increase in caregiver confidence and a decrease in depression levels and fatigue. Use of these models support the caregiver in the

FIGURE 15.6. Over time, caregiving roles may shift. In this setting, a well 92-year-old is assisted by her daughter for transportation needs.

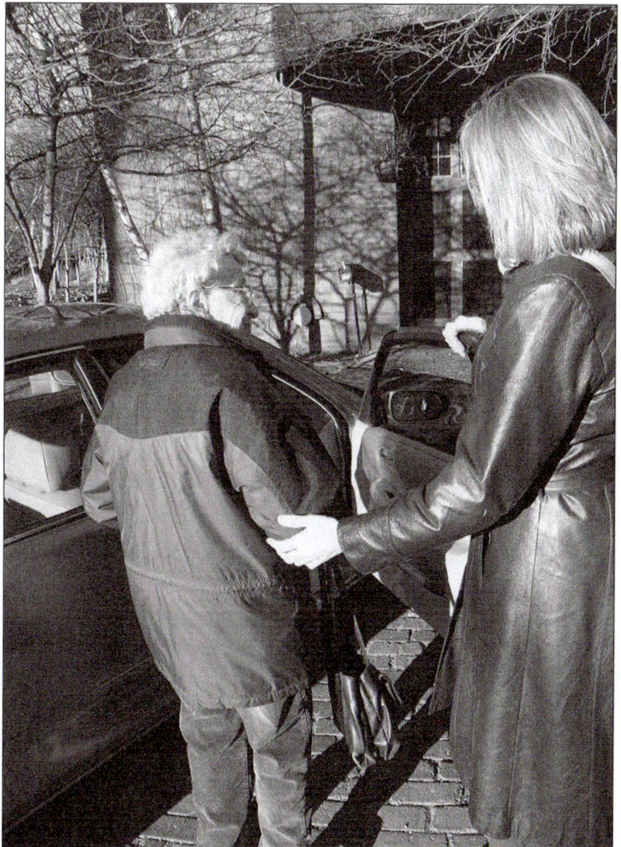

Source. K. Haertl. Used with permission.

FIGURE 15.7. Within the same relationship, this mother cared for her daughter during a serious illness.

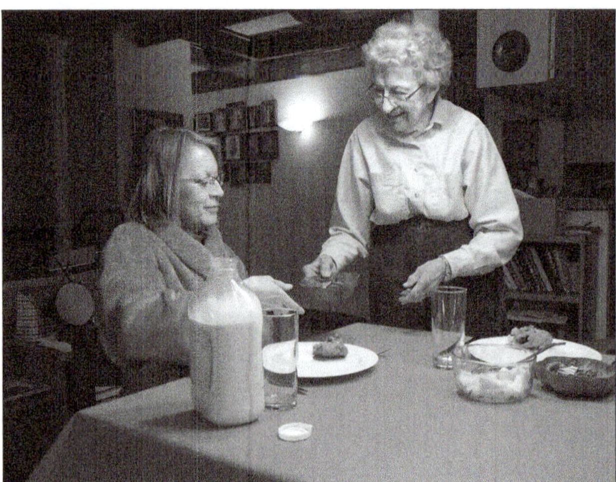

Source. K. Haertl. Used with permission.

home and facilitate services for both the caregiver and the care receiver.

Care Transition

Clinicians are instrumental in the facilitation of ***care transition*** (i.e., moving from one setting to another). Families may have to cope with feelings of guilt, ambivalence, and loss around decisions of, for example, placing a child with disabilities in a group home or an elderly spouse in a nursing home. Kellet (1999) identified five themes common to family caregivers after nursing home placement:

- perceived loss of control
- a feeling of disempowerment
- perceived sense of failure
- feelings of simultaneous sadness, guilt, and relief
- feeling of being forced to make a negative choice.

It is important for practitioners to support the family through such transitions and to include the family in decisions regarding the extent and nature of their involvement after placement. Families and caregivers can be supported in maintaining contact and staying involved with their family member's care in several ways through visits, involvement with the care team, and ongoing communication.

EXERCISE 15.5. Long-Term-Care Facility

Consider the effects of having a family member placed in a long-term-care facility (e.g., nursing home, group home). Answer the following questions:

- What is the impact on the family and on the person placed in the facility?
- As an occupational therapy practitioner, what strategies can you use to facilitate family involvement after placement?
- How can the family maintain meaningful occupational and social engagement with the person placed in the facility?
- As an occupational therapy practitioner, how can you support families in working through these transitions?

Hospice Care

Palliative and hospice models of care fulfill specific needs for caregivers and care receivers. ***Palliative care*** refers to reducing pain and distress during an illness and may occur at any stage of the illness, whereas ***hospice care*** focuses on the last months of life (Lowey, 2015). Note that many of the goals of hospice care are applicable to all caregiving situations. Hospice models were developed through charitable organizations to provide a compassionate, homelike atmosphere in the end stages of life, and in recent years, guidelines around hospice care have evolved surrounding care requirements and reimbursement (Grant & Scott, 2015).

Hospice models focus on dignity, comfort, and quality of life throughout the dying process. Four key values of these models identified by Lattanzi-Licht (2001) are (1) worth of the person, (2) importance of choice and self-determination, (3) provision for whole-person care, and (4) family-centered care. Hospice also aims to enhance dignity through holistic individualized approaches that focus on comfort, pain management, and care. Such care may include the community, neighbors, and those who care about the client to provide education and support throughout the hospice experience (e.g., Poroch, 2012). This support continues for the family after their loved one's death, with grieving, recognition of the loss, and a period of mourning being part of the process.

During the transition into hospice, daily patterns and activities may shift, yet the preservation of self-worth, dignity, and meaning is imperative. In studying people in hospice, occupational therapists Jacques and Hasselkus (2004) found that throughout the dying process, occupational engagement takes on new meaning even in ordinary and familiar everyday activities. Provision for daily routines that support meaningful occupational engagement and co-occupation between caregivers and care receivers throughout all phases of care appears to mediate stress brought on by daily requirements of caregiving and the transition to hospice or other caregiving facilities.

The role of the rehabilitation practitioner in the hospice environment includes working to maintain function in the end-of-life process and serving to preserve and enhance overall quality of life for the entire family (Javier & Montagnini, 2011). Thus, practitioners serving all client populations may benefit from understanding the goals and values of the hospice model in supporting quality of life throughout all phases of habilitation, rehabilitation, and caregiving.

Role of Occupational Therapy in Caregiving

As the demographic profiles of many industrialized nations shift toward increasing numbers of elderly people, the occupational therapy profession must work to meet the needs of more family members who are informal caregivers for those with illness and disability. Although many health professions adhere to models of caregiving, occupational therapy holds a unique viewpoint in its emphasis on the use of occupation-based evaluation and intervention. A comprehensive review of the need for occupational therapy services in caregiving families revealed key themes:

- importance of emphasizing meaning and motivation in the caregiving relationship
- emphasis on caregiver–care receiver occupations and the use of meaningful occupation in therapy
- acknowledgment of gender roles, which often influence occupational engagement
- importance of developing positive caregiving–care receiving routines and habits
- management and development of environmental structures and modifications to support meaningful occupation and improve outcomes
- use of Person–Environment–Occupation models to facilitate positive adaptation (Coutinho et al., 2006).

The *OTPF–4* cites an overarching assertion of occupational therapy's domain in "achieving health, well-being, and participation in life through engagement in occupation" (AOTA, 2020b, p. 5). Within the realm of caregiving, occupational therapy practitioners work with families to ensure that caregiving skills are supported to maximize client participation, meaning, and engagement in occupations. The primary client may include the caregiver (e.g., a client with mental health concerns who is learning parenting skills), the care receiver (e.g., a client with dementia whose family must be educated in the client's caregiving needs), or an entire system (e.g., facilitating positive environments for seniors). When considering environmental and caregiver supports to maximize occupational engagement, Haertl (2011) emphasized the importance of including the family and the extended care network (additional people involved with a client's care and daily activities) throughout the evaluation and intervention process. Key questions regarding family identified by Haertl included:

- What is the role of the family in the client's life?
- Are there conflicts within the family, and what is the client's view of the family?
- To what extent is, and should, the family be involved in the therapy process?
- Will the client return to live with the family (or spouse)? If not, where will the client live?
- Is there agreement regarding the course of intervention among the family, health professionals, and other care providers?
- What are the family's strengths, resources, and needs? How can the strengths be most effectively used, and how can the needs be most successfully met?

Key questions regarding the extended care network included:

- Who are the important people in the client's life, and how will they be involved in the therapy process?
- Are the caregivers adequately trained, prepared, and willing to follow through with the intervention plan? What training needs exist?
- What extended care network resources are available, and how can they best be used?
- What are the strengths and needs of the extended care network, and how are they used?

Practitioners providing family and caregiver occupational therapy services assess strengths and needs and provide supports necessary for maximal occupational function. Such support may include the use of direct models of intervention, education, and adaptation or home modification. Evaluation and intervention methods may be delivered at the client, family, or systems level and may include virtual or telehealth models as well as coaching to deliver services to both the client and caregiver (Fortuna, 2020).

Evaluation

Although childrearing, care of others, and care of pets are listed in the *OTPF–4* as IADLs in occupational therapy's domain of practice (AOTA, 2020b), limited options are available pertaining to direct occupational therapy–based standardized assessment tools for parenting and caregiving. Evaluation involves identifying the client's current state, the contextual influences of the setting in which the caregiving takes place, assessing the care receiver–caregiver relationship, and identifying the role of the occupational therapist throughout the evaluation and intervention process. Most of the formalized instruments designed for assessing ADLs and IADLs focus on self-care skills rather than care of others. Within occupational therapy, observation, interviews, and the Canadian Occupational Performance Measure (COPM; Law et al., 1994, 2019) are client-based tools that are used to identify client and caregiver needs and priorities. There are also some interdisciplinary parenting and caregiver assessments that are useful in practice.

The updated COPM is available in 36 languages and may be used with both clients and families to identify priorities, goals, and client–caregiver perceptions of change over time. In addition, a family-based tool in occupational therapy, the Life Participation for Parents, assesses parental satisfaction and participation in daily occupations (Fingerhut, 2013). Therapists may also use formal and informal occupation-based self-reports, interviews, and observations to assess the caregiver relationship and to identify strengths and needs regarding priorities for therapy. Clymer et al. (2020) assessed caregivers of people who have had a stroke and found that although occupational therapists believe formal caregiving assessment is important, productivity, availability, time, and other barriers often led them to use informal means of assessment.

Several interdisciplinary tools regarding parenting and caregiving can be used in occupational therapy evaluation. From an interdisciplinary perspective, Gordon (2012) identified the use of questionnaires, observation, clinical expertise, and interviews as integral to the parenting evaluation process. Evaluations may be conducted to determine actual skills in parenting or caregiving or for court-related purposes; for instance, to ascertain whether a person is fit to parent or a client needs an appointed guardian or conservator. Regardless of the purpose, the therapist must take care to consider the appropriate selection of assessment tools and evaluation methods. The following are a few options used across disciplines.

The Parenting Stress Index (Abidin, 1995) is a self-report instrument often used in high-risk families to identify parents' stress levels. The inventory was designed for parents of children with physical and emotional problems, for families at risk of failing to promote normal development, and for parents at risk for dysfunctional parenting. Measurements are rated on a Likert 5-point scale that ranges from *strongly agree* to *strongly disagree* regarding child characteristics, parent personality, and contextual variables. In recent years, this tool has had increased international use, including in Japan (Tachibana et al., 2012) and India (Gupta et al., 2012), and has been translated into several languages for use throughout the world (Toucheque et al., 2016). The short form of this evaluation is also heavily used and was recently validated for use with minority populations in the United States (Lee et al., 2016). Note that when considering use of this index in families with children with autism spectrum disorder (ASD), studies suggest caution because certain items may not fully replicate psychometric properties when compared with families without children with disabilities (Zaidman-Zait et al., 2010).

For families who have a child with ASD, the Autism Parenting Stress Index is identified as an effective measure for determining parents who need extra supports (Silva & Schalock, 2012). Similar to other tools, the instrument has parents self-report on a Likert scale from 0 (*not stressful*) to 5 (*so stressful we can't cope*). Research indicates that two other questionnaires, the Parent Behavior Importance Questionnaire–Revised and the Parenting Behavior Frequency Questionnaire–Revised appear to have sound psychometric properties and may be useful measures before, during, and after parental training programs (Mowder & Shamah, 2011a, 2011b). Another interview-based tool, the Structured Problem Analysis of Raising Kids, has been shown to be effective in identifying risks and needs in families of toddlers (Staal et al., 2011). A widely used tool in research, the Alabama Parenting Questionnaire (Frick, 1991), includes both child and parent versions to assess five dimensions of parenting, including positive involvement with children, supervision and monitoring, use of positive discipline, consistency with discipline, and use of corporal punishment. Although it has been used extensively in research (e.g., Elgar et al., 2007; Hawes & Dadds, 2006; Scott et al., 2011), it has practical application in both clinical and research settings.

In addition to self-questionnaires, observation and task assessment are helpful in parenting and caregiving evaluation. The Keys to Interactive Parenting Scale (Comfort & Gordon, 2005) is an observational tool designed to measure parent behaviors with children ages 2 months through preschool. A videotaped observation is conducted in a familiar environment, and parents are rated on 12 behaviors in areas such as sensitivity, involvement in child activities, reasonable expectations, and responsiveness to the child. Additional use of informal play and parent–child interaction observation can also determine strengths and needs for planning intervention. In addition, several newer tools, available on the U.S. Department of Health and Human Services, Child Welfare Information Gateway (n.d.), are designed to examine the family system and identify strengths, resources, and needs. Although assessments designed to measure parenting skills can be valuable, occupational therapists must consider results in a larger context because the psychometric properties of these tools vary (Hurley et al., 2014). Therefore, clinical reasoning skills must be used in applying the results within the larger evaluation process.

Evaluation of caregivers for elderly people and for people with disabilities often includes a survey of the strengths and needs of the caregiving situation and a review of the caregiving environment. Instruments fall into both general and illness-specific categories. Several tools, including the Carers' Checklist (Hodgson et al., 1998), Caregiving Activity Survey (Davis et al., 1997), Caregiver Burden Inventory (Novak & Guest, 1989), and Caregiver Reaction Assessment (Given et al., 1992), are specifically designed to assess caregiving situations for elderly people and people with cognitive disorders and dementia.

The Carers' Checklist is designed for people with dementia and their caregivers. It assesses the caregiving situation, symptoms of dementia, burden of care, strengths and needs of the caregiving situation, and impact of services. This tool may be used to facilitate intervention planning and monitor change over time. The Caregiving Activity Survey monitors use of time within the daily occupations of the caregiving relationship, including communication, transportation, dressing, eating, appearance and grooming, and supervision. An updated version (McCarron et al., 2002) includes bathing, toileting, housekeeping, and nursing activities. The Caregiver Burden Inventory reviews five dimensions of burden: time-dependent, developmental, physical, social, and emotional. The Caregiver Reaction Assessment measures caregiver reaction to caring for an elderly relative with an illness. Dimensions measured include esteem; lack of family support; and impact on schedules, finances, and health. Research suggests that a Chinese version of the instrument also has sound psychometrics (Ge et al., 2011).

Another tool, the American Medical Association's Caregiver Self-Assessment, has been shown useful in improving health services to families and in early identification of caregiver depression (Epstein-Lubow et al., 2010). Additional general tools such as the Appraisal of Caregiving Scale (Oberst, 1991; Oberst et al., 1989), Caregiver Burden Scale (Elmstahl et al., 1996), Caregiving Self-Efficacy (Zeiss et al., 1999), and the modified version of the Caregiving Appraisal Scale (Hughes & Caliandro, 1996) may be used to assess perceived burden, self-efficacy, and personal satisfaction in a variety of caregiving situations. In addition, the Kingston Caregiver Stress Scale (Kilik & Hopkins, 2006) and Kingston Standardized Behavior Scale (Hopkins et al., 2006) can be used with caregivers of people with chronic conditions regardless of age. Research has demonstrated that with these tools, caregivers are able to identify sources of stress, particularly when there are changes in the caregiving situation or in the behavior of the person being cared for (Iacob et al., 2021; Kilik & Hopkins, 2019).

In addition to surveys and interviews, it is advantageous if the caregiver evaluation process includes an informal assessment that involves observation and a review of the environment. Occupational therapists identify supports and barriers in the environment in which the daily routine typically occurs. They analyze occupational engagement in the environment and recommend adaptations to enhance occupational performance.

Formal assessments serve to identify resources needed for the client and caregiver to maximize occupational performance as well as opportunities for meaningful engagement in daily activities. Formal tools such as the Home Observation for Measure of the Environment (Caldwell & Bradley, 1984) and the Environmental Rating Scales (Burgess & Burowsky, 2010; Harms, Cryer, & Clifford, 2003, 2007; Harms et al., 1996, 1998) are useful in pediatric populations to assess environmental factors that support healthy development. For adults and seniors, the Home Assessment Profile (Chandler et al., 2001), a newer version of the Functional Environment Assessment (Chandler et al., 1991), and the Safe at Home (Anemaet & Moffa-Trotter, 1997, 1999) tools may be used to consider environmental needs in the home. In addition, the I-Hope In-Home Occupational Performance Evaluation can monitor change in the client–environment fit (Stark et al., 2010). A newer collaborative effort between Rebuilding Together and AOTA (n.d.) is the Safe At Home Checklist (n.d.), which is available at the AOTA website. This checklist identifies safety hazards in the home and areas for potential change.

Many of the tools discussed in this section provide a review of the home environment in which caregiving takes place, identify the extent of assistance needed and barriers to performance, and give suggestions for resources and equipment. Formal assessment tools in conjunction with informal observations are used to develop an occupational profile and priorities for intervention.

As the evaluation process is completed, the creation of an occupational profile results in a greater understanding of the client's past and current occupational performance, patterns of daily living, strengths, and needs (AOTA, 2020b). The development of an occupational profile in a caregiving relationship should include client and contextual factors pertaining to the caregiver, the care receivers, and the systems that influence the delivery of care. The resulting analysis of occupational performance should identify key priorities and outcomes for intervention.

Intervention

Therapeutic approaches to caregiving should be client centered and occupation based. In the context of the caregiving relationship, the client may include the caregiver and the care receiver along with additional family members, practitioners, aides, or assistants (e.g., a personal care attendant), and even organizations involved in care. The *OTPF–4* emphasizes the importance of guiding the intervention plan through the client's goals, values, interests, and occupational needs; health and well-being; performance skills and patterns; context, activity demands, and client factors; and best available evidence (AOTA, 2020b). In the practitioner–client relationship, emphasis is placed on maximizing quality of life for the caregiver and the care receiver while fostering occupational performance and participation throughout the lifespan.

General Recommendations for Intervention

Working with caregivers and families in a client-centered model may be a challenge because of the potential for disagreement regarding priorities for therapy. Family members and primary caregivers have been shown to question health professionals' decisions regarding care (Hasselkus, 1988). Therefore, communication and discussion of priorities are critical before the onset of intervention.

To move beyond the occupational therapy practitioner's priorities and work toward a collaborative relationship, the practitioner may have to suspend personal ideals and come to understand the client family's dynamics, priorities, and values. Research supports the use of collaborative and educational approaches to support clients in working on their priorities (Piersol et al., 2017; Smallfield, 2017). More recently, the use of coaching models and telehealth has provided new opportunities for working with families (Graham et al., 2017; Zahoransky & Lape, 2020). Partnerships in therapy should engage "parents, families and other paid/formal and unpaid/informal caregivers to develop strategies that support occupational engagement and participation, health, and well-being, as well as support caregivers as they cope with the complex demands inherent in the caregiving role" (Gray et al., 2007, p. CE1).

Within the occupational requirements of caregiving, Hasselkus (1988) outlined three broad goals identified by caregivers: getting things done, promoting the care receiver's health and well-being, and maintaining the caregiver's health and well-being. To achieve these goals, the practitioner uses intervention strategies that include education, skill training, adaptation, and modification. Figures 15.8 and 15.9 give examples of modifications. Determining the specific requirements for intervention involves understanding the dynamic interaction of the caregiver and care receiver while considering the contextual factors of the environment, occupational routines and requirements, and priorities. Schumacher et al. (2000, 2006) identified nine core skills important in the caregiving process:

- monitoring—ensuring that everything is going well
- interpreting—making sense of observations
- making decisions—considering options for the best course of action

FIGURE 15.8. Home modifications can facilitate aging in place.

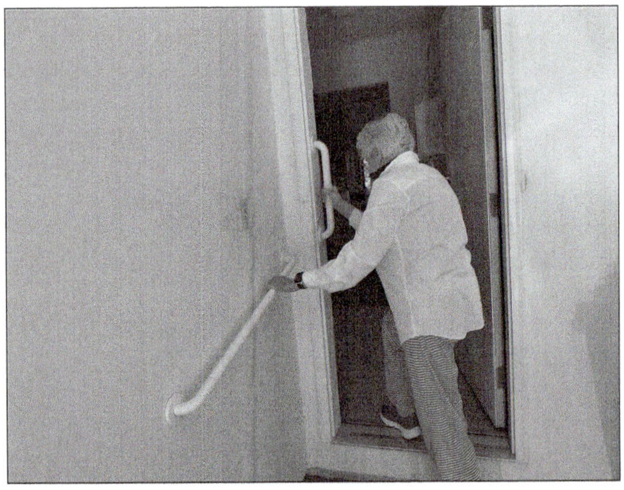

Source. K. Haertl. Used with permission.

FIGURE 15.9. Shower modifications.

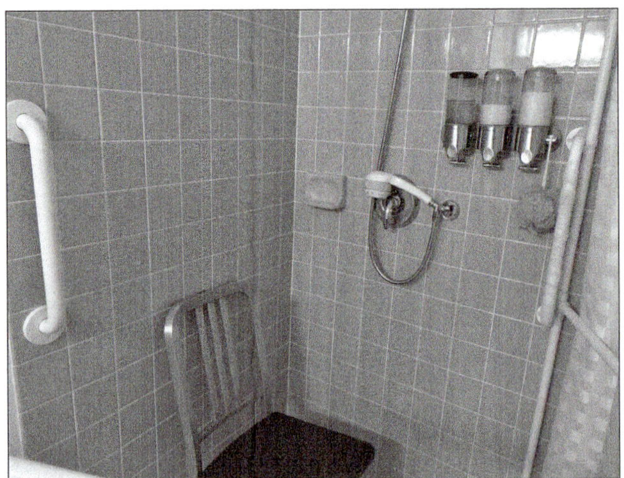

Source. K. Haertl. Used with permission.

- taking action—carrying out daily caregiver tasks and requirements
- providing hands-on care—ensuring safety and comfort while providing care
- making adjustments—considering the best strategies
- accessing resources
- working together with the ill person and considering the personhood of both the caregiver and the care receiver
- negotiating the health care system.

Occupational therapy practitioners can assist clients by helping them apply these core skills while maximizing their quality of life and enhancing opportunities for meaningful engagement in daily activities.

According to Cohn and Henry (2009), occupational therapy services for caregivers are categorized into skills training, adaptations, and support services. Skills training includes providing education about the condition of the care receiver, helping organize schedules and ensure meaningful personal and family occupations, teaching parenting and caregiver skills, and facilitating communication within the caregiving relationship. Adaptations include teaching compensatory techniques and implementing environmental modifications. Support services include connecting clients to support groups and to community and health services organizations. Practitioner roles and interactions within the caregiving relationship shift over time. In early stages, practitioners serve to educate the care receiver and caregiver and to facilitate adaptation to roles and responsibilities in the caregiving relationship. Perkinson et al. (2004) outlined the roles and responsibilities of the practitioner and family through the application of Aneshensel et al.'s (1995) three stages of caregiving: (1) role acquisition stage, (2) role enactment stage, and (3) role disengagement stage. Within each stage, the practitioner and family interact in a unique manner according to contextual needs. During the initial stage of role acquisition, given the challenge of a newly acquired illness, the family must adjust to new roles, functions, and routines. The practitioner serves as an educator about the illness, helps the family identify resources, and anticipates future needs.

In the role enactment stage, the family may need additional training in direct care skills and advice about available resources. Particularly in cases of progressive illness or disease, this stage may also involve discussion of future needs for environmental or housing modifications or housing transitions. During this phase, the occupational therapy practitioner may be called on to expand skills training in the use of special devices, make home modifications, and provide guidance for community placement.

For people with a terminal illness, or perhaps children with disabilities who reach adulthood, the third stage, role disengagement, involves major transition. Although the original model was patterned around elders and coping with death, there are also emotional stresses if a grown child is placed in a residential facility or moves away from home. During this stage, caregivers often must work through grief, loss, and bereavement. The practitioner's role is to facilitate support for family members in coping with loss and transition. Families may require assistance to find support groups, to identify new roles should the loved one move into a community facility or group home, and to deal with grief in times of death and loss. Throughout each of these stages, the practitioner works with the family to promote skills and routines that preserve time for meaningful activity and promote quality of life for all people in the caring relationship.

Caregivers With Special Needs

Much of the literature on caregiving is aimed at those caring for people with illness or disability; however, caregivers can also have special needs. For example, parents with disabilities and populations unaccustomed to providing caregiving (e.g., children) may require training and support to fulfill caregiving roles. Questions surrounding a person's competence to provide parenting or take on a caregiving role may arise, particularly in instances of cognitive or psychological impairment such as major mental illness or a severe traumatic brain injury. Similarly, people already in a caregiver role may develop challenges, such as an elderly woman caring for her spouse who later experiences a stroke or a parent who becomes physically disabled after an illness or severe injury.

A ***family systems approach*** to working with all people in a caregiving situation takes into account caregivers' and care receivers' needs. Using family-centered care involves a dynamic whereby families and occupational therapy practitioners create, negotiate, and modify perceptions regarding caregiving and intervention practices (Lawlor & Mattingly, 2020). The Social Care Institute for Excellence (2007) identified general principles of good practice for services to parents with special needs, and these principles are applicable to all caregiving situations:

- Needs arising from people who have special needs or considerations are addressed before making judgments about their capacity for caregiving.

EXERCISE 15.6. A Family Affected by Alzheimer's Disease

Case Example

You have been working with **George,** a 61-year-old real estate agent diagnosed during the past year with Alzheimer's disease. Over time, George's wife, **Elizabeth,** has had to take on some of the higher-level daily occupations such as managing finances and paying the bills. George has continued to place high importance on his work of selling homes. His position requires him to drive clients around town. Elizabeth reports that he frequently gets lost and at times disobeys traffic laws. She has expressed sincere concern about the safety of his driving.

What would be your role as their occupational therapist? As Elizabeth gradually takes on a caregiving role, how can you support the two of them in this process? How would you address the disagreement about driving? What supports and barriers do you see in this situation?

Discussion

An important area of consideration in this case example is clarification of the occupational therapist's role in working with the caregiver. The therapist's primary therapeutic relationship is usually with the care receiver or person in need. Thus, patient privacy and the needs of the family and all those involved in the client's care must be considered in determining priorities. In addition, as the therapist works with the family, they must understand that this newly formed caregiver situation is likely to require a period of transition for both the caregiver and the care receiver. The therapist can serve this client by using appropriate strategies to address the identified needs while simultaneously working with the family to implement occupational adaptations and environmental modifications that will maximize occupational performance and enhance the caregiver–care receiver relationship. Therefore, in this case, the occupational therapist must address George's competency to continue with work, transportation alternatives, available resources for both George and Elizabeth, and future plans.

For the occupational therapist to apply the key questions presented earlier in the chapter, they would need to consider the relationship between George and Elizabeth, the context in which he will continue to live, and the current and future prognosis. A comprehensive evaluation of George's current cognitive status and ability to complete ADLs must be done, along with an evaluation of his living environment. The use of the Canadian Occupational Performance Measure (Law et al., 2019) may prove valuable to attain input from both George and Elizabeth about their priorities, current routines and habits, and areas of meaningful engagement.

For people in the middle to late stages of Alzheimer's disease, driving is often contraindicated because although they may remember how to turn on and steer the car, they have trouble navigating signs, safety situations, and unfamiliar environments because of a decline in higher level cognitive skills. Therefore, if George continues to have some level of knowledge about his vocation, a meeting with his employer to consider driving alternatives may be suggested. If George and Elizabeth have to adapt to his transition out of work, the therapist can help them identify daily routines and meaningful activities to promote quality of life. To assist with the ability to carry out daily routines and meaningful activities, the therapist can recommend home modifications, in-home services, or special programs (e.g., daily adult day care). The family's resources and needs should be addressed, along with the health and well-being of Elizabeth and her ability to meet her own and George's daily needs in her caregiving role. Education for the family regarding Alzheimer's disease, prognosis, and caregiving concerns should be another focus. Preservation of meaning and family education are important, as is close work with the multidisciplinary team.

- The rights of the caregivers and the responsibilities of service organizations should be clear and transparent.
- There should be positive working relationships among service organizations, service disciplines, and the people receiving services.
- There should be a prevention–intervention continuum.

For practitioners, consideration of daily occupational patterns in caregiving situations, current skills and resources, and barriers to performance facilitate a foundation for the therapeutic relationship. The practitioner generally works with an interdisciplinary team to develop strategies to ensure that caregivers' and care receivers' needs are met.

The roles and functions of the occupational therapist working with caregivers who have special needs may include evaluating skills and competence as well as intervention that involves training, modification, and procuring resources. People who experience an alteration of caregiving roles caused by a traumatic event have differing needs than those with chronic conditions (Fasoli, 2008). Services for children or teens assisting in the caregiving of a parent or sibling should include not only skills training but also consideration of student roles and peer relationships. Families with parents with disabilities may have role shifts as the parent with a disability parents the child and the child provides extra care and assistance to the parent (Frank & Kasnitz, 2011).

In some situations, it is helpful to have outside assistance for the family unit, such as services of therapists or personal care attendants. People with mental illness have often found that providing care and maintaining a parenting role are motivating factors in agreeing to services because maintaining such roles provides a connection to the community and a way to acknowledge themselves as "normal" (Bassett & Lloyd, 2005). For people with cognitive deficits, given potential difficulties with generalization, it is often best for evaluation and intervention to occur in the natural environment (Cohn & Henry, 2009). In addition, people with major physical and motor impairments often need adaptive strategies and home modification to facilitate caregiving. The use of ergonomic techniques to facilitate lifting and carrying, energy conservation techniques to minimize fatigue, and environmental modification such as adaptive cribs and changing tables helps preserve the parent–child bond and facilitate maximal occupational performance in the parenting role (Fasoli, 2008).

In instances in which the client is deemed unable to fully carry out caregiving roles, the occupational therapy practitioner, multidisciplinary team, client, and family work together to identify available supports. In-home care and supportive services may be advantageous. When possible, efforts should be made to facilitate the bond between the caregiver and the care receiver amid the presence of external supports. AOTA (2016) has developed a comprehensive toolkit aimed at caregivers of children and adults. The toolkit provides a compilation of information and resources that may be useful in occupational therapy practice.

Applying Evaluation and Intervention and Determining the Role of the Therapist

Exercise 15.6 describes a case example of a caregiver and a care receiver with Alzheimer's disease to explore evaluation and intervention, as well as the role of the therapist, in occupational therapy practice. Use the information detailed in this chapter on these areas of occupational therapy practice to answer the questions in this exercise. A discussion of important elements to consider follows the case example.

Summary

This chapter provided an overview of the definitions of *care* and *caregiver,* a description of gender and cultural influences on caregiving, a review of current models, and discussion of the roles and functions of the occupational therapy practitioner. Occupational therapy serves a unique and vital role in providing services to caregivers and care receivers. Using client-centered occupation-based evaluation and intervention, therapists work to enhance meaning and quality of life for the caregiver and the care receiver. Service delivery includes the micro (individual and family) approach and the macro (systems) approach. Unique to occupational therapy is its focus on evaluation and intervention through assessment of the client–environment fit; daily caregiving occupational patterns; supports and barriers to health, well-being, and daily occupational performance; and the development of strategies to enhance quality of life for both the caregiver and the care receiver.

References

Abidin, R. R. (1995). *Parenting Stress Index* (3rd ed.). Psychological Assessment Resources.

Abrahamy, M., Finkelson, E. B., Lydon, C., & Murray, K. (2003, spring). Caregivers' socialization of gender roles in a children's museum. *Perspectives in Psychology,* pp. 19–25.

American Occupational Therapy Association. (2016). *Caregivers toolkit: How occupational therapy can help you.* https://www.aota.org/About-Occupational-Therapy/Patients-Clients/Caregivers.aspx

American Occupational Therapy Association. (2020a). *AOTA's statement on family caregivers.* Author.

American Occupational Therapy Association. (2020b). Occupational therapy practice framework: Domain and process (4th ed.). *American Journal of Occupational Therapy, 74*(Suppl. 2), 7412410010. https://doi.org/10.5014/ajot.2020.74S2001

Anemaet, W. K., & Moffa-Trotter, M. E. (1997). *The user-friendly home care handbook.* LEARN.

Anemaet, W. K., & Moffa-Trotter, M. E. (1999). Promoting safety and function through home assessments. *Topics in Geriatric Rehabilitation, 15,* 26–55.

Aneshensel, C. S., Pearlin, L. I., Mullan, J. T., Zarit, S. H., & Whitlatch, C. J. (1995). *Profiles in caregiving: The unexpected career.* Academic Press.

Ashdown, B. K., & Faherty, A. N. (2020). Introduction: What do we mean when we talk about good parenting? In B. K. Ashdown & A. N. Faherty (Eds.), *Parents and caregivers across cultures: Positive development from infancy to adulthood* (pp. 1–8). Springer.

Awad, A. G., & Voruganti, L. N. (2008). The burden of schizophrenia on caregivers: A review. *Pharmacoeconomics, 26,* 149–162. https://doi.org/10.2165/00019053-200826020-00005

Ayalong, L. (2004). Cultural variants of caregiving or the culture of caregiving. *Journal of Cultural Diversity, 11,* 131–138.

Bao, J., & Kato, M. (2020). Determinants of maternal emotion socialization: Based on Belsky's process of parenting model. *Frontiers in Psychology, 11,* 2044. https://doi.org/10.3389/fpsyg.2020.02044

Bassett, H., & Lloyd, C. (2005). At-risk families with mental illness: Partnerships in practice. *New Zealand Journal of Occupational Therapy, 52,* 31–37.

Baumrind, D. (1967). Childcare practices anteceding three patterns of preschool behavior. *Genetic Psychology Monographs, 75,* 43–88.

Baumrind, D. (1971). Current patterns of parental authority. *Developmental Psychology Monograph, 4,* 1–103.

Baumrind, D. (1996). The discipline controversy revisited. *Family Relations, 45,* 405–414.

Belsky, J. (1984). The determinants of parenting: A process model. *Child Development, 55,* 83–96.

Belsky, J., Fearon, R. M., & Bell, B. (2007). Parenting, attention, and externalizing problems: Testing mediation longitudinally, repeatedly and reciprocally. *Journal of Child Psychology and Psychiatry, 48,* 1233–1242. https://doi.org/10.1111/j.1469-7610.2007.01807.x

Belsky, J., Vandell, D. L., Burchinal, M., Clarke-Stewart, K. A., McCartney, K., & Owen, M. T. (2007). Are there long-term effects of early child care? *Child Development, 78,* 681–701. https://doi.org/10.1111/j.1469-7610.2007.01807.x

Bhattarai, L. P. (2013). Reviving the family model of care: Can it be a panacea for the new century? *Indian Journal of Gerontology, 27,* 202–218.

Bowlby, J. (1982). *Attachment and loss. Volume 1: Attachment* (2nd ed.). Basic Books.

Broese van Groenou, M. I., de Boer, A., & Iedema, J. (2013). *European Journal of Aging, 10,* 301–311. https://doi.org/10.1007/s10433-013-0276-6

Burgess, A. M., & Burowsky, I. W. (2010). Health and home environments of caregivers investigated by child protective services. *Pediatrics, 125,* 273–281. https://doi.org/10.1542/peds.2008-3814

Caldwell, B., & Bradley, R. H. (1984). *Home Observation for Measure of the Environment* (Rev. ed.). University of Arkansas.

Cardemil, E. V. (2010). The complexity of culture: Do we embrace the challenge or avoid it? *Scientific Review of Mental Health Practice, 7*(2), 41–47.

Cardosa, J. B., Padilla, Y. C., & Sampson, M. (2010). Racial and ethnic variation in the predictors of maternal parenting stress. *Journal of Social Service Research, 36,* 429–444. https:/doi.org/10.1080/01488376.2010.510948

Caregiver Action Network. (2021). *Caregiving statistics.* http://caregiveraction.org/statistics/

Castellanos, E. H., Dietrich, M. S., Bond, S. M., Wells, N., Schumacher, K., Ganti, A. K., & Murphy, B. A. (2019). Impact of patient symptoms and caregiving tasks on psychological distress in caregivers for head and neck cancer (HNC). *Psycho-Oncology, 28,* 511–517. https:/doi.org/10.1002/pon.4968

Centers for Disease Control and Prevention. (2019). *Caregiving for family and friends: A public health issue.* https://www.cdc.gov/aging/caregiving/caregiver-brief.html#:~:text=22.3%25%20of%20adults%20reported%20providing,in%20five%20(18.9%25)%20men

Chandler, J. M., Duncan, P. W., Weiner, D. K., & Studenski, S. A. (2001). Special feature: The Home Assessment Profile—A reliable and valid assessment tool. *Topics in Geriatric Rehabilitation, 16,* 77–88.

Chandler, J. M., Prescott, B., Duncan, P. W., & Studenski, S. (1991). Reliability of a new instrument: The Functional Environment Assessment. *Physical Therapy, 71,* 574.

Clymer, D. R., Fields, H. A., & Kniepmann, K. (2020). Assessing unmet needs of caregivers after stroke: Occupational therapist practice and perspectives. *Open Journal of Occupational Therapy, 8,* 1–13. https://doi.org/10.15453/2168-6408.1653

Cohn, E. S., & Henry, A. D. (2009). Caregiving and childrearing. In E. B. Crepeau, E. S. Cohn, & B. A. Schell (Eds.), *Willard and Spackman's occupational therapy* (11th ed., pp. 579–591), Lippincott Williams & Wilkins.

Collins Essential English Dictionary. (n.d.). Care. In *collinsdictionary.com dictionary.* https://www.collinsdictionary.com/us/dictionary/english/care

Comfort, M., & Gordon, P. (2005). *Keys to Interactive Parenting Scale.* Comfort Consultants.

Corey Magan, K., McCurry, M. K., Sethares, K. A., Bourbonniere, M., Meghani, S. H., & Hirschman, K. B. (2020). The Post-Caregiving Health Model: A theoretical framework for understanding the health of former family caregivers of persons with dementia. *Advances in Nursing Science, 43,* 292–305. https://doi.org/10.1097/ANS.0000000000000316

Coutinho, F., Hersch, G., & Davidson, H. (2006). The impact of informal caregiving in occupational therapy. *Physical and Occupational Therapy in Geriatrics, 25,* 47–61. https://doi.org/10.1300/J148v25n01_04

Cruz, D., & Caro, C. (2017). Correlation between poststroke patients' independence and cognition and their family caregivers' burden and quality of life. *American Journal of Occupational Therapy, 71,* 7111500022. https://doi.org/10.5014/ajot.2017.71S1-PO1139

Davis, K. L., Marin, D. B., Kane, R., Patrick, D., Peskind, E. R., Raskind, M. A., & Puder, K. L. (1997). The Caregiver Activity Survey (CAS): Development and validation of a new measure for caregivers of persons with Alzheimer's disease. *International Journal of Geriatric Psychiatry, 12,* 978–988. https://doi.org/10.1002/(SICI)1099-1166(199710)12:10<978::AID-GPS659>3.0.CO;2-1

Dehyadegary, E., Yaacob, S. N., & Juhari, R. B. (2012). Relationship between parenting style and academic achievement among Iranian adolescents in Sirjan. *Asian Social Science, 8,* 156–160. https://doi.org/10.5539/ass.v8n1p156

Drentea, P. (2007). Caregiving. In G. Ritzer (Ed.), *Blackwell encyclopedia of sociology.* www.blackwellreference.com/public/tocnode?id=g9781405124331_chunk_g97814051243319_ss1-7

Elgar, F. J., Waschbusch, D. A., Dadds, M. R., & Sigvaldason, N. (2007). Development and validation of a short form of the Alabama Parenting Questionnaire. *Journal of Child and Family Studies, 16,* 243–259. https://doi.org/10.1007/s10826-006-9082-5

Elmstahl, S., Malmberg, B., & Annerstedt, L. (1996). Caregiver's burden of patients 3 years after stroke assessed by a novel caregiver burden scale. *Archives of Physical Medicine and Rehabilitation, 77,* 177–182. https://doi.org/10.1016/S0003-9993(96)90164-1

Epstein-Lubow, G., Guadiano, B. A., Hinkley, M., Salloway, S., & Miller, I. W. (2010). Evidence for the validity of the American Medical Association's Caregiver Self-Assessment Questionnaire as a screening measure for depression. *Journal of the American Geriatrics Society, 58,* 387–388. https://doi.org/10.1111/j.1532-5415.2009.02701.x

Ergh, T. C., Rapport, L. J., Coleman, R. D., & Hanks, R. A. (2002). Predictors of caregiver and family functioning following traumatic brain injury: Social support moderates caregiver stress. *Journal of Head Trauma Rehabilitation, 17,* 155–174. https://doi.org/10.1097/00001199-200204000-00006.

European Commission. (2018). *Informal care in Europe: Exploring formalisation, availability, and quality.* Author. https://doi.org/10.2767/78836

Family Equality Council. (2017). *LGBTQ family fact sheet.* Author.

Farnfield, S. (2008). A theoretical model for the comprehensive assessment of parenting. *British Journal of Social Work, 38,* 1076–1079. https://doi.org/10.1093/bjsw/bcl395

Fasoli, S. E. (2008). Restoring competence for homemaker and parent roles. In M. V. Radomski & C. A. Trombly (Eds.), *Occupational therapy for physical dysfunction* (6th ed., pp. 854–874). Lippincott Williams & Wilkins.

Fingerhut, P. E. (2013). Life Participation for Parents: A tool for family-centered occupational therapy. *American Journal of Occupational Therapy, 67,* 37–44. https://doi.org/10.5014/ajot.2013.005082

Fortuna, J. (2020). *The role of the OT in caregiver coaching over telehealth.* Medbridge. https://www.medbridgeeducation.com/

blog/2020/07/the-role-of-the-ot-in-caregiver-coaching-over-telehealth/

Frank, G., & Kasnitz, D. (2011). The meaning of self-care occupations. In C. H. Christiansen & K. M. Matuska (Eds.), *Ways of living: Adaptive strategies for special needs* (4th ed., pp. 27–43). AOTA Press.

Frick, P. J. (1991). *Alabama Parenting Questionnaire.* Author.

Ge, C., Yang, X., Fu, J., Chang, Y., Wei, J., Zhang, F., . . . Wang, L. (2011). Reliability and validity of the Chinese version of the Caregiver Reaction Assessment. *Psychiatry and Clinical Neurosciences, 65,* 254–263. https://doi.org/10.1111/j.1440-1819.2011.02200.x

Geisler, M. (2012). Gay fathers' negotiation of gender role strain: A qualitative inquiry. *Fathering, 10,* 119–139. https://doi.org/10.3149/fth.1002.119

Given, C. W., Given, B., Stommel, M., Collins, C., King, S., & Franklin, S. (1992). The Caregiver Reaction Assessment (CRA) for carers to persons with chronic physical and mental impairments. *Research in Nursing Health, 15,* 271–273.

Gordon, P. (2012). *Choosing the right parenting assessment tool to delight your funders.* http://comfortconsults.com/blog/bid/243638/Choosing-the-Right-Parenting-Assessment-Tool-to-Delight-Your-Funders

Graham, F., Boland, P., Ziviani, J., & Rodger, S. (2017). Occupational therapists' and physiotherapists' perceptions of implementing occupational performance coaching. *Disability and Rehabilitation, 40,* 1386–1392. https://doi.org/10.1080/09638288.2017.1295474

Grant, H., & Scott, K. K. (2015). An introduction and overview of social model hospice care. *Journal of Hospice and Palliative Nursing, 17,* 466–471. https://doi.org/10.1097/NJH.0000000000000186

Gray, K., Horowitz, B. P., O'Sullivan, A., Behr, S. K., & Abreu, B. C. (2007). Occupational therapy's role in the occupation of caregiving. *OT Practice, 12*(15), CE-1–CE-8.

Gupta, V. B., Mehrota, P., & Mehrota, N. (2012). Parental stress in raising a child with disabilities in India. *Disability, CBR, and Inclusive Development, 23,* 41–52. https://doi.org/10.5463/DCID.v23i2.119

Haertl, K. H. (2011). Strategies for adults with developmental disabilities. In C. H. Christiansen & K. M. Matuska (Eds.), *Ways of living: Adaptive strategies for special needs* (4th ed., pp. 171–205). AOTA Press.

Harding, R., Gao, W., Jackson, D., Pearson, C., Murray, J., & Higginson, I. J. (2015). Comparative analysis of informal caregiver burden in advanced cancer, dementia and acquired brain injury. *Journal of Pain and Symptom Management, 50,* 445–452. https://doi.org/10.1016/j.jpainsymman.2015.04.005

Harms, T., Clifford, R., & Cryer, D. (1998). *Early Childhood Environment Rating Scale–Revised (ECERS–R).* Teachers College Press.

Harms, T., Cryer, D., & Clifford, R. (2003). *Infant/Toddler Environment Rating Scale–Revised (ITERS–R).* Teachers College Press.

Harms, T., Cryer, D., & Clifford, R. (2007). *Family Child Care Environment Rating Scale–Revised (FCCERS–R).* Teachers College Press.

Harms, T., Jacobs, E. V., & White, D. R. (1996). *School-Age Care Environment Rating Scale.* Teachers College Press.

Hasselkus, B. R. (1988). Meaning in family caregiving: Perspectives on caregiver/professional relationships. *Gerontologist, 28,* 686–691. https://doi.org/10.1093/geront/28.5.686

Hasselkus, B. R., & Murray, B. J. (2007). Everyday occupation, well-being, and identity: The experience of caregivers in families with dementia. *American Journal of Occupational Therapy, 61,* 9–20. https://doi.org/10.5014/ajot.61.1.9

Hawes, D. J., & Dadds, M. R. (2006). Assessing parenting practices through parent-report and direct observation during parent-training. *Journal of Child and Family Studies, 15,* 555–568. https://doi.org/10.1007/s10826-006-9029-x

Hayes, K. (2021). *Caregiving sourcebook: First edition.* Omnigraphics.

Hodgson, C., Higginson, I., & Jeffreys, P. (1998). *Carers' Checklist: An outcome measure for people with dementia and their carers.* Mental Health Foundation.

Hoffman, F., & Rodrigues, R. (2010). *Informal carers: Who takes care of them?* [Policy brief]. *European Centre.* https://www.euro.centre.org/downloads/detail/1256

Hopkins, R., Kilik, L., Day, D., Bradford, L., & Rows, C. (2006) Kingston Standardized Behavioural Assessment. *American Journal of Alzheimer's* Disease *and Other Dementias, 21,* 339–346. https://doi.org/10.1177/1533317506292576

Hughes, C. B., & Caliandro, G. (1996). Effects of social support, stress, and level of illness on caregiving of children with AIDS. *Journal of Pediatric Nursing, 11,* 347–358. https://doi.org/10.1016/S0882-5963(96)80079-0

Hurley, K. D., Huscroft-D'Angelo, J., Trout, A., Griffith, A., & Epstein, M. (2014). Assessing parenting skills and attitudes: A review of the psychometrics of parenting measures. *Journal of Child and Family Studies, 23,* 812–823. https://doi.org/10.1007/s10826-013-9733-2

Iacob, C. I., Avram, E., & Burtaverde, V. (2021). Psychometric properties of the Kingston Caregiver Stress Scale in Romanian caregivers of children and adults with disabilities. *Research in Developmental Disabilities, 112,* 103921. https://doi.org/10.1016/j.ridd.2021.103921

Jacques, N. D., & Hasselkus, B. R. (2004). The nature of occupation surrounding dying and death. *OTJR: Occupation, Participation and Health, 24,* 44–53.

Jahoda, G. (2012). Critical reflections on some recent definitions of culture. *Culture and Psychology, 18,* 289–303. https://doi.org/10.1177/1354067X12446229

Javier, N. S., & Montagnini, M. L. (2011). Rehabilitation of the hospice and palliative care patient. *Journal of Palliative Medicine, 14,* 638–648. https://doi.org/10.1089/jpm.2010.0125

Johns Hopkins Medicine. (2021). *What is a caregiver?* https://www.hopkinsmedicine.org/about/community_health/johns-hopkins-bayview/services/called_to_care/what_is_a_caregiver.html

Jones, A. L., Harris-Cojetin, L., & Valverde, R. (2012). Characteristics and use of home health care by men and women aged 65 and over. *National Health Statistics Report, 52,* 1–8.

Kazemi, A., Azimian, J., Mafi, M., Allen, K. A., & Motalebi, S. A. (2021). Caregiver burden and coping strategies in caregivers of older patients with stroke. *BMC Psychology, 9,* http://dx.doi.org.pearl.stkate.edu/10.1186/s40359-021-00556-z

Kellet, U. M. (1999). Transition in care: Family carer's experience of nursing home placement. *Journal of Advanced Nursing, 29,* 1474–1481. https://doi.org/10.1046/j.1365-2648.1999.01035.x

Kennedy Root, A., & Denham, S. A. (2010). The role of gender in the socialization of emotion: Key concepts and critical issues. *New Directions for Child and Adolescent Development, 128,* 1–9. https://doi.org/10.1002/cd.265

Kiff, C. J., Lengua, L. J., & Zalewski, M. (2011). Nature and nurturing: Parenting in the context of child temperament. *Clinical Child and Family Psychology Review, 14,* 251–301. https://doi.org/10.1007/s10567-011-0093-4

Kilik, L. A., & Hopkins, R. (2006). *The Kingston Caregiver Stress Scale.* http://www.kingstonscales.org/caregiver-stress-scale.html

Kilik, L. A., & Hopkins, R. W. (2019). The relationship between caregiver stress and behavioural changes in dementia. *OBM Geriatrics, 3*(2), 052. https://doi.org/10.21926/obm.geriatr.1902052

Klein, J., & Liu, L. (2010). Family–therapist relationships in caring for older adults. *Physical and Occupational Therapy in Geriatrics, 28,* 259–270. https://doi.org/10.3109/02703181.2010.494822

Kooraneh, A. E., & Amirsardari, L. (2015). Predicting early maladaptive schemas using Baumrind's parenting styles. *Iranian Journal of Psychiatric and Behavioral Sciences, 9,* E952. https://doi.org/10.17795/ijpbs952

Kuipers, E., Onwumere, J., & Bebbington, P. (2018). Cognitive models of caregiving in psychosis. *British Journal of Psychiatry, 196,* 259–265. https://doi.org/10.1192/bjp.bp.109.070466

Lackey, N. R., & Gates, M. F. (2001). Adults' recollections of their experiences as young caregivers of family members with chronic mental illness. *Journal of Advanced Nursing, 34,* 320–328. https://doi.org/10.1046/j.1365-2648.2001.01761.x

Lattanzi-Licht, M. (2001). Hospice as a model for caregiving. In K. J. Doka & J. D. Davidson (Eds.), *Caregiving and loss: Family needs, professional responses* (pp. 19–31). Hospice Foundation of America.

Law, M., Baptiste, S., Carswell, A., McColl, M. A., Polatajko, H., & Pollock, N. (1994). *Canadian Occupational Performance Measure* (2nd ed.). Toronto: CAOT Publications.

Law, M., Baptiste, S., Carswell, A., McColl, M. A., Polatajko, H., & Pollock, N. (2019). *Canadian Occupational Performance Measure* (5th ed., rev.). COPM, Inc.

Lawlor, M. C., & Mattingly, C. (2020). Family perspectives on occupation, health and disability. In B. A. Boyt Schell & G. Gillen (Eds.), *Willard and Spackman's occupational therapy* (13th ed., pp. 196–211). Wolters Kluwer.

Leaper, C. (2002). Parenting girls and boys. In M. H. Bornstein (Ed.), *Handbook of parenting. Volume 1: Children and parenting* (2nd ed., pp. 189–225). Erlbaum.

Lee, E., Bristow, J., Faircloth, C., & Macvarish, J. (2014). *Parenting culture studies.* Macmillan.

Lee, S. J., Gopalan, G., & Harrington, D. (2016). Validation of the Parenting-Stress Index–Short Form with minority caregivers. *Research on Social Work Practice, 26,* 429–440. https://doi.org/10.1177/1049731514554854

Lee, Y., & Hofferth, S. L. (2017). Gender differences in single parents' living arrangements and childcare time. *Journal of Child and Family Studies, 26,* 3439–3451. https://doi.org/10.1007/s10826-017-0850-1

Leininger, M. (1988a). Cross-cultural hypothetical functions of caring and nursing care. In M. Leininger (Ed.), *Caring—an essential human need: Proceedings of the three National Caring Conferences* (pp. 95–102). Wayne State University Press.

Leininger, M. (1988b). The phenomenon of caring: Importance, research questions and theoretical considerations. In M. Leininger (Ed.), *Caring—an essential human need: Proceedings of the three National Caring Conferences* (pp. 3–16). Wayne State University Press.

Leininger, M. (1996). Culture care theory, research, and practice. *Nurse Science Quarterly, 9*(2), 71–78. https://doi.org/10.1177/089431849600900208.

Lindsay, E. W., & Mize, J. (2001). Contextual differences in parent–child play: Implications for children's gender role development. *Sex Roles, 44,* 155–176. https://doi.org/10.1023/A:1010950919451

Liu, H., & Huang, L. (2018). The relationship between family functioning and caregiving appraisal of dementia family caregivers: Caregiving self-efficacy as a mediator. *Aging and Mental Health, 22,* 558–567. https://doi.org/10.1080/13607863.2016.1269148

Lowey, S. E. (2015). *Nursing care at the end of life.* Open SUNY textbooks.

Lynch, S. H., & Lobo, M. L. (2012). Compassion fatigue in family caregivers: A Wilsonian concept analysis. *Journal of Advanced Nursing, 68,* 2125–2134. https://doi.org/10.1111/j.1365-2648.2012.05985.x

Mak, W. W. (2005). Integrative model of caregiving: How macro and micro factors affect caregivers of adults with severe and persistent mental illness. *American Journal of Orthopsychiatry, 75,* 40–53. https://doi.org/10.1037/0002-9432.75.1.40

McCarron, M., Gill, M., Lawlor, B., & Beagly, C. (2002). A pilot study of the reliability and validity of the Caregiver Activity Survey–Intellectual Disability (CAS–ID). *Journal of Intellectual Disability Research, 46,* 605–612. https://doi.org/10.1046/j.1365-2788.2002.00437.x

McCleary, L., & Blain, J. (2013). Cultural values and family caregiving for persons with dementia. *Indian Journal of Gerontology, 1,* 178–201.

McKinney, C., & Renk, K. (2011). A multi-variable model of parent–adolescent relationship variables in early adolescence. *Child Psychiatry and Human Development, 42,* 442–462. https://doi.org/10.1007/s10578-011-0228-3

Meidenbauer, J., Lynch, K., Thill, J., Gantz, L., & Tomita, M. (2019). Effects of OT intervention to reduce caregiving stress of informal caregivers of older adults with dementia: A pilot study [Poster Presentation]. *American Journal of Occupational Therapy, 73*(Suppl. 1), 7311515368. https://doi.org/10.5014/ajot.2019.73S1-PO6027

Merriam-Webster. (n.d.). Care. In *Merriam-Webster.com dictionary.* https://www.merriam-webster.com/dictionary/care

Mironenko, I. A., & Sorokin, P. S. (2018). Seeking for the definition of "culture": Current concerns and their implications. A comment on Gustav Jahoda's article: "Critical reflections on some recent definitions of 'culture'". *Integrative Psychological and Behavioral Science, 52,* 331–340. https://doi.org/10.1007/s12124-018-9425-y

Mowder, B. A., & Shamah, R. (2011a). Parent Behavior Importance Questionnaire Revised: Scale development and psychometric properties. *Journal of Child and Family Studies, 20,* 295–302. https://doi.org/10.1007/s10826-010-9392-5

Mowder, B. A., & Shamah, R. (2011b). Test–retest reliability of the Parent Behavior Importance Questionnaire–Revised and the Parent Behavior Frequency Questionnaire–Revised. *Psychology in the Schools, 48,* 843–854. https://doi.org/10.1002/pits.20593

Murray, L., Tarren-Sweeny, M., & France, K. (2011). Foster carer perceptions of support and training in the context of high burden of care. *Child and Family Social Work, 16,* 149–158. https://doi.org/10.1111/j.1365-2206.2010.00722.x

Napoles, A. M., Chadiha, L., Eversley, R., & Moreno-John, G. (2010). Developing culturally sensitive caregiving interventions: Are we there yet? *American Journal of Alzheimer's Disease and Other Dementias, 25,* 389–406. https://doi.org/10.1177/1533317510370957

National Alliance for Caregiving. (2021). *Unified state strategy.* Author.

Novak, M., & Guest, C. (1989). Application of a multi-dimensional caregiver burden inventory. *Gerontologist, 29,* 798–803.

Oberst, M. T. (1991). *Appraisal of Caregiving Scale: Manual.* Wayne State University.

Oberst, M. T., Gass, K. A., & Ward, S. E. (1989). Caregiving demands and appraisal of stress among family caregivers. *Cancer Nursing, 12,* 209–215. https://doi.org/10.1097/00002820-198908000-00003

Perkinson, M. A., La Vesser, P., Morgan, K., & Perlmutter, M. (2004). Therapeutic partnerships: Caregiving in the home setting. In C. H. Christiansen & K. M. Matuska (Eds.), *Ways of living: Adaptive strategies for special needs* (3rd ed., pp. 445–461). AOTA Press.

Pharr, J. R., Francis, C. D., Terry, C., & Clark, M. C. (2014). Culture, caregiving and health: Exploring the influence of culture on family caregiving experiences. *International Scholarly Research Notices, 2014,* 1–8. https://doi.org/10.1155/2014/689826

Piersol, C. V., Canton, K., Connor, S. E., Giller, I., Lipman, S., & Sager, S. (2017). Effectiveness of interventions for caregivers of people with Alzheimer's disease and related major neurocognitive disorders: A systematic review. *American Journal of Occupational Therapy, 71,* 7105180020. https://doi.org/10.5014/ajot.2017.027581

Pioli, M. F. (2010). Global and caregiving mastery as moderators in the caregiving stress process. *Aging and Mental Health, 14,* 603–612. https://doi.org/10.1080/13607860903586193

Pinquart, M., & Rubina, K. (2018). Do the associations of parenting styles with behavior problems and academic achievement vary by culture? Results from a meta-analysis. *Cultural Diversity and Ethnic Minority Psychology, 24,* 75–100. https://doi.org/10.1037/cdp0000149

Poroch, N. C. (2012). Karunpa: Keeping spirit on country. *Health Sociology Review, 21,* 383–395. https://doi.org/10.5172/hesr.2012.21.4.383

Post University. (2020). *Madeline Leininger, founder of culture care theory.* Author. https://www.americansentinel.edu/blog/2020/10/08/madeleine-leininger-founder-of-culture-care-theory/

Rebuilding Together and American Occupational Therapy Association. (n.d.). *Safe at Home Checklist.* https://www.aota.org/-/media/Corporate/Files/Practice/Aging/rebuilding-together/RT-Aging-in-Place-Safe-at-Home-Checklist.pdf

Riina, E. M., & Feinberg, M. E. (2012). Involvement in childrearing and mothers' and fathers' adjustment. *Family Relations, 61,* 836–850. https://doi.org/10.1111/j.1741-3729.2012.00739.x

Roskam, I., & Mikolajczak, M. (2020). Gender differences in the nature, antecedents and consequences of parental burnout. *Sex Roles, 83,* 485–498. https://doi.org/10.1007/s11199-020-01121-5

Rote, S. M., & Moon, H. (2018). Racial ethnic differences in caregiving frequency: Does immigrant status matter? *Journals of Gerontology, Series B, 73,* 1088–1098. https://doi.org/10.1093/geronb/gbw106

Sarkisian, N., Gerena, M., & Gerstel, M. (2007). Extended family integration among Euro and Mexican Americans: Ethnicity, gender and class. *Journal of Marriage and Family, 69,* 40–54. https://doi.org/10.1111/j.1741-3737.2006.00342.x

Schumacher, K. L., Beidler, S. M., Beeber, A. S., & Gambino, P. (2006). A transactional model of cancer family caregiving skill. *Advances in Nursing Science, 29,* 271–286.

Schumacher, K. L., Stewart, B. J., Archbol, P. G., Dodd, M. J., & Dibble, S. L. (2000). Family caregiving skill: Development of the concept. *Research in Nursing and Health, 23,* 191–203. https://doi.org/10.1002/1098-240X(200006)23:33.0.CO;2-B

Scott, S., Briskman, J., & Dadds, M. R. (2011). Measuring parenting in community and public health research: Using brief child and parenting reports. *Journal of Child and Family Studies, 20,* 343–352. https://doi.org/10.1007/s10826-010-9398-z

Sellick, J. (2005). *Traditions: Improving quality of life in caregiving.* Venture.

Sharma, N., Chakrabarti, S., & Grover, S. (2016). Gender differences in caregiving among family: Caregivers of people with mental illness. *World Journal of Psychiatry, 6,* 7–17. https://doi.org/10.5498/wjp.v6.i1.7

Silva, L. M., & Schalock, M. (2012). Autism Parenting Stress Index: Initial psychometric evidence. *Journal of Autism and Developmental Disorders, 42,* 566–574. https://doi.org/10.1007/s10803-011-1274-1

Smallfield, S. (2017). Supporting adults with Alzheimer's disease and related major neurocognitive disorders and their caregivers: Effective occupational therapy interventions. *American Journal of Occupational Therapy, 71,* 7105170010. https://doi.org/10.5014/ajot.2017.715002

Social Care Institute for Excellence. (2007). *The adult services resource guide 9: Working together to support disabled parents.* Author.

Sorkhabi, N. (2005). Applicability of Baumrind's parent typology to collective cultures: Analysis of cultural explanations of parent socialization effects. *International Journal of Behavior Development, 29,* 552–563. https://doi.org/10.1080/01650250500172640

Staal, I. I. E., van den Brink, H. A. G., Hermanns, J. M. A., Shrijvers, A. J. P., & van Stel, H. F. (2011). Assessment of parenting and developmental problems in toddlers: Development and feasibility of a structured interview. *Childcare, Health and Development, 37,* 503–511. https://doi.org/10.1111/j.1365-2214.2011.01228.x

Stark, S. L., Sommerville, E. K., & Morris, J. C. (2010). In-Home Occupational Performance Evaluation (I–HOPE). *American Journal of Occupational Therapy, 64,* 580–589. https://doi.org/10.5014/ajot.2010.08065

Statistics Canada. (2018). *Caregivers in Canada 2018.* https://www150.statcan.gc.ca/n1/daily-quotidien/200108/dq200108a-eng.htm

Swindle, T. M., Patterson, Z., & Boden, C. J. (2017). A qualitative application of the Belsky model to explore early care and education teachers' mealtime history, beliefs and interactions. *Journal of Nutrition Education and Behavior, 49,* 568–578. https://doi.org/10.1016/j.jneb.2017.04.025

Swinkels, J., van Tilburg, T., Verbakel, E., & Broese van Groeneu, M. (2019). Explaining the gender gap in caregiving burden in partner caregivers. *Journals of Gerontology: Series B, 74,* 309–317. https://doi.org/10.1093/geronb/gbx036

Tachibana, Y., Fukushima, A., Saito, H., Yoneyama, S., Ushida, K., Yoneyama, S., & Kawashima, R. (2012). A new mother–child play activity program to decrease parenting stress and improve child cognitive abilities: A cluster randomized controlled trial. *PLOS One Journal, 7,* e3828. https://doi.org/10.1371/journal.pone.0038238

Taraban, L., & Shaw, D. S. (2018). Parenting in context: Revisiting Belsky's classic process of parenting model in early childhood. *Developmental Review, 48,* 55–81. https://doi.org/10.1016/j.dr.2018.03.006

Toucheque, M., Etienne, A., Stassart, C., & Catale, C. (2016). Validation of the French version of the Parenting Stress Index short form (fourth edition). *Journal of Community Psychology, 44,* 419–425. https://doi.org/10.1002/jcop.21778

Tsai, Y., & Pai, H. (2016). Burden and cognitive appraisal of stroke survivors' informal caregivers: An assessment of depression model with mediating and moderating effects. *Archives of Psychiatric Nursing, 30,* 237–243. https://doi.org/10.1016/j.apnu.2015.11.007

Upton, N., & Reed, V. (2006). The influence of social support on caregiver coping. *International Journal of Psychiatric Nursing Research, 11,* 1256–1267.

U.S. Department of Health and Human Services, Child Welfare Information Gateway. (n.d.) *Assessing parent strengths and family connections.* https://www.childwelfare.gov/topics/systemwide/assessment/family-assess/parentalneeds/strengthsandconnections/

Vellone, E., Piras, G., Talucci, C., & Cohen, M. Z. (2008). Quality of life for caregivers of people with Alzheimer's disease. *Journal of Advanced Nursing, 61,* 222–231. https://doi.org/10.1111/j.1365-2648.2007.04494.x

Weierbach, F. M., & Cao, Y. (2016). A model of health for family caregivers of elders. *Healthcare, 5.* https://doi.org/10.3390/healthcare5010001

Wells, R., Dywan, J., & Dumas, J. (2005). Life satisfaction and distress in family caregivers as related to specific behavioural changes after traumatic brain injury. *Brain Injury, 19,* 1105–1115. https://doi.org/10.1080/02699050500150062

Woolfsen, L., & Grant, E. (2006). Authoritative parenting and parental stress in parents of preschool and older children with developmental disabilities. *Child: Care, Health and Development, 32,* 177–184. https://doi.org/10.1111/j.1365-2214.2006.00603.x

Zahoransky, M. A., & Lape, J. E. (2020). Telehealth and home health occupational therapy: Clients' perceived satisfaction with and perception of occupational performance. *International Journal of Telerehabilitation, 12,* 105–124. https://doi.org/10.5195/ijt.2020.6327

Zaidman-Zait, A., Mirenda, P., Zumbo, B. D., Wellington, S., Dua, V., & Kalynchuk, K. (2010). An item response theory analysis of the Parenting-Stress Index Short Form with parents of children with autism spectrum disorder. *Journal of Child Psychology and Psychiatry, 51,* 1269–1277. https://doi.org/10.1111/j.1469-7610.2010.02266.x

Zeiss, A. M., Gallagher-Thompson, D., Lovett, S., Rose, J., & McKibbin, C. (1999). Self-efficacy as a mediator of caregiver coping: Development and testing of an assessment model. *Journal of Clinical Geropsychology, 5,* 221–230.

16

Spirituality and Occupation

KRYSTAL ROBINSON-BERT, OTD, OTR/L, CSRS, C/NDT, CBIS, CKTP, CAPS, AND WESLEY BLOUNT, SHRM-CP

CHAPTER HIGHLIGHTS

- Brief history of spirituality in occupational therapy
- Occupational therapy practice and spirituality
- Assessment of spirituality and perceived barriers
- Personal spirituality of occupational therapy practitioners
- Spirituality intervention
- Religious observation and practices

KEY TERMS AND CONCEPTS

- religion • spirituality • therapeutic use of self

The previous edition of *The Texture of Life* (Hinojosa & Blount, 2014) introduced a chapter on occupations in the context of spirituality. The chapter's examination followed the addition of spirituality into the *Occupational Therapy Practice Professional Framework: Domain and Process* (2nd ed.; *OTPF–2;* American Occupational Therapy Association [AOTA], 2008). Since the *OTPF–2's* inclusion of spirituality as a client factor, other articles, chapters, and texts developed rationales and reasoning for looking at spirituality as part of occupation and its therapeutic role in client treatment (Cadge & Bandini, 2015; Csontó, 2009; Morris et al., 2014; Waite, 2014).

Although the spiritual aspect of the human experience may seem like new and uncharted territory for occupational therapy, much of it has served to revive a foundational aspect of the profession itself. Adolf Meyer, who brought together the founders of occupational therapy in upstate New York, believed that the therapeutic benefit of occupation was a renewal of the human spirit. The idea that we derive benefits from activity beyond physical or mental improvements was the basis of using occupation and activity as a therapeutic treatment. What we have also come to understand is that treating the spiritual aspect specifically is part of the role of occupational therapy, too.

A Brief History of Spirituality in Occupational Therapy

Historically, some of the early focus on the emotional and spiritual satisfaction of being occupied—of performing useful activities with purpose—was gradually sidelined as the occupational therapy profession adopted a more medically based, clinical model of practice. Achieving goals around function and form—enhancing performance—overtook looking at the holistic, individualized improvements achieved by the client as their own reward. With the return of the concept of holistic improvements to the forefront of practice, such improvements have become not just an added benefit but the goal of the treatment itself.

The idea of spirituality in the context of occupational therapy practice has moved beyond the initial phase of understanding spirituality and its role in practice and more toward making it part of actual practice. It is important for students, educators, and occupational therapy practitioners to be familiar and comfortable with the foundational literature around spirituality. Equally important is for them to take those learnings into practice. This is the expectation of the profession, clients, and the community of care.

After more than 10 years of relevant scholarship (Espiritu et al., 2020; Milliken, 2020; Pizzi & Richards, 2017; Thompson et al., 2018) and an even longer period of popular cultural interest, bringing spiritual support, treatment, and care to clients is neither controversial nor mysterious. That does not mean that discussions of appropriate interventions may not lead to or require examination of personal opinions and biases—conversations that, in some ways, may seem overdue. Such examinations are necessary and vital as the relationship between client and therapist becomes more holistic; they also are essential to developing a personalized treatment plan for each client.

Spirituality is not religion. *Spirituality* is

> the personal quest for understanding answers to ultimate questions about life, about meaning, and about relationship with the sacred or transcendent, which may (or may not) lead to or arise from the development of religious rituals and the formation of community. (Moreira-Almeida & Koenig, 2006, p. 844)

Definitions of *spirituality* similar to that by Moreira-Almeida and Koenig (2006) exist (see, e.g., Csontó, 2009; Egan & DeLaat, 1997; Engquist et al., 1997; Schulz, 2004; Urbanowksi & Vargo, 1994). One's sense of connection, of having a purpose, and of believing that, as individuals, we have something to contribute to society are the ways in which we can understand the role of spirituality in each person's life. ***Religion*** can be defined as "an organized system of beliefs, practices, rituals, and symbols designed to facilitate closeness to the sacred or transcendent" (Moreira-Almeida & Koenig, 2006, p. 844). The point here is not to set up an "either/or" or "this or that" contrast between spirituality and religion. Understanding how spirituality stands as its own, unique concept helps to gain a clearer understanding of a client's needs and promotes a comprehensive way of thinking about the role occupational therapy can play in meeting those needs.

In this chapter, we discuss spiritual practice both in the context of its role in treatment and in the ways in which an occupational therapy practitioner can integrate spiritual aspects in a respectful, unbiased, and supportive manner. This means that, in part, the practitioner will need to examine and rethink the use of common terms to give them proper context. In addition, integrating spiritual aspects into treatment means understanding how to assist clients with the religious and spiritual practices they want and need. Together, the practitioner and the client can collaboratively find the right balance of therapeutic intervention that provides spiritual satisfaction.

Occupational Therapy Practice and Spirituality

Occupational therapy practitioners hold diverse perspectives on what role occupational therapy has in addressing spirituality; many disagree that it is an area that should be addressed by an occupational therapy practitioner (Belcham, 2004; Collins et al., 2002; Csontó, 2009; Engquist et al., 1997). Engquist et al. (1997) found that a large percentage of occupational therapists believe that spirituality is an important client factor that can affect overall health and well-being, but only 36.6% of therapists felt that addressing spirituality was within the scope of occupational therapy practice. Although many years have passed, this feeling among practitioners may remain, contradicting the inclusion of spirituality within frameworks, guidelines, and theories, including the fourth edition of the *OTPF* (AOTA, 2020), the Canadian Association of Occupational Therapists' Occupational Therapy Guidelines (Canadian Association of Occupational Therapists, 1991) and the Canadian Model of Occupational Performance and Engagement (Polatajko et al., 2007).

If spirituality is explicitly documented as an important aspect of the domain of occupational therapy (AOTA, 2020), why is it consistently reported that practicing occupational therapists are not addressing this client factor in practice (see, e.g., Brémault-Phillips, 2018; Espiritu et al., 2020; Milliken, 2020; Pham et al., 2020; Pizzi & Richards, 2017; Thompson et al., 2018)? Many occupational therapy practitioners have expressed discomfort with addressing the topic of spirituality and are not incorporating spirituality into practice for these reasons:

- Lack of one concrete definition of spirituality (Brémault-Phillips, 2018; Csontó, 2009; Espiritu et al., 2020; Milliken, 2020; Morris et al., 2014; Pham et al., 2020), even though the definition of spirituality has been included in the *OTPF* since 2008 (AOTA, 2008)
- Confusion regarding the meaning of "spirituality" versus "religion" (Csontó, 2009; Engquist et al., 1997; Morris et al., 2014)
- Fear of crossing unspoken and often poorly defined "boundaries" with a client or damaging therapeutic rapport because of cultural norms of avoiding "religious" or "controversial" subjects (Collins et al., 2002; Kroeker, 1997; Milliken, 2020; Udell & Chandler, 2000)
- Lack of time (Collins et al., 2002)
- Lack of education and training as well as a perceived self-competence in addressing spirituality in practice (Belcham, 2004; Collins et al., 2002; Csontó, 2009; Egan & Swedersky, 2003; Engquist et al., 1997).

Because of this lack of preparedness and discomfort, occupational therapy practitioners may omit the client factor of spirituality from practice, and rarely assess or address it through the intervention process (Brémault-Phillips, 2018; Csontó, 2009; Espiritu et al., 2020; Milliken, 2020; Morris et al., 2014; Pham et al., 2020). For a profession that emphasizes the importance of client-centered practice and the design of goals and intervention plans that prioritize client needs and desires, "glossing over" the client factor of spirituality is a disservice to clients.

The professional literature points to a strong client desire that spirituality be addressed within hospital settings. Koenig (2013 as cited in Milliken, 2020) completed a study reporting that

> 75%–90% of seriously ill patients identify themselves as spiritual or religious, yet 75% of hospitalized patients state that their spiritual needs are minimally or not addressed at all by their healthcare providers. Furthermore, emotional and spiritual support is rated among the "lowest for patient satisfaction and highest in need of improvement." (p. 4)

Koenig (2004) also reported that hundreds of research studies have elucidated the role that spirituality or religion has in allowing clients to cope with various physical and mental conditions. Spirituality and religion do not just affect the client's subjective experience as they journey through a medical condition or disability; they provide tangible objective outcomes, including "less depression and faster recovery from depression (60 of 93 studies), lower suicide rates (57 of 68), less anxiety (35 of 69), and less substance abuse (98 of 120)" (Koenig, 2004, p. 1195). In one study (Silvestri et al., 2003), individuals with lung cancer were asked to rank the importance of seven factors in their cancer treatment decisions; this ranking was then compared to the ranking of the client's family and the client's oncologist. The study found that all groups ranked the expertise and recommendations of their oncology physician as the most important factor in their treatment decision making and then ranked faith in God as the second most important factor. Oncologists, though, ranked faith in God as the least important factor in cancer treatment decisions (Silvestri et al., 2003). This research illustrates health care professionals' underestimation of the value that clients place on spirituality and religion during their health care journey.

The occupational therapy profession needs to continue to critically examine and reflect on the lack of consideration of spirituality in practice. As Christiansen (1997) asserted, "If occupational therapy is to be complete and genuine in its consideration of humans as occupational beings, it must acknowledge spirituality as an important dimension of everyday life" (p. 169). When the occupational therapy profession was created during World War I, the focus was explicitly on the mind, body, and spirit of wounded soldiers. This triumvirate of aspects—mind, body, and spirit—was further exemplified by a triangle patch that the first occupational therapists wore (Friedland, 2011). Since then, much has changed in the profession, including trends toward a more medical model approach, a more outcome-focused approach, and less emphasis on issues of mental health. Additionally, theorists continue to assert that an occupational therapist is "holistic" and "client centered" (Christiansen, 1997; Finlay, 2000; Hemphill-Pearson & Hunter, 1997; Waite, 2014). And, more recently, the *OTPF–4* (AOTA, 2020) emphasizes the broader view of the profession.

Assessment of Spirituality and Perceived Barriers

Although occupational therapy practitioners often agree that spirituality as a client factor and its effect on health are important, spirituality is rarely assessed within practice (Collins et al., 2002; Egan & Swedersky, 2003; Engquist et al., 1997). When surveying practicing occupational therapists regarding their views and perspectives of spirituality in practice, Morris et al. (2014) found that

> 85% of the respondents indicated that they are not utilizing assessments of spirituality to evaluate their clients' spiritual needs. Only six percent of the study respondents indicated that they were even aware of instruments that they might use to measure spiritual need in their clients. (p. 31)

The discomfort that health care providers feel assessing and addressing spirituality in practice can be likened to the historical discomfort of assessing, within the health care setting, sexuality and addressing sexual practices and relationships (Espiritu et al., 2020).

Assessing spirituality is best completed as part of an initial evaluation to better understand the occupational profile of the client. The initial evaluation, which consists of the occupational profile and analysis of occupational performance, can too often focus on the perceived physical impairments of the client, such as in body functions, body structures, or performance skills (Low, 1997). This focus within the evaluation often drives the intervention plan and targeted outcomes of the occupational therapy process.

Making Formal Spirituality Assessments

Many formal spirituality assessments are available within the literature (Cadge & Bandini, 2015). Consequently, some individuals have called for the continued creation of spirituality assessments to cease and, instead, a renewed focus on what to do with the results of a spirituality assessment (Cadge & Bandini, 2015).

Each structured spirituality assessment asks questions through a different lens and perspective. Some of the assessments focus on religion—and frequently a single religion—whereas some aim to capture the full scope of spirituality as a whole. For example, the FICA Spiritual History Tool© (Puchalski & Romer, 2000; see Exhibit 16.1), which is designed to be used within a health care setting, asks the client questions about their personal spiritual and faith beliefs, attached meaning and importance of those beliefs, whether they're connected to a broader spiritual community, and how they would like to address their spirituality throughout the health care process.

The HOPE assessment (Anandarajah & Hight, 2001) includes various questions targeted at the broad idea of spirituality, including sources of hope (H), organized religion (O), spiritual or religious practices (P), and their effects on the client's health care decisions (E). The assessments SPIRIT (Maugans, 1996)—spiritual belief system (S), personal

EXHIBIT 16.1. FICA Spiritual History Tool

The acronym FICA—Faith, Importance, Community, and Address—can help to structure questions for health care professionals who are taking a spiritual history.

F—Faith, Belief, Meaning

- "Do you consider yourself to be spiritual?" or "Is spirituality important to you?"
- "Do you have spiritual beliefs, practices, or values that help you to cope with stress, difficult times, or what you are going through right now?"
- "What gives your life meaning?"

I—Importance and Influence

- "What importance does spirituality have in your life?"
- "Has your spirituality influenced how you take care of yourself, particularly regarding your health?"
- "Does your spirituality affect your health care decision making?

C—Community

- "Are you part of a spiritual community?"
- "Is your community of support to you and how?"
- And, for people who do not identify with a community: "Is there a group of people you really love or who are important to you?"
  (*Note.* Communities, such as churches, temples, mosques, family, groups of like-minded friends, or yoga, can serve as strong support systems for some patients.)

A—Address/Action in Care

- "How would you like me, as your health care provider, to address spiritual issues in your health care?"
  (*Note.* With newer models, including the diagnosis of spiritual distress, "A" also refers to the "Assessment and Plan" for patient spiritual distress, needs, or resources within a treatment or care plan.)

Source. Puchalski and Romer (2000). Adapted with permission from Christina Puchalski, MD.

spirituality (P), integration with a spiritual community (I), ritualized practices and restrictions (R), implications for medical care (I), and terminal events planning (T)—and FAITH (King, 2002)—Faith (F), Application (A), Involvement (I), Treatment (T), and Hope (H)—also aim to capture religion and religious practices, spirituality and spiritual practices, and personal beliefs and effects on health care decisions. Csontó (2009) reported that approximately half of occupational therapists are not assessing spirituality in part because of a lack of inclusion of spirituality within assessments frequently used in practice. Two occupational therapy–specific assessments that include a spiritual component are the (1) Qual-OT (Robnett & Gliner, 1995) and (2) Mayers' Lifestyle Questionnaire (Mayers, 1995). Each broadly assesses quality of life, health and wellness, and well-being with an inclusion of a subset of spirituality.

Addressing Time Constraints

A frequently cited barrier to assessing and addressing spirituality in practice is the lack of time to do so within the constraints of the health care system (Collins et al., 2002; Koenig, 2004). The time available to an occupational therapist for client assessment is precious. The therapist must carefully select and prioritize the use of standardized and nonstandardized assessments and screenings that will provide the most information to have an effect on the client's intervention planning and targeted outcomes. An occupational therapist does not always have the luxury of time to use a standardized or nonstandardized assessment or screening for every client factor that appears to be affected by disability, illness, or trauma. Low (1997) wrote that

> in this era of fast-paced schedules and limited patient visits it is ludicrous to recommend interactions with the patient that demand the luxury of extended time. However, sensitivity to factors other than the physical may prevent ineffective or prolonged treatment. There are ways that the occupational therapist can, within the time allotted for physical treatment, address spiritual needs as well. (pp. 218–219)

In a world of insurance reimbursement and productivity requirements, it is often unrealistic to expect occupational therapy practitioners to complete a comprehensive and wide-ranging spirituality assessment with a client during an initial evaluation. What is realistic is that, during the initial evaluation as part of the client's occupational profile, the therapist can ask one or two questions that target the client's spirituality or religion. In that initial evaluation, the client is often asked multiple questions by multiple disciplines; therefore, the client would be less likely to be surprised or even resistant to an additional question or two because they are generally cognizant that multiple disciplines are attempting to get to know all applicable information that could affect their medical or rehabilitative services and outcomes (Koenig, 2004).

An occupational therapist could select a couple of these questions to better assess a broad picture of their client's spirituality. If therapists continue to focus purely on ADLs during an occupational profile but omit other areas of the *OTPF–4* (AOTA, 2020), such as spirituality and religious expression, they are doing a disservice to the client. If occupational therapists continue to omit assessment of these occupations and client factors, they are missing important information that could guide intervention and selection of outcomes, build therapeutic rapport, motivate the client, and assist in goal setting. It should be as feasible to ask a client during an initial evaluation about their spiritual or religious beliefs as it is to ask the number of steps in their home environment or if they are the one to complete the laundry or pet care in the home. As reported by Koenig (2007), the literature shows that collecting a spiritual history of a client only adds 1 to 2 minutes to the initial evaluation. Thus, it should not be an unrealistic step for practicing occupational therapists because this information can have a powerful impact on intervention planning and the client's functional outcomes.

The Joint Commission on Accreditation of Healthcare Organizations (now referred to as The Joint Commission) requires that a spiritual history be documented in the medical record for all individuals admitted to an acute care hospital, nursing home, or home health agency (The Joint Commission, 2022). However, this history is often reduced to a single question regarding religion or if hospital staff should contact a religious leader (Koenig, 2007). This reduced documentation is akin to an occupational therapy practitioner asking only one or two questions regarding previous functional abilities, home environment, or support system during the occupational profile or initial evaluation. Such practice is rarely done or accepted because it does not provide a full enough picture of the client to assist in the occupational therapy process. In addition to the available variety of formal standardized and nonstandardized spirituality and religious assessments with structured questions, the occupational therapist could ask individual questions within a traditional evaluation. Koenig (2006) recommended inclusion of any of the following type of questions within an initial evaluation:

- "Are spiritual or religious beliefs important to you?"
- "Does spirituality or religion cause you increased stress, or does it provide you with comfort?"
- "Do you have spiritual or religious beliefs that may affect your medical decisions or care?"
- "Do you have a spiritual community?"

Occupational therapists should take time to review the wealth of available spirituality assessments for incorporation into practice and perhaps select one or two questions from one assessment that they find to be the most helpful. To ease the therapist's discomfort with addressing spirituality, it would be wise for them to select one trial spirituality question as part of the occupational profile with their clients. As the practitioner becomes more comfortable with continued practice of spirituality assessment, they could add more questions into their individual practice.

EXERCISE 16.1. Spirituality Assessment Reflection

Read and review one of the following spirituality assessments: HOPE, FICA, SPIRIT, or FAITH.

- In an initial occupational therapy evaluation, could you envision yourself asking one or more specific questions from the assessment you reviewed?
- Would it be feasible to integrate the assessment you reviewed in an initial evaluation with clients?
- Based on your own understanding of spirituality and religion, write your own assessment question(s) that you believe would capture an understanding of a client's spirituality and could be helpful in guiding intervention and targeting outcomes.

Personal Spirituality of Occupational Therapy Practitioners

Important elements for an occupational therapy practitioner to consider in assessing spirituality or religion for a client is having an understanding and an awareness of their own personal spirituality. The *OTPF–4* states that *spirituality* is "a deep experience of meaning brought about by engaging in occupations that involve the enacting of personal values and beliefs, reflection, and intention within a supportive contextual environment" (Billock, 2005, p. 887 as cited in AOTA, 2020). It is important to recognize spirituality as "dynamic and often evolving" (Humbert, 2016, p. 12).

Questions occupational therapy practitioners may consider asking include:

- "What are the most important values and beliefs that I hold as true in my life?"
- "How do I personally engage in occupations that align with my personal values and beliefs and provide me with deep life meaning?"
- "Can I separate my own values and beliefs from those of a client and work wholeheartedly to assist them in their personal spirituality goals?"
- "How do I feel about assisting a client in fully participating in their religious and spiritual practices if those practices appear to contradict my own religious and spiritual practices?"
- "Can I withhold judgment for a client who practices spiritual and religious experiences different than my own?"

Anandarajah and Hight (2001) stated that an occupational therapy practitioner is required to "understand his or her own spiritual beliefs, values and biases in order to remain patient-centered and nonjudgmental" (p. 84). This is easier said than done if you are working with an individual who practices spiritual or religious beliefs that contradict your own. It is important for occupational therapy practitioners and students to take time to both reflect on their own personal spirituality and religion as well as consider how they would respond in various spiritual and religious scenarios that could and often do happen in practice. As Pain (2005) noted, unless a practitioner has explored his or her own spiritual nature, the challenge of assessing spiritual need would be akin to a blind occupational therapist assessing the lighting levels in a client's home" (p. 583).

Spirituality Intervention

After an occupational therapist assesses spirituality or religion during an initial evaluation, it is important to use that information to guide and inform intervention.

Using the Evaluation

How do practitioners aim to "treat" spirituality? Occupational therapists should use the spirituality information in the initial

EXERCISE 16.2. Exploring Your Personal Beliefs

Consider each of the following situations:

Situation 1: You are the primary occupational therapist for a client who has experienced a stroke and has significant motor impairment of the right side of their body. Whenever you go to visit the client, the client is unmotivated to participate and repeatedly states, "Don't worry, dear. God is going to heal me. God will fix me. We don't want to take it out of His hands."

- How would you deal with or manage this situation?
- What would you say?
- How do you feel about this situation?
- Do you believe that medical miracles happen? Why or why not?

Situation 2: You walk into your client's room in an acute care hospital as a husband tells his wife, "We obviously aren't praying hard enough because you're not better yet."

- How do you feel about this situation?
- What would you do (or not do?)

Situation 3: Your client asks you to pray with them.

- Would you?
- How would you feel about it?

Situation 4: A parent refuses treatment for their child because they are waiting for a miracle to occur.

- How do you think that would affect your interactions with the family?
- How would you handle the situation?

Situation 5: You have a client who has been diagnosed with the terminal illness of amyotrophic lateral sclerosis, or ALS. You are working with them consistently in the home health setting. The client tells you that they have hope that they will be healed.

- What do you say?
- How do you feel about this?

Situation 6: You are working with a client in an acute care hospital who is a member of the Jehovah's Witnesses. The client has been declining in independence during occupational therapy and physical therapy sessions, and the physician is recommending that the client undergo significant blood transfusions secondary to their medical status. In the interdisciplinary team meeting, you are informed that the client has declined this intervention. You are required to continue to attempt therapy with this client.

- How do you feel about this situation?
- Would you say anything to the client during therapy sessions?
- Say the client states, "I wish I could get stronger. I'm so weak." How would you respond?

Situation 7: You are working with a client who has a different faith or cultural worldview than you. The client asks you, "Who should I put hope in?"

- What do you say?

Personal reflections:

- How would you define *hope?*
- Is "hope" a spiritual thing to you?
- Can hope be irrational? Why or why not?
- How would you define *faith?*
- Is "faith" a spiritual thing to you?
- Do you believe that prayer can help to heal someone? Why or why not?
- Do you have any experiences with miracles involving you or someone close to you?
- What are hope-inspiring strategies for people in a variety of life circumstances?
- What are some ways that hope or optimism can be taught to a client?
- Do you see your personal faith influencing or affecting your practice as an occupational therapy practitioner? Why or why not?
- How would your answer affect your practice?

After you have explored your own feelings about each of these situations, discuss them with your peers to explore potentially different views.

evaluation to determine if a spiritual or religious goal is appropriate for the client.

The occupational therapy practitioner has numerous ways to look at how to potentially intervene in the realm of spirituality. Could a spiritual therapeutic activity address various impaired body functions, performance skills, or performance patterns within an intervention that provides meaning, purpose, and motivation to the client? Is spirituality infused throughout intervention to enhance meaning, purpose, and motivation? Is increased occupational performance in engagement of spiritual or religious practices the targeted outcome of the intervention plan? Are health or well-being targeted outcomes of the occupational therapy process that would emphasize incorporating interventions that focus on spirituality or religion within the occupational therapy process (AOTA, 2020)?

Differentiating Between Religion and Spirituality

Using the definition of spirituality in the *OTPF-4* (AOTA, 2020; Billock, 2005) provided earlier in the section "Personal Spirituality of Occupational Therapy Practitioners" to guide interventions can seem overwhelming because of the definition's broad nature. Occupational therapy practitioners should not combine the client factor of "spirituality" with "religion" because each is distinct from the other. Religious observation and practice are expressions of spirituality and thus are always a part of the client factor of spirituality, but spirituality is not always expressed through religion and religious practices.

This confusion by occupational therapy practitioners is evident in the literature: The few practitioners who have reported that they incorporate spirituality interventions into the occupational therapy process reduced the examples to only meet the client's religious-based spiritual needs (Udell & Chandler, 2000). These intervention examples included assisting a client to participate in religious services, assisting a client in the ability to pray, or assisting a client in preparing food related to religious holidays (Udell & Chandler, 2000). Johnston and Mayers (2005) contended that spirituality interventions can be much broader, such as assisting a client to explore the beauty in the world, including nature and art, and to enjoy time with family and close friends. As they put it, "Although it is not always easy to interpret secular expressions of spirituality, occupational therapists should be developing an awareness of what is important to clients and not limiting spiritual needs to religious traditions" (Johnston & Mayers, 2005, p. 389).

Meeting Clients' Spiritual Needs Through Occupation

Udell and Chandler (2000) categorized the spiritual needs that occupational therapy practitioners should be aware of or address with a client as "meeting the practical spiritual needs of a client, acknowledg[ing] spiritual aspects of a client, and spiritual counseling" (p. 493). However there is sparse occupational therapy literature on spiritual interventions that a practitioner could use in daily practice to meet a client's practical spiritual needs (Engquist et al., 1997; Johnston & Mayers, 2005), which may contribute to the lack of intervention planning focused on spirituality. There is confusion about what spiritual interventions might look like with clients; however, any chosen occupation can play a role in meeting the client's spiritual needs (Johnston & Mayers, 2005). This is the foundation of occupational therapy as a whole: selecting personal, meaningful, and important occupations or activities as a type of intervention with the client. The ability to transfer out of bed or cook a meal may be a very personal and important occupation to the client, but neither occupation may meet the client's spiritual needs. It is important for occupational therapists to assess what occupations of the client facilitate "deep experience of meaning," "reflection," or "intention," as stated by Billock (2005, p. 887). This is a different type of question to ask a client rather than this frequently used one: "What occupations do you need or want to do?"

As is true of all attached meanings to occupations, spiritual occupation is subjective and personal to the client. This highlights the importance of conducting an in-depth occupational profile with a client to determine which occupations fill them in the way that spirituality interventions are meant to do. The occupational profile and relationship building with a client are key to assessing spirituality and subsequently incorporating spirituality interventions into the occupational therapy process. This could be why Urbanowski and Vargo (1994) stated that "the prime therapeutic tool for addressing the spirituality of the individual is the therapeutic use of self" (p. 93). Without ***therapeutic use of self***—in which practitioners "develop and manage their therapeutic relationship with clients by using professional reasoning, empathy, and a client-centered, collaborative approach" (AOTA, 2020, p. 20)—a client will not feel comfortable enough to open up during a spirituality assessment that is included in the occupational profile of an initial evaluation. Therefore, the occupational therapist will not be equipped to incorporate spirituality into future intervention sessions.

A client may want to go to their granddaughter's dance recital, walk the dog, or clean their home, but these occupations may not meet the spiritual criterion of facilitating a deep experience of meaning, reflection, or intention. Occupations that meet spiritual needs are personalized from client to client as evidenced by an Unruh et al. (2002) article in which the authors found that all three occupational therapy clients enjoyed gardening as part of their intervention, but only two of those clients identified the gardening intervention as being "spiritual" to them. One client could find walking or meditating to be an important and enjoyable occupation, yet another client could find walking or meditating to be an important, enjoyable, *and* spiritual occupation because of the significant sense of meaning experienced through participation in the occupation.

Although the occupations that meet the spiritual criteria of facilitating deep experience of meaning, reflection, or intention are specifically based on the individual client, the literature does provide examples of occupations that clients have frequently reported as meeting their spiritual needs (Billock, 2005). Walking, gardening, reading, tai chi, yoga, meditation, charity projects, crafts, prayer, singing, food preparation, and religious rituals are all occupations that may promote deep meaning and reflection for a client (Rose, 1999; Rosenfeld, 2000; Udell & Chandler, 2000). Occupational therapy practitioners frequently cite their fear of crossing boundaries with a client as one of the primary barriers to assessing or addressing spirituality with clients (Collins et al., 2002; Kroeker, 1997; Udell & Chandler, 2000). This fear appears to be unsubstantiated because clients have indicated their desire for health care personnel to discuss spirituality and involve it in their plan of care (Milliken, 2020). In one study, clients were asked explicitly about their desire to include spiritual occupations within the occupational therapy process. They reported a desire to participate in the following self-perceived "spiritual" activities: journaling, playing music, engaging in gratitude practice, having therapy take place in nature, using spiritual or inspiring quotes, having an increased ability to transfer into a vehicle to attend religious activities, focusing on increasing client factors to enable riding a motorcycle, and talking about spirituality during therapy sessions (Milliken, 2020).

Religious Observation and Practices

Spiritual health and wellness might not be just an ancillary benefit of occupational therapy treatment; it could be a goal in itself. When a spiritual practice or intervention intersects with faith or religious practice, the occupational therapy practitioner will need to be able to look inclusively across various faiths and faith practices. If an occupational therapy intervention can allow an individual to resume participation in society, the goal of the intervention may mean participation in a religious service or resumption of other traditional practices. For practitioners and caregivers, facilitating participation is the goal—just as with any other activity or occupation.

Occupational therapy practitioners also know that being active is part of developing and maintaining a healthy spirit. Activity and occupation help calm the mind, focus our thinking, and maintain our physical well-being. When those activities also provide spiritual satisfaction, allow one to feel useful, are part of one achieving a larger purpose, or fulfill a sense of destiny, we as practitioners know that the potential for therapeutic benefit is that much greater. It is vital that practitioners understand what activities and occupations will address a client's spiritual needs in addition to addressing the physical and mental health components.

Although spirituality is not synonymous with religious expression and observation, religious practices are often the way in which individuals express their personal spirituality, thus making it important for occupational therapy practitioners to understand the specific religion of the clients they serve. McColl (2003) stated, "If we are to serve all clients with regard to spirituality, we must accept that religious participation is a legitimate means of spiritual expression" (p. 12). Christiansen (1997) argued, "One cannot discuss spirituality without recognizing its relationship to religion" (p. 197). Again, practitioners have historically expressed a discomfort in discussing religion or designing an intervention specifically to meet the goals of increasing the client's ability to participate in religious practices (Engquist et al., 1997).

Having an understanding of a client's specific religion and religious observation and practices is of utmost importance for any health care provider; that understanding allows them to assess, be mindful of, and to incorporate client practices into interactions with the client and the therapeutic process. Practitioners can use this information to provide more effective client-centered practice, using the knowledge as both a means and an end in the occupational therapy process. Such practices can also be important to clients as a coping strategy and a motivational tool to increase therapeutic rapport and facilitate the client's participation. Practitioners can use their knowledge of the client's religion to build therapeutic rapport by facilitating the continued expression and observation of religion while the client receives therapy services.

Occupational therapists can incorporate goals into the therapeutic process so that the client is able to meaningfully participate in religious practices, such as participating in communion, kneeling at the mosque, holding a Bible while standing in a temple, and navigating the choir loft. Occupational therapy practitioners' knowledge of the client's religion can also facilitate an understanding of how the client views their illness, disability, injury, or even pain; that information can assist the practitioner in facilitating increased participation, motivation, and functional outcomes of the occupational therapy process. Williams et al. (1994) emphasized that "while knowledge of a person's beliefs cannot perfectly predict future behavior, assessing [the] sufferer's beliefs can provide insight into how one understands what they are experiencing and what needs to be done to remedy the experience" (p. 77).

Intervention for Religious Observation

On surveying practicing occupational therapists to assess how they are assessing and intervening for religious observation in practice, Thompson et al. (2018) reported that "more than 25% of the respondents indicated that they never assess a client's ability to participate in religious observance. Approximately 29% never wrote interventions related to religious observance in their plans of care" (p. 5). Of the practitioners who did report constructing interventions to target increased client participation in religious observation, methods largely focused on indirect interventions that targeted remediating the client's body functions or performance skills that are required to successfully participate in religious observation and practices. Although more direct interventions were reported, including actively using the occupation of religious observation within practice, such as attending a religious ceremony with a client, indirect interventions were the most frequently selected type of intervention to focus on this area of occupation.

It is important for occupational therapy practitioners to ask the client about any religious practices or observations that the client feels are important to maintain or return to after illness, disability, or trauma. Indirect interventions for the client could include focusing on the body functions and performance skills required to pass an offering plate; stand while holding a Bible, prayer book, or hymn book; kneel to participate in salat, participate in meal preparation for Shabbat or Rosh Hashanah; or climb the stairs to the designated area to worship at the mosque. Analysis of occupational performance is an important aspect of the occupational therapy process and should be applied to the occupation of religious observation. A client may desire to hold and read the hymn book at church with both hands while standing; therefore, the occupational therapist could design interventions that target the required body functions to complete this task successfully, such as bilateral integration, balance, proprioception, visual acuity and stability, visual fields, bilateral upper-extremity muscle strength, and overall endurance. Performance skills to target within intervention could include motor skills like reaches, stabilizes, lifts, grips, coordinates, bends or manipulates; process skills such as attends, initiates, sequences, or terminates; or social skills such as looks, replies, or empathizes (AOTA, 2020).

Milliken (2020) assessed clients' personal perspectives of spirituality as reported to occupational therapy students during fieldwork. When clients were asked if they considered themselves a spiritual individual, 257 out of 281 respondents said yes. When those same clients were asked how occupational therapy could help them to meet their spiritual goals, most respondents reported a desire for the occupational therapist to provide emotional support or mental or physical intervention, or they had specific spiritual goals (Milliken, 2020). A number of stated spiritual goals focused on religious observation, such as "Help me learn new ways to kneel so I don't look like I'm not participating in church" or "I'd really like to read my Bible, but my eyes cannot see well enough anymore. Can you help with that?" or "Teach me some techniques to hold my Bible" (Milliken, 2020, p. 13). The literature clearly demonstrates a significant desire of clients to have their spiritual and religious observation goals met by a health care provider. As occupational therapy practitioners, we strive to increase or enhance occupational performance for all occupations, which includes the IADLs of religious observation and participation.

Understanding Religious Beliefs

Occupational therapy practitioners should strive to gain basic knowledge of major religions to better understand clients' perspectives. An understanding of how a client's religious beliefs may affect their occupations and overall participation in therapy can facilitate increased therapeutic rapport and increased outcomes. One area that may affect participation in therapy services is the client's perceived pain and belief in pain management. Various religions view the experience of pain differently, and not understanding those perspectives could limit participation in therapy or limit the therapeutic relationship (Lynn, 1993). Clients may decline pain management even though they are be in severe pain. Lynn (1993) documented a client declining pain management even during excruciating wound dressing changes because their religious affiliation did not condone the use of narcotics. In Buddhism, pain is viewed as an unescapable aspect of life and is to be "endured in a matter-of-fact manner" (Lynn, 1993, p. 217).

Religious beliefs may also dictate the client's performance patterns, such as habits, routines, and roles. A Hindu client, in observance of their beliefs, may want to complete the ADLs of grooming and hygiene as the first activity after waking because oral hygiene is of utmost importance (Abbato, 2011). A Hindu client completing the ADL of bathing may desire to complete this activity with continual running water, such as a shower, rather than through sponge bathing at the sink (Abbato, 2011). For a Muslim client, bathing before prayers is extremely important, in addition to doing so after voiding or having a bowel movement. A Muslim client may also desire more modest clothing than a hospital gown offers if admitted to an acute care or rehabilitation hospital (Islamic Council of Queensland, 1999). Occupational therapy practitioners understand that performance patterns affect occupational performance, but increased time may be required to determine how the client's religion delegates the rhythm of their performance patterns.

A client's religion often includes celebrations and holidays, and it will be important to facilitate client participation in the occupations and activities that accompany the religion's celebratory rituals. Religious rituals, holidays, and celebrations may provide a valuable motivational tool for an occupational therapist to incorporate into intervention planning and to provide increased client-centered care. For example, facilitating a Jewish client's occupational performance to participate in preparations for Rosh Hashanah provides excellent client-centered and occupation-based care rather than using therapeutic exercise to increase upper-extremity range of motion and strength. Egan and DeLaat (1994) stated it well: "An increase in muscle strength is not important, a tub seat is not important, unless these materials things allow the individual self-expression and connection" (p. 101).

Importantly, it is not solely within the scope of an occupational therapy practitioner to be responsible for a client's spiritual and religious crises. It is helpful for an occupational therapist to assess spirituality and religious practices and use that information appropriately to provide the most support possible for the client throughout the occupational therapy process. In a hospital setting, chaplaincy is often available to

EXERCISE 16.3. Spirituality Action Steps for an Occupational Therapy Student

- Get to know your own spirituality. Reflect on your spiritual and religious beliefs and clarify your own values and how they infuse your identity and will likely infuse your future practice.
- Practice "assessing" spirituality through targeted questions to be incorporated into an occupational profile. Review the available spirituality assessments and select a minimum of one question to incorporate into an initial evaluation with a client.
- Attempt to understand a client's specific religion, how it may affect the client's occupational performance, and how activity analysis of religious observation and spiritual practices can create client-centered intervention planning that targets required body functions and performance skills.

meet with the client to discuss spiritual matters. Contacting the client's spiritual or religious leader may also increase the client's occupational performance and enhance the occupational therapy process (Denham & Humbert, 2016).

Summary

Integrating spiritual practices into treatment may initially seem challenging or uncomfortable. It takes time to adjust, adapt, and grow into understanding different and important areas of practice. We are in a period of rapid cultural shifts with a new awareness of cultural implications on our practice and interventions. As occupational therapy practitioners, we have learned the importance of being open to unfamiliar ideas, beliefs, and activities. How we approach a client from a different or unfamiliar background can be important to the effectiveness of our interventions. Changing a word choice or embracing an unfamiliar cultural idea can have a significant effect on our clients. It is critical that we explore our own perspectives, beliefs, and potential biases so we can be better at understanding and intervening with our clients. When we are confronted by client needs in an unfamiliar spiritual practice, looking to colleagues, mentors, teachers, and leaders can make a tremendous difference and expand our shared knowledge and understanding. Similarly, our own spiritual connections can deepen and grow as we learn and study the beliefs and practices of others as well as what gives those practices meaning and value.

Like many other aspects of occupational therapy, what we know and understand about the spiritual aspect of the individual has deepened since the early days of the occupational therapy profession, when we focused solely on the positive benefits of useful activities. As the *OTPF-4* (AOTA, 2020) suggests, addressing spiritual considerations is an important aspect of therapeutic interventions. It can improve the sense of personal fulfillment and can foster an improved sense of self for the client. These are important values in occupational therapy and relate to the roots of the profession.

References

Abbato, S. (2011). *Community profiles for health care providers*. https://www.health.qld.gov.au/__data/assets/pdf_file/0033/158775/profiles-complete.pdf

American Occupational Therapy Association. (2008). Occupational therapy practice framework: Domain and process (2nd ed.). *American Journal of Occupational Therapy, 62*(6), 625–683. https://doi.org/10.5014/ajot.62.6.625

American Occupational Therapy Association. (2020). Occupational therapy practice framework: Domain and process (4th ed.). *American Journal of Occupational Therapy, 74*(Suppl. 2), Article 7412410010. https://doi.org/10.5014/ajot.2020.74s2001

Anandarajah, G., & Hight, E. (2001). Spirituality and medical practice: Using the HOPE questions as a practical tool for spiritual assessment. *American Family Physician, 63*(1), 81–88.

Belcham, C. (2004). Spirituality in occupational therapy: Theory in practice? *British Journal of Occupational Therapy, 67*(1), 39–46. https://doi.org/10.1177/030802260406700106

Billock, C. (2005). *Delving into the center: Women's lived experience of spirituality through occupation* (Publication No. AAT 3219812) [Doctoral dissertation, University of Southern California]. ProQuest Dissertations and Theses Global.

Brémault-Phillips, S. (2018). Spirituality and the metaphorical self-driving car. *Canadian Journal of Occupational Therapy, 85*(1), 4–6. https://doi.org/10.1177/0008417417751143

Cadge, W., & Bandini, J. (2015). The evolution of spiritual assessment tools in health care. *Society, 52*(5), 430–437. https://doi.org/10.1007/s12115-015-9926-y

Canadian Association of Occupational Therapists. (1991). *Occupational therapy guidelines for client-centred practice*. CAOT/L'ACE Publications.

Christiansen, C. (1997). Acknowledging a spiritual dimension in occupational therapy practice. *American Journal of Occupational Therapy, 51*(3), 169–172. https://doi.org/10.5014/ajot.51.3.169

Collins, J. S., Paul, S., & West-Frasier, J. (2002). The utilization of spirituality in occupational therapy: Beliefs, practices, and perceived barriers. *Occupational Therapy in Health Care, 14*(3–4), 73–92. https://doi.org/10.1080/J003v14n03_05

Csontó, S. (2009). Occupational therapy students' consideration of clients' spirituality in practice placement education. *British Journal of Occupational Therapy, 72*(10), 442–449. https://doi.org/10.1177/030802260907201005

Denham, P., & Humbert, T. (2016). Spirituality through the lens of healthcare chaplaincy. In T. Humbert (Ed.), *Spirituality and occupational therapy: A model for practice and research* (pp. 59–75). AOTA Press.

Egan, M., & DeLaat, M. D. (1994). Considering spirituality in occupational therapy practice. *Canadian Journal of Occupational Therapy, 61*(2), 95–101. https://doi.org/10.1177/000841749706400307

Egan, M., & DeLaat, M. D. (1997). The implicit spirituality of occupational therapy practice. *Canadian Journal of Occupational Therapy, 64*(3), 115–121. https://doi.org/10.1177/000841749706400307

Egan, M., & Swedersky, J. (2003). Spirituality as experienced by occupational therapists in practice. *American Journal of Occupational Therapy, 57*(5), 525–533. https://doi.org/10.5014/ajot.57.5.525

Engquist, D. E., Short-DeGraff, M., Gliner, J., & Oltjenbruns, K. (1997). Occupational therapists' beliefs and practices with regard to spirituality and therapy. *American Journal of Occupational Therapy, 51*(3), 173–180. https://doi.org/10.5014/ajot.51.3.173

Espiritu, E. W., TenHaken-Riedel, J. P., Brown, R., Frame, T. R., Adam, J., Koch, A., . . . Owens, A. (2020). Incorporating spirituality into graduate health professions education. *Christian Higher Education, 19*(4), 254–271. https://doi.org/10.1080/15363759.2019.1687050

Finlay, L. (2000). Holism in occupational therapy: Elusive fiction and ambivalent struggle. *American Journal of Occupational Therapy, 55*(3), 268–276. https://doi.org/10.5014/ajot.55.3.268

Friedland, J. (2011). *Restoring the spirit: The beginnings of occupational therapy in Canada, 1890–1930*. McGill-Queen's University Press.

Hemphill-Pearson, B., & Hunter, M. (1997). Holism in mental health practice. *Occupational Therapy in Mental Health, 13*(2), 35–49. https://doi.org/10.1300/J004v13n02_03

Hinojosa, J., & Blount, M.-L. (Eds.). (2014). *The texture of life* (4th ed.). AOTA Press.

Humbert, T. (Ed.). (2016). *Spirituality and occupational therapy: A model for practice and research*. AOTA Press.

Islamic Council of Queensland. (1999). *Health care provider's handbook on Muslim patients*.

Johnston, D., & Mayers, C. (2005). Spirituality: A review of how occupational therapists acknowledge, assess and meet spiritual needs. *British Journal of Occupational Therapy, 68*(9), 386–392. https://doi.org/10.1177/030802260506800902

Joint Commission on Accreditation of Healthcare Organizations. (2022). *The Joint Commission guide to patient and family education*. Joint Commission Resources.

King, D. E. (2002). Spirituality and medicine. In M. B. Mengel, W. L. Holleman, & S. A. Fields (Eds.), *Fundamentals of clinical practice: A text book on the patient, doctor and society* (pp. 651–670). Springer. https://doi.org/10.1007/0-306-47565-0_29

Koenig, H. G. (2004). Religion, spirituality, and medicine: Research findings and implications for clinical practice. *Southern Medical Journal, 97*(12), 1194–1200. https://doi.org/10.1097/01.SMJ.0000146489.21837.CE

Koenig, H. G. (2006). The spiritual history. *Southern Medical Journal, 99*(10), 1159–1160. https://doi.org/10.1097/01.smj.0000242751.31841.35

Koenig, H. G. (2007). *Spirituality in patient care: Why, how, when, and what.* Templeton Press.

Kroeker, P. T. (1997). Spirituality and occupational therapy in a secular culture. *Canadian Journal of Occupational Therapy, 64*(3), 122–126. https://doi.org/10.1177/000841749706400308

Low, J. F. (1997). Religious orientation and pain management. *American Journal of Occupational Therapy, 51*(3), 215–219. https://doi.org/10.5014/ajot.51.3.215

Lynn, J. (1993). Travels in the valley of the shadow. In H. M. Spiro, M. G. Curnen, E. Peschel, & D. St. James (Eds.), *Empathy and the practice of medicine* (pp. 40–53). Yale University Press.

Maugans, T. A. (1996). The SPIRITual history. *Archives of Family Medicine, 5*(1), 11–16.

Mayers, C. A. (1995). Defining and assessing quality of life. *British Journal of Occupational Therapy, 58*(4), 144–150. https://doi.org/10.1177/030802269505800402

McColl, M. A. (2003). *Spirituality and occupational therapy.* Canadian Association of Occupational Therapy Publications ACE.

Milliken, B. E. (2020). Clients' perspectives of spirituality in occupational therapy: A retrospective study. *Open Journal of Occupational Therapy, 8*(4), 1–19. https://doi.org/10.15453/2168-6408.1666

Morris, D. N., Stecher, J., Briggs-Peppler, K. M., Chittenden, C. M., Rubira, J., & Wismer, L. K. (2014). Spirituality in occupational therapy: Do we practice what we teach? *Journal of Religion and Health, 53*(1), 27–36. https://doi.org/10.1007/s10943-012-9584-y

Pain, H. (2005). Spirituality [Letter]. *British Journal of Occupational Therapy, 68*(12), 583.

Pham, L., Sarnicola, R., Villasenor, C., & Vu, T. (2020). Spirituality in OT practice: Where is our spirituality now? *American Journal of Occupational Therapy, 74*(Suppl. 1), 7411505108. https://doi.org/10.5014/ajot.2020.74S1-PO2309

Pizzi, M. A., & Richards, L. G. (2017). Promoting health, well-being, and quality of life in occupational therapy: A commitment to a paradigm shift for the next 100 years. *American Journal of Occupational Therapy, 71*(4), Article 7104170010. https://doi.org/10.5014/ajot.2017.028456

Polatajko, H. J., Townsend, E. A., & Craik, J. (2007). Canadian Model of Occupational Performance and Engagement (CMOP–E). In E. A. Townsend & H. J. Polatajko (Eds.), *Enabling occupation II: Advancing an occupational therapy vision of health, well-being, & justice through occupation* (pp. 22–36). CAOT Publications ACE.

Puchalski, C., & Romer, A. L. (2000). Taking a spiritual history allows clinicians to understand patients more fully. *Journal of Palliative Medicine, 3*(1), 129–137. https://doi.org/10.1089/jpm.2000.3.129

Robnett, R. H., & Gliner, J. A. (1995). Qual-OT: A quality of life assessment tool. *Occupational Therapy Journal of Research, 15*(3), 198–213. https://doi.org/10.1177/153944929501500304

Rose, A. (1999). Spirituality and palliative care: The attitudes of occupational therapists. *British Journal of Occupational Therapy, 62,* 307–312. http://doi.org/10.1177/030802269906200707

Rosenfeld, M. S. (2000). Spiritual agent modalities for occupational therapy practice. *OT Practice, 5*(2), 17–21.

Schulz, E. K. (2004). Spirituality and disability: An analysis of select themes. *Occupational Therapy in Health Care, 18*(4), 57–83. https://doi.org/10.1080/J003v18n04_05

Silvestri, G. A., Knittig, S., Zoller, J. S., & Nietert, P. J. (2003). Importance of faith on medical decisions regarding cancer care. *Journal of Clinical Oncology, 21*(7), 1379–1382. https://doi.org/10.1200/JCO.2003.08.036

Thompson, K., Gee, B. M., & Hartje, S. (2018). Use of religious observance as a meaningful occupation in occupational therapy. *Open Journal of Occupational Therapy, 6*(1). https://doi.org/10.15453/2168-6408.1296

Udell, L., & Chandler, C. (2000). The role of the occupational therapist in addressing the spiritual needs of clients. *British Journal of Occupational Therapy, 63*(10), 489–494. https://doi.org/10.1177/030802260006301006

Unruh, A. M., Versnel, J., & Kerr, N. (2002). Spirituality unplugged: A review of commonalities and contentions, and a resolution. *Canadian Journal of Occupational Therapy, 69*(1), 5–19. https://doi.org/10.1177/000841740206900101

Urbanowski, R., & Vargo, J. (1994). Spirituality, daily practice, and the occupational performance model. *Canadian Journal of Occupational Therapy, 61*(2), 88–94. https://doi.org/10.1177/000841749406100204

Waite, A. (2014, August 25). Have faith: How spirituality is a regular part of occupational therapy practice. *OT Practice, 19,* 13–16.

Williams, D. A., Robinson, M. E., & Geisser, M. E. (1994). Pain beliefs: Assessment and utility. *Pain, 59*(1), 71–78. https://doi/10.1016/0304-3959(94)90049-3

17

Meaningful Occupation: Critical Literature

SUSAN LIN, ScD, OTR/L, FAOTA, FACRM

CHAPTER HIGHLIGHTS

- Defining *meaningful*
- Meaning and the *Occupational Therapy Practice Framework*
- Reviews of research about meaning in occupation
- Measuring meaningfulness
- Research on occupation and health
- Activity, brain health, and cognitive functions
- Situating meaning in group and population health
- Meaningful occupation and the environment
- Meaning making from different perspectives
- Future research
- Historical views of meaning

KEY TERMS AND CONCEPTS

• affordance • belonging • client factors • doing, being, and becoming • life balance • meaning • meaning in life • meaning salience • meaning structure method • occupation • personal factors

> *"To make life a little better for people less fortunate than you, that's what I think a meaningful life is. One lives not just for oneself but for one's community."*
>
> —Ruth Bader Ginsburg (2017), Stanford Rathbone Lecture

In this chapter, I discuss meaningful occupations and examine their defining qualities, as well as recent reviews of the literature focused on meaningful occupational engagement. Meaningfulness plays a central role in occupation-based and client-centered practice, but how do practitioners identify and measure what is meaningful to clients? Instruments that have been cited in recent literature are also described. Although their inclusion in this chapter does not serve as an endorsement, it may spark interest in exploring their potential use in research and practice.

In the early years of occupational therapy, the founders noted that meaningful occupation has an effect on health and mood (Meyer, 1922; Tracy, 1910). However, does research support this long-held tenet? If evidence supports the health-inducing effects of meaningful occupational engagement, what are some of its specific benefits? Thought-provoking results regarding occupation's effects on physical health, mental health, quality of life, and even brain health are presented, offering many potential research questions to ponder. Research on population health and environment is then discussed, as it relates to meaning. Finally, the chapter concludes with ideas for future research and a brief reflection on the views of occupational therapy's founders regarding meaningful occupation.

Defining Meaningful

Meaning—"everybody wants it, but nobody quite knows what it is" (Baumeister & Landau, 2018, p. 1). Its complexity can partly be attributed to the fact that meaning represents a combination of affective, motivational, and cognitive factors (Reker, 2000). Although a special issue of *Review of General Psychology* was devoted to meaning, delineating the varied nature of meaning, this chapter will focus on the aspect of meaning most applicable to occupational therapy: how meaning affects behavior (Baumeister & Landau, 2018).

Meaning is often cited in definitions of occupational therapy. A recent definition of *occupation* refers to "personalized and meaningful engagement in daily life events by a specific client" (American Occupational Therapy Association [AOTA], 2020c, p. 7). Occupations ranging from the ordinary to the extraordinary bring meaning and purpose to life (World Federation of Occupational Therapists, 2021). In this context, meaning is derived from occupations.

In her Eleanor Clarke Slagle lecture, Trombly (1995) cited meaningfulness, which she termed *occupation-as-means,* as an integral aspect of therapeutic occupation when used to remediate impaired abilities. The meaning of the occupation and its relevance serve as a motivator, activating a propensity to act or to do. With respect to occupation-as-end, meaningfulness may stem from the person's values, family and cultural experiences, prioritization of important occupations and how they are performed, and perception of consequences (i.e., pleasure, negative repercussions; Trombly, 1995). In best practice, practitioners verify clients' perceptions of the meaning of occupations and avoid making assumptions (Goldstein-Lohman et al., 2003; Trombly, 1995). The meaning of an occupation, as means or an end, can motivate people to engage in that occupation. For example, a client could perceive baking as a meaningful activity because of its therapeutic value (e.g., addressing cognitive functions) or because it accomplishes a goal (e.g., providing a cake for a relative's birthday). Thus, meaning can precede occupational engagement as well as be influenced during and after occupational engagement (see Figure 17.1).

What makes an occupation meaningful to a person? Learning which activities and relationships a person values is often helpful in identifying individual meanings (Eschenfelder, 2005). One way to determine what a person finds meaningful is to inquire about their current roles and, if necessary, their past and anticipated future roles. Roles have unique and specific meanings to a person, with associated tasks and activities and in particular contexts (Trombly, 1993). Occupational therapists can then focus interventions on helping clients fulfill their valued roles.

Meaning is more likely to be ascribed to activities if they provide pleasure and enjoyment and fulfill basic psychological needs through choice, control, and belonging (Eakman, 2012). In addition, having social relationships is correlated with meaning in life (King et al., 2016). A mixed-methods study of people with mental illness reported that the most meaningful occupations were those that provided opportunities for social connection and being valued by others (Hancock et al., 2015).

FIGURE 17.1. Relationship between meaning and occupational engagement.

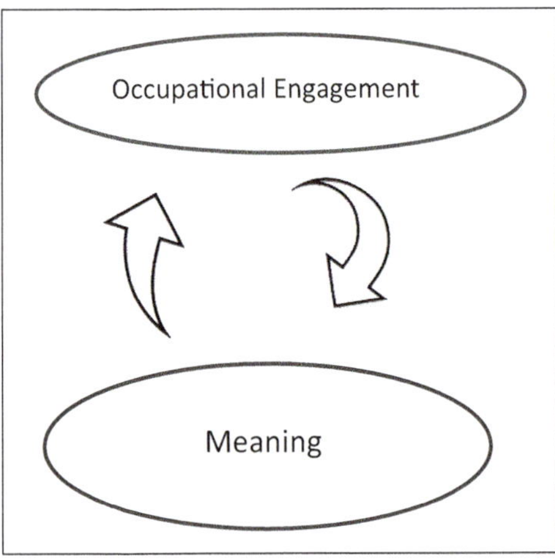

Relatively recent literature reflects a greater emphasis on understanding the dimensions of how one interprets activity engagement (Atler et al., 2017). Pierce (2003) proposed that people's well-being is correlated with three dimensions of subjective experience: pleasure, productivity, and restoration (a sense of renewal). What one person finds enjoyable, another might find onerous. For example, a middle-aged woman with rheumatoid arthritis commented on her new medication's effectiveness, saying, "I knew I was feeling better when I could vacuum again." Another person might put vacuuming last on their list of enjoyable occupations. Other aspects to consider are the values (Eakman & Eklund, 2011) and assumptions (Goldstein-Lohman et al., 2003) associated with occupations.

Broadening Categories of Meaning

By and large, occupational therapy has focused on occupations that are framed in a positive light, but such a narrow view may mean that practitioners are not capturing the full breadth of occupations. White et al. (2013) posited that by focusing only on occupations that elicit positive subjective meaning and are socially approved, the profession has not acknowledged other potential categories of meaning. White et al. used grounded theory, a qualitative research methodology, to investigate the activities and occupations of 16 adults living with chronic conditions in Australia. They defined ***occupation*** as "doing activities and actions with meaning, in the context of one's life, health condition(s), and world" (White et al., 2013, p. 61). All participants ascribed meaning to their activities and occupations, but they drew a distinction between "my world," including their environment and chronic condition, and "the world," referring to the external physical, social, and cultural environment. White et al. (2013) summarized the meaning of participants' occupations by creating three two-dimensional categories: (1) connecting–reconnecting and disconnecting activities, (2) caring and harming activities, and (3) contributing and detracting activities. These researchers noted that two categories, disconnecting activities and detracting activities (i.e., activities that detract people from reaching their potential), have not been discussed in the occupational therapy literature. However, the aspects of connecting and reconnecting are included in the *Occupational Therapy Practice Framework: Domain and Process* (4th ed.; *OTPF–4;* AOTA, 2020c) in the occupations of health management (i.e., social and emotional health and maintenance) and IADLs (i.e., care of others, care of pets or animals, child rearing, communication management). A deeper understanding of the subjective experience of engagement in occupations will undoubtedly add to the foundation of occupational science and inform client-centered occupational therapy practice.

Doing, Being, Belonging, and Becoming

Building on Wilcock's (1998) well-known conceptualization of occupation, ***doing, being, and becoming,*** Hammell (2004) called on the profession to recognize four dimensions of meaning in occupation: doing, being, ***belonging,*** and becoming. *Doing* provides a purpose, occupies time, and leads to feelings of competence and positive self-worth. *Being* refers to being introspective or meditative, (re)discovering the self, and experiencing the moment and environment. *Belonging* highlights the social connections and sense of being included in groups and communities. Finally, *becoming* is the process of reimagining future selves positively, as a capable being who can enjoy life and find meaning (Hammell, 2004). These four dimensions of meaning in occupation were identified in a qualitative study of the meaning of dance as an occupation from the perspective of undergraduate occupational therapy students in South Africa (Lingah & Paruk, 2021). In fact, Lingah and Paruk (2021) offered this formula for meaning: "Doing (an occupation) + Being (immersing oneself within the occupation, a state in which all else ceases to be) + Becoming (growth and self-actualization) + Belonging (the formation of connections with others and the wider world) = Meaning" (p. 97).

Hammell (2014) urged occupational therapy practitioners to focus on occupations concerned with belonging, connecting, and contributing to others because of their associations with well-being. For example, a qualitative study of Israeli mothers revealed that giving (investing values related to the roles) and receiving (needs being fulfilled) were important to well-being and connecting with others (Avrech Bar et al., 2016). Some occupations associated with being a mother were meaningful but disliked; still, mothers did them because of their values (e.g., the occupations are important). Mothers also indicated that their needs were met by performing mothering and nonmothering occupations—that is, when receiving. The give-and-take aspect of the occupation of mothering highlights how values and needs shape the meaning of an occupation (Avrech Bar et al., 2016). This trio of innate needs—belonging, connecting, and contributing to others—suggests that the social aspect of meaningful occupational engagement is salient across cultures and time.

Neurophysiology of Meaningful Activities

Despite the complexity of determining what is meaningful to people, occupational therapy practitioners need to understand the neurophysiology of doing meaningful activities. Different types of meanings include biological, social, psychological, personal, and social (G. Fidler, personal communication, April 12, 1997), and it is important to identify what is meaningful to the individual. Understanding these different meanings can enable occupational therapy practitioners' ability to choose the most appropriate theoretical approaches, create tailored interventions, measure outcomes, and disseminate findings.

Meaning and the *OTPF–4*

The *OTPF–4* identifies client factors and personal factors that may influence the meaning of activities and occupations to a client (AOTA, 2020c). Listed under ***client factors*** are people's values, beliefs, and spirituality, which can shape how they perceive and perform occupations. Many of the personal factors included may, in context, influence how people construct meaning through activities and occupations. Some of these ***personal factors*** include cultural identification and cultural attitudes; upbringing and life experiences; race and ethnicity; social background, social status, and socioeconomic status; lifestyle; health conditions and fitness; and individual psychological assets (e.g., temperament, coping styles; AOTA, 2020c).

Each of these factors can be likened to a lens through which people view and interpret the world around them. Just as no two people are alike, no two people have the same number and colors of lenses through which to see life events and contexts; rather, each has an individualized kaleidoscope.

The evaluation process focuses on obtaining a variety of information, such as the client's history, wants and needs, abilities, supports, and barriers (AOTA, 2020c). As part of the evaluation process, the occupational profile provides valuable information about a client's occupational history and experiences, patterns of daily living, interests, values, goals, and relevant contexts. Practitioners can use AOTA's free Occupational Profile Template (AOTA, 2020a) to gain a better understanding of the client's background and current needs (AOTA, 2020b). The occupational therapy profile helps practitioners determine what is most important and meaningful to the client, which is an essential step in planning meaningful occupational therapy interventions.

In the process of obtaining information, occupational therapy practitioners can establish therapeutic rapport with clients and their caregivers or significant people in their lives. Using a client-centered approach, practitioners should always ask clients or their family members about the occupations and roles that are most important to the client. "Only clients can identify the occupations that give meaning to their lives and select the goals and priorities that are important to them" (AOTA, 2020c, p. 22). Upon completing the occupational profile and formal and informal interviews, practitioners can continue with personalizing the evaluation and the intervention planning and implementation stages. If the occupational profile can be incorporated into the client's electronic medical record, it can help the interprofessional team to understand the client as a person, not merely a patient, and help to facilitate client-centered practice. The AOTA Occupational Profile Template is available to download at https://bit.ly/3dE65SH.

Review of Research on Meaning in Occupation

Recent research on meaning in occupation has highlighted the complexity of meaning and reinforced occupational therapy's tenet that engaging in meaningful occupations is inextricably associated with health and well-being. Two qualitative research syntheses, one from Roberts and Bannigan (2018) in the United Kingdom and the other from Eakman et al. (2018) in the United States, offer slightly different organizations of themes relating to personal meaning.

Roberts and Bannigan (2018) searched multiple electronic databases in 2016 and identified 20 studies that met the inclusion criteria for their metasynthesis. Using a process of meta-aggregation, they identified four predominant themes of meaning: (1) Occupations provide a sense of fulfillment; (2) occupations provide a sense of restoration; (3) occupations shape personal and sociocultural identity; and (4) occupations provide social, cultural, and intergenerational family connection. They also identified subthemes for each of the main themes. For example, "Occupations provide a sense of restoration" included the following subthemes: "structuring the day" and "sense of health and wellness and negative feelings." The latter refers to occasions when engaging in occupations confers a sense of wellness, such as keeping the mind engaged and active (Scheerer et al., 2004), or negative feelings, such as sadness or frustration.

Eakman et al.'s (2018) qualitative research synthesis differed from Roberts and Bannigan's (2018) metasynthesis in its methods and approach. Most notably, Eakman et al.'s review was narrower than Roberts and Bannigan's because Eakman et al. limited their search to qualitative studies published between 1993 and 2010 in the *Journal of Occupational Science.* Also, their review of 11 qualitative studies focused only on positive subjective experiences in occupation (forms of meaning), whereas Roberts and Bannigan considered negative and positive meanings associated with engagement in occupations. Eakman et al. used content analysis to guide their interpretation of their framework's synthesis data, producing an occupational meaning system. They identified three higher order themes—social, selfhood, and pleasure meanings—which were associated with 12 underlying forms of meaning: belonging and helping (social); autonomy, mastery, continuity, self-esteem, health and well-being, purposes, and identity (selfhood); and enjoyment, stimulation, and satisfaction (pleasure; see Table 17.1).

Although both reviews focused on the occupational science literature and found similar themes, they differed slightly in methodology and interpretation. Many of Eakman et al.'s (2018) themes and subthemes overlap in concept with those of Roberts and Bannigan (2018). Social and cultural connections emerge as salient themes in both reviews, highlighting belonging, helping, and connecting to families and communities. Another important dimension of occupational meaning is pleasure or, more specifically, enjoyment, satisfaction, and stimulating (Eakman et al., 2018). Roberts and Bannigan also included enjoyment, pleasure, and emotional and sensory feelings but added relaxation, being in the moment, sense of health and wellness, and structuring the day. Thus, Roberts and Bannigan called their theme "Occupations provide a sense of restoration." Both reviews acknowledged mastery and purpose, but Roberts and Bannigan identified this as fulfillment, whereas Eakman et al. included these forms of meaning under the higher order theme of selfhood. Another difference between the two reviews is that Roberts and Bannigan's fourth overarching theme was occupation's influence on personal and sociocultural identity, whereas Eakman et al. included identity as one of the forms of meaning under selfhood. Finally, Roberts and Bannigan included negative feelings associated with engagement in occupation, whereas although Eakman et al. acknowledged that negative emotions occur within occupational engagement, their review focused only on positive subjective experiences.

A related scoping review by Black et al. (2019) on occupational engagement reinforced the key concepts of meaning outlined in Eakman et al. (2018) and Roberts and Bannigan (2018). This scoping review analyzed 26 journal articles (12 qualitative, 11 quantitative, and 3 scoping reviews) published from 1993 to 2017, 15 of which referred to meaning, value, or personal significance when discussing occupational engagement. Aspects of meaning included the actual doing of meaningful things, deriving meaning from occupational engagement, and using occupational engagement to construct a meaningful life (Black et al., 2019).

To summarize, two independent reviews of qualitative research, one from the United Kingdom and one from the United States, offer similar interpretations of meaning associated with occupation (Eakman et al., 2018; Roberts & Bannigan, 2018). Common themes associated with meaningful occupation are enjoyment, purpose, satisfaction, identity, and social and cultural connections. A scoping review by Black et al. (2019) corroborated the findings of these two qualitative research reviews, noting that value and personal significance are frequently associated with meaningful occupational engagement (see Case Example 17.1).

TABLE 17.1. THEMES AND SUBTHEMES IDENTIFIED IN TWO REVIEWS OF QUALITATIVE RESEARCH ON MEANING FROM OCCUPATIONAL ENGAGEMENT

ROBERTS & BANNIGAN (2018)	EAKMAN ET AL. (2018)
Occupations provide a sense of fulfillment • Learning and personal development • Achieving mastery and establishing future goals • Pride and satisfaction • Making a contribution to community and others	Selfhood • Autonomy • Mastery • Continuity • Self-esteem • Health and well-being • Purposes • Identity
Occupations provide a sense of restoration • Enjoyment, pleasure, and happiness • Emotional, spiritual, and sensory feelings • Relaxation and stress relief • Being in the moment • Sense of health and wellness and negative feelings • Structuring the day	Pleasure • Enjoyment • Stimulating • Satisfaction
Occupations shape personal and sociocultural identity • Personal identity • Sociocultural identity	
Occupations provide social, cultural, and intergenerational family connection • Social/community support • Connection to one's culture • Intergenerational family connection	Social • Belonging • Helping

CASE EXAMPLE 17.1. Katie: Coping With Illness

Shortly after **Katie** celebrated her 40th birthday, she was diagnosed with breast cancer (invasive ductal carcinoma, Stage 2B). Staging of cancer is based on the size and location of the primary tumor, whether cancer cells have spread to lymph nodes or other parts of the body, tumor grade, and whether certain biomarkers are detected. Katie had a positron emission tomography (PET) scan to determine whether the cancer cells had spread, and indeed they had, to her spine and liver. In an instant, her diagnosis changed to Stage 4 metastatic breast cancer.

Her routine now had to accommodate chemotherapy infusions on a regular basis as well as PET scans every 4 to 6 months to monitor abnormal cell activity and the effectiveness of treatment. Side effects of chemotherapy include extreme fatigue, joint pain, gastrointestinal issues, and peripheral neuropathy. Katie struggled with mental stamina and word recall, and she matter-of-factly stated, "Chemo brain is real."

In the beginning, Katie's side effects were manageable, and she continued working as a pediatric occupational therapist. Over time, however, the side effects became more intrusive, affecting her short-term memory and word recall.

Katie had no control over getting a cancer diagnosis, but she did have control over her response and attitude. Spiritually, she focused on faith, not fear. By visualizing that she was sleeping in God's hands surrounded in white light, she was able to sleep soundly. "Fear does not get you anywhere. It just sucks up the space in your heart where faith lives," Katie recounted.

Coping with anxiety, worry, and sadness is also part of Katie's new normal, especially because she has two children. Katie said, "You have to let the feelings come. Honor them. Accept how you are feeling, and then let it go. Experience it all, the good and the bad. There is no right or wrong. When you feel it all, still try to choose joy."

Katie lives by that mantra, "Choose joy," and finds solace in preparing for the future. She has created scrapbooks, greeting cards for special occasions, and personal letters for her children. Katie is grateful for this time to prepare, saying "Preparedness is peaceful. It makes me feel less anxious about the future."

(Continued)

CASE EXAMPLE 17.1. Katie: Coping With Illness (*Cont.*)

Participating in Crowns of Courage in 2017 enabled Katie to share her story through art. Amanda Gilbert, a henna tattoo artist, started the program to help women with cancer feel empowered and beautiful. Although it was difficult to publicly share her story, Katie also felt stress relief and viewed the experience as cathartic. Katie's henna tattoo featured a large sunflower with the phrase "You are my sunshine" in the center. Katie relates to cheerful sunflowers because "even though I am going through dark times, I can stand tall." She added, "Sunflowers have deep roots. They are grounded, and turn to follow the sun."

After participating in Crowns of Courage, Katie started writing a blog and then began watercolor painting. Writing was a cathartic experience for her, allowing her to express her feelings about living with cancer, but painting offered something different. "When I am painting, I do not think about cancer. I can just create and find joy in that space." Katie experienced *flow,* described by Csikszentmihalyi (1990) as the experience of being so immersed in an activity that you lose track of time. Katie now paints for her family and friends, favoring night skies. She also painted bookmarks to give as Christmas gifts, calling them "small pictures of joy." An encouraging personal message on the back of each painting allows Katie to communicate across space and time. Katie said, "For me, it's therapeutic."

Over time, Katie became a patient advocate, helping other patients who might not have the knowledge, expertise, and energy to advocate for themselves. Her perspective as an occupational therapist has helped her make informed decisions and communicate with doctors and researchers. To advocate for the broader community of people with breast cancer, she has served on patient advocacy committees and testified at a Senate Health Policy Committee hearing in support of a bill introduced in the Michigan legislature.

What makes life worth living for Katie? Helping others in need and leaving a legacy makes life meaningful. Living with intention, she chooses joy and life experiences that create joy. Engagement in meaningful occupations, such as watercolor paintings and patient advocacy, helps Katie cope and find new purpose in life. Painting provides moments of flow in which Katie does not have to think about cancer; she experiences pleasure and satisfaction in the process and product. Everything she paints has meaning and brings joy to her life.

Case adapted from "Creating a New Normal Through Engagement in Meaningful Occupation," by J. K. Fortuna, 2021, *Open Journal of Occupational Therapy, 9*(1), 1–6 (https://doi.org/10.15453/2168-6408.1828).

EXERCISE 17.1. Reflecting on Katie's Story

Read Case Example 17.1 and answer the following questions:

1. Using either Roberts and Bannigan's (2018) or Eakman et al.'s (2018) themes and subthemes (see Table 17.1), which themes resonate in Katie's story? Explain the connections.
2. To Katie, is painting a therapeutic occupation-as-means, occupation-as-end (Trombly, 1995), or both? Justify your answer with information from the case.
3. Hammell (2014, p. 46) asserted, "If occupational therapy is to address meaningful occupations, attention should be paid to occupations concerned with belonging, connecting, and contributing to others." Do you agree with Hammell's statement? Do any of Katie's meaningful occupations address these three needs: belonging, connecting, and contributing to others? If yes, which ones and in what ways?

Reflection:

Think of an activity and time in your life when you have experienced flow.

1. What was the context of the activity?
2. Describe the meaning of the activity.
3. Did you experience feelings similar to or different from Katie's experience of flow?

Measuring Meaningfulness

Over the past decade, instruments have been developed to measure aspects of meaningfulness and participation in meaningful activities that may help occupational therapy practitioners design therapeutic occupations. Although the list of instruments described in this section is by no means exhaustive, it is intended to give the reader an idea of the tools available to assess the meaningfulness of occupations.

Engagement in Meaningful Activities Survey

The Engagement in Meaningful Activities Survey (EMAS), developed by Goldberg et al. (2002), consists of 12 items that measure the extent of engagement in meaningful activities. Respondents rate items on a 5-point Likert scale ranging from 1 (*never*) to 5 (*always*). To capture a person's activity involvement, the EMAS includes an interview schedule with open-ended questions that ask about the person's top three activities associated with positive feelings about themselves. With respect to psychometrics, the EMAS demonstrates good face validity (Goldberg et al., 2002), moderate test–retest reliability ($r = .56$), and good internal consistency ($\alpha = .89$; Eakman et al., 2010a).

An increasing amount of research using the EMAS has demonstrated its positive relationship to measures of life satisfaction and health-related quality of life (Eakman, 2012). Goldberg et al. (2002) reported a relationship between the extent of engagement in meaningful activities and quality of life, as measured with the Quality of Life Interview, among a sample of adults with mental illness. Using Rasch analysis, Eakman (2012) found that eliminating the "never" response option improved the category functioning of the EMAS in an age-diverse sample. In conclusion, the EMAS is a valid, unidimensional measure of meaningful activity participation.

Meaningful Activity Participation Assessment

The Meaningful Activity Participation Assessment (MAPA) is a self-report instrument designed to measure older adults' frequency of participation in and the meaningfulness of 28 activities (Eakman et al., 2010b). It measures subjective and objective aspects of activity engagement. The activities in the MAPA include IADLs such as driving, home making and maintenance, and social activities (e.g., helping others). Respondents rate each activity's meaningfulness on a 5-point Likert scale ranging from 0 (*not at all meaningful*) to 4 (*extremely meaningful*) and their frequency of participation on a 7-point scale ranging from 0 (*not at all*) to 6 (*every day*). On the basis of data from a sample of 154 older adults, the MAPA has demonstrated adequate construct validity, internal consistency, and test–retest reliability (Eakman et al., 2010b). Greater participation in meaningful activities, as indicated by higher scores on the MAPA, is associated with better psychological well-being and health-related quality of life (Eakman et al., 2010b).

Meaningful Activities Checklist

Another self-report measure, the Meaningful Activities Checklist, measures the meaningfulness of daily activities (Hooker et al., 2020). The checklist includes 46 items, such as sleeping, cleaning, taking care of others, spending time in nature, and talking or texting on a device. Of these 46 activities, 28 are also included in the MAPA (Eakman et al., 2010b). Respondents rate their meaningfulness on a 5-point scale ranging from 0 (*not at all meaningful*) to 4 (*extremely meaningful*).

Occupational Value Assessment with Predefined Items

The Occupational Value Assessment with predefined items (OVal–pd) is a 26-item Likert-like questionnaire designed to provide a global assessment of occupational experience and well-being (Eakman & Eklund, 2011). Raters report how they have experienced different forms of activity value in their daily life over the past month. The items cover three forms of activity value: concrete, symbolic, and self-reward. Response options range from 4 (*very often*) to 1 (*very seldom;* Eklund et al., 2017). On the basis of the responses of 277 randomly selected graduate and undergraduate students in the northwestern United States, test–retest and internal consistency reliability coefficients were found to be very good for the improved 22-item American English version of the OVal–pd. In addition, the structural validity of this version was partly confirmed through exploratory factor analysis (Eakman & Eklund, 2011).

Meaningful and Psychologically Rewarding Occupations Rating Scale

The Meaningful and Psychologically Rewarding Occupations Rating Scale (MPRORS) was developed to identify meaningful and psychologically rewarding occupations for therapeutic purposes (Ikiugu et al., 2019). Internal consistency reliability was higher for the Psychologically Rewarding scale (Cronbach's $\alpha = .73$) than for the Meaningfulness scale (Cronbach's $\alpha = .65$). Designed to complement the occupational profile, the MPRORS helps to identify occupations that are meaningful and mentally stimulating to clients, as well as psychologically rewarding and fun. Ikiugu et al. (2019) posited that when meaningful and enjoyable interventions are delivered to or incorporated into a client's lifestyle, the client will demonstrate improved health and well-being.

Daily Experiences of Pleasure, Productivity, and Restoration Profile

The Daily Experiences of Pleasure, Productivity, and Restoration Profile (PPR Profile) is a time-use diary designed to measure the subjective experience of engaging in daily occupations (Atler et al., 2016). It provides occupation-specific information about pleasure (enjoyment), productivity (accomplishment), and restoration (energy renewal). By recounting occupational experiences and contextual variables (e.g., social, geographical, and temporal) within a 24-hour time period, the PPR Profile provides knowledge about the meaning of specific occupations to the client. Evidence of its convergent validity was provided by Atler et al. (2016). Clinical use of the PPR Profile increases clients' awareness of their occupations and experiences, but its use with stressed or vulnerable populations, such as caregivers, may need careful consideration (Atler et al., 2017).

Aid for Decision-making in Occupation Choice for Hand

As mobile health technologies are developed, more apps to assess clients' interests and meaningful occupations may become available. For example, the Aid for Decision-making in Occupation Choice for Hand (ADOC–H) is an iPad (Apple Corp., Redmond, WA) application developed in collaboration with ADOC in Japan to promote shared decision making in hand therapy (Tomori et al., 2012). Clients choose from illustrations depicting daily activities that represent activities and participation, such as IADLs and leisure, included in the World Health Organization's (2001) *International Classification of Functioning, Disability and Health*. Feedback from 100 clients and 37 occupational therapists in Japan was positive. After clients identify and prioritize their most important occupations, they rate their satisfaction with engaging in those occupations on a scale ranging from 1 to 5. An interesting feature is the app's documentation feature; occupational therapy practitioners can store and print the client's profile, prioritized occupations, and intervention plans as PDF files. Preliminary results indicate that the ADOC–H is useful and acceptable to both hand therapy clients and occupational therapists in shared decision making for occupation-based goal setting (Ohno et al., 2020). The ADOC–H is available for purchase in Apple's App Store.

Possibilities for Activity Scale

The Possibilities for Activity Scale (PActS) is a slightly different instrument because it focuses on older adults' beliefs about occupational possibilities (Pergolotti & Cutchin, 2015). In the activity expectations section, questions relate to older adults' beliefs with respect to what they should be doing (e.g., physical exercise, creative activities). In the activity self-efficacy section of the instrument, questions focus on older adults' feelings concerning self-efficacy and their confidence level in doing certain activities (e.g., physical exercise, getting around town). Response options range from 1 (*very little*) to 5 (*quite a lot*). Higher scores therefore indicate greater perceived possibilities for participation in select activities. With regard to psychometrics, the PActS has shown evidence of internal consistency reliability (stratified coefficient $\alpha = .77$), construct-related validity, convergent validity, and known-groups validity (Pergolotti & Cutchin, 2015). In a study of 71 older adults with cancer, the PActS was the strongest predictor of meaningful activity participation (Pergolotti et al., 2015). These findings highlight the importance of measuring what older adults feel they should and could do and their expectations of and self-efficacy associated with engagement in meaningful activities.

Meaning Awareness Scale

The Meaning Awareness Scale (MAS) is a 6-item scale designed to measure *meaning salience,* the daily awareness of what makes life meaningful, because empirically supported measures of meaning salience are lacking (Vagnini, 2020). Two categories of items were developed to capture how individual meanings of life can be experienced during daily life activities. To determine the frequency with which a person experiences and senses meaningfulness throughout the day, the first category includes items such as "My day-to-day tasks felt meaningful" (Vagnini, 2020, p. 63). To assess cognitive awareness of personal meaning in life throughout the day, the second category features items such as "I was aware of when my activities aligned with my meaning in life" and "Meaning influenced the decisions I made." Respondents rate the items on a 7-point Likert-type scale ranging from 1 (*very rarely*) to 7 (*very often*) on the basis of their experiences in the past day or moment. The MAS has evidence of adequate preliminary internal consistency reliability and criterion-related validity (Vagnini, 2020).

Research on Occupation and Health

With the flourishing of occupational science, a renewed focus on the relationship between engagement in meaningful occupations and health and well-being has emerged (Reed et al., 2013). AOTA's (2020b) fact sheet on occupational therapy's role in health promotion states that practitioners enable "clients to maximize their capacity to participate in life activities that are important and meaningful to them, to promote overall health and wellness" (p. 1). Meaningful occupation is often linked to doing well, well-being, and becoming what people are best suited to become (Wilcock, 1998). In this section, I describe some selected studies to answer the following questions:

- Does recent evidence support the tenet that participation in meaningful occupations leads to improved health and well-being?
- Does research offer insights into understanding meaning across the lifespan?
- Does engagement in certain activities promote brain health?

Relationship of Participation in Meaningful Occupations to Health and Well-Being

Research has reinforced the long-held assumption that participation in meaningful occupations is associated with health and well-being. A meta-analysis of eight studies by Ikiugu et al. (2019) found that engagement in meaningful and psychologically rewarding occupations had a small to medium effect in promoting perceived health and well-being. Although the findings should be interpreted with caution because of the small sample and evidence of publication bias, Ikiugu et al. (2019) found that meaningful occupations involving community and social participation were effective in promoting well-being.

Evidence from psychology also supports the belief that engagement in personally meaningful activities is associated with better health and well-being. Research has suggested that meaning in life is associated with reduced stress, more adaptive coping, and greater engagement in health-promoting behaviors (Hooker et al., 2018). To examine the relationships among daily engagement in meaningful activity, mood, vitality, life satisfaction, meaning in life, purpose in life, and ***meaning salience*** (i.e., awareness of personal meaning in life throughout the day), Hooker et al. (2020) randomized 160 adults to either a control group or a self-monitoring group that completed daily surveys of positive mood, physical activity, and meaning salience for 4 weeks via the Meaning in Life Questionnaire. On 8 random days during those 4 weeks, all participants reported their activities in the past 24 hours. Meaning salience was measured with the 10-item Thoughts of Meaning Scale; participants responded on a 7-point Likert scale ranging from 1 (*none*) to 7 (*absolutely or quite a bit*) to questions such as "How much have you thought about your purpose in life today?" The Meaningful Activities Checklist was used to measure the level of meaningfulness of 46 daily activities, including the 28 MAPA items (Eakman et al., 2010b). Hooker et al. conducted multiple linear regression models with demographics and participation in meaningful activities predicting vitality, life satisfaction, presence of meaning, purpose, and depressive symptoms at 4 weeks.

What did Hooker et al. learn? First, participants who engaged in more meaningful activities on average reported greater *meaning salience,* the awareness of personal meaning in life at any given moment. Moreover, when demographic variables were controlled, greater engagement in meaningful activities was positively correlated with greater purpose in life, life satisfaction, and vitality at follow-up. Because participants who reported greater vitality, life satisfaction, purpose in life, and fewer depressive symptoms at the start of the study went on to engage in more meaningful activities, and those who engaged in more meaningful activities during the study later reported more vitality, life satisfaction, and purpose in life at follow-up, these findings collectively underscore the importance of meaning to health and well-being. Hooker et al. (2020) posited that those who report greater well-being may engage in more meaningful activities, may experience more meaning from routine daily activities, or both.

In addition, participation in meaningful activities was not related to negative mood or depressive symptoms at 4 weeks (Hooker et al., 2020). As one might expect, depressive symptoms at baseline were correlated with engagement in less meaningful activities, which is in keeping with observations that depressed people often withdraw from activities, even ones that hold meaning or importance. When participants engaged in more meaningful activities than usual, they reported a more positive mood and greater meaning salience (the extent to which they were aware of what makes their lives meaningful at that moment). However, participation in meaningful activities was not associated with ***meaning in life*** (i.e., the extent to which participants interpreted their lives as meaningful); the construct measured by the Meaning in Life Questionnaire may be too disconnected from engagement in daily activities because it asks respondents to reflect on the meaning of their life, a long-term view. One of the strengths of Hooker et al.'s (2020) study was its longitudinal design with a 4-week follow-up survey. Although the study could not establish causality, it established temporal precedence and provides evidence for the relationship between participation in meaningful activities and well-being.

Insights Into Understanding Meaning Throughout the Lifespan

Childhood

Although determining children's meaningful activities is sometimes challenging, depending on their age and abilities, researchers can use creative methods to identify meaningful activities. One study (Coussens et al., 2020) used photographs taken by 16 children with developmental disabilities to capture their meaningful activities. After analyzing the data from 47 interviews by means of inductive thematic analysis, the researchers found four themes: playing together, learning, family gatherings, and barriers to and facilitators of participation. Younger children were surprisingly quite satisfied with their participation, which may reflect the facilitating support of their mothers and teachers. Participation is therefore optimized when the confluence of constructs such as activity, body functions, and environmental factors enables it.

What do practitioners do if they cannot determine what is meaningful to a client? With a nonverbal client, practitioners can ask their family and caregivers. Sometimes, however,

CASE EXAMPLE 17.2. Tyrone: 18-Month-Old Boy With Burn Injury

As an occupational therapist at Children's National Medical Center, I was used to seeing children with a variety of conditions. All the occupational therapists at the center were generalists in the sense that we all covered the intensive care, burn, oncology, orthopedics, cardiac, and neurology units, as well as outpatients. Some of us with training or experience also covered the neonatal intensive care unit, a specialized practice. Our daily schedule was a mix of inpatients and outpatients and was subject to change if an inpatient was unavailable because of a procedure or an outpatient did not show up or canceled at the last minute.

Because of a scheduling conflict, a colleague asked me to cover one of her outpatients, an 18-month-old toddler named **Tyrone**, and I agreed. Tyrone had second- and third-degree burns on his right palm and had been an inpatient on the burn unit. My colleague reported that she had been working on increasing functional use of Tyrone's right hand (fine motor skills) and bimanual activities. I added a few toddler-appropriate toys to my large canvas tote and headed to the colorful L-shaped waiting area, which included a play structure. Lined along the wall were chairs where parents or caregivers would sit and watch their children play in the play structure or wait for their child to return from the occupational and physical therapy treatment rooms. The play structure was brilliantly designed; it included a few carpeted low walls of varying heights that surrounded spaces filled with large, colorful foam blocks of various sizes. Some children would stack the blocks into towers, and others would jump onto them from one of the low walls.

(Continued)

CASE EXAMPLE 17.2. Tyrone: 18-Month-Old Boy With Burn Injury (*Cont.*)

As I walked toward the waiting area, I spotted Tyrone, who had climbed onto one of the low walls. He jumped off purposefully, eyeing his destination, the pit filled with foam blocks. Tyrone's protective extension reflex was elicited as he fell in prone position, but to my surprise, before landing, he withdrew his right hand, flexing his right elbow. I marveled at how his instincts to protect his right palmar burn overrode his protective reflex.

Normally, I would escort a client to the outpatient clinic, which was large and open, with a suspended swing, cabinets of toys, and a child-sized table with chairs, but Tyrone shook his head and refused my extended hand. I chalked up his reluctance to the fact that he was used to his primary therapist and I was new to him. Tyrone's caregiver had waved and departed when she saw me starting to work with him. The waiting area was not crowded, so I tried to engage him in play; after all, treatment can be delivered almost anywhere. I started with a small toy truck and then a small inflatable ball, but neither drew his interest. I then tried some switch toys—surely, a dancing, music-playing switch toy would interest him. But that and my go-to squeezable bubble-bear toy also failed to capture his attention. As my toy options rapidly dwindled, I had the sinking feeling that there would be no progress to report in his progress note. I pictured myself reluctantly recounting this unproductive session to my colleague and questioned my abilities as a therapist.

At least I could say that I tried everything, I told myself, as I reached for one of the last toys in my bag, a fabric tiger cub puppet. It did not have the high-tech allure of the switch toys or the magical aspects of translucent floating bubbles that dared clients to pop them, so my hopes that it would interest Tyrone were not high. I slipped my hand into the puppet and made it come to life in front of Tyrone, waving one of its paws in a silent but friendly greeting. What happened next was nothing short of miraculous.

Tyrone's expression immediately softened, and his eyes widened with interest. His invisible shield of resistance was deactivated by a soft, furry, black-striped, marigold-yellow tiger cub with rounded ears and innocent black eyes. I was momentarily stunned but quickly reacted, not wanting to lose his attention. "If he likes this puppet," I thought, "wait until he sees this." I shifted my fingers to squeeze a small rubber bulb behind the puppet's inner mouth, and the tiger cub squeaked as a 3-inch thin strip of red plastic tongue unfurled. As expected, Tyrone reacted positively, opening his mouth in amazement and a smile of wonder. I told Tyrone, "Uh-oh. Tiger says he's hungry. Do you want to feed him?"

Tyrone nodded eagerly, and I reached for a small tin where I kept a stash of Cheerios™ just for fine motor activities. I grabbed one and held it over his right hand. "Can you hold the food with this hand?" To my surprise, he supinated and opened his burned hand, an instant receptacle for tiger food. Without prompting, Tyrone used his nonburned left hand to pluck the Cheerio from his right hand and deposit it into the tiger's mouth. The tiger chewed it with exaggerated head and mouth movements, akin to Cookie Monster's voracious chewing of cookies. There was a method to my masticating madness: I had mastered the art of making the Cheerio drop from the puppet's mouth during his overenthusiastic chewing, depositing it discreetly onto my lap or the floor, to ensure that it looked like the tiger had eaten it. Seeing the tiger's messy chewing made Tyrone chuckle and he looked toward my tin for another Cheerio. Although I was pleased that Tyrone was willing to hold the cereal with his burned hand, I wanted him to use the hand functionally. I took a chance; the tiger touched Tyrone's right hand and then looked at Tyrone with an open mouth. "He's still hungry," I explained to Tyrone. "Can you feed him with this hand?" I pointed to his right hand and held a Cheerio right over it. While Tyrone thought about my request, I positioned the tiger's open mouth to be just under his right hand; gravity-assisted feeding to a puppet counts as an activity of daily living. Tyrone opened his burned hand to accept the Cheerio from my hand. I do not know whether Tyrone mentally calculated that he could perform this activity without pain or difficulty or if he just responded to the tiger's empty mouth, the occupational form awaiting his volitional choice, but he flexed his fingers around the piece of cereal, pronated his right forearm, and after a momentary pause extended his fingers to release it right into tiger's not-so-ferocious mouth. Of course, Tiger and I celebrated this accomplishment. Tiger clapped his front paws together silently and then squeaked and unfurled his tongue again. I decided not to compliment Tyrone

(Continued)

CASE EXAMPLE 17.2. Tyrone: 18-Month-Old Boy With Burn Injury (*Cont.*)

on his movement (my goal). Instead, I said, "Tiger said that one was very yummy! Can you feed him another one, with this hand again?" Tyrone seemed pleased with the tiger's reaction and nodded. I reached for the container of Cheerios again and sighed with relief.

Later, when writing the progress note, I wondered why Tyrone did not like any of the toys I had thought would interest him. Had he seen them before and tired of them? Although it was a possibility, I doubted that explanation. Tyrone had been an inpatient and had suffered pain from his injury, whether it was during wound debridement or recovering from surgery. Maybe he did not trust the many health care professionals he encountered in this hospital, although we were all trying to help him recover.

Sometimes practitioners do not know what a client will find meaningful, but they can do their best to find out in advance and keep trying different activities. An interesting fact is that I had not purchased the puppet; it was given to me by my 8-year-old cousin when I had visited Taiwan a year earlier. I was taken with the puppet because I had never seen one that simultaneously emitted a noise and stuck out its tongue, and when I departed, my cousin bestowed it upon me as a parting gift. Who knew that a puppet that was meaningful to me would be meaningful to Tyrone, too?

It then occurred to me that maybe Tyrone's distrust in me had been temporarily displaced by his fascination with feeding the puppet. In other words, he did not trust me, but he could trust the puppet. Did the activity give him purpose or meaning or both? I am not sure, but I hope it did. There was something he could do to help the puppet not feel so hungry. The act of doing nourishes people's identities and souls. Part of what makes an occupation therapeutic is how it reminds clients of what they can do, even as they function to the best of their abilities, despite injury or illness.

EXERCISE 17.2. Tyrone's Story

Read Case Example 17.2 and answer the following questions:

1. Occupation as a means or ends of intervention should be understood from the person's perspective—how did the person perceive it and value it (Pierce, 2003)? What do you think were Tyrone's assumptions about or meanings associated with the tiger puppet?
2. In occupation-based practice, the therapist's viewpoint may often function silently in the background. In this case, the therapist consciously refrained from praising Tyrone for using his right (burned) hand successfully. What do you think might have happened if she had given feedback on his performance rather than feedback within the occupation of play, feeding the tiger puppet?
3. Have you ever been in a situation in which someone was not able to communicate their values, meaningful occupations, or preferences? How did you respond? What, if anything, would you do differently if faced with a similar situation?

caregivers are not readily available. Case Example 17.2 depicts such a situation and how the occupation of play can be used to engage a pediatric client and engender meaning.

Working years

The SARS-CoV-2 virus (COVID-19) pandemic has underscored the need to focus on health care professionals' health and well-being, including prevention of burnout. An Australian study explored the relationships among job satisfaction, burnout, professional identity, and meaningfulness of work activities for occupational therapy practitioners working in mental health (Scanlan & Hazelton, 2019). Scanlan and Hazelton (2019) found that higher levels of meaningfulness of work activities were associated with higher job satisfaction, lower burnout, and stronger sense of professional identity. Of the components of work activities' meaningfulness, value to self had the strongest correlation with each measure of work well-being. Therefore, to optimize the work well-being of occupational therapy practitioners in mental health, work allocations should be based on personal preferences (Scanlan & Hazelton, 2019).

Although some adults are able to engage in meaningful occupations, others experience a *meaning gap,* in which their occupational engagement is not aligned with what they enjoy or find meaningful. For example, 82 caregivers of orphaned children in India, Kenya, and Cambodia reported that they spent most of their time cooking and cleaning despite those being their least enjoyable activities (Liu et al., 2020). Most caregivers highly enjoyed providing educational activities such as teaching about religion or letters and numbers, but they spent the least amount of time on these educational activities, creating a meaningful activity gap. Knowing which occupations are most meaningful and enjoyable can help guide efforts to support workers.

Helping veterans transition to civilian life has been an area of focus for several occupational therapy researchers. A cross-sectional study of 389 veterans attending college examined whether meaningful activity, coping ability, and social support mediate the relationship between participation and veterans' psychological and subjective well-being (Kinney et al., 2020). For this study, *meaningful activity* was defined as engagement in activity that is congruent with one's values and interests, and it was measured with the EMAS (Eakman, 2012; Goldberg et al., 2002). Using multiple mediation models, Kinney et al. (2020) found that meaningful activity was the only mechanism that mediated the relationship between participation and both psychological and subjective well-being. The relationships were still evident when the researchers accounted for service-related health conditions (i.e., posttraumatic stress disorder, depression). These findings suggest that occupational therapy interventions designed for engagement in meaningful activities could promote veterans' well-being.

Older adults

Because the number of Americans age 65 and older is estimated to nearly double from 52 million in 2018 to 95 million by 2060, many studies and programs strive to keep older adults as healthy and happy for as long as possible (Mather et al., 2019). To understand how older adults live meaningful lives, Bonder (2018) proposed four main themes: instrumental meanings (occupations supporting daily life), evaluative meanings (subjective assessments of satisfaction with life, such as quality of life and well-being), existential meanings (whether life is worth living or whether one is living a life of meaning), and self-identity.

Although retirement is associated with fewer work-related activities and more leisure activities, whether leisure activities help older adults maintain purposefulness in retirement has not been determined with a large sample. Lewis and Hill (2020) analyzed data from 7,277 participants, representing three waves of the Health and Retirement Study (2008–2016), a biennial national longitudinal study of American adults older than age 50 and their spouses. Activity engagement was measured using an 18-item list of activities in four domains: cognitive, physical, social, and supportive (Jopp & Hertzog, 2010). Sense of purpose was assessed with the 7-item version of the Ryff Psychological Well-Being Scale, which includes items such as "I have a sense of direction and purpose in my life," on which higher scores indicate agreement. Multilevel modeling with robust maximum likelihood estimation was used to determine the association between participation in leisure activity and changes in sense of purpose over time. Is engagement in leisure activities associated with being purposeful in older adulthood? Research has suggested that the answer is yes; participants reported a higher sense of purpose when they performed more leisure activities, and more active participants' purposefulness was less likely to decline over time. Engaging more frequently in leisure activities appeared to have a greater influence on the purpose of retired adults than on that of adults who were still working (Lewis & Hill, 2020). Moreover, the effects of engaging in leisure activity remained significant after adjusting for age, sex, education, race, and number of chronic health conditions.

If people older than age 50 years retire or cut back on work hours, should they volunteer? To determine whether changes in volunteering were associated with 34 indicators of physical health, health behaviors, and psychological well-being, data from 12,998 participants in the Health and Retirement Study (a prospective, nationally representative cohort of U.S. adults) were analyzed using multiple logistic, linear, and generalized linear regression models (Kim et al., 2020). During the 4-year follow-up, people who had volunteered 100 or more hours per year showed a lower risk of mortality and limitations in physical functioning, higher physical activity, and better psychosocial outcomes (greater positive affect, optimism, and purpose in life; lower depressive symptoms, hopelessness, loneliness, and infrequent socialization) than people who did not. Thus, encouraging older adults to volunteer at least 2 hours per week would not only bestow health benefits, it would also benefit society (Kim et al., 2020).

Even though retirement may differ across cultures, meanings of some social activities remain salient, suggesting cross-cultural themes of older adults' social engagement. As an example, retired older men living in an urban area of Japan cited these five values of social activities: "feeling I am still useful," "feeling that something is my responsibility," "finding interest through interactions," "feeling of time well spent," and "health as a resource and reward for social activities" (Takashima et al., 2020, p. 17). Having a purpose in life means having a strong sense of meaning and an ability to identify future-oriented goals (Bartrés-Faz et al., 2018). Older adults want to still play a role in their communities, whether they are contributing to something larger or connecting with others; social activities reinforce their self-identity and provide personal fulfillment.

The benefits of meaningful activity for older adults in care homes include physical and mental health as well as quality of life. Residents with dementia in care homes who engaged in meaningful activities showed reduced levels of challenging behavior and improved mood and function (Wenborn, 2017). One study investigated why older adults in six nursing homes in England did not engage in meaningful activities (Smith et al., 2018). The researchers attributed the lack of participation in meaningful activities to two issues: insufficient staffing to offer and supervise activities; and the opinion that meaningful occupations, even leisure activities, are not part of everyday routines. Because additional staff training is often insufficient to improve residents' quality of life, other strategies, such as changing the culture in care homes, could address staff attitudes about older adults' lack of motivation or capability to engage in meaningful activities (Smith et al., 2018).

A study of Swedish older adults found statistically significant improvements in general health variables such as vitality and mental health after 4 months of community-based occupational therapy intervention, compared with a control group (Johansson & Björklund, 2016). The intervention group participated in group activities for 2 hours per week for 4 months and received a maximum of 4 hours of individual treatment, whereas the control group received only occasional occupational therapy. Each group selected the themes and topics (e.g., mobility, mental well-being, eating) as well as what they considered meaningful. The group intervention was therapeutic because it facilitated positive relationships, self-acceptance and personal growth, and communication and ideas about adapting (Johansson & Björklund, 2016).

The beneficial effects of engagement in meaningful occupations can be extended to community health care. For example, Lithuanian women with breast cancer who participated in a 6-week community-based occupational therapy program scored significantly higher on the EMAS than women in the control group (Petruseviciene et al., 2018). The therapeutic activities included replanting and donating saplings, making origami cranes, increasing hand amplitude (the extent, range, and quality of hand movements), preventing or reducing lymphedema, art therapy and music therapy, fatigue and energy conservation, knitting and donating socks for preterm newborns, and socializing (e.g., sharing positive experience and emotions; Petruseviciene et al., 2018). These activities exemplify Roberts and Bannigan's (2018) four dimensions of meaning (fulfillment; restoration; personal and sociocultural identity; and social, cultural, and intergenerational family connection). Greater engagement in meaningful activities was associated with better emotional functioning, a component of health-related quality of life, and less insomnia. The moderate to large effect sizes for global quality of life, fatigue, systemic side effects of therapy, and cognitive functions suggest that the effects of meaningful activities for women with breast cancer can be wide ranging and highly influential on health-related quality of life. Overall, participating in meaningful activities is associated with better health, well-being, and quality of life for older adults.

Engagement in Activity, Brain Health, and Cognitive Functions

MRI studies have advanced understanding of the relationships between activity engagement and brain functioning, especially in older adulthood. Research has shown that exercise and aerobic physical activity are beneficial to cognitive functioning and brain structure (Erickson et al., 2011). But do other activities confer benefits to brain structure and functioning?

Hashimoto et al. (2017) examined the relationship among physical activity, hippocampal atrophy, and memory in 213 community-dwelling elderly participants in Japan. They found that hippocampal atrophy was associated with leisure-time physical inactivity, age, and less education. Because the hippocampus is vital for learning, memory, spatial navigation, and other functions (Anand & Dhikav, 2012), this finding suggests that leisure activities involving physical activity could represent a modifiable risk factor to prevent cognitive decline. Moreover, low-intensity walking, which would not usually be characterized as exercise, was associated with larger hippocampal volume among older women. Given the important role the hippocampus plays in the process of storing and retrieving memory, Hashimoto et al. (2017) suggested that leisure-time physical activity could be used to thwart Alzheimer's disease.

If leisure-time physical activity can be health promoting, could other types of activities enhance cognitive functions in older adults? In the Synapse Project, Park et al. (2014) hypothesized that older adults who learned new skills in activities that required working memory, episodic memory, and reasoning over 3 months would demonstrate better cognitive function. Participants were randomly assigned to one of six lifestyle conditions, five of which required 15 hours of weekly participation. Activities were classified as *productive engagement* (requires active learning and sustained activation of working memory, long-term memory, and other executive functions or receptive engagement) or *receptive engagement* (requires passive observation, activation of existing knowledge, and familiar activities). Participants were assigned to the three productive engagement conditions: the digital photography and photo-editing software condition, the quilt designing and sewing condition, or the dual condition, half the time in digital photography and the other half in quilt making. The receptive engagement conditions consisted of a social engagement condition (facilitator-led field trips, watching movies) and a placebo condition (tasks at home, such as listening to music and completing word-meaning puzzles). The last condition was a no-treatment control condition, which did not require a 15-hour time commitment per week.

Park et al. (2014) analyzed the 221 participants' data and found that productive engagement (i.e., the digital photography, quilt making, and dual conditions) resulted in better episodic memory than the receptive engagement conditions, and these differences were statistically significant. Moreover, participants who learned digital photography, either alone or in combination with quilting, showed improved episodic memory, and this difference was also statistically significant, whereas the effect approached significance for those who learned quilting. In terms of activity analysis, quilting required more of a procedural component, consisting of repetitive tasks, after the initial skills were taught. In contrast, digital photography required a large amount of cognitive processing regarding cameras, computers, and editing software, and the occupation of taking digital photos is more complex; one has to consider multiple variables such as lighting and composition. Thus, the results may reflect the different cognitive demands of each activity. Surprisingly, the social engagement control group did not demonstrate cognitive benefits. These findings highlight the dynamic interplay between cognitive functions and productive engagement activities (Park et al., 2014). It is never too late to learn a new activity, and some cognitively challenging activities may be self-reinforcing, leading to a lifelong leisure activity and better brain health.

In a follow-up to Park et al.'s (2014) study, McDonough et al. (2015) examined the functional neuroimaging data from a subset of participants in the Synapse Project to assess whether productive engagement activities (digital photography, quilting, or dual conditions) can increase modulation of brain activity. Previous research found that older adults showed less modulation in the lateral frontal, parietal, and temporal regions, and these reductions were a function of age. In the functional MRI (*f*MRI) task, older adults were asked to judge whether words represented living or nonliving objects; the words varied from easy (concrete) to difficult (ambiguous). McDonough et al. (2015) classified the 39 participants into either the High-Challenge group (n=23), consisting of the photo, quilting, or dual groups, or the Low-Challenge group (n=16), consisting of the social and placebo groups. Of the 39 participants, 26 consented to *f*MRI scans 1 year later.

The high-challenge group showed significant increases in modulation in 11 regions, most notably in the frontal, temporal, and parietal lobes of the cerebral cortex (McDonough et al., 2015). The low-challenge group showed an increase in modulation only in the precentral gyrus. Further analyses suggested that the increased modulation observed in the high-challenge group was the result of the participants using fewer neural resources in the easy condition of the *f*MRI task. The researchers concluded that engaging in a novel, cognitively challenging task over a sustained period (i.e., 3 months) led to more fluent retrieval of semantic information.

If engaging in new cognitively challenging tasks is beneficial for brain health, is more engagement, in terms of time, better? Participants were allowed to spend more than the requisite 15 hours per week in the Synapse Project space, and their hours were collected. Greater modulation changes were associated with more hours of engagement in the high-challenge group but not in the low-challenge group (McDonough et al., 2015). Thus, participants who spent more time learning new skills (i.e., digital photography, quilting, or dual condition) were more likely to demonstrate increased modulation of brain activity. This dose–response effect between time spent in high-challenge engagement and increased brain modulation is intriguing because it raises the question, "Would a longer period of Synapse Project intervention result in more participants benefitting from the program?" This question, among others, deserves further research.

Does age matter when considering the potential influence of activities on modulation of brain activity? By correlating pretest-to-posttest changes in modulation of brain activity with age at pretest, researchers found that the older the participant at the start of the Synapse Project, the greater the brain changes (McDonough et al., 2015). The researchers hypothesized that the oldest participants had the most potential to improve, and correlations of pretest-to-posttest changes and age at pretest were significantly negative in the high-challenge group (in all but the midcingulate gyrus). Thus, learning a new activity is always beneficial; in fact, there is actually more potential for increased brain modulation.

How long do the effects of engagement in cognitively challenging activities last? After conducting a Group × Time analysis of variance on the five significant brain clusters (left midcingulate gyrus, right precuneus, left intraparietal sulcus, right inferior temporal gyrus, left middle temporal gyrus), McDonough et al. (2015) found that the effects of engagement were maintained for 1 year, primarily in the left midcingulate gyrus. Although a similar pattern was observed for the right precuneus, the interaction did not reach significance. Because many of the other brain regions showed a return to their pretest levels of brain modulation, this could signify that engagement must continue over longer periods to maintain effects.

Critics may assert that whether participants in the Synapse Project found their assigned high- and low-challenge activities meaningful is unknown. Granted, there are trade-offs when conducting randomized controlled trials; however, is there a way to balance client-centeredness with rigorous scientific methods? In an effort to ensure that the novel activity was of some interest to participants, Park et al. (2014) allowed participants to veto one of the three high-challenge conditions before their random assignment. Studies such as these need to include a large enough sample to ensure enough participants in each condition.

In summary, the findings from the Synapse Project demonstrate that engagement in novel, cognitively challenging activities for a sustained period of time increases neural efficiency, particularly in regions associated with attention and semantic processing. McDonough et al. (2015) posited that the underlying mechanism for the engagement effects is

> via a restoration of brain activity to more youth-like states, thus facilitating the efficiency of neural resources that is a direct consequence of participation in a demanding learning environment. (p. 880)

Imagine if additional research supported the hypothesis that engagement in novel cognitively challenging occupations can restore certain regions of the brain to a more youthlike state. Might occupational therapy play a role in designing and structuring such occupations for the general population or subsets of the population? Does the profession have a portfolio of health-promoting intervention programs for different populations? If occupational therapy practitioners assert their skills in activity analysis, person-centered treatment planning, and knowledge of mind–body–activity transactions during engagement in meaningful occupations, we could be partners in future research and health promotion program planning initiatives.

Situating Meaning in Group and Population Health

The Institute for Healthcare Improvement's Triple Aim framework to improve health care has influenced many health organizations because of its focus on three important aspects of health care: better outcomes, lower costs, and improved patient experiences (Obucina et al., 2018). A fourth aim, to improve the clinician experience, was cited as an urgent need even before the COVID-19 pandemic (Rathert et al., 2018). This emphasis on a broader view of improving the value and experience of health care has influenced occupational therapy as well.

The *OTPF–4* broadens the possibilities for occupational therapy's influence on group and population health. Occupational therapy practitioners possess the knowledge and skills to utilize "occupation-based health approaches to enhance occupational performance and participation, quality of life, and occupational justice for populations" (AOTA, 2020b, p. 3). In addition to including performance skills for groups and performance patterns for groups and populations, the *OTPF–4* describes the occupational therapy process for groups and populations.

Although some occupational therapy practitioners are accustomed to providing meaningful occupations at the population level, there is room for many more to aid in public health initiatives. Similar to working with a client, practitioners can determine what a group or population finds meaningful. For example, occupational therapy practitioners have helped COVID-19 vaccination sites be more inclusive and accessible to people with varying abilities and mobility challenges. From environmental considerations to accommodations, occupational therapy practitioners can safely and more expediently facilitate vaccination for people with disabilities or varying abilities. Another example is occupational therapy practitioners' work with groups of residents in skilled nursing facilities to create safe opportunities to socialize during the pandemic, especially when visits from family and friends were restricted.

As the profession broadens its scope to include population health, it behooves practitioners to consider the language used to communicate occupational therapy concepts. For example, terms such as *activity* and *doing* are readily understood by people outside of occupational therapy (White et al., 2020). Practitioners can also think creatively about translating occupational therapy's principles and concepts to their communities' needs, values, and preferences.

Meaningful Occupation and the Environment

As the more complex nature of the meaning of occupation has emerged in the past few decades, scholars have described how occupational performance is influenced by context, including sociocultural factors and competing demands (Reed et al., 2013). For example, the Person–Environment–Occupation Model (Law et al., 1996) and the Ecology of Human Performance framework (Dunn, 2007) have emphasized the transactional nature of occupation between a person and varied contexts.

Although it is known that the meanings associated with everyday activities depend on context, how these meanings are attributed and how they vary by different environments is less clear. A conceptual framework showing the interrelations among person, activity, and environment is presented in Figure 17.2, which shows three kinds of meanings, represented by the arrows (Meesters, 2009). Meaning from an activity that is performed in a specific environment, or feature, is called an ***affordance.*** One example of an affordance is sitting outside on a porch or deck, which affords pleasure. A second type of meaning is derived from the activity itself. For example, eating with friends means that a person can catch up and share things with others. The third type of meaning is attached to features of the environment. An example is having a garden, which offers a connection to nature and results in enjoyment. The relationship among people, their environment, and their activities is reciprocal; the meanings from either activities or features of the environment should not be viewed separately. These types of meanings are related and may overlap.

Meesters (2009) studied how everyday activities are related to residential environmental features and the meanings of those activities to people. Network analysis and logistic regression models were used to analyze survey data from

FIGURE 17.2. Conceptual framework: Interrelations among people, activity, and environments.

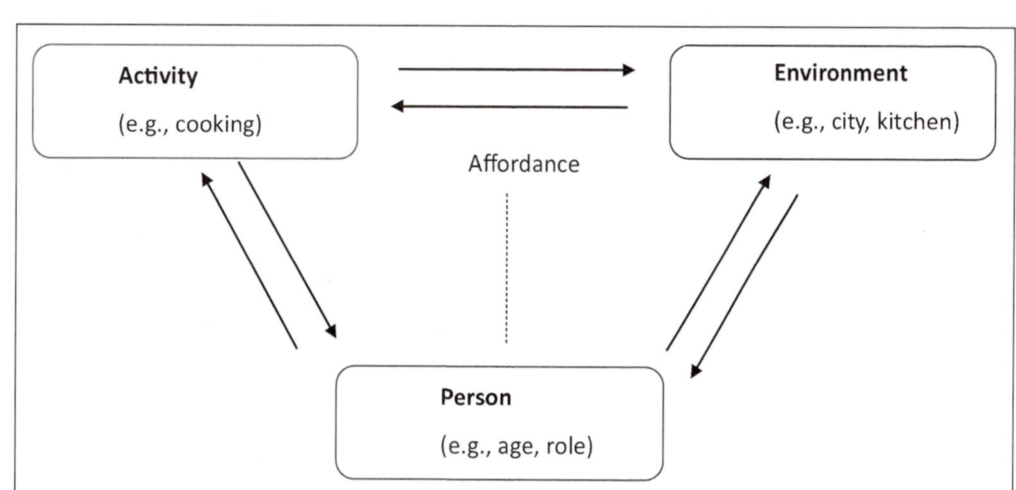

Source. Meesters (2009). Copyright 2009 by IOS Press. Adapted with permission.

1,495 residents of the Netherlands, classified by city, suburban, or rural residence. Meesters found that places within one's residence differ in meaning depending on the setting of the residence. For example, private outdoor space was associated with activities of gardening and being outside, and meanings ascribed to outdoor space included relaxation, keeping busy, pleasure, and nature. However, only people who lived in suburban and rural environments cited outdoor space as being important. People who lived in the city identified working at home and the home office or study as important, ascribing to it meanings of saving time, concentrated work in one place, and doing what they wanted. However, those who lived in suburban and rural homes identified the home office or study as where they did hobbies, with an associated meaning of creativity. Other everyday activities have the same meaning no matter where the residence is located; cooking, for example, fulfills the need for social interaction and is associated with eating together with family or friends. Some people associated eating together with the meaning of health because they believe sharing a meal with others positively contributes to their health (Meesters, 2009). Thus, an everyday activity can have multiple meanings, and these meanings may vary by person and environment.

An interesting finding was that meaning significantly increased the logistic regression model's ability to estimate everyday activities; adding general meaning as an independent variable contributed additional information (besides the sociodemographic variables, environmental dwelling, and residential features) and accounted for more of the variance in activities (Meesters, 2009). This study provided insight into people–environment relations, which is called a ***meaning structure method*** or approach.

Meaning Making From Different Perspectives

People's culture and past experiences make the transaction between person and environment quite complex. Belonging, connectedness, and interdependence should be considered by occupational therapy practitioners because they can inform the meanings associated with the occupations of culturally diverse people (Hammell, 2014). For example, an elderly female immigrant from an Asian country who is hospitalized in the United States may feel heightened anxiety (compared with an immigrant from another country) simply because of what she sees around her. In Asian culture, white symbolizes

CASE EXAMPLE 17.3. Rima: Difficulties With Child Care

Rima is a 41-year-old married woman who was referred to outpatient occupational therapy because she has significant edema throughout her body, and the edema in her hands is limiting her functional abilities. Rima has private insurance, which will cover 12 sessions of outpatient occupational therapy. She is seeing a rheumatologist who has not yet diagnosed Rima's condition but is considering a diagnosis of sero-negative rheumatoid arthritis.

Rima is an adjunct professor of psychology at a local university and reports that she is still able to type on her computer. However, she reports that she has difficulty opening baby food jars for her infant daughter, who is 7 months old. Rima also has difficulty opening and manipulating small items. "I couldn't open a Capri Sun straw package for my 3-year-old daughter at a birthday party. My fingers felt like fat sausages, and I struggled with sticking the skinny straw into the pouch. All the other mothers could do it, but I couldn't."

The occupational therapist, Yolanda, takes range-of-motion (ROM) measurements and observes that Rima has decreased ROM in flexion and extension of most finger joints. Strength measurements for grip and pinch are slightly weak. Rima reports that she is taking prednisone and meloxicam, a nonsteroidal anti-inflammatory drug, daily.

Rima reports difficulty with some activities, such as cooking, child care, dressing, bathing, and sleeping. Her husband assists when he can but travels frequently for his work as a software consultant. When asked about an activity that she would like to do but has difficulty with, Rima replies, "I'd like to do my baby daughter's hair. It's long enough for ponytails, but I can't twist the elastic around her tiny hair bundles."

Yolanda makes a note of Rima's meaningful activity and starts thinking about activities to try. But she is also worried about the lack of a diagnosis. Another task Rima finds difficult is feeding her infant daughter. "When I hold her to feed her with the bottle, my left arm, supporting her head, will turn purplish after a few minutes, and if I don't shift positions, it becomes painful." Rima becomes teary-eyed as she recounts this story. "I don't know what's going on with my body, but I hate the fact that I have to constantly switch positions to feed my daughter."

(Continued)

CASE EXAMPLE 17.3. Rima: Difficulties With Child Care (*Cont.*)

As Yolanda provides Rima's fingers with passive ROM and determines that Rima lacks full finger flexion and extension, particularly in her interphalangeal joints. After performing some aggressive stretches, Yolanda asks, "Does this hurt?" Rima shrugs and replies, "Not really." Yolanda shows Rima how to passively stretch her fingers, adding that Rima's husband could do this when he is home.

Yolanda wonders if teaching Rima self-lymphatic drainage for the arm would be helpful; she wants to reduce the edema in Rima's hands, but she does not know what is causing the edema and, apparently, neither does Rima's rheumatologist. Yolanda does not think Rima has rheumatoid arthritis because Rima did not report much pain, but she leaves it to the physicians to come up with a diagnosis. Yolanda decides to talk with her colleagues about self-lymphatic drainage before teaching it to Rima. Without a diagnosis or prognosis, Yolanda is mindful of how she documents her sessions with Rima, and she decides the next session will focus on adaptations for opening jars and containers and adaptive equipment for cooking.

In the meantime, Yolanda shows Rima two alternative positions for bottle feeding her baby that do not require that Rima support the baby's weight on her arm. Rima likes the position in which she is face-to-face with her daughter, who sits on Rima's abdomen with her back resting on Rima's flexed legs, which can control the angle of her daughter's sitting. Yolanda also shows Rima how to position a pillow between the baby and her thighs to provide a little more support or comfort.

death; thus, when she sees the white lab coats worn by health professionals and white bed linens, she assumes that she is dying. Hospital staff report that she is noncompliant with ADL training, but this noncompliance may just be due to her different (and frightening) interpretation of the situation. Meaning making is dependent on one's past experiences, culture, and environment.

If meaning is highly individualistic, who judges and approves the meaningfulness of a person's occupations? The answer lies with the various stakeholders and contexts influencing practice, policies, and reimbursement. Occupational therapy practitioners must abide by licensure requirements and a code of ethics; thus, an occupation or goal that involves harm to the client or others would not be appropriate for therapy, even if the client claims it is highly meaningful. To illustrate that meaning is in the eye of the beholder, Case Example 17.3 is offered for contemplation and discussion.

EXERCISE 17.3. Rima's Story

Read Case Example 17.3 and answer the following questions:

1. What is a meaningful occupation that Rima has difficulty doing?
2. What do you think the private health insurance company cares about? What is a meaningful occupation from their perspective?
3. How does Yolanda navigate the space between health insurance or payer and Rima's challenges and concerns? If Yolanda addresses Rima's goal of styling her daughter's hair, should she document it?
4. What questions would you ask Rima if you wanted to create an occupational therapy profile?

Future Research

Research on meaningful occupations has reinforced the observations of occupational therapy's founders that meaningful occupation is health promoting in many populations. Additional longitudinal studies may offer insights into the process of formulating meaning, ascribing meaning to occupations, and adapting meanings. Occupational science has enhanced understanding of the dimensions of meaningful engagement in occupations, and such research needs to continue (e.g., in different contexts, cultures, and populations). Similarly, great strides have been made with regard to measuring meaning and constructs associated with meaningful engagement. Further instrument development and investigation of those instruments' utility in predicting health and well-being would be of interest to audiences both within and external to occupational therapy.

Considering the dynamic variables associated with the effect of illness or injury on everyday occupations, breadth of possible occupations, complexity of environments, and uniqueness of meanings across cultures, it may be daunting to study the mechanisms by which engagement in meaningful occupations influences health and well-being. Nevertheless, it is a worthwhile endeavor. Take, for example, a person who is a workaholic and prioritizes work as an important and meaningful occupation that possibly contributes to self-identity and self-esteem. Even though this person can identify purpose and meaning in life (i.e., work), this occupation may not translate to physical and psychological health if the person lacks ***life balance,*** defined as having a high level of meaningful activity and a low need for meaningful activity experiences (Eakman, 2016). The person may choose to forego health behaviors (e.g., physical activity, nutritious meals) and neglect social relationships, which could negatively influence physical and psychological health.

Although studies have strengthened the assumptions between meaning and positive health outcomes, many are observational or quasi-experimental. Research is needed to systematically test causal relationships in models. Hooker et al.'s (2018) conceptual model of meaning salience, or one's awareness of meaning in the moment, is intriguing because it posits that meaning salience enhances self-regulation, which subsequently influences physical and psychological health. Enhanced self-regulation is theorized to improve stress buffering, promote adaptive coping, and improve engagement in health behaviors. Their framework offers assumptions and mechanisms that can be tested, which could offer new insights into the relationships between meaning and health.

Although Hooker et al.'s (2018) model is conceptually sound, and self-regulation (controlling one's emotions, thoughts, and behaviors) is worth studying as a causal mechanism, other variables may also be important. Occupational therapy practitioners often work with populations who have lost the ability to participate in meaningful occupational engagement, and self-efficacy may play an intermediary role between meaning salience and psychological or physical health. Self-efficacy, the belief in one's capacity to do tasks successfully (Bandura, 1997), may change as a result of occupational therapy intervention. Occupational therapy practitioners enable people to participate in an occupation, either again or for the first time. They recognize these victories in the smiles and positive statements of their clients. The opportunity may be challenging but still feasible, and a successful result, in turn, serves as a motivator to repeat the activity that they did not believe they could do.

As models evolve, they must be empirically tested and refined. Occupational therapy practitioners need models for wellness and prevention for a variety of populations, but these models must hold to the basic constructs of occupational therapy. A grounding in occupational therapy will also serve practitioners when they study the art and science of doing meaningful occupations. Table 17.2 lists selected studies pertaining to meaningful engagement in activities or occupations.

TABLE 17.2. SELECTED EVIDENCE FOR MEANINGFUL OCCUPATION

AUTHOR/DATE	DESCRIPTION	PARTICIPANTS	TYPE OF STUDY
	General meaning		
Heintzelman & King (2019)	Having found a positive relationship between preference for routine and meaning in life in Study 1, Study 2 found that routines are positively correlated with a feeling that life is meaningful.	*N* = 85 undergraduates	Experience sampling method, hierarchical analyses
Royeen (2020)	The researcher posited that the meta-emotion of occupation provides the restorative qualities of occupational engagement, and almost any aspect of occupational engagement and its unique meaning is correlated with the value (positive feelings and arousal) produced by the occupational engagement.	N/A	Narrative review
	Pediatric clients		
Dür et al. (2018)	Parents reported that the meaning of certain activities (e.g., bathing baby) changed because of preterm birth. Meaningful activities could help parents transition from a feeling of parental immaturity to one of maturity. Occupational therapists could help parents gain skills and a better balance of activities.	*N* = 36 parents of very low–birth-weight preterm infants	Focus group interviews using Steinar Kvale's meaning condensation method
Rosenberg & Avrech Bar (2020)	Meanings associated with children's everyday activities are slightly correlated with their socioemotional characteristics and executive functions.	*N* = 80 children (ages 6–13 years) and their parents	Cross-sectional study

(Continued)

TABLE 17.2. **SELECTED EVIDENCE FOR MEANINGFUL OCCUPATION *(Cont.)***

AUTHOR/DATE	DESCRIPTION	PARTICIPANTS	TYPE OF STUDY
Lindsay et al. (2019)	Youths with Duchenne muscular dystrophy engaged in a wide variety of meaningful occupations (e.g., school, social and recreational activities, work).	*N* = 26 participants (11 parents, 8 youth with Duchenne muscular dystrophy, and 7 practitioners)	Qualitative thematic analysis of interviews
	Adult clients		
Lingah & Paruk (2021)	Explored 5 themes for the meaning of dance: factors motivating engagement, beneficial effects of dance, individual journey, role of relationships, and time available for engagement.	*N* = 12 undergraduate OT students	Focus groups, semistructured interviews, thematic analysis
Kinney et al. (2020)	Veterans' participation is correlated with meaningful activity and social support, which subsequently influence psychological and subjective well-being.	*N* = 389 community-based veterans attending college	Explanatory cross-sectional design
Tate et al. (2020)	Programme for Engagement, Participation and Activities intervention increased meaningful activity for 6 of the 7 participants with sTBI. Effect sizes were large for 5 participants. These results add to the evidence for the effectiveness of goal-directed interventions.	*N* = 7 participants with sTBI (4 with cognitive and functional impairments, 3 with neurobehavioral impairments and functional disability)	Single-case experiment with replication (Australia)
White et al. (2020)	Data from adults with chronic conditions engaged in human occupations were used to develop 3 2-dimensional categories: connecting/reconnecting–disconnecting, caring–harming, and contributing–detracting	*N* = 16 adults with multiple chronic conditions	Grounded theory
Eklund et al. (2017)	Balancing Everyday Life group improved significantly more than usual-care group on activity engagement, activity level, and activity balance after 16-week group- and activity-based lifestyle intervention.	*N* = 133 activity-based lifestyle intervention, *n* = 93 usual-care control	Cluster RCT
Petruseviciene et al. (2018)	Women in the experimental group showed significantly greater engagement in meaningful activities, as measured with the Engagement in Meaningful Activities Survey. Greater engagement in meaningful activities was associated with better emotional functions and a lower level of insomnia ($p < .05$).	*N* = 22	RCT
Yokoi et al. (2020)	High self-rated health was significantly correlated with high occupational performance scores.	*N* = 675 community-dwelling Japanese adults	Multiple logistic regression analysis

(Continued)

TABLE 17.2. **SELECTED EVIDENCE FOR MEANINGFUL OCCUPATION *(Cont.)***

AUTHOR/DATE	DESCRIPTION	PARTICIPANTS	TYPE OF STUDY
Bradley et al. (2021)	Acute-care patients perceived a reductionist version of rehabilitation; value was placed on physical improvement, achieving safety, and rehabilitation being led by PT. This version of rehabilitation was unsatisfactory to OTs and PTs and differed from their ideals.	*N* = 5 older patients in acute care in the United Kingdom	Focused ethnography
Takashima et al. (2020)	Retired older men living in an urban area of Japan cited these 5 values of social activities: "feeling I am still useful," "feeling that something is my responsibility," "finding interest through interactions," "feeling of time well spent," and "health as a resource and reward for social activities."	*N* = 15 older men	Semistructured interviews, grounded theory
Lewis & Hill (2020)	Older adults who engage more frequently in leisure-time activities reported a higher sense of purpose, which had a greater impact on the purpose of retired adults.	*N* = 7,277 American adults older than age 50 and their spouses	Secondary data; Health and Retirement Study, 2008–2016
Maruta et al. (2021)	Characteristics of activities that are most meaningful to people with MCI may be similar, regardless of the presence of apathy. Logistic regression analysis showed that activity satisfaction was significantly associated with apathy after adjusting for age, sex, education, IADLs, depressive symptoms, and MCI subtype. The prevalence of apathy in MCI was 23.8%.	*N* = 235 older adults with MCI in Tarumizu, Japan	Cross-sectional study
Yeh et al. (2018)	One theme: valued occupations might be doing, being, becoming, or belonging occupations. OT's unique contribution to palliative care could be its focus on valued occupations.	70 articles	Scoping review

Note. MCI = mild cognitive impairment; N/A = not applicable; OT = occupational therapy/therapist; PT = physical therapist; RCT = randomized controlled trial; sTBI = severe traumatic brain injury.

The following list of questions, by no means exhaustive or comprehensive, is offered to stimulate thinking about potential research:

- Is engagement in meaningful occupations associated with reduced risk of age-related chronic conditions (e.g., cognitive impairment, cardiovascular disease)?
- To what extent is meaningful occupational engagement associated with health-promoting behaviors?
- How does one's perspective on meaning in life and meaning salience influence health behavior?
- What is the role of meaning in life in the process of turning a health behavior into a habit?
- Does engagement in meaningful physical activities promote a sense of purpose? If so, by what mechanism does it do so (e.g., promoting physical health, promoting self-efficacy; Lewis & Hill, 2020)?
- Does meaning influence self-efficacy and self-regulation, which thereby influence health and well-being?
- Do people who report having a higher positive meaning feel that they have better life satisfaction and health-related quality of life and well-being?
- Does the process of engaging in meaningful occupations in different contexts vary across time?
- What is the chronological process of the interactions between affective mood states and meaningfulness (e.g.,

meaning salience) preceding, during, and after occupational engagement?

- How do people with chronic conditions perceive meaning and participation in meaningful activities? How do their perceptions compare with those of the general population or people with acute conditions (methods that could be used include ecological momentary assessments, or qualitative research)?
- Is the transition process to retirement linear or nonlinear with respect to activity engagement and sense of purpose (Lewis & Hill, 2020)?
- Which dimensions of meaningful occupational engagement predict satisfying retirement or semiretirement?

Historical Views of Meaning

Adolph Meyer (1922), one of the proponents of occupational therapy in its formative years, emphasized the importance of meaningful and successful occupations in the treatment of adults with psychiatric illness. Susan Elizabeth Tracy, a nurse, also emphasized the quality and purposefulness of the end product. She observed that patients on surgical wards who were occupied with handicrafts seemed happier (Tracy, 1910). Occupational therapy outcomes should strive to be achievable, and the product of treatment should provide the patient with an emotional value, such as satisfaction and pride (Meyer, 1922).

The founders of occupational therapy observed the effects of occupation on temporal organization. By engaging in pleasurable occupations, patients experienced a sense of reality, and their time was engaged and more balanced. A professor of psychiatry at Johns Hopkins University, Meyer believed that balancing the "big four"—work, play, rest, and sleep—helped to create an orderly rhythm of life. Eleanor Clarke Slagle (1922) underscored habit training through occupational engagement, "to the end that habit reaction will be favourable to the restoration and maintenance of health" (p. 14).

One of the characteristics that distinguishes occupational therapy from other health care disciplines is that occupational therapy practitioners give "opportunities rather than prescriptions" (Meyer, 1922, p. 641). These opportunities enable clients "to do and to plan and create, and to learn to use material" (Meyer, 1922, p. 641). Providing customized therapeutic opportunities to patients with a variety of ailments was not an easy task. In fact, after touring an occupational therapy department at a large institution, Meyer (1922) remarked, "It takes, above all, resourcefulness and ability to respect at the same time the native *capacities and interests* of the patient" (p. 641). He cited the tact and skills of occupational therapists in their encouragement of patients' efforts. Tapping into the clients' interests facilitated motivation and meaning making from occupational engagement. The uniqueness of occupational therapy is the result of its holistic viewpoint and core values, including "pleasure and fulfillment in activity or tasks" (Engelhardt, 1977, p. 672).

Even in occupational therapy's early years, the link between occupation and health was well described, first in psychiatry and then later in physical rehabilitation. At the 1976 AOTA Annual Conference, Tristram Engelhardt Jr. (1977) acknowledged the risk to the profession's standing among health care professions but nevertheless urged the profession to embrace broader values of fulfillment through activity. He asserted that occupational therapy's perspective of "viewing humans as engaged in activities, realizing themselves through their occupations" (p. 166) is essential in health care because no other profession links meaningful engagement in activities to adaptation, health, and well-being. After all, isn't the aim of health care to help people do things? If so, then occupational therapy has a deserved role in the ever-evolving health care system. Although it may be a burden to espouse a holistic and humanistic view of therapy and health, "the virtue of occupational therapy is engagement in the world" (Engelhardt, 1977, p. 672).

Summary

In this chapter, I have presented findings from recent research on meaningful occupation to enhance occupational therapy practitioners' knowledge and ability to apply it in a variety of contexts. The multidimensional nature of meaning has been validated by recent systematic reviews of qualitative research. Roberts and Bannigan's (2018) metasynthesis identified themes on meaning from occupational engagement (fulfillment; restoration; personal and sociocultural identity; and social, cultural, and intergenerational family connection) that were similar to those identified by Eakman et al. (2018; social, selfhood, and pleasure). Many of the themes from these two reviews were described by occupational therapy founders. For example, Meyer (1922) acknowledged that there is pleasure in the process of making or doing, as well as satisfaction and achievement from the product or end result of the occupation.

The dynamic and fluid aspects of meaning coupled with the individualized perceptions of meaning across occupations and contexts may present challenges in measurement variables. However, many instruments have been developed, or are in stages of development, in occupational therapy and psychology. Overall, these instruments assess the wide range of aspects associated with meaning, such as value (Eakman & Eklund, 2011), extent of engagement (Eakman, 2012), pleasure and restoration (Atler et al., 2016), interests and meaningful occupations for hand therapy (Tomori et al., 2012), mental stimulation and fun (Ikiugu et al., 2019), beliefs and self-efficacy (Pergolotti & Cutchin, 2015), and meaning salience (Vagnini, 2020).

A growing number of studies have indicated that meaningful occupational engagement is positively associated with measures of health, quality of life, well-being, and brain health. Participation in meaningful activities is correlated with vitality, greater life satisfaction, and purpose in life (Hooker et al., 2020); higher job satisfaction, decreased burnout, and a stronger sense of professional identity (Scanlan & Hazelton, 2019); and psychological and subjective well-being (Kinney et al., 2020). Although exercise and physical activity improve cognitive functioning and brain structure and function (Erickson et al., 2011), research has now shown that leisure-time physical activity increases hippocampal volume (Hashimoto et al., 2017), and novel leisure activities result in better episodic memory (Park et al., 2014). Moreover, those who experienced leisure activities with higher cognitive demands demonstrated significantly more modulation in the frontal, temporal, and parietal lobes (McDonough et al., 2015).

Continued study of health outcomes is needed to understand occupational therapy's effects on individuals, groups, and populations. Meanings of occupations develop and shift over time and are influenced by a wide array of factors, such as personal events and contexts. A person may ascribe multiple meanings to an occupation; a person from a rural area may regard gardening as a chore, whereas someone from a suburban area may find gardening enjoyable.

Closing Thoughts

Now more than ever, people and populations need occupational therapy services and care. Can practitioners translate occupational therapy's principles and concepts, including meaningful occupation, to serve their communities? Can interventions be scaled up to promote the health and well-being of groups and populations? If so, society will recognize the value of occupational therapy for years to come.

The magic of occupational therapy lies in practitioners' ability to put together the pieces of a multidimensional human puzzle. Practitioners assess multiple variables affecting occupational performance, such as abilities and strengths, problems or concerns, contextual supports and barriers, roles, interests, and goals. After assessment, they have a more complete picture of the individual and a better sense of which dimensions of the puzzle are missing. Occupational therapy practitioners address people's physical and psychological well-being in the form of meaningful activity and function.

What makes occupational therapy so different from other health care professions? Occupational therapy practitioners engage people in occupations, matching them to meaningful therapeutic activities, which can provide, among many things, a sense of empowerment and self-efficacy. "In our knowledge and understanding of the meaning of activities and in their uses lies our unique and distinguishing characteristic as occupational therapists" (Fidler, 1981, p. 570).

References

American Occupational Therapy Association. (2020a). AOTA Occupational Profile Template. *American Journal of Occupational Therapy, 71*(Suppl. 2), 7112420030. https://doi.org/10.5014/ajot.2017.716S12

American Occupational Therapy Association. (2020b). Occupational therapy in the promotion of health and well-being. *American Journal of Occupational Therapy, 74,* 7403420010. https://doi.org/10.5014/ajot.2020.743003

American Occupational Therapy Association. (2020c). Occupational therapy practice framework: Domain and process (4th ed.). *American Journal of Occupational Therapy, 74*(Suppl. 2), 7412410010. https://doi.org/https://doi.org/10.5014/ajot.2020.74S2001

Anand, K. S., & Dhikav, V. (2012). Hippocampus in health and disease: An overview. *Annals of Indian Academy of Neurology, 15,* 239–246. https://doi.org/10.4103/0972-2327.104323

Atler, K. E., Barney, L., Moravec, A., Sample, P. L., & Fruhauf, C. A. (2017). The daily experiences of pleasure, productivity, and restoration profile: A case study. *Canadian Journal of Occupational Therapy, 84,* 262–272. https://doi.org/10.1177/0008417417723119

Atler, K. E., Eakman, A., & Orsi, B. (2016). Enhancing construct validity evidence of the Daily Experiences of Pleasure, Productivity and Restoration Profile. *Journal of Occupational Science, 23,* 278–290. https://doi.org/10.1080/14427591.2015.1080625

Avrech Bar, M., Forwell, S., & Backman, C. L. (2016). Ascribing meaning to occupation: An example from healthy, working mothers. *OTJR: Occupation, Participation and Health, 36,* 148–158. https://doi.org/10.1177/1539449216652622

Bandura, A. (1997). *Self-efficacy: The exercise of control.* W. H. Freeman/Times Books/Henry Holt.

Bartrés-Faz, D., Cattaneo, G., Solana, J., Tormos, J. M., & Pascual-Leone, A. (2018). Meaning in life: Resilience beyond reserve. *Alzheimer's Research and Therapy, 10,* 47. https://doi.org/10.1186/s13195-018-0381-z

Baumeister, R. F., & Landau, M. J. (Eds.). (2018). Meanings of meaning [Special issue]. *Review of General Psychology, 22*(1).

Black, M. H., Milbourn, B., Desjardins, K., Sylvester, V., Parrant, K., & Buchanan, A. (2019). Understanding the meaning and use of occupational engagement: Findings from a scoping review. *British Journal of Occupational Therapy, 82,* 272–287. https://doi.org/10.1177/0308022618821580

Bonder, B. (2018). Meaningful occupation in later life: Occupation and meaning. In B. Bonder & V. Dal Bello-Haas (Eds.), *Functional performance in older adults* (4th ed., pp. 62–66). F. A. Davis.

Bradley, G., Baker, K., & Bailey, C. (2021). The meaning of rehabilitation: A qualitative study exploring perspectives of occupational therapists and physiotherapists working with older people in acute care. *Disability and Rehabilitation, 43,* 2295–2303. https://doi.org/10.1080/09638288.2019.1697762

Coussens, M., Destoop, B., De Baets, S., Desoete, A., Oostra, A., Vanderstraeten, G., . . . Van de Velde, D. (2020). A qualitative photo elicitation research study to elicit the perception of young children with developmental disabilities such as ADHD and/or DCD and/or ASD on their participation. *PLoS ONE, 15*(3), 1–20. https://doi.org/10.1371/journal.pone.0229538

Csikszentmihalyi, M. (1990). *Flow: The psychology of optimal experience.* Harper & Row.

Dunn, W. (2007). Ecology of Human Performance Model. In S. B. Dunbar (Ed.), *Occupational therapy models for intervention with children and families* (pp. 127–156). SLACK.

Dür, M., Brückner, V., Oberleitner-Leeb, C., Fuiko, R., Matter, B., & Berger, A. (2018). Clinical relevance of activities meaningful to parents of preterm infants with very low birth weight: A focus group study. *PLoS ONE, 13*(8), e0202189. https://doi.org/10.1371/journal.pone.0202189

Eakman, A. M. (2012). Measurement characteristics of the Engagement in Meaningful Activities Survey in an age-diverse sample. *American Journal of Occupational Therapy, 66,* e20–e29. https://doi.org/10.5014/ajot.2012.001867

Eakman, A. M. (2013). Relationships between meaningful activity, basic psychological needs, and meaning in life: Test of the Meaningful Activity and Life Meaning Model: Occupation, participation and health. *OTJR: Occupation, Participation and Health, 33,* 100–109. https://doi.org/10.3928/15394492-20130222-02

Eakman, A. M. (2016). A subjectively-based definition of life balance using personal meaning in occupation. *Journal of Occupational Science, 23,* 108–127. https://doi.org/10.1080/14427591.2014.955603

Eakman, A. M., Atler, K. E., Rumble, M., Gee, B. M., Romriell, B., & Hardy, N. (2018). A qualitative research synthesis of positive subjective experiences in occupation from the Journal of Occupational Science (1993–2010). *Journal of Occupational Science, 25,* 346–367. https://doi.org/10.1080/14427591.2018.1492958

Eakman, A. M., Carlson, M. E., & Clark, F. A. (2010a). Factor structure, reliability, and convergent validity of the Engagement in Meaningful Activities Survey for older adults. *OTJR: Occupation, Participation and Health, 30,* 111–121. https://doi.org/10.3928/15394492-20090518-01

Eakman, A. M., Carlson, M. E., & Clark, F. A. (2010b). The Meaningful Activity Participation Assessment: A measure of engagement in personally valued activities. *International Journal of Aging and Human Development, 70,* 299–317. https://doi.org/10.2190/AG.70.4.b

Eakman, A. M., & Eklund, M. (2011). Reliability and structural validity of an assessment of occupational value. *Scandinavian Journal of Occupational Therapy, 18,* 231–240. https://doi.org/10.3109/11038128.2010.521948

Eklund, M., Tjörnstrand, C., Sandlund, M., & Argentzell, E. (2017). Effectiveness of Balancing Everyday Life (BEL) versus standard occupational therapy for activity engagement and functioning among people with mental illness—A cluster RCT study. *BMC Psychiatry, 17,* 1–12. https://doi.org/10.1186/s12888-017-1524-7

Engelhardt, H. T. (1977). Defining occupational therapy: The meaning of therapy and the virtues of occupation. *American Journal of Occupational Therapy, 31,* 666–672.

Erickson, K. I., Voss, M. W., Prakash, R. S., Basak, C., Szabo, A., Chaddock, L., . . . Kramer, A. F. (2011). Exercise training increases size of hippocampus and improves memory. *Proceedings of the National Academy of Sciences of the United States of America, 108,* 3017–3022. https://doi.org/10.1073/pnas.1015950108

Eschenfelder, V. G. (2005). *Individual meaning and its role in occupational therapy* (Publication No. 3188013) [Doctoral dissertation, Texas Woman's University]. ProQuest Dissertations and Theses Global.

Fidler, G. S. (1981). From crafts to competence. *American Journal of Occupational Therapy, 35,* 567–573. https//dx.clin.org/10.5014/ajot.35.9.567

Fortuna, J. K. (2021). Creating a new normal through engagement in meaningful occupation. *Open Journal of Occupational Therapy, 9,* 1–6. https://doi.org/10.15453/2168-6408.1828

Goldberg, B., Brintnell, E. S., & Goldberg, J. (2002). The relationship between engagement in meaningful activities and quality of life in persons disabled by mental illness. *Occupational Therapy in Mental Health, 18,* 17–44. https://doi.org/10.1300/J004v18n02_03

Goldstein-Lohman, H., Kratz, A., & Pierce, D. (2003). A study of occupation-based practice. In D. Pierce (Ed.), *Occupation by design: Building therapeutic power* (pp. 239–262). F. A. Davis.

Hammell, K. W. (2004). Dimensions of meaning in the occupations of daily life. *Canadian Journal of Occupational Therapy, 71,* 296–305. https://doi.org/10.1177/000841740407100509

Hammell, K. R. W. (2014). Belonging, occupation, and human well-being: An exploration. *Canadian Journal of Occupational Therapy, 81,* 39–50. https://doi.org/10.1177/0008417413520489

Hancock, N., Honey, A., & Bundy, A. C. (2015). Sources of meaning derived from occupational engagement for people recovering from mental illness. *British Journal of Occupational Therapy, 78,* 508–515. https://doi.org/10.1177/0308022614562789

Hashimoto, M., Araki, Y., Takashima, Y., Nogami, K., Uchino, A., Yuzuriha, T., & Yao, H. (2017). Hippocampal atrophy and memory dysfunction associated with physical inactivity in community-dwelling elderly subjects: The Sefuri study. *Brain and Behavior, 7*(2), e00620. https://doi.org/https://doi.org/10.1002/brb3.620

Heintzelman, S. J., & King, L. A. (2019). Routines and meaning in life. *Personality and Social Psychology Bulletin, 45,* 688–699. https://doi.org/10.1177/0146167218795133

Hooker, S. A., Masters, K. S., & Park, C. L. (2018). A meaningful life is a healthy life: A conceptual model linking meaning and meaning salience to health. *Review of General Psychology, 22,* 11–24. https://doi.org/10.1037/gpr0000115

Hooker, S. A., Masters, K. S., Vagnini, K. M., & Rush, C. L. (2020). Engaging in personally meaningful activities is associated with meaning salience and psychological well-being. *Journal of Positive Psychology, 15,* 821–831. https://doi.org/10.1080/17439760.2019.1651895

Ikiugu, M. N., Lucas-Molitor, W., Feldhacker, D., Gebhart, C., Spier, M., Kapels, L., . . . Gaikowski, R. (2019). Guidelines for occupational therapy interventions based on meaningful and psychologically rewarding occupations. *Journal of Happiness Studies: An Interdisciplinary Forum on Subjective Well-Being, 20,* 2027–2053. https://doi.org/10.1007/s10902-018-0030-z

Johansson, A., & Björklund, A. (2016). The impact of occupational therapy and lifestyle interventions on older persons' health, well-being, and occupational adaptation. *Scandinavian Journal of Occupational Therapy, 23,* 207–219. https://doi.org/10.3109/11038128.2015.1093544

Jopp, D. S., & Hertzog, C. (2010). Assessing adult leisure activities: An extension of a self-report activity questionnaire. *Psychological Assessment, 22,* 108–120. https://doi.org/10.1037/a0017662

Kim, E. S., Whillans, A. V., Lee, M. T., Chen, Y., & VanderWeele, T. J. (2020). Volunteering and subsequent health and well-being in older adults: An outcome-wide longitudinal approach. *American Journal of Preventive Medicine, 59,* 176–186. https://doi.org/10.1016/j.amepre.2020.03.004

King, L. A., Heintzelman, S. J., & Ward, S. J. (2016). Beyond the search for meaning: A contemporary science of the experience of meaning in life. *Current Directions in Psychological Science, 25,* 211–216. https://doi.org/10.1177/0963721416656354

Kinney, A. R., Graham, J. E., & Eakman, A. M. (2020). Participation is associated with well-being among community-based veterans: An investigation of coping ability, meaningful activity, and social support as mediating mechanisms. *American Journal of Occupational Therapy, 74,* 7405205010. https://doi.org/10.5014/ajot.2020.037119

Law, M., Cooper, B., Strong, S., Stewart, D., Rigby, P., & Letts, L. (1996). The Person–Environment–Occupation Model: A transactive approach to occupational performance. *Canadian Journal of Occupational Therapy, 63,* 9–23. https://doi.org/10.1177/000841749606300103

Lewis, N. A., & Hill, P. L. (2020). Does being active mean being purposeful in older adulthood? Examining the moderating role of retirement. *Psychology and Aging, 35,* 1050–1057. https://doi.org/10.1037/pag0000568

Lindsay, S., Cagliostro, E., & McAdam, L. (2019). Meaningful occupations of young adults with muscular dystrophy and other neuromuscular disorders. *Canadian Journal of Occupational Therapy, 86,* 277–288. https://doi.org/10.1177/0008417419832466

Lingah, T., & Paruk, J. (2021). The meaning that undergraduate occupational therapy students at the University of KwaZulu-Natal attach to the occupation of dance. *South African Journal of Occupational Therapy, 51,* 91–98. https://doi.org/10.17159/2310-3833/2021/vol51n2a12

Liu, X., Whetten, K., Prose, N. S., Eagle, D., Parnell, H. E., Amanya, C., . . . Proeschold-Bell, R. J. (2020). Enjoyment and meaning in daily activities among caregivers of orphaned and separated children in four countries. *Children and Youth Services Review, 116,* 105103. https://doi.org/10.1016/j.childyouth.2020.105103

Maruta, M., Makizako, H., Ikeda, Y., Miyata, H., Nakamura, A., Han, G., . . . Tabira, T. (2021). Association between apathy and satisfaction with meaningful activities in older adults with mild cognitive impairment: A population-based cross-sectional study. *International Journal of Geriatric Psychiatry, 36,* 1065–1074. https://doi.org/10.1002/gps.5544

Mather, M., Scommegna, P., & Kilduff, L. (2019, July 15). *Fact sheet: Aging in the United States*. https://www.prb.org/resources/fact-sheet-aging-in-the-united-states/

McDonough, I. M., Haber, S., Bischof, G. N., & Park, D. C. (2015). The Synapse Project: Engagement in mentally challenging activities enhances neural efficiency. *Restorative Neurology and Neuroscience, 33,* 865–882. https://doi.org/10.3233/rnn-150533

Meesters, J. (2009). *The meaning of activities in the dwelling and residential environment: A structural approach in people–environment relations*. IOS Press. https://doi.org/10.3233/978-1-60750-012-4-i

Meyer, A. (1922). The philosophy of occupational therapy. *American Journal of Physical Medicine and Rehabilitation, 1,* 1–10.

Obucina, M., Harris, N., Fitzgerald, J. A., Chai, A., Radford, K., Ross, A., . . . Vecchio, N. (2018). The application of Triple Aim framework in the context of primary healthcare: A systematic literature review. *Health Policy, 122,* 900–907. https://doi.org/10.1016/j.healthpol.2018.06.006

Ohno, K., Saito, K., Matsumoto, H., Tomori, K., & Sawada, T. (2020). The clinical utility of a decision-aid to facilitate the use of the hand in real-life activities of patients with distal radius fractures: A case study. *Journal of Hand Therapy, 34,* P341–347. https://doi.org/https://doi.org/10.1016/j.jht.2020.03.002

Park, D. C., Lodi-Smith, J., Drew, L., Haber, S., Hebrank, A., Bischof, G. N., & Aamodt, W. (2014). The impact of sustained engagement on cognitive function in older adults: The Synapse Project. *Psychological Science, 25,* 103–112. https://doi.org/10.1177/0956797613499592

Pergolotti, M., & Cutchin, M. P. (2015). The Possibilities for Activity Scale (PActS): Development, validity, and reliability. *Canadian Journal of Occupational Therapy, 82,* 85–92. https://doi.org/10.1177/0008417414561493

Pergolotti, M., Cutchin, M. P., & Muss, H. B. (2015). Predicting participation in meaningful activity for older adults with cancer. *Quality of Life Research, 24,* 1217–1222. https://doi.org/10.1007/s11136-014-0849-7

Petruseviciene, D., Surmaitiene, D., Baltaduoniene, D., & Lendraitiene, E. (2018). Effect of community-based occupational therapy on health-related quality of life and engagement in meaningful activities of women with breast cancer. *Occupational Therapy International, 2018,* 6798697. https://doi.org/10.1155/2018/6798697

Pierce, D. (2003). *Occupation by design: Building therapeutic power*. F. A. Davis.

Rathert, C., Williams, E. S., & Linhart, H. (2018). Evidence for the quadruple aim: A systematic review of the literature on physician burnout and patient outcomes. *Medical Care, 56,* 976–984. https://doi.org/10.1097/MLR.0000000000000999

Reed, K., Hocking, C., & Smythe, L. (2013). The meaning of occupation: Historical and contemporary connections between health and occupation. *New Zealand Journal of Occupational Therapy, 60,* 38–44.

Reker, G. T. (2000). Theoretical perspective, dimensions, and measurement of existential meaning. In G. T. Reker (Ed.), *Exploring existential meaning: Optimizing human development across the life span* (pp. 39–55). Sage.

Roberts, A. E. K., & Bannigan, K. (2018). Dimensions of personal meaning from engagement in occupations: A metasynthesis. *Canadian Journal of Occupational Therapy, 85,* 386–396. https://doi.org/10.1177/0008417418820358

Rosenberg, L., & Avrech Bar, M. (2020). The perceived meaning of occupations among children: Correlations with children's socio-emotional characteristics and executive functions. *Australian Occupational Therapy Journal, 67,* 572–580. https://doi.org/10.1111/1440-1630.12690

Royeen, C. B. (2020). Meta-emotion of Occupation with Wissen (MeOW): Feeling about feeling while doing with meaning. *Journal of Occupational Science, 27,* 460–473. https://doi.org/10.1080/14427591.2020.1742196

Scanlan, J. N., & Hazelton, T. (2019). Relationships between job satisfaction, burnout, professional identity and meaningfulness of work activities for occupational therapists working in mental health. *Australian Occupational Therapy Journal, 66,* 581–590. https://doi.org/10.1111/1440-1630.12596

Scheerer, C. R., Cahill, L. G., Kirby, K., & Lane, J. (2004). Cake decorating as occupation: Meaning and motivation. *Journal of Occupational Science, 11,* 68–74. https://doi.org/10.1080/14427591.2004.9686533

Slagle, E. C. (1922). Training aides for mental patients. *American Journal of Physical Medicine and Rehabilitation, 1,* 11–17.

Smith, N., Towers, A.-M., Palmer, S., Beecham, J., & Welch, E. (2018). Being occupied: Supporting "meaningful activity" in care homes for older people in England. *Ageing and Society, 38,* 2218–2240. https://doi.org/10.1017/S0144686X17000678

Takashima, R., Onishi, R., Saeki, K., & Hirano, M. (2020). The values and meanings of social activities for older urban men after retirement. *PLoS ONE, 15*(11), 0242859. https://doi.org/http://dx.doi.org/10.1371/journal.pone.0242859

Tate, R. L., Wakim, D., Sigmundsdottir, L., & Longley, W. (2020). Evaluating an intervention to increase meaningful activity after severe traumatic brain injury: A single-case experimental design with direct inter-subject and systematic replications. *Neuropsychological Rehabilitation, 30,* 641–672. https://doi.org/10.1080/09602011.2018.1488746

Tomori, K., Uezu, S., Kinjo, S., Ogahara, K., Nagatani, R., & Higashi, T. (2012). Utilization of the iPad application: Aid for Decision-making in Occupation Choice. *Occupational Therapy International, 19,* 88–97. https://doi.org/10.1002/oti.325

Tracy, S. (1910). *Studies in invalid occupation: A manual for nurses and attendants*. Whitcomb & Barrows.

Trombly, C. (1993). Anticipating the future: Assessment of occupational function. *American Journal of Occupational Therapy, 47,* 253–257. https://doi.org/10.5014/ajot.47.3.253

Trombly, C. A. (1995). Occupation: Purposefulness and meaningfulness as therapeutic mechanisms. *American Journal of Occupational Therapy, 49,* 960–972. https://doi.org/10.5014/ajot.49.10.960

Vagnini, K. M. (2020). *The Meaning Awareness Scale (MAS): Development and initial psychometric analysis of a measure of meaning salience* (Publication No. 27964020) [Master's thesis, University of Colorado at Denver]. ProQuest Dissertations & Theses Global.

Wenborn, J. (2017). Meaningful activities. In S. Shussler & C. Lohrmann (Eds.), *Dementia in nursing homes* (pp. 5–20). Springer International. https://doi.org/10.1007/978-3-319-49832-4_2

White, C., Lentin, P., & Farnworth, L. (2013). An investigation into the role and meaning of occupation for people living with on-going health conditions. *Australian Occupational Therapy Journal, 60,* 20–29. https://doi.org/10.1111/1440-1630.12023

White, C., Lentin, P., & Farnworth, L. (2020). "I know what I am doing": A grounded theory investigation into the activities and occupations of adults living with chronic conditions. *Scandinavian Journal of Occupational Therapy, 27,* 56–65. https://doi.org/10.1080/11038128.2019.1624818

Wilcock, A. A. (1998). Reflections on doing, being and becoming. *Canadian Journal of Occupational Therapy, 65,* 248–256. https://doi.org/10.1177/000841749806500501

World Federation of Occupational Therapists. (2021). *About occupational therapy*. https://wfot.org/about/about-occupational-therapy

World Health Organization. (2001). *International classification of functioning, disability and health*.

Yeh, H.-H., McColl, M. A., & Huang, L.-J. (2018). A model for client-centered, occupation-based palliative care: A scoping review. *American Journal of Occupational Therapy, 72*(4, Suppl.1), 7211505084. https://doi.org/10.5014/ajot.2018.72S1-PO1015

Yokoi, K., Miyai, N., Utsumi, M., Hattori, S., Kurasawa, S., Uematsu, Y., & Arita, M. (2020). The relationship between meaningful occupation and self-rated health in Japanese individuals: The Wakayama Study. *Occupational Therapy in Health Care, 34,* 116–130. https://doi.org/10.1080/07380577.2020.1746469